PATHOLOGY ILLUSTRATED

The late Alasdair D.T. Govan PhD FRCP(Glas) FRCP(Edin) FRCOG
Late Consultant Pathologist, Glasgow Royal Maternity Hospital, Glasgow, UK

Peter S. Macfarlane MBChB FRCP(Glas) FRCP(Edin) FRCPath
Formerly Consultant Pathologist and Honorary Clinical Lecturer,
University of Glasgow at the Western Infirmary;
Visiting Professor of Pathology, University of California, Los Angeles, USA

Robin Callander FFPh FMAA AIMI
Formerly Director, Medical Illustration Unit, University
of Glasgow, Glasgow, UK

FOURTH EDITION

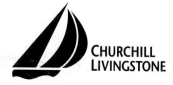

CHURCHILL
LIVINGSTONE

EDINBURGH LONDON MADRID MELBOURNE NEW YORK AND TOKYO 1995

CHURCHILL LIVINGSTONE
Medical Division of Pearson Professional Ltd

Distributed in the United States of America by Churchill
Livingstone Inc., 650 Avenue of the Americas, New York, N.Y.
10011, and by associated companies, branches and representatives
throughout the world.

First edition 1981
Second edition 1986
Third edition 1991
Fourth edition 1995
    Reprinted 1995
    Reprinted 1996

ISBN 0 443 05068 6

British Library Cataloguing in Publication Data
A catalogue record for this book is available from the British
Library.

Library of Congress Cataloging in Publication Data
A catalog record for this book is available from the Library of
Congress.

The
publisher's
policy is to use
**paper manufactured
from sustainable forests**

Produced by Longman Singapore Publishers (Pte) Ltd.
Printed in Singapore

CONTENTS

PREFACE

In the preface to the first edition we stated our motive as follows: "We believe that communication by verbal and written methods is the fundamental basis for study and learning. Nevertheless, in the modern setting where knowledge is increasing so rapidly and in a subject such as pathology where morphological changes are a major component, we consider that the visual image has an important facilitating role. We therefore offer this book as a companion to its predecessors in the Illustrated Series on medical subjects".

In this fourth edition the general layout and style have been retained; we have attempted, with no little difficulty, to accommodate, but at the same time keep in perspective, the important advances arising from the continuing explosive growth of knowledge of cellular and subcellular activities. The role of genetic influences on disease processes has been elaborated.

We are greatly indebted to our colleagues, Professor F.D. Lee and Doctors A.K. Foulis and R.P. Reid, for their help in the preparation of this edition: they offered detailed criticism and advice. They share in any credits for improvement: the short-comings are our responsibility.

It is with regret and sadness that we have to record the death of Alasdair Govan during the preparation of this edition. He has been greatly missed.

P.S. Macfarlane
R. Callander

INTRODUCTION

Students of pathology have already studied anatomy and physiology which represent the scientific study of the structure and function of the body in the process of normal living. At every level of measurement a range is established within which normal structure and function are defined. They have learned the relationship between form and function and must now enter the world of clinical medicine and the concept of disease.

Disease occurs when there are variations of structure and/or function outside the normal range.

PATHOLOGY is the scientific study of DISEASE. It is concerned with the causes and mechanisms by which disease is produced, with the descriptions of the manifestations of disease and with its progress and sequels. It is therefore one of the important sciences on which the practice of clinical medicine and surgery is based.

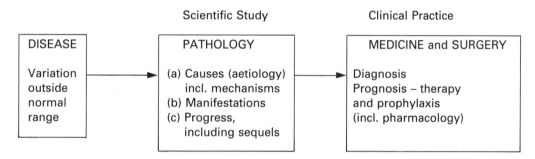

Because of the close relationship between the subjects, anatomical and physiological resumés are given throughout the book.

MANIFESTATIONS of DISEASE are essentially a summation of the damage done by a harmful agent and the body's response to it.

DAMAGE done by *HARMFUL AGENT + BODY'S REACTION = DISEASE*

The components of this simple equation are themselves so very diverse and subject to modification by many factors that the spectrum of disease process is very broad. Nonetheless scientific study demands analysis followed by resynthesis in the form of CLASSIFICATION.

The important broad groups of disease are:

INFLAMMATORY	DEGENERATIVE	NEOPLASTIC
(incl. infections)	(excl. ageing)	(tumours)

Streptococcal sore throat is an example of a disease process caused by a single harmful agent.

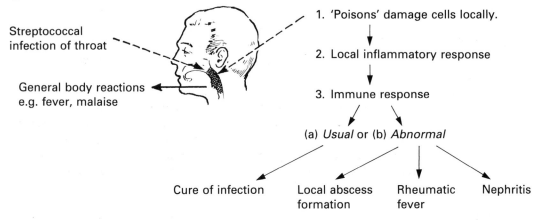

However in many diseases the harmful agents are multiple and the manifestations and progress of the disease are very complex.

Causes of Disease
The various factors involved are considered in 2 broad groups:
(1) Environmental factors and (2) Genetic factors.
ENVIRONMENTAL FACTORS are many and are classified under the following general headings:

Physical agents Among these are trauma, radiations, extremes of heat and cold, electrical power, i.e. the application to the body of an excess of physical energy in any form.

Chemical poisons These are increasing in number particularly with the advances in industrial processing. Some act in a general manner, such as cyanide which is toxic to all cells. Others act locally, for example strong acids and caustics. Another group exhibit a predilection for certain organs – paraquat affects the lungs, phosphorus and organic solvents cause damage especially in the liver and kidneys.

Iatrogenic disease is an important subgroup, not uncommon in present times due to the development of powerful drugs, many of which have undesirable side-effects.

Nutritional deficiencies and excesses They may arise as a result of poor supply, interference with absorption, inefficient transport within the body or defective utilisation. In addition, the effects may be of a general nature as in starvation or lack of oxygen or they cause specific damage, for example, in vitamin deficiencies. Dietary excess plays an important role in diseases in Western countries.

Infections and infestations Viruses, bacteria, fungi, protozoa and metazoa all cause disease. They may do so by causing cell destruction directly as in certain virus infections, for example poliomyelitis, or protozoal infections, for example malaria. In many cases, however the damage is done by toxins elaborated by the infecting agent as in diphtheria and tetanus. As with poisons they may have a general effect or show a predilection for certain tissues.

Environmental factors (continued)

Abnormal immunological reactions The immune process is normally protective but in certain circumstances the reaction may become deranged. Hypersensitivity to various substances can lead to alarming shock-like conditions – anaphylaxis or to more localised lesions such as asthma. In other circumstances the immune process may act against the body cells – autoimmunity. This can be seen in certain endocrine diseases such as thyroiditis.

Psychological factors cause and influence disease processes in several ways: (a) psychological stress may lead to mental illness; (b) their influence on the individual's symptoms and reaction to established somatic disease is apparent; (c) they are important components in disease caused by addiction, for example alcohol, tobacco; (d) finally it is thought that psychogenetic factors, by as yet ill-defined mechanisms, may be causally related to such diseases as hypertension, peptic ulcer, coronary arterial thrombosis and ulcerative colitis.

GENETIC FACTORS are essentially the results of activities of single genes and groups of genes. Both normal and abnormal genes influence SUSCEPTIBILITY and RESISTANCE to disease.

Normal genes
1. *Susceptibility* of fair skin to damage (e.g. skin cancer) by the ultraviolet rays in sunlight is well known and the mechanism – the lack of protective pigment melanin – is obvious.
2. The blood group A is associated with an increased incidence of pernicious anaemia and gastric cancer, and blood group B with duodenal ulcer.
3. The Human Leucocyte Antigen (HLA) [syn: Major Histocompatibility Complex (MHC)] is associated with *susceptibility* and *resistance* to infection and also to the occurrence of auto-immune disorders.
4. The blood group Duffy negative confers *resistance* to infection by *Plasmodium Vivax* (a type of malaria).

Abnormal genes
Mutations give rise to abnormalities of chromosomes and component genes: the majority occur spontaneously (or without known cause): in some cases radiation, chemical or infective agents are incriminated.

Hereditary diseases, where the genetic abnormality *directly* determines a disease, are relatively rare: in contrast there is a genetic *component* in many diseases. Thus although the factors composing the cause of a disease have been divided into the above 2 main groups many common diseases are multifactorial and elements of both groups are operative.

Abnormal genes (continued)

The new technologies, particularly the use of genetic probes, which allow the identification of individual genes and their specific functions have increased our knowledge of the genetic component in many acquired diseases, for example where there is a high familial incidence of a particular disease it is now possible in some to identify the abnormal genes which may be contributing to the disorder. Another example is the discovery of acquired specific genetic abnormalities in stem cells, which potentiate the development of malignant tumours. The genes involved are proto-oncogenes (and virus oncogenes) which control cell proliferation and antioncogenes which control differentiation. The agents causing the abnormalities include chemicals, radiations and viruses.

Congenital disease is present at birth. It can either be genetically determined or acquired. An example of the latter type are the deformities caused by thalidomide taken by the mother during early pregnancy and it is becoming clear that environmental factors, for example nutritional factors and smoking, are very important environmental causes of congenital disease.

Age and disease

In young subjects a single harmful agent may cause disease leading to death if a vital organ is affected. With increasing age the chances of several harmful agents each causing separate diseases are enhanced and death is often due to the cumulative effect of such independent disease processes.

Physiological ageing implies a gradual loss of cellular and body vitality usually associated with atrophy of tissues and organs. This process is accentuated and mimicked by the degenerative diseases of old age (particularly arterial disease) so that the physiological and pathological states tend to merge. Nevertheless the student should try to identify the distinctions between ageing and disease although in some instances they may prove difficult to define.

Investigation of disease In practice the objectives of the study of disease are twofold:
1. To determine the nature of the disease process and its causation i.e. make a diagnosis.
2. To monitor the extent and progress of the disease and provide a prognosis.

Historically the study of disease was based on morphological observations, first at a gross level and from the nineteenth century at cellular level, and morbid anatomy and histology remain the corner stones of pathological study. The emergence of subspecialities, for example biochemistry and haematology, has led to greater understanding in depth. But it is important that such knowledge should not be compartmentalised and the task of the modern student is to integrate information from various sources and thus acquire a breadth of pathological knowledge.

Methods in pathology

The traditional methods of careful naked eye and light microscope examination of organs and tissues at autopsy have been supplemented by the much wider use in clinical practice of *biopsy* which is the removal of tissue during life for diagnostic purposes. With the development of modern instrumentation biopsies are obtained from many parts of the body.

In addition, numerous technological advances have been applied to pathological methods at various levels with advantage. The following is a brief outline of these levels:

Level A. Morbid anatomy reveals the gross changes in diseased organs and indicates the secondary effects in other parts of the body.

Level B. Histology: diseases generally have a distinct pattern which can be recognised using the light microscope. Extensions of the methods are histochemistry and immunohistochemistry by which the presence of various chemicals can be revealed.

Level C. Cytology: the study of cellular details is, of course, a part of histology but the study of individual cells in detail is now important particularly in the diagnosis of cancer.

Level D. Electron-microscopy (EM) reveals the cellular organelles and various patterns of change found in disease.

Level E. The ultimate level, which is as yet beyond the scope of pathology in most cases, is in the field of molecular biology where form and function become one. At this level important advances in pathological knowledge have been made for example in the understanding of the roles of many chemical messengers and receptors.

These increasingly sophisticated methods tend to influence the student to focus on detailed mechanisms occurring at microscopic level. Without discouraging such an approach to the subject it must not be forgotten that the observations obtained over many years by simple methods of gross examination and histological assessment of routinely stained specimens are fundamental.

The following descriptions therefore begin with gross pathology and proceed stepwise to the detailed cellular changes where these are known. The students will find that such an approach is the basis of their learning and progress in clinical practice.

CHAPTER 1

CELL AND TISSUE DAMAGE
Degenerations and Depositions

CELLULAR PHYSIOLOGY AND PATHOLOGY

The complexity and detail of intra-cellular structure and function and their disorders, as revealed by recent research, is such that only the basic principles can be illustrated.

In many respects, cellular pathology mimics organ and tissue pathology, e.g. (a) the various cellular components and activities are closely interdependent (it is of course convenient to describe them separately) (b) all activities are conducted with balancing control mechanisms and (c) very efficient compensation and repair mechanisms exist to minimise damage.

Energy

Source	Production		Utilisation
O_2 + Glucose $\longrightarrow$	Via MITOCHONDRIA $\longrightarrow$	Release $\longrightarrow$	For all cellular
	ADP ATP	of energy	activities
	(Oxidative phosphorylation)		

Defects in source, production and utilisation can be reflected in all aspects of cellular function.

Plasma membranes

Main functions
(1) Contact with extra-cellular environment — e.g. recognition receptors antigenicity

(2) Passage of complex chemicals in and out of cell by
(a) pinocytosis or phagocytosis
(b) selective permeability

Any disorder may initiate a chain reaction leading to disease.

Lysosomes These membrane-bound organelles contain hydrolytic enzymes and are responsible for digestion and disposal of complex substances. $\longrightarrow$ Disorder may lead to enzyme escape or to cellular overloading, e.g. storage disorders.

Nucleus

The nucleus contains at least 50,000 genes and through them exercises control of all cellular activities. Each gene is responsible for a single specific chemical product, e.g. a protein, an enzyme or a complex lipid.

Nuclear damage occurs usually during cell replication and is greatly potentiated by ionising radiation. Repair mechanisms are very effective.

Germ cell nuclear damage
(1) Severe damage to chromosomal structure $\longrightarrow$ Prevention of conception.
$\longrightarrow$ Early abortion.

(2) Less severe damage affecting groups of genes, single genes or DNA sequences within genes $\longrightarrow$ Developmental and HEREDITARY DISEASES and SUSCEPTIBILITY to disease.

Stem cell nuclear damage
This is acquired during life.
The development of cancer is the best example — nuclear changes induced by carcinogens — activation of oncogenes — chain of events leading to malignancy.

CELL DAMAGE

Visible changes occur in cells as a result of noxious agents, the degree of change varying with the severity of the damaging process: with minor damage the repair mechanisms within the cell reverse the changes: more severe damage results in cell death.

CAUSES OF CELL DAMAGE

These are innumerable but are grouped as follows (the individual diseases mentioned are illustrative examples):

1. **Reduced oxygen supply** — respiratory disease, cardiovascular disease, anaemia
2. **Physical agents** — mechanical trauma, excessive heat or cold, radiations
3. **Chemical agents** — these continue to increase enormously with the complexity of industrial processes
4. **Toxins** — bacteria, plants, animals e.g. snakes
5. **Viruses**
6. **Abnormal immunological reaction** — hypersensitivity states, glomerulonephritis
7. **Nutritional deficiencies** — vitamin deficiency and malabsorption syndromes
8. **Genetic abnormalities** — Down's syndrome

NECROSIS

When, as a result of damage by the various agents mentioned above, cells or groups of cells die while still part of the living body the term **necrosis** is used. Death of the cell is associated with rapid depletion of intracellular energy systems. Initially there are no morphological changes. What we describe as necrosis is the result of the liberation of intracellular enzymes following upon the disruption of cytoplasmic organelles with the production of oxygen free radicals, disintegration of the nucleus and changes in the plasma membrane.

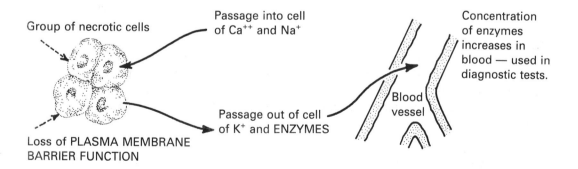

Group of necrotic cells

Passage into cell of Ca^{++} and Na^+

Passage out of cell of K^+ and ENZYMES

Loss of PLASMA MEMBRANE BARRIER FUNCTION

Blood vessel

Concentration of enzymes increases in blood — used in diagnostic tests.

Necrosis is associated with visible changes:

1. **Coagulative necrosis** is the classical appearance.
2. Several other descriptive forms where the appearances are modified by additional local factors, particularly the action of released enzymes.

NECROSIS

COAGULATIVE NECROSIS
This type of necrosis is frequently caused by lack of blood supply and is exemplified well in infarcts of solid organs, e.g. heart, spleen and kidney.

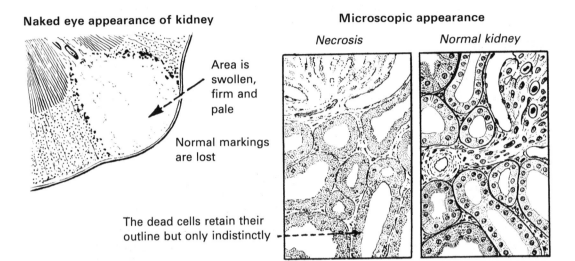

Naked eye appearance of kidney

Area is swollen, firm and pale

Normal markings are lost

The dead cells retain their outline but only indistinctly ◄- - -

Microscopic appearance

Necrosis *Normal kidney*

At *light microscopic level* the following changes in the cell are seen:
1. The nucleus shows one of two changes (a) Karyolysis (b) Karyorrhexis.
2. The cytoplasm becomes opaque and strongly eosinophilic (affinity for the red dye, eosin).

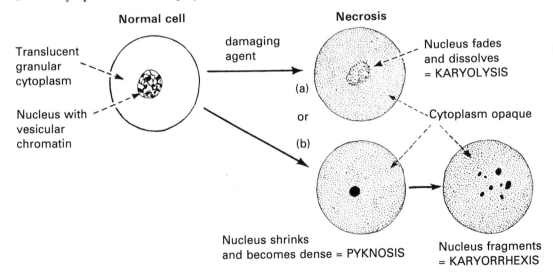

Normal cell   **Necrosis**

Translucent granular cytoplasm

damaging agent

Nucleus with vesicular chromatin

(a)

or

(b)

Nucleus fades and dissolves = KARYOLYSIS

Cytoplasm opaque

Nucleus shrinks and becomes dense = PYKNOSIS

Nucleus fragments = KARYORRHEXIS

At *electron microscope (E.M.) level*, in addition to the above nuclear changes, disorganisation and disintegration of the cytoplasmic organelles and severe damage to the plasma membrane are seen.

NECROSIS

COLLIQUATIVE NECROSIS

In the brain consistently, and in other tissues when they contain a large amount of fluid and enzyme activity is marked, necrotic areas undergo softening and are filled with pigmented or turbid fluid, with complete loss of structure.

An **abscess** (see p. 42, 43) is an example of colliquative necrosis caused by the enzymatic action of polymorphonuclear leucocytes.

GANGRENE

This is a complication of necrosis. In certain circumstances necrotic tissue is liable to be invaded by putrefactive organisms which are both saccharolytic and proteolytic. Foul-smelling gases are produced and the tissue becomes green or black due to breakdown of haemoglobin. Obstruction of the blood supply to the bowel is almost inevitably followed by gangrene, e.g.:

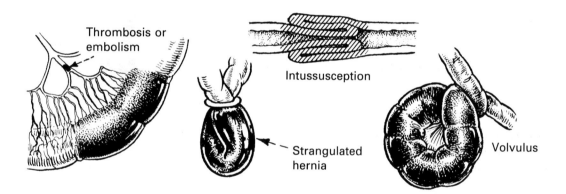

Gangrene also occurs on the skin surface following arterial obstruction. It is particularly liable to affect the limbs, especially the toes in diseases such as diabetes.

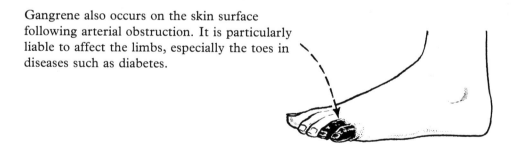

A special type of gangrene follows infection with clostridial organisms (gas gangrene; see p. 76).

NECROSIS

CASEOUS NECROSIS (CASEATION)

The necrotic tissue assumes a cream-cheesy appearance, slightly greasy to the touch. It is commonly seen in tuberculosis (see p. 78).

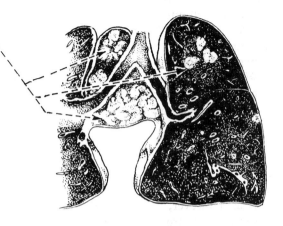

FAT NECROSIS

Adipose tissue is damaged in pancreatitis and occasionally due to trauma. The special appearances are due to the action of lipases on triglycerides as follows:

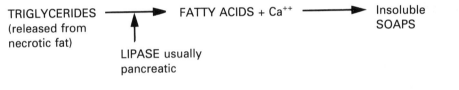

TRIGLYCERIDES (released from necrotic fat) ⟶ FATTY ACIDS + Ca⁺⁺ ⟶ Insoluble SOAPS

LIPASE usually pancreatic

E.g. Appearances in omentum and mesenteries.

Naked eye   **Microscopic**

Normal fatty tissue   *Necrotic*

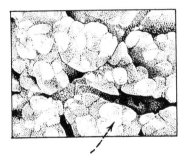

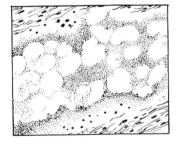

Opaque white patches

Note loss of nuclei and cell structure, and deposition of insoluble **soaps**.

FIBRINOID NECROSIS

This is a descriptive term in which connective tissues and especially arterial walls are infiltrated by a strongly eosinophilic hyaline material which shows some of the characteristics of fibrin. Any actual necrosis is usually inconspicuous (see p. 221).

NECROSIS – AUTOLYSIS

SEQUELS OF NECROSIS

1. When small numbers of cells are involved, the cellular debris is removed by PHAGOCYTOSIS (see p. 38).
2. With larger numbers of dead cells, there is an inflammatory response with **organisation** and fibrous repair (see p. 44).
3. When the necrotic tissue cannot be completely removed or organised, deposition of **calcium** may be an additional feature, for example in TUBERCULOUS CASEOUS NECROSIS and the ARTHEROMATOUS AORTA. This feature is important in radiological diagnosis.

AUTOLYSIS

The process of 'self-digestion' begins after the death of the cell (as described above) and proceeds at a rate dependent on the local enzyme content; it is an inevitable sequel of necrosis. However, the term is more commonly applied to the changes which take place in tissues removed from the body and in the whole body after death.

In practice, autolysis can be modified or inhibited as follows:

(1) by REFRIGERATION
↓
ENZYME activity
slowed down
↓
Whole body
'preserved'
↓
AUTOPSY performed
without undue
haste

(2) by FIXATION
↓
CHEMICALS added
(e.g. formalin)
or HEAT
↓
ENZYMES and PROTEINS
DENATURED
↓
AVAILABLE for PATHOLOGICAL
PROCESSING

CELL DAMAGE – FATTY CHANGE

This is accumulation of fat in non-fatty tissues, especially the parenchymatous organs, skeletal muscles and the heart, which have a high metabolic rate.

The essential problem is the inability of the non-fatty tissues to metabolise the amount of lipid presented to them, resulting in its accumulation within the cells. The most important causes range from direct cell poisons through clinical conditions associated with reduced cellular energy.

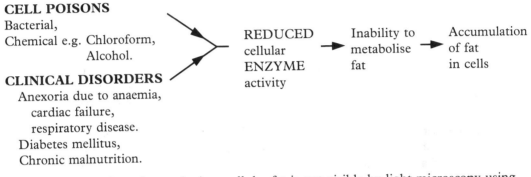

CELL POISONS
Bacterial,
Chemical e.g. Chloroform,
      Alcohol.

CLINICAL DISORDERS
Anexoria due to anaemia,
   cardiac failure,
   respiratory disease.
Diabetes mellitus,
Chronic malnutrition.

REDUCED cellular ENZYME activity → Inability to metabolise fat → Accumulation of fat in cells

In normal non-fatty tissues the intracellular fat is not visible by light microscopy using conventional fat stains.

In fatty change, the accumulated fat is visualised using frozen sections and fat-soluble dyes: in routine paraffin sections the fat has been dissolved and is indicated by clear vacuoles.

For example, in the **LIVER**, the increase of deposited fat causes enlargement of the organ. Its distribution varies with the cause, e.g. —

(1) Lack of Oxygen — in anaemia and cardiac failure

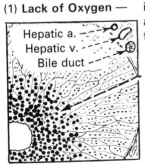

Hepatic a.
Hepatic v.
Bile duct

Fats tend to be deposited furthest from the arterial blood supply (hepatic arteriole) around the efferent vein (hepatic venule)

(2) Poison, Toxins etc — alcohol, infections, organic solvents

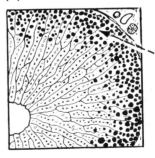

Fat is found nearest the afferent blood supply (portal venule and hepatic arteriole)

CELL DAMAGE – FATTY CHANGE

EFFECTS OF FATTY CHANGE

Impairment of cellular function is usually due to the pathological process causing the fatty change (e.g. anoxia in severe anaemia) and not to the physical presence of fat within the cell. In the liver, for example, very large accumulations of fat do not impair basic liver functions.

A possible exception is the myocardium in certain circumstances.

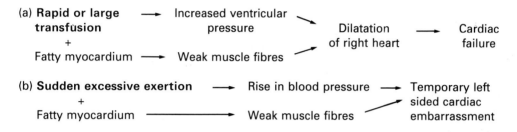

(a) **Rapid or large transfusion** → Increased ventricular pressure ↘
Dilatation of right heart → Cardiac failure
+
Fatty myocardium → Weak muscle fibres ↗

(b) **Sudden excessive exertion** → Rise in blood pressure → Temporary left sided cardiac embarrassment
+
Fatty myocardium → Weak muscle fibres ↗

OBESITY must be distinguished from intra-cellular fatty change described above.

Gross degrees of obesity lead to increased **adipose tissue** in abnormal sites, e.g. between myocardial fibres. In addition, parenchymal cells are unable to deal with the excessive intake of fat and a degree of fatty change occurs in them. The myocardium is under strain due to the circulatory resistance in the excessive adipose tissues.

The main controllable cause of obesity is increased intake of food, but other factors, both genetic and environmental, exert an influence. The diagram illustrates how the Food/Energy balance may be upset.

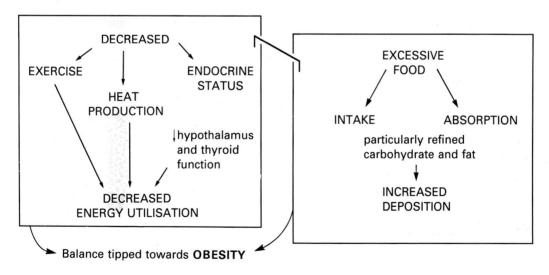

Effects: Obesity reduces life expectancy mainly due to its association with cardiovascular disease, including HYPERTENSION and CORONARY ATHEROMA.
Type II diabetes, osteoarthritis of the lower limb joints, and gall stones are closely associated.

11

CELL DAMAGE – RADIATION

High energy (ionising) radiation, particularly in the form of gamma (γ) or X-rays can cause serious cellular and tissue damage.

At cellular level there are 2 mechanisms involving:

1. The cell **CYTOPLASM**

A large dose of radiation hydrolyses water producing damaging hydroxyl radicals: acute cell death follows

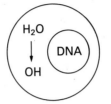

2. The cell **NUCLEUS**

Lower doses damage DNA with 2 results:
(a) failure to replicate
(b) mutation with variable genetic abnormalities

These effects will be considered under 3 headings:

1. The **localised effects** complicating radiotherapy in the tissues adjacent to the therapeutic field.

Following any reparable acute damage a latent period precedes persistent injury. This is caused by:

(a) damage to blood vessels ⎫ leading to   (a) *ischaemia*
(b) damage to fibroblasts ⎭   (b) *dense fibrosis*

Injury to organs which are difficult to shield is seen, for example, in skin, eyes, alimentary tract, bladder, lungs, gonads and spinal cord.

In surgical practice, wound healing is seriously impaired.

2. Some of the mutations may lead to cancer, particularly leukaemias and lymphomas. (About 2% of all malignancies are associated with radiation.)

The mechanisms are described on page 158.

3. **Whole body radiation** is usually the result of atomic explosion. The acute effects which are related to large doses are summarised below.

Dose (Grays)	Result	Mechanism
above 50	Death in a few hours	All cells damaged but particularly **CNS**: CEREBRAL OEDEMA ↓ COMA
5 – 10	Death 3–7 days	Mucous lining of **intestine** destroyed: DIARRHOEA: SEPTICAEMIC SHOCK
2 – 5	Death 2–3 weeks	**Bone marrow** destroyed: LEUCOPENIA THROMBOCYTOPENIA ↓ INFECTION: HAEMORRHAGE
0.2 – 1	Damage to fetus in early pregnancy	Embryonal cell mutation

ATROPHY

This is a simple decrease in cell size or number, resulting in a shrinkage of affected tissues and organs. The most common example is atrophy of old age (see p. 14)

Causes

(1) **Gradual diminution**   ⟶   Reduction in   ⟶   General fall in cell
     in blood supply   oxygen supply   activity and shrinkage,
                               and nutrients   e.g. narrowing of coronary
                                                arteries ⟶ myocardial
                                                           atrophy

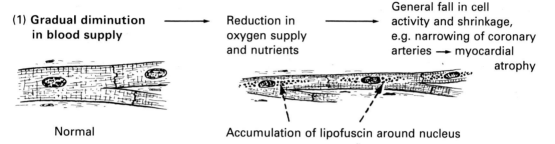

        Normal   Accumulation of lipofuscin around nucleus

Lipofuscin ("wear and tear" pigment) is a golden yellow pigment representing undigested lipid material derived from cellular metabolism.

(2) **Reduced functional activity**   ⟶   Diminished demand   ⟶   Atrophy
     (disuse atrophy)   for nutrition   of cells

       E.g. Obstruction of gland duct   ⟶   Atrophy of gland

(3) **Interrupted nerve supply** ⟶ Reduced reflex and metabolic activities, e.g. atrophy of skeletal muscles after destruction of motor nerves as in poliomyelitis.

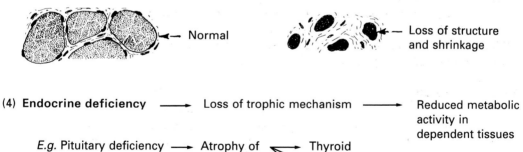

                         ⟵ Normal   Loss of structure
                                                     and shrinkage

(4) **Endocrine deficiency**   ⟶   Loss of trophic mechanism   ⟶   Reduced metabolic
                                                                  activity in
                                                                   dependent tissues

       E.g. Pituitary deficiency ⟶ Atrophy of ⟵ Thyroid
                                                  Adrenals
                                                  Gonads and genital organs

(5) **Pressure** ⟶ Interruption of blood supply and interference with function, e.g. neoplasm pressing on surrounding tissues.

Atrophy is reversible provided the cause is eliminated or deficiencies restored.

AGEING

The distinction between 'true' ageing and ageing complicated by disease processes may be difficult; since therapy can be directed at the latter the distinction is important in clinical practice.

The changes associated with *true* ageing would be seen in a theoretical 'ideal' environment (minimal stress).

The following diagram is illustrative. The main controlling factors are *intrinsic*, i.e. genetic: ? associated with ageing changes in mitochondrial DNA.

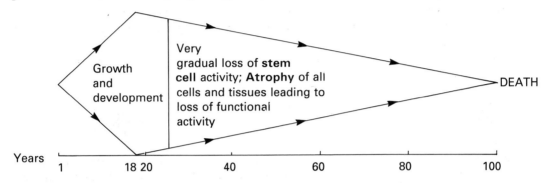

In the real environment this theoretical concept of ageing is accelerated and aggravated by two groups of *extrinsic* factors:

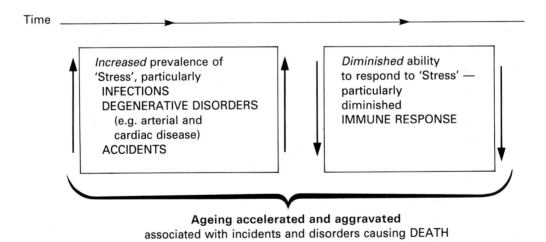

Ageing accelerated and aggravated
associated with incidents and disorders causing DEATH

N.B. Death is only very rarely, if ever, due to 'pure' ageing. It is the result of disease — either a single process or, with increasing age, more often several causes.

HEREDITY, GENES AND DISEASE

CELL NUCLEUS AND CHROMOSOMES

Knowledge of the GENETIC influence on disease is expanding very rapidly. The following can only be a brief outline of basic facts:

The cell **NUCLEUS** contains structures, CHROMOSOMES, which transmit hereditary traits from one generation to the next and also control the synthesis of all the proteins in the body.

The 46 chromosomes which most human nuclei contain are not identifiable in differentiated cells or cells in the non-proliferating phase of the cell cycle (G_o).

The different morphological appearances of nuclei in histological sections indicate to some extent the amount of nuclear activity.

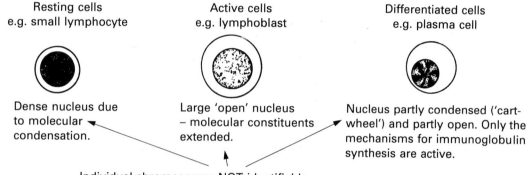

Resting cells
e.g. small lymphocyte

Active cells
e.g. lymphoblast

Differentiated cells
e.g. plasma cell

Dense nucleus due to molecular condensation.

Large 'open' nucleus – molecular constituents extended.

Nucleus partly condensed ('cartwheel') and partly open. Only the mechanisms for immunoglobulin synthesis are active.

Individual chromosomes NOT identifiable.

CHROMOSOMES

During MITOSIS the chromosomes condense into specific morphological forms which are identifiable by light microscopy: when colchicine is added to a cell culture, mitosis is arrested at the metaphase: chromosomes are then separable and can be studied.

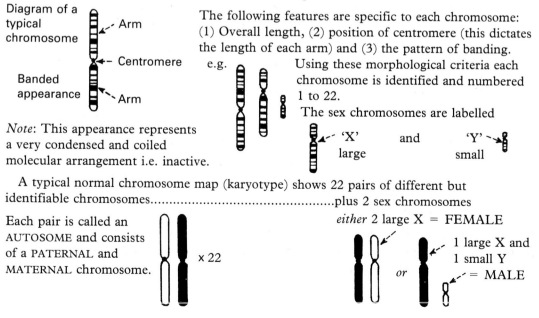

Diagram of a typical chromosome

Arm

Centromere

Banded appearance

Arm

Note: This appearance represents a very condensed and coiled molecular arrangement i.e. inactive.

The following features are specific to each chromosome: (1) Overall length, (2) position of centromere (this dictates the length of each arm) and (3) the pattern of banding.

e.g. Using these morphological criteria each chromosome is identified and numbered 1 to 22.

The sex chromosomes are labelled

'X' and 'Y'
large small

A typical normal chromosome map (karyotype) shows 22 pairs of different but identifiable chromosomes..plus 2 sex chromosomes

Each pair is called an AUTOSOME and consists of a PATERNAL and MATERNAL chromosome.

x 22

either 2 large X = FEMALE

or

1 large X and 1 small Y = MALE

15

HEREDITY, GENES AND DISEASE

DEOXYRIBONUCLEIC ACID (DNA)

Since Watson and Crick defined the molecular structure of DNA in 1963 there has been a great increase in knowledge of the 'genetic code'.

Each chromosome is a very long single molecule of DNA, condensed during mitosis.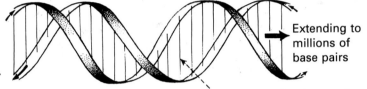

It is extended to its characteristic structure when active:

The **DOUBLE HELIX**

Diagram of a very small part of a very long molecule.

2 long spirals of nucleotides [consisting of a ribose (sugar) + phosphate] around a central axis, complementary but running in opposite directions.

Extending to millions of base pairs

Joined by purine and pyrimidine base pairs

The essential function is to initiate and control the synthesis of proteins from amino-acids. All types of protein (structural proteins, hormones, receptors, intra-cellular messengers etc.) are ENCODED along the molecule.

A GENE is the unit of the chromosome responsible for the synthesis of a single SPECIFIC PROTEIN. Genes vary in length but on average occupy about 20,000 base pairs of the molecule.

There are about 50,000 genes in all the 46 human chromosomes, not all are active: some are repetitive: some form clusters subserving related activities (e.g. MHC (HLA) locus, see p. 100).

There is a complex REGULATION of gene activity involving stop and start signals, promoter and enhancer functions all within the DNA structure.

Modern techniques of 'gene mapping', in which genes and their functions are identified, are proceeding very rapidly (some 2,000 have now been identified).

Diagram of Protein Synthesis

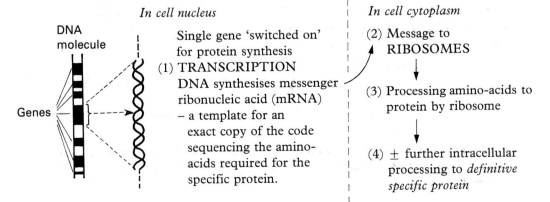

In cell nucleus

DNA molecule

Genes

Single gene 'switched on' for protein synthesis

(1) TRANSCRIPTION DNA synthesises messenger ribonucleic acid (mRNA) – a template for an exact copy of the code sequencing the amino-acids required for the specific protein.

In cell cytoplasm

(2) Message to RIBOSOMES

(3) Processing amino-acids to protein by ribosome

(4) $\pm$ further intracellular processing to *definitive specific protein*

MITOSIS AND MEIOSIS

MITOSIS is the process by which SOMATIC cells proliferate ensuring *exact replication of the daughter cells.* Following the stimulus to proliferate, the chromosomes condense and replicate exactly.

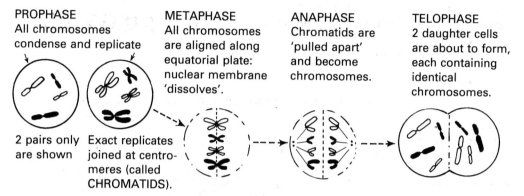

PROPHASE
All chromosomes condense and replicate

2 pairs only are shown Exact replicates joined at centromeres (called CHROMATIDS).

METAPHASE
All chromosomes are aligned along equatorial plate: nuclear membrane 'dissolves'.

ANAPHASE
Chromatids are 'pulled apart' and become chromosomes.

TELOPHASE
2 daughter cells are about to form, each containing identical chromosomes.

MEIOSIS is a complex process occurring during GAMETOGENESIS: it involves the reduction and division of chromosomes in such a way that (1) a random mixture of both parental genes is present in the gamete and that (2) the chances are equal for fertilisation to result in either sex.

This simple diagram shows the important results of meiosis.

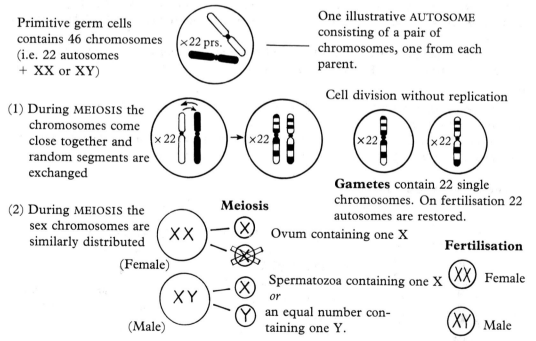

Primitive germ cells contains 46 chromosomes (i.e. 22 autosomes + XX or XY)

One illustrative AUTOSOME consisting of a pair of chromosomes, one from each parent.

(1) During MEIOSIS the chromosomes come close together and random segments are exchanged

Cell division without replication

Gametes contain 22 single chromosomes. On fertilisation 22 autosomes are restored.

(2) During MEIOSIS the sex chromosomes are similarly distributed

Meiosis

(Female)

(Male)

Ovum containing one X

Spermatozoa containing one X
or
an equal number containing one Y.

Fertilisation

Female

Male

Note: In this simplified diagram a preliminary replication before meiosis and mitotic divisions after meiosis are omitted. The chances of error can be seen to be greatly increased.

17

GENETIC ABNORMALITIES AND ASSOCIATED DISORDERS

It is not surprising that errors arise during these complex genetic activities. GERM CELLS and proliferating SOMATIC CELLS (including STEM CELLS) are susceptible to such errors.

They may occur spontaneously or be potentiated by external influences (see carcinogenesis, p. 158).

It is important to distinguish between germ cell and somatic cell abnormalities.

GERM CELL ABNORMALITIES

Errors which have arisen during germ cell development are transferred to the fertilised ovum and thence to all cells including the germ cells of the new individual.

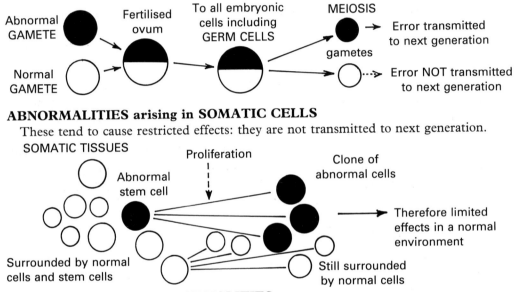

ABNORMALITIES arising in SOMATIC CELLS

These tend to cause restricted effects: they are not transmitted to next generation.

TYPES OF GENETIC ABNORMALITIES

They range from large, involving whole chromosomes, through parts of chromosomes, to gene clusters and single genes.

CHROMOSOMAL ABNORMALITIES

(1) *Polyploidy* — when the chromosomal numbers are increased by an exact multiple of the normal (23) e.g. 23 × 3 = 69 chromosomes. Such nuclei are seen in hypertrophied muscle cells and ageing liver cells (i.e. somatic cell polyploidy).

Such gross chromosomal abnormalities occurring during gametogenesis or at fertilisation are usually incompatible with life and are a common cause of spontaneous abortion.

(2) *Aneuploidy* — where the number of chromosomes is increased usually by one (TRISOMY) or decreased by one (MONOSOMY). Early spontaneous abortion is again common: survivors show mental retardation and varied physical abnormalities.

Down's syndrome is a good example of AUTOSOMAL TRISOMY and is due to an extra chromosome (i.e. Trisomy 21 — karyotype 47XX + 21 or 47XY + 21).

The abnormality occurs in utero after fertilisation of the ovum and is therefore autosomal. Increasing maternal age is a potentiating factor in Down's syndrome and many other genetic defects.

GENETIC ABNORMALITIES AND ASSOCIATED DISORDERS

CHROMOSOMAL ABNORMALITIES (continued)

(3) *Structural abnormalities*

Despite the existence of efficient repair mechanisms structural errors do arise when the long DNA molecules are accidentally broken during the dramatic physical changes occurring at replication. They include, for example, duplication and deletion of gene clusters and single genes: and translocation of fragments of DNA between chromosomes.

SINGLE GENE DISORDERS

Factors regulating the production of the final specific protein are extremely complex and interacting:

1. *In the nucleus*   *In the cytoplasm*

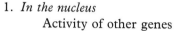

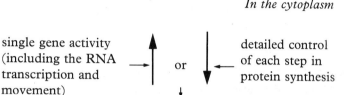

Therefore GENETIC EXPRESSION very VARIABLE

2. The corresponding genes on each parental chromosome exert important influences on each other. The inheritance of the Rhesus blood group D is illustrative: there are two possibilities at the D locus on the chromosome — 'D' or 'd'. The 3 possible combinations give rise to the actual blood group (phenotype) as follows:

	Homozygous		Heterozygous	
Genotype	DD	dd	Dd	⟶ The presence of one D confers the
Blood group (phenotype)	D	d	D	blood group D i.e. D is DOMINANT.

The presence of two d's is required to confer the blood group d, i.e. d is RECESSIVE.

This concept is important in *inherited single gene disorders*.

(1) In DOMINANT inheritance any HETEROZYGOUS offspring bearing the abnormal trait will be affected: mating with a normal partner statistically produces 50% of normal offspring and 50% affected.

(2) In RECESSIVE inheritance only HOMOZYGOTES for the trait are affected. Such cases usually arise from the mating of 2 heterozygous CARRIERS who, by definition, are themselves unaffected.

The results of mating are as follows: (A = affected gene, N = normal gene)
NN = normal individual: NA = carrier: AA = affected individual.

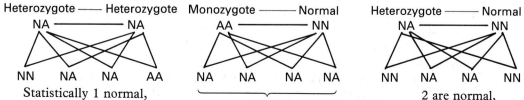

Heterozygote —— Heterozygote: NA × NA → NN NA NA AA. Statistically 1 normal, 2 carriers, 1 affected.

Monozygote —— Normal: AA × NN → NA NA NA NA. All offspring are carriers.

Heterozygote —— Normal: NA × NN → NN NA NA NN. 2 are normal, 2 are carriers.

19

GENETIC ABNORMALITIES AND ASSOCIATED DISORDERS

The concept of dominant and recessive traits is useful in genetic counselling. Long lists of dominant and recessive disorders are available: only a few important examples are given.

Autosomal dominant – neurofibromatosis, Huntington's disease: polyposis coli: congenital spherocytosis.

Autosomal recessive – cystic fibrosis, congenital deafness, mucopolysaccharidoses.

Sex-linked disorders are usually recessive and are carried on the X-chromosome: males are affected and females are carriers. Important disorders are haemophilia and muscular dystrophy.

METABOLIC DISORDERS (inborn errors of metabolism)

These are inherited disorders of single genes which code for the enzymes concerned in many metabolic pathways. The clinical effects show considerable variation in severity.

Examples are: disorders of carbohydrate (including glycogen storage), lipid and amino-acid metabolism: lysosomal storage: and membrane transport (including cystic fibrosis).

Note: Not all single gene abnormalities cause, by themselves, significant pathological effects. As indicated above, the controlling factors are complex and include the important effects of 'modifying genes'. It seems likely that abnormal recessive genes exist in the normal population but only present as clinical disorders in rare special circumstances.

MULTIFACTORIAL DISORDERS

Most human diseases have a genetic component but environmental factors usually play a very important part in the pathogenesis.

$$\text{COMBINED ACTIVITY of SEVERAL GENES (both normal and abnormal)} + \text{ENVIRONMENTAL FACTORS} \longrightarrow \text{DISEASE}$$

Examples are: atopic (allergic) disorders: diabetes mellitus, hypertension, rheumatoid arthritis and various infections.

SOMATIC CELL GENETIC DISORDERS

When mutation occurs after fertilisation of the ovum and at any stage throughout life the effects are limited to the disordered cell(s) and progeny. The clinical effects tend to be localised.

Neoplasms and hamartomas are examples of somatic cell disorders (see carcinogenesis).

Note: In the systematic section of this book significant genetic contribution to the pathogenesis of diseases will be recorded.

DEPOSITIONS

AMYLOID DEPOSITION

In this condition, a 'waxy' substance composed essentially of an abnormal protein is deposited in the extracellular tissues, particularly around the supporting fibres of blood vessels and basement membranes. Amyloid is resistant to degradation and removal by the usual process so that the deposition progresses relentlessly.

Detection

Amyloid may be suspected when the organs are pale and enlarged and have a firm waxy texture at post-mortem, but in clinical practice, chemical tests on microscopic preparations and even electron microscopy are required using biopsy material.

Post-mortem organs

LUGOL'S IODINE ⟨ Amyloid — deep brown
Normal tissue — yellow

Biopsy materials 1. Light microscopic sections

CONGO RED ⟨ Amyloid — red and specific apple green fluorescence in polarised light
Normal tissue — pale pink or yellow: no fluorescence

2. E.M. — specific appearance: closely packed interlacing fibrils 70 to 100 Å in diameter

Nature of amyloid

Chemical — the fibrils are composed of one major and two minor components:
1. Protein — variable (see p. 23)
2. (a) Protein — constant normally found in serum:
        called SERUM AMYLOID PROTEIN (SAP).
   (b) Carbohydrate — a glycosaminoglycan (e.g. heparin sulphate) — this gives the iodine stain.

Physical — the fibrils are organised uniquely — β-pleated.

   This accounts for the specific staining properties and the inability of the body to degrade the substance.

Pathological effects

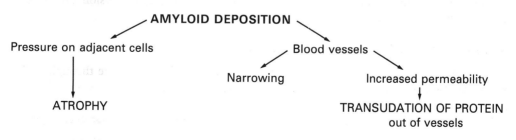

AMYLOID DEPOSITION

Pressure on adjacent cells

ATROPHY

Blood vessels

Narrowing   Increased permeability

TRANSUDATION OF PROTEIN
out of vessels

AMYLOID DEPOSITION

Almost any tissue in the body may be affected by amyloid deposition, but the most important changes occur in the kidney, gastrointestinal tract and the heart. Other organs, such as the liver and spleen, may also be grossly affected without serious functional impairment.

KIDNEY

In severe cases the kidneys are pale, firm and waxy, and with the iodine test the glomeruli stand out as brown dots to the naked eye.

Renal biopsy is useful in the diagnosis of amyloidosis.

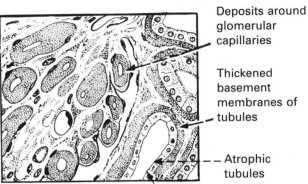

Deposits around glomerular capillaries

Thickened basement membranes of tubules

Atrophic tubules

Effects: Glomerular capillary permeability altered:

GROSS PROTEINURIA ⟶ NEPHROTIC SYNDROME

GASTROINTESTINAL TRACT

Due to altered permeability of the capillaries, the patient suffers from diarrhoea and protein loss. There may also be malabsorption, nutritional deficiencies and electrolyte imbalance.

Rectal biopsy is useful in the diagnosis of amyloidosis.

HEART

Amyloid deposition occurs around the cardiac muscle fibres and the capillary basement membranes. The heart is enlarged with apparently thick muscular walls but much of the thickness is due to amyloid deposition.

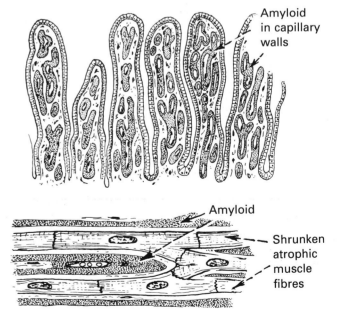

Amyloid in capillary walls

Amyloid

Shrunken atrophic muscle fibres

Effects: Cardiac failure develops mainly due to the mechanical effect of amyloid, preventing proper muscular contraction, and partly to malnutrition of the muscle fibres caused by poor blood supply.

AMYLOID DEPOSITION

MECHANISMS OF AMYLOID DEPOSITION

The essential element in amyloid deposition is the production of a protein which is either amyloidogenic itself or can be modified to become amyloidogenic.

Amyloidogenic proteins

1. Amyloid A protein (AA)
This protein is closely related to acute phase reactive protein which appears in the serum in many inflammatory conditions.

2. Amyloid Light Chain derived protein (AL)
This protein is derived from fragments of immunoglobulin molecules (particularly lambda light chains) and is essentially a product of plasma cells.

The important facts about these proteins is that they form specific amyloid fibrils in which the molecules of constituent polypeptides are arranged in a most unusual fashion, called β-pleating. This imparts to amyloid its specific chemical staining characteristics and accounts for its resistance to degradation.

The mechanism of amyloid deposition is shown thus:

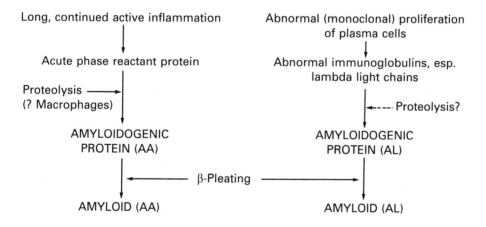

Amyloidogenic proteins and polypeptides may also occur in other circumstances, e.g. in tumours of endocrine glands producing polypeptide hormones (e.g. calcitonin, insulin) and in cases of rare familial amyloidosis.

In old age, minor deposits of amyloid may occur in the heart and brain; the amyloidogenic protein in these cases is related to prealbumin.

AMYLOID DEPOSITION

CLASSIFICATION

Amyloidosis was previously classified into two main types, and the distribution of amyloid among various organs was observed to be different in these types, although considerable overlapping occurred.

1. **Primary**, i.e. without known cause.
2. **Secondary**, i.e. associated with chronic inflammatory diseases such as tuberculosis, osteomyelitis, rheumatoid arthritis.

Modern knowledge of the mechanisms underlying amyloid deposition have made this classification obsolete. The classification which emerges from knowledge of the mechanisms of amyloid deposition and the more usual associated precursor diseases is shown as follows:

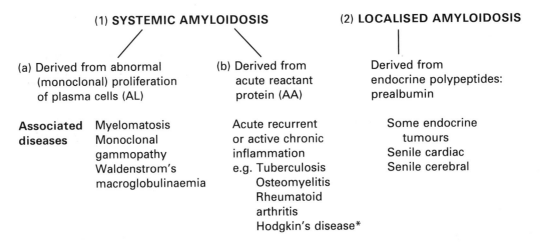

(1) SYSTEMIC AMYLOIDOSIS   **(2) LOCALISED AMYLOIDOSIS**

(a) Derived from abnormal (monoclonal) proliferation of plasma cells (AL)

(b) Derived from acute reactant protein (AA)

Derived from endocrine polypeptides: prealbumin

Associated diseases

Myelomatosis
Monoclonal gammopathy
Waldenstrom's macroglobulinaemia

Acute recurrent or active chronic inflammation e.g. Tuberculosis
Osteomyelitis
Rheumatoid arthritis
Hodgkin's disease*

Some endocrine tumours
Senile cardiac
Senile cerebral

Note: Not all cases of these diseases are associated with amyloid; e.g. certain chronic inflammatory diseases are not associated with amyloid, such as ulcerative colitis and systemic lupus erythematosus, since the serum acute reactant protein is minimally raised.

*Hodgkin's disease is considered to be a tumour with a marked inflammatory reaction (see p. 585).

CALCIFICATION

Abnormal deposits of calcium salts occur in two circumstances: dystrophic calcification and metastatic calcification.

1. DYSTROPHIC CALCIFICATION

Local deposits of calcium may occur in:

(a) Necrotic tissue which is not absorbed,

e.g. old caseous lesions of tuberculosis; old infarcts; old collections of pus; dead parasites; old thrombi.

An important variation of this is the accumulation of calcium around dead cells in ducts, leading to stone formation.

(b) Tissues undergoing slow degeneration,

e.g. hyaline areas in simple tumours; tissues in old age, especially fibrous tissue, cartilage and in arteries due to atheromatous degeneration.

The mechanism may be as follows:

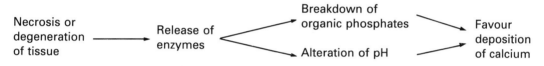

Note: The presence of radio-opaque Ca^{++} is of diagnostic use particularly in old healed disease (e.g. tuberculosis) and also in some tumours, e.g. breast cancer where very small deposits of calcium may be present.

2. METASTATIC CALCIFICATION

In this case the essential feature is an increase in the blood calcium. The 2 usual mechanisms are as follows:

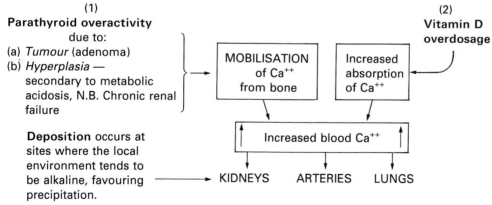

About 5% of MALIGNANCY cases — particularly with carcinoma of the breast and lung — have HYPERCALCAEMIA, although most do not live long enough to have significant systemic deposition.

The mechanisms are (1) secretion by the tumour of a protein which mimics the action of parathormone and (2), of less importance, the local release of bone resorbing cytokines by tumour metastases in bones.

25

ENDOGENOUS PIGMENTATION

MELANIN PIGMENTATION

Melanin is a normal pigment found in the form of fine brown granules in the skin, choroid of the eye, adrenal medulla and sometimes in the meninges. It is produced by melanocytes embryologically derived from the neural crest and which have a dendritic branching form. After secretion of the pigment, it is taken up by adjacent epidermal cells and phagocytic melanophores in the underlying dermis.

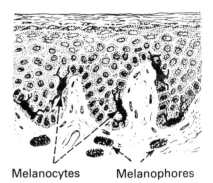

Melanocytes   Melanophores

Local melanin pigmentation

This is seen in tumours derived from the melanocytes of the skin and choroid coat of the eye.

Generalised melanin pigmentation

Suntan is a temporary general melanin pigmentation of the skin due to ultraviolet rays. The mechanism and its control are as follows:

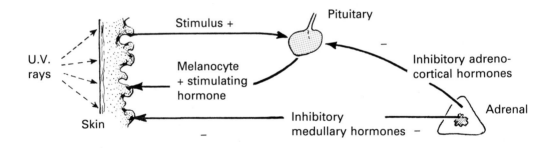

Melanocyte-stimulating hormone (MSH) stimulates production of melanin in the skin and probably also an increase of melanocytes. The secretion of MSH is monitored by adreno-cortical hormones. In addition, the adrenal catecholamines appear to inhibit the formation of pigment at a local skin level.

Addison's disease. Generalised melanosis is a characteristic of this condition which involves the destruction of the adrenals, thus removing the inhibitory adrenal control. Secretion of MSH proceeds unopposed. Pigmentation is seen on exposed skin surfaces, and those subject to local irritation including squamous mucous surfaces such as the mouth.

Chloasma. Patches of melanotic pigmentation appear on the skin of the face, breasts and genitalia due to increased secretion of MSH. It is most common in pregnancy.

ENDOGENOUS PIGMENTATION

Haemoglobin is broken down and the main products, haem and its derivatives and the protein fraction GLOBIN, are re-used or excreted as follows:

(A) Destruction of effete red cells by the MACROPHAGES in the SPLENIC RETICULUM (also in other tissues, e.g. bone marrow and liver)

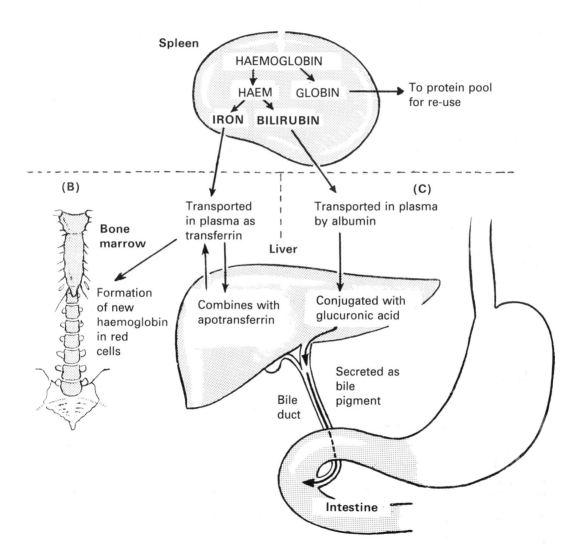

Abnormalities arising at various stages may be associated with the accumulation of pigments as illustrated in the following examples.

ENDOGENOUS PIGMENTATION

JAUNDICE due to BILIRUBIN (IRON-FREE PIGMENT)

When the bilirubin content of the serum rises above 34μmol/l, jaundice appears. This can be brought about by an abnormality in one of 3 main ways:

1. **Post-hepatic (obstructive) Jaundice**

    OBSTRUCTION OF BILE DUCTS is commonly due to gall stones in the major ducts, tumour compression or, very occasionally, fibrosis involving the small intrahepatic ducts. The bile canaliculi become distended with conjugated bilirubin which is reabsorbed. Conjugated bilirubin is water-soluble and is excreted in the urine.

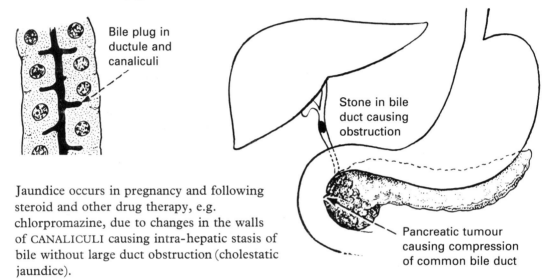

Bile plug in ductule and canaliculi

Stone in bile duct causing obstruction

Pancreatic tumour causing compression of common bile duct

Jaundice occurs in pregnancy and following steroid and other drug therapy, e.g. chlorpromazine, due to changes in the walls of CANALICULI causing intra-hepatic stasis of bile without large duct obstruction (cholestatic jaundice).

2. **Pre-hepatic Jaundice**

    INCREASED DESTRUCTION OF RED CELLS as in haemolytic anaemia, e.g. acholuric jaundice or haemolytic anaemia of the newborn. In these conditions the excessive amount of pigment has not passed through the liver for conjugation. It is held in solution in the plasma in combination with albumin. In adults the pigment may have little effect, but in the newborn it can crystallise out in the tissues and, in the brain, may cause necrosis. Because of the size of the bilirubinalbumin molecule, the pigment does not appear in the urine (Acholuric jaundice, see p. 515).

3. **Hepato-cellular Jaundice**

    LIVER CELL DAMAGE (occurring most commonly in HEPATITIS) is the essential feature. The mechanisms are complex:

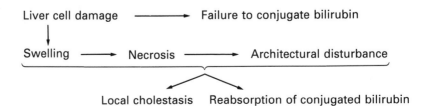

Liver cell damage ⟶ Failure to conjugate bilirubin

Swelling ⟶ Necrosis ⟶ Architectural disturbance

Local cholestasis   Reabsorption of conjugated bilirubin

ENDOGENOUS PIGMENTATION

IRON-CONTAINING PIGMENT

Haemosiderin

The iron derived from red cell breakdown is held in the spleen, liver and marrow, combined with apoferritin. In the plasma it is transported by transferrin. The two mechanisms maintain an equilibrium between the iron contents in these three sites. When the amount of iron within the cells becomes excessive and overloads the ferritin system, it is deposited in a brown granular form — haemosiderin.

This occurs in two situations:-

1. **Local breakdown of red cells in tissues e.g. in**

The colour changes in a 'black' eye exemplify this mechanism

Internal haemorrhage

Extravasated red cells
↓
Phagocytosis of red cells by macrophages

Haemosiderin   Iron free pigments

RED
↓
GREENISH BLUE
↓
YELLOW

2. **Visceral siderosis**

This is seen in the liver, spleen and sometimes the kidneys in cases of haemolytic anaemia, and in patients requiring repeated blood transfusion. The change is most strikingly seen in the liver, which becomes deep brown. Iron is found in the liver parenchyma, in cells and in liver cells. Easily demonstrated by the Prussian Blue reaction.

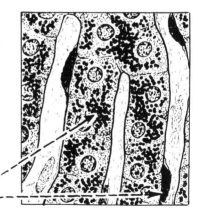

Granules of haemosiderin in liver cells and Kupffer cells

ENDOGENOUS PIGMENTATION

Haemosiderin (continued)

Haemochromatosis (Bronzed diabetes)

The absorption of iron from the intestine is controlled by the ferritin-transferrin mechanism already mentioned.

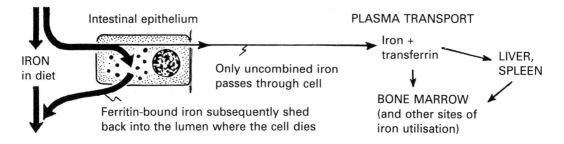

IRON in diet

Intestinal epithelium

Only uncombined iron passes through cell

Ferritin-bound iron subsequently shed back into the lumen where the cell dies

PLASMA TRANSPORT

Iron + transferrin

LIVER, SPLEEN

BONE MARROW (and other sites of iron utilisation)

The ferritin content of the intestinal epithelium, iron saturation of the plasma, stores of iron in the liver and spleen and the demand for iron by the bone marrow form a balancing mechanism preventing overloading of any part of the system.

In haemochromatosis, a genetic disorder, the absorption of iron is virtually uncontrolled. The system becomes overloaded and iron is deposited as haemosiderin in many sites, the main ones being:

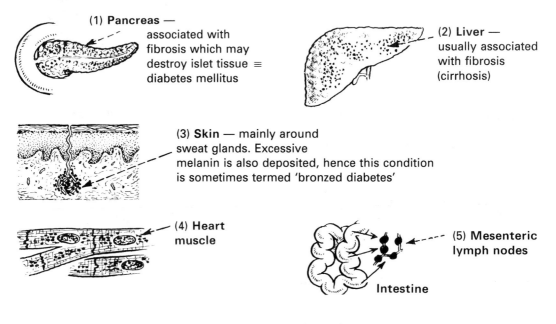

(1) Pancreas — associated with fibrosis which may destroy islet tissue ≡ diabetes mellitus

(2) Liver — usually associated with fibrosis (cirrhosis)

(3) Skin — mainly around sweat glands. Excessive melanin is also deposited, hence this condition is sometimes termed 'bronzed diabetes'

(4) Heart muscle

(5) Mesenteric lymph nodes

Intestine

Haemosiderin may be found in almost any site in the body.

ENDOGENOUS PIGMENTATION

Haemoglobin

Occasionally, intravascular haemolysis occurs. Haemoglobin appears in the urine, giving it a dull red colour — in the severe acute situation (e.g. incompatible blood transfusion) acute renal tubular necrosis occurs. If the condition is chronic, as in paroxysmal haemoglobinuria, some of the haemoglobin is reabsorbed and subsequently broken down so that iron, as haemosiderin, appears in the renal tubular epithelium. — — — — —

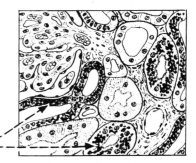

(Demonstrated by the Prussian blue reaction)

Haematin (or haemazoin)

This is a brown pigment produced by malarial parasites from haemoglobin. It is taken up by the monocytes in the blood and subsequently deposited in the liver and spleen.

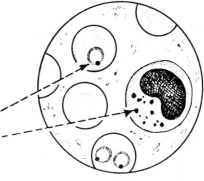

Red-cell — containing malarial parasite

Monocyte — containing haematin

Lipofuscin

This is a yellowish brown pigment having a high lipid content, often found in the atrophied cells of old age — 'wear and tear' pigment. It is particularly common in the heart muscle, and the term 'brown atrophy' is often applied.

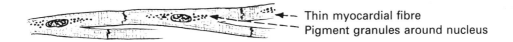

Thin myocardial fibre
Pigment granules around nucleus

It is also found in liver cells, testes and nerve cells.

EXOGENOUS PIGMENTATION – DEGENERATIONS

EXOGENOUS PIGMENTATION

Pigments may be introduced by inhalation, ingestion or injection. The most important are those introduced by inhalation of dusts in industrial processes.

Inhalation

The commonest substances inhaled are COAL DUST (carbon) — black, and STONE DUST (silica) — grey.

The particles reach the alveoli especially if the bronchial ciliary action is disturbed by chronic bronchitis.

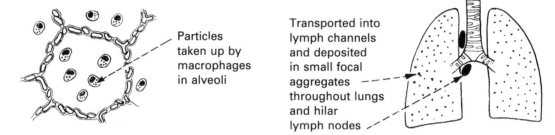

Particles taken up by macrophages in alveoli

Transported into lymph channels and deposited in small focal aggregates throughout lungs and hilar lymph nodes

The effects are described in detail under PNEUMOCONIOSIS (p. 335).

Ingestion

Pigmentation can be caused by chronic ingestion of metals such as silver or lead. In both, the skin has a metallic hue, and in the case of lead a blue line appears on the gums due to interaction between lead and sulphuretted hydrogen. Excessive intake of carrots can lead to yellowish red skin pigmentation caused by carotene.

Injection

Tattooing is the most striking example of pigmentation following injection.

DEGENERATIONS

1. **Hyaline**

   This is a descriptive term meaning a glossy, refractile appearance, seen in sections stained with haematoxylin and eosin. It does not denote any specific substance. It is most commonly encountered in the form of dense collagen, particularly in simple tumours such as fibromyomata where the collagen may replace muscle fibres. Cytoplasmic hyaline substance is sometimes seen when cells are severely damaged, e.g. in alcoholic hepatitis.

   The term 'hyaline' is used in many situations where degeneration is not a feature, e.g. old fibrin thrombi often assume a glossy appearance.

2. **Mucoid**

   This is a common change in epithelial tumours which secrete mucin. In these cases the epithelial cells undergo degeneration and appear to dissolve in the mucin.

   Occasionally connective tissue appears to secrete mucin. Spaces filled with mucopolysaccharides appear between the fibres. The change is not uncommon in some tumours. In these cases the term 'myxomatous' may be used.

32

INFLAMMATION

INFLAMMATION

Inflammation is the dynamic processes by which living tissues react to injury. They concern vascular and connective tissues particularly.

Causes:
Various agents may kill or damage cells:

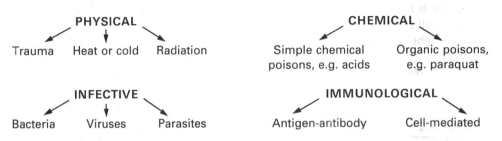

PHYSICAL			CHEMICAL	
Trauma	Heat or cold	Radiation	Simple chemical poisons, e.g. acids	Organic poisons, e.g. paraquat

INFECTIVE			IMMUNOLOGICAL	
Bacteria	Viruses	Parasites	Antigen-antibody	Cell-mediated

. . . and any other circumstance leading to tissue damage, e.g. VASCULAR or HORMONAL DISTURBANCE.

The inflammatory reaction takes place in the surviving adjacent vascular and connective tissues; the specialised parenchymal cells do not directly participate.

The initial stages are known as the **acute** inflammatory reaction. Where the process is prolonged the inflammation may be **subacute** or **chronic**.

ACUTE INFLAMMATION
The classical signs are:

REDNESS (rubor)
HEAT (calor)
SWELLING (tumor)
PAIN (dolor)
LOSS OF FUNCTION (functio laesa).

e.g. Boil

These gross signs are explained by changes occurring at microscopic level.
Three essential features are:

1. **HYPERAEMIA**
2. **EXUDATION**
3. **EMIGRATION OF LEUCOCYTES**

ACUTE INFLAMMATION

HYPERAEMIA

The hyperaemia in inflammation is associated with the well known microvascular changes which occur in Lewis' triple response — a FLUSH, a FLARE and a WEAL. It occurs when a blunt instrument is drawn firmly across the skin and illustrates the vascular changes occurring in acute inflammation.

The stroke is marked momentarily by a white line due to VASOCONSTRICTION.

The flush, a dull red line, immediately follows and is due to CAPILLARY DILATATION.

The flare, a bright red irregular surrounding zone, is due to ARTERIOLAR DILATATION.

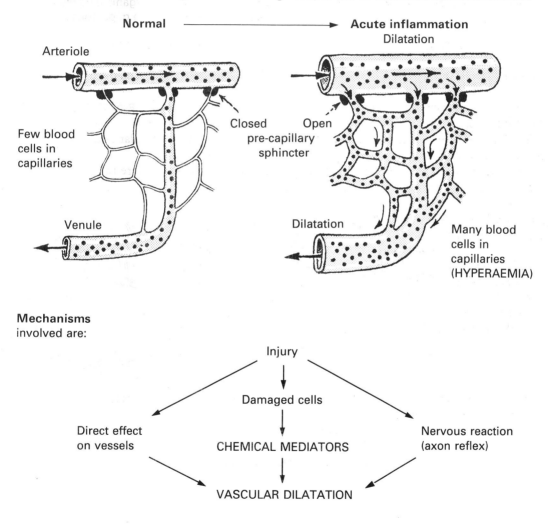

Mechanisms
involved are:

HYPERAEMIA explains the classical signs of REDNESS and HEAT.

ACUTE INFLAMMATION

EXUDATION

Exudation is the increased passage of protein — rich fluid through the vessel wall into the interstitial tissue. It explains the **weal** in Lewis' triple response.

Advantageous results

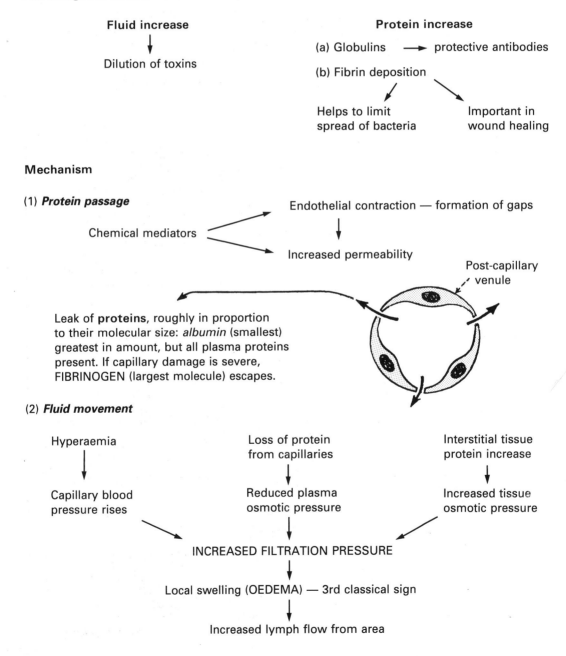

Fluid increase

↓

Dilution of toxins

Protein increase

(a) Globulins ⟶ protective antibodies

(b) Fibrin deposition

Helps to limit
spread of bacteria

Important in
wound healing

Mechanism

(1) *Protein passage*

Chemical mediators

Endothelial contraction — formation of gaps

↓

Increased permeability

Post-capillary
venule

Leak of **proteins**, roughly in proportion
to their molecular size: *albumin* (smallest)
greatest in amount, but all plasma proteins
present. If capillary damage is severe,
FIBRINOGEN (largest molecule) escapes.

(2) *Fluid movement*

Hyperaemia

↓

Capillary blood
pressure rises

Loss of protein
from capillaries

↓

Reduced plasma
osmotic pressure

Interstitial tissue
protein increase

↓

Increased tissue
osmotic pressure

INCREASED FILTRATION PRESSURE

↓

Local swelling (OEDEMA) — 3rd classical sign

↓

Increased lymph flow from area

ACUTE INFLAMMATION

EMIGRATION OF LEUCOCYTES

Neutrophils and mononuclears pass between the endothelial cell junctions by amoeboid movement through the venule wall into the tissue spaces.

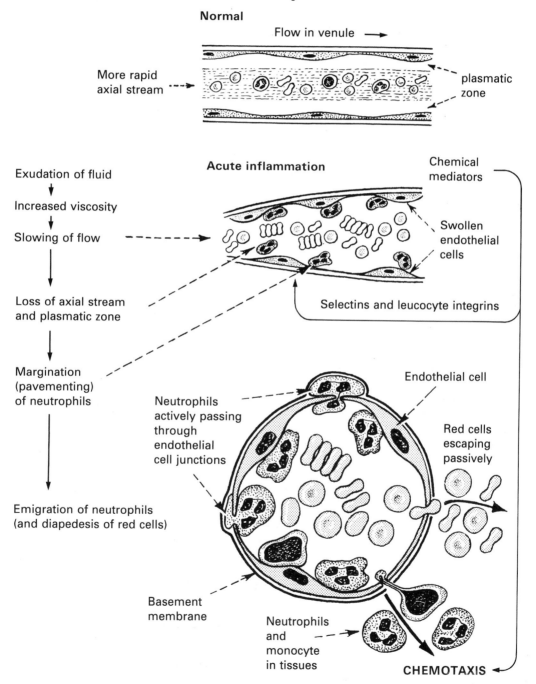

Normal

Flow in venule →

More rapid axial stream ·-·→

plasmatic zone

Acute inflammation

Exudation of fluid
↓
Increased viscosity
↓
Slowing of flow - - - →
↓
Loss of axial stream and plasmatic zone
↓
Margination (pavementing) of neutrophils
↓
Emigration of neutrophils (and diapedesis of red cells)

Chemical mediators

Swollen endothelial cells

Selectins and leucocyte integrins

Neutrophils actively passing through endothelial cell junctions

Endothelial cell

Red cells escaping passively

Basement membrane

Neutrophils and monocyte in tissues

CHEMOTAXIS ←

37

ACUTE INFLAMMATION

CHEMOTAXIS

The initial margination of neutrophils and mononuclears is potentiated by slowing of blood flow and by increased 'stickiness' of the endothelial surface.

After penetration of the vessel wall, the subsequent movement of the leucocytes is controlled by CHEMOTAXIS. The cell moves in response to an increasing concentration gradient of the particular chemotactic agent, usually a protein or polypeptide.

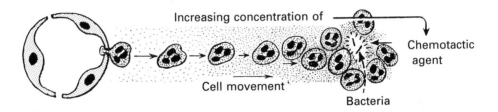

Important examples of chemotactic agents are:

Fractions of the COMPLEMENT system (esp. C5a)
Factors derived from arachidonic acid by the neutrophils — LEUKOTRIENES
Factors derived from pathogenic BACTERIA
Factors derived from sensitised lymphocytes — LYMPHOKINES.

The process helps to explain the apparently purposeful movement of leucocytes and their aggregation in large numbers in inflammation.

PHAGOCYTOSIS

This is the process by which neutrophils and macrophages ingest debris and 'foreign' particles. It is similar to the feeding process of the amoeba.

It is an important defence mechanism in bacterial infections particularly.

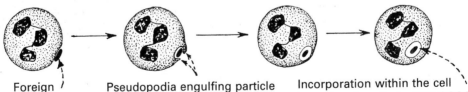

Factors influencing the efficiency of phagocytosis:

(1) OPSONINS — antibodies of both natural and specific immune type (see p. 107)
(2) Fractions of the COMPLEMENT system
(3) The PHYSICAL STATE of the cellular environment

The opsonic activity is enhanced when it is confined within a solid organ or rigid medium such as a fibrin network; where the conditions are looser and more fluid, activity is diminished.

ACUTE INFLAMMATION

Sequels of phagocytosis

NEUTROPHIL (*natural life span 1 — 3 days*)

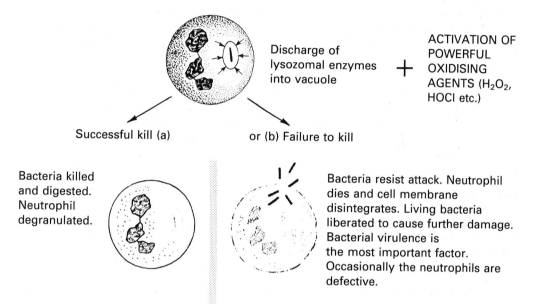

Discharge of
lysozomal enzymes
into vacuole

$+$

ACTIVATION OF
POWERFUL
OXIDISING
AGENTS (H_2O_2,
HOCl etc.)

Successful kill (a)

or (b) Failure to kill

Bacteria killed
and digested.
Neutrophil
degranulated.

Bacteria resist attack. Neutrophil
dies and cell membrane
disintegrates. Living bacteria
liberated to cause further damage.
Bacterial virulence is
the most important factor.
Occasionally the neutrophils are
defective.

MACROPHAGE (*natural life span — months to several years*)

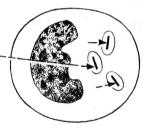

(a) Successful kill may be accomplished.
(b) Failure to kill may allow bacteria to continue to live within
the cell which may move via lymphatics to adjacent parts.
This partly explains the spread of tuberculosis in the body.

(c) All debris (including dead polymorphs) which has been ingested by macrophages is
gradually removed from the site of the inflammation.
(d) Antigenic material from bacteria available for presentation to the immune system.

Side effects: The liberation of enzymes and oxidising agents into adjacent tissues
contributes in varying degree to the tissue damage seen in several diseases, e.g. rheumatoid
arthritis, progressive pulmonary emphysema.

ACUTE INFLAMMATION

THE ROLE OF CHEMICAL FACTORS

Various substances are credited with roles in the inflammatory process; they have complex overlapping actions, many of which are only imprecisely defined. Regulatory mechanisms prevent uncontrolled progression of the inflammatory process.

Agents associated with vascular dilatation and increased permeability include:
1. *Vaso-active* AMINES — these appear early and their action is short.

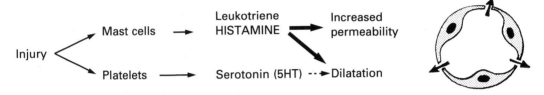

2. *Vaso-active* POLYPEPTIDES formed by specific enzyme action (breakdown products of proteins and tissues).

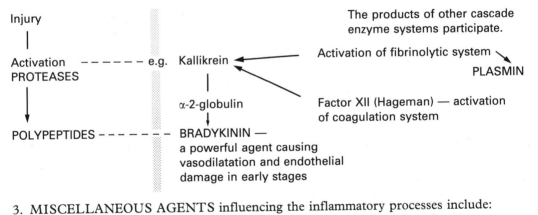

3. MISCELLANEOUS AGENTS influencing the inflammatory processes include:
- Toxins from bacteria
- Complement factors C3a and C5a
- Prostaglandins
- Leukotrienes ⎫
- Lysosomal enzymes ⎬ (from leucocytes)
- Interleukins (macrophages)
- Globulin permeability factor
- Lymph node permeability factor
- Products of DNA and RNA breakdown
- Antigen-antibody complexes
- Tumour necrosis factor
- Nitric oxide (from endothelial cells)

SEQUELS OF ACUTE INFLAMMATION

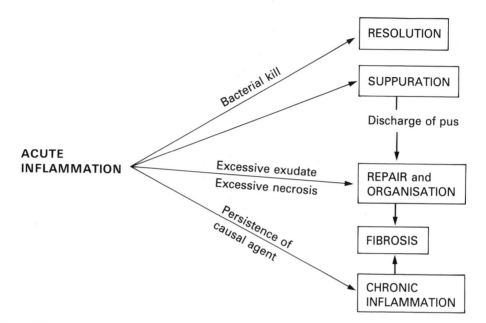

RESOLUTION

This means the complete restoration of normal conditions after the acute inflammation.
The three main features which potentiate this sequel are:
1. minimal cell death and tissue damage
2. rapid elimination of the causal agent, e.g. bacteria
3. local conditions favouring removal of fluid and debris.

Resolution of lobar pneumonia (bacterial inflammation of lung alveoli) is a good example:

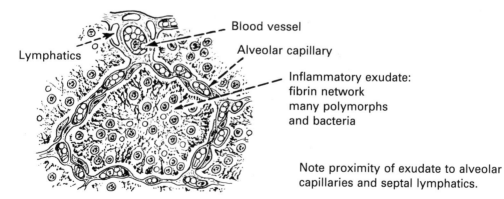

Note proximity of exudate to alveolar capillaries and septal lymphatics.

Following bacterial kill the mechanism is as follows:
1. Solution of fibrin by enzyme action (polymorphs and fibrinolysin)
2. Removal of fluid by blood vessels and lymphatics
3. Removal of all debris by phagocytes to hilar lymph nodes
4. The capillary hyperaemia diminishes and restoration to normal is complete

41

SEQUELS OF ACUTE INFLAMMATION

SUPPURATION

This means this formation of PUS; where pus accumulates an ABSCESS forms.

Infection by pyogenic (pus-forming) bacteria is the usual cause, e.g. staphylococcal abscess (or boil). The pus in this case is a thick, creamy yellow fluid which, on centrifugation, separates thus:

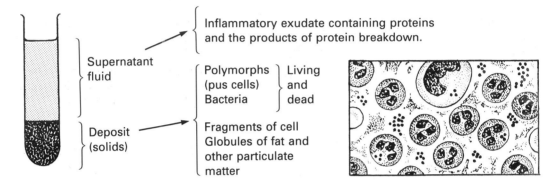

Supernatant fluid → Inflammatory exudate containing proteins and the products of protein breakdown.

Polymorphs (pus cells) | Living and
Bacteria | dead

Deposit (solids) → Fragments of cell Globules of fat and other particulate matter

Evolution of an abscess

The usual evolution of an abscess is as follows:

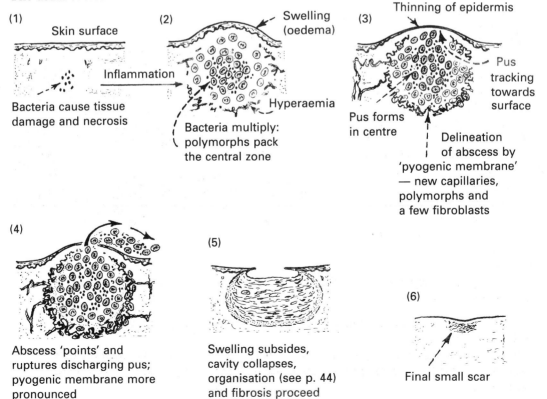

(1) Skin surface

Bacteria cause tissue damage and necrosis

Inflammation →

(2) Swelling (oedema)

Hyperaemia

Bacteria multiply: polymorphs pack the central zone

(3) Thinning of epidermis

Pus tracking towards surface

Pus forms in centre

Delineation of abscess by 'pyogenic membrane' — new capillaries, polymorphs and a few fibroblasts

(4) Abscess 'points' and ruptures discharging pus; pyogenic membrane more pronounced

(5) Swelling subsides, cavity collapses, organisation (see p. 44) and fibrosis proceed

(6) Final small scar

42

SEQUELS OF ACUTE INFLAMMATION

Evolution of an abscess (continued)

When the abscess is deep-seated, the process may be modified as follows:

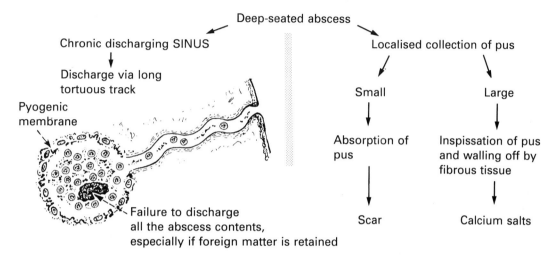

Deep-seated abscess

Chronic discharging SINUS

Discharge via long tortuous track

Pyogenic membrane

Failure to discharge all the abscess contents, especially if foreign matter is retained

Localised collection of pus

Small → Absorption of pus → Scar

Large → Inspissation of pus and walling off by fibrous tissue → Calcium salts

CHRONIC INFLAMMATION

This follows the acute inflammatory reaction if the causal agent is not removed.

The essential changes superimposed upon and replacing the acute reaction are:

1. Diminution in numbers of polymorphs; appearance of *lymphocytes* and *plasma cells*. *Macrophages* play an increasingly important role (see Granulomas, p.47). In some cases, *giant cells* form.
2. Proliferation of vascular endothelium by 'budding' — formation of *new capillaries*.
3. Proliferation of *fibroblasts* with *collagen* production –
4. **Fibrosis**.

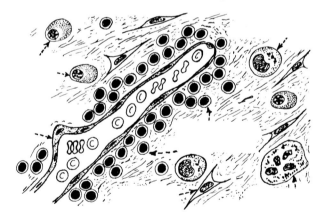

Frequently the local vessels show thickening of their walls with diminution in the lumina, due to intimal proliferation — endarteritis and endophlebitis (see p.47).

Commonly chronic inflammation is *primary*, i.e. there is no preceding acute inflammatory reaction.

The pathological processes following abscess formation and chronic inflammation are very closely allied to and merge with those occurring when repair of damaged tissue commences.

INFLAMMATION – SPECIAL TYPES

EXUDATIVE INFLAMMATION (continued)
Fibrinous exudation

In this type, the formation of fibrin
is striking. An example is acute pleurisy,
complicating pneumonia, where the fibrin can
be seen as an amorphous dull deposit on the
pleural surface. Note that the presence of
solid fibrin tends to inhibit resolution,
and *organisation* with *adhesion formation*
often follows.

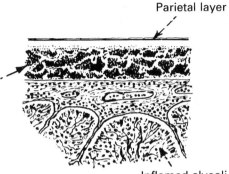

Parietal layer

Inflamed alveoli

A membranous film consisting mainly of fibrin with necrotic cells admixed sometimes
forms on a MUCOSAL surface (esp. respiratory and alimentary tracts.) The classical
example is DIPHTHERIA affecting the pharynx and adjacent areas.

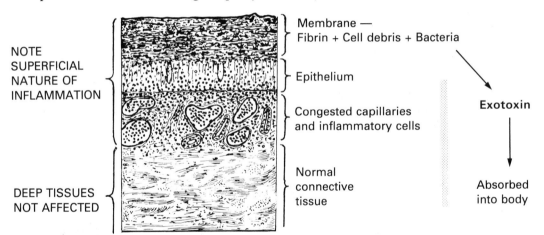

NOTE
SUPERFICIAL
NATURE OF
INFLAMMATION

DEEP TISSUES
NOT AFFECTED

Membrane —
Fibrin + Cell debris + Bacteria

Epithelium

Congested capillaries
and inflammatory cells

Normal
connective
tissue

Exotoxin

Absorbed
into body

This is often referred to as pseudo-membranous inflammation (see p.386).

SUPPURATIVE (PURULENT — PYOGENIC) INFLAMMATION

In this type (usually caused by infection with pyogenic bacteria), production of pus is the
main characteristic. Good examples are (a) an abscess, where an enclosed collection of pus
forms (see p.42), and (b) acute appendicitis (see p.401), where a purulent exudate forms on
the peritoneal surface.

HAEMORRHAGIC INFLAMMATION

Where the damage is severe, actual rupture of all blood vessels occurs, with haemorrhage
the most striking feature. An example is the acute haemorrhagic pneumonia occasionally
occurring in fatal cases of influenza.

These are not rigid compartments into which every inflammation can be conveniently
placed; overlaps and combinations of the various types are common, e.g. sero-sanguinous,
muco-purulent.

CHRONIC INFLAMMATION

GRANULOMATOUS INFLAMMATION

This is the term given to forms of chronic inflammation in which modified macrophages (epithelioid cells) accumulate in small clusters (follicles) surrounded by lymphocytes. The small clusters are called GRANULOMAS. The basic lesion in TUBERCULOSIS is a good example.

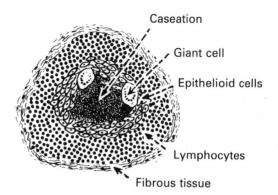

Caseation
Giant cell
Epithelioid cells
Lymphocytes
Fibrous tissue

Similar follicles are seen in:

Sarcoidosis — a rare inflammatory disease of unknown aetiology affecting especially the lymph nodes and lungs, but also many other organs

'Talc' granuloma — where particular silicates introduced into the tissues evoke an inflammatory reaction after a latent period (usually years)

Crohn's disease — a chronic inflammatory disease affecting the terminal ileum and colon (see p.387),

Lymph nodes draining ulcerated areas in which breakdown of lipid is occurring.

N.B. In all of these follicular granulomatous diseases the basic lesion may be identical, but CASEATION only occurs in tuberculosis.

The epithelioid cells of the follicular granulomas are modified macrophages, and giant cells are derived from macrophages usually by cell fusion but occasionally by nuclear division without cytoplasmic separation.

The Langhan's giant cell — seen in chronic granulomata, e.g. tuberculosis and sarcoidosis.

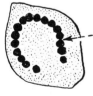

Nuclei in horse-shoe arrangement

The foreign body giant cell — seen in association with particulate insoluble material.

Nuclei scattered throughout cytoplasm

INFLAMMATORY ENDARTERITIS

The small arteries adjacent to a chronic inflammatory site often show **fibrous proliferation** of the **intima** with serious diminution of the lumen causing ischaemic effects, e.g. *atrophy* of specialised tissues, *necrosis* and *delayed healing*.

Occasionally the results are beneficial, e.g. in chronic peptic ulceration bleeding may be minimal.

Similar changes — ENDOPHLEBITIS — may affect veins.

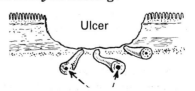

Ulcer

Lumen obliterated by endarteritis

ULCERATION – SIMPLE

ULCERATION is a complication of many disease processes.

An **ulcer** is formed when the surface covering of an organ or tissue is lost due to necrosis and replaced by inflammatory tissue.

The most common sites are the alimentary tract and the skin.

Ulcers are divided into two main groups: (1) SIMPLE (inflammatory) and (2) MALIGNANT (cancerous).

The word 'simple' is used here in the limited sense of contrasting with 'malignant': 'simple' ulcers may have serious consequences.

Evolution of a simple ulcer

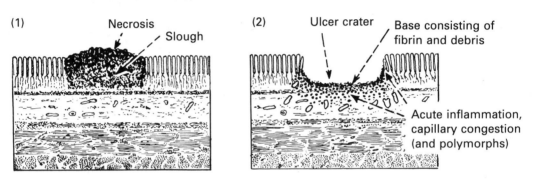

Healing can occur at this stage with restoration to normal, but if irritation (e.g. bacterial action, slight trauma, digestive juices and acid) continues, a CHRONIC ULCER forms.

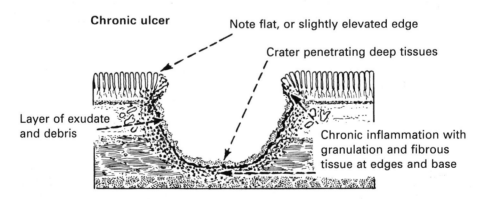

Healing of a chronic ulcer may be impeded by the secondary obliterative changes in the blood vessels due to the chronic inflammation, and it is inevitably associated with a variable amount of scarring.

ULCERATION – MALIGNANT

Evolution of a malignant ulcer (ulcerated tumour)

Such an ulcer is the result of the growth of a malignant tumour.

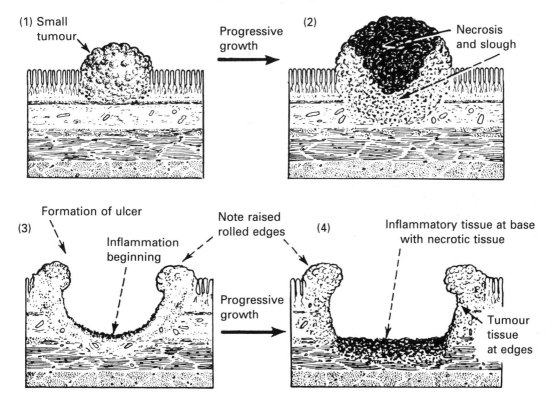

The differences between simple and malignant ulcers are most prominent at the edges — from which a diagnostic biopsy should be taken.

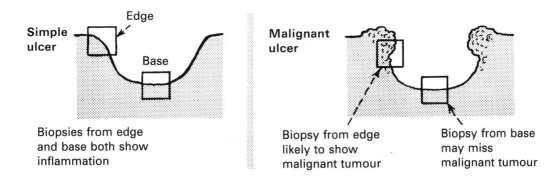

49

INFLAMMATION – ANATOMICAL VARIETIES

SINUS

A sinus is a tract lined usually by granulation tissue leading from a chronically inflamed cavity to a surface. In many cases the cause is the continuing presence of 'foreign' or necrotic material.

Examples include:

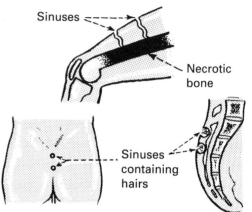

- **Sinuses associated with osteomyelitis** (inflammation of bone). Where necrosis of bone occurs, chronic sinuses form over it.
- **Pilonidal sinus** (pilonidal = nest of hairs). Seen in the mid-line over the sacrum (natal cleft) where hairs which have penetrated deeply under the skin are associated with chronic relapsing inflammation.

FISTULA

A fistula is a track open at both ends, through which abnormal communication between two surfaces is established.

There are two main types:

1. **Congenital** — due to developmental abnormality: any inflammation is superimposed.
2. **Acquired** — due to:

(a) Trauma	(b) Inflammation	(c) Necrosis — particularly of tumour

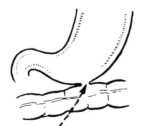

Biliary fistula following operation

Gastrocolic fistula in Crohn's disease (p.388)

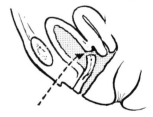

Vesicovaginal fistula following radionecrosis in treatment of cancer of cervix

An **EMPYEMA** is a collection of pus in a body cavity or hollow organ. The term refers usually to the pleural cavity or the gall bladder.

CELLULITIS occurs when inflammation spreads in the connective tissue planes.

CHAPTER 3

HEALING

WOUND HEALING

In almost all situations repair is brought about by the formation of 'granulation tissue'. **WOUND HEALING** is a good example of this process.

Healing by first intention (primary union)
This occurs in clean, incised wounds with good apposition of the edges — particularly planned surgical incisions.

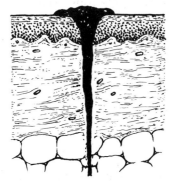

Immediately: Blood clot and debris fill the small cleft.

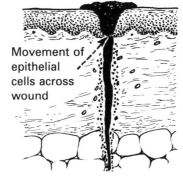

Movement of epithelial cells across wound

2–3 hours: Early inflammation close to edges.
Mild hyperaemia and a few polymorphs.

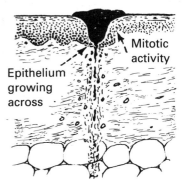

Mitotic activity

Epithelium growing across

2–3 days: Macrophage activity removing clot. Fibroblastic activity.

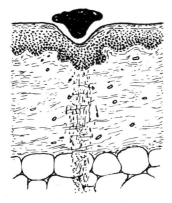

10–14 days: Scab loose and epithelial covering complete. Fibrous union of edges, but wound is still weak.

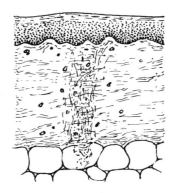

Weeks: Scar tissue still slightly hyperaemic. Good fibrous union, but not full strength.

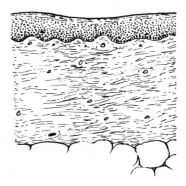

Months — years: Devascularisation. Remodelling of collagen by enzyme action. Scar is now minimal and merges with surrounding tissues.

WOUND HEALING

WOUND HEALING (continued)

Healing by second intention (secondary union)

This occurs in open wounds, particularly when there has been significant loss of tissue, necrosis or infection.

Early

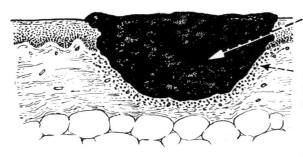

Cavity fills with blood and fibrin clot

Acute inflammation commences at junction of living tissue

A few days

Scab dries out

Note contraction of wound size due to action of myofibroblasts at edges

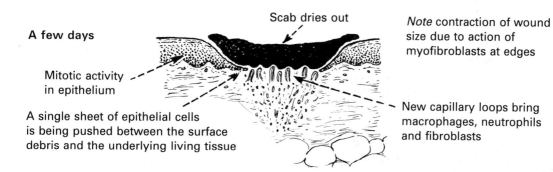

Mitotic activity in epithelium

A single sheet of epithelial cells is being pushed between the surface debris and the underlying living tissue

New capillary loops bring macrophages, neutrophils and fibroblasts

1 week approximately

Note contraction continuing

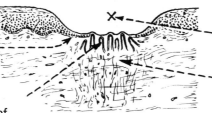

Epithelium continues to grow across

Surface debris has been shed

Loose connective tissue formed by fibroblasts

Capillary loops form small 'granulations' in the base of the wound. These can be seen by the naked eye and, historically, are the origin of the term 'granulation tissue'. This term is now used in a wider context to describe tissue consisting of newly formed capillaries with fibroblasts and macrophages and occurring in many circumstances in addition to wounds.

WOUND HEALING

Healing by second intention (continued)

2 weeks onwards

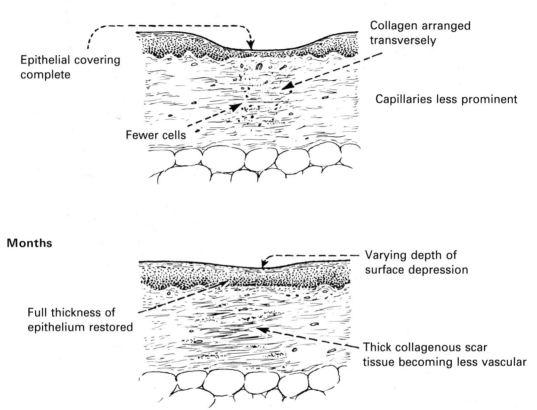

Epithelial covering complete

Collagen arranged transversely

Capillaries less prominent

Fewer cells

Months

Varying depth of surface depression

Full thickness of epithelium restored

Thick collagenous scar tissue becoming less vascular

Note that the differences in the two types of wound healing are quantitative: the essential pathological processes are the same.

Wound contraction

Wound contraction which is beneficial and begins early, is due mainly to the young, specialised 'myofibroblasts' in the granulation tissue exerting a traction effect at the wound edges. The exposed surface is reduced by gradual regeneration of the surface epithelium. The remodelling of the collagen continues for many months.

WOUND HEALING – COMPLICATIONS

Contracture

Later CONTRACTURE with distortion due to thickening and shortening of collagen bundles may cause serious cosmetic and functional disability, particularly in deep and extensive skin burns and around joints if muscles are seriously damaged.

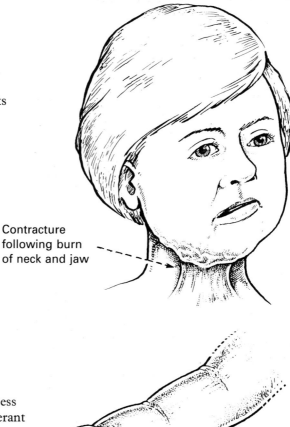

Contracture
following burn
of neck and jaw

Occasional complications

1. At the edges and base of a wound granulation tissue may form in excess and prevent proper healing ('exuberant granulations': 'proud flesh').

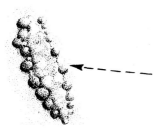

2. The formation of excess collagen in the form of thick interlacing bundles which causes marked swelling at the site of the wound is known as a KELOID.
   The essential cause is unknown but it may be due to deficient polymerisation of fibrin (factor XIII deficiency).

HEALING – FIBROSIS

FIBROSIS is the end result of WOUND HEALING, CHRONIC INFLAMMATION and ORGANISATION.

Formation of fibrous tissue

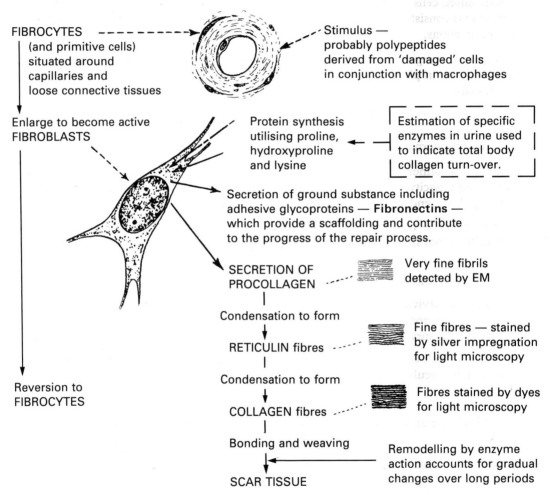

FIBROCYTES ----------> (and primitive cells) situated around capillaries and loose connective tissues

Stimulus — probably polypeptides derived from 'damaged' cells in conjunction with macrophages

Enlarge to become active **FIBROBLASTS**

Protein synthesis utilising proline, hydroxyproline and lysine

Estimation of specific enzymes in urine used to indicate total body collagen turn-over.

Secretion of ground substance including adhesive glycoproteins — **Fibronectins** — which provide a scaffolding and contribute to the progress of the repair process.

SECRETION OF PROCOLLAGEN ---- Very fine fibrils detected by EM
|
Condensation to form
↓
RETICULIN fibres ---- Fine fibres — stained by silver impregnation for light microscopy
|
Condensation to form
↓
COLLAGEN fibres ---- Fibres stained by dyes for light microscopy
|
Bonding and weaving ← Remodelling by enzyme action accounts for gradual changes over long periods
↓
SCAR TISSUE

Reversion to FIBROCYTES

Factors influencing wound healing by fibrosis

1. Local
   INFECTION, a POOR BLOOD SUPPLY, excessive movement and presence of foreign material DELAY HEALING.
2. General
   DEFICIENCY of VITAMIN C
   DEFICIENCY of AMINO ACIDS (in malnutrition)   } Failure of proper collagen
   DEFICIENCY of ZINC   synthesis with delayed
   EXCESS of ADRENAL GLUCOCORTICOIDS   healing and weak scars.
   DEBILITATING CHRONIC DISEASES

HEALING

REGENERATION

In the examples of wound healing, the restoration of the epithelial surface of the skin was effected by movement and proliferation of the surviving epithelial cells. Such regeneration of the specialised cells occurs in most organs and tissues to a varying degree, and the healing process consists of combinations of regeneration and repair by granulation tissue in varying proportions.

The capacity to regenerate is related to the amount of proliferation and replacement which takes place in physiological conditions. It is convenient to consider three broad groups of cells:

1. *Labile cells* — normally a continuous process of active replacement is occurring; the chances of restoration by regeneration are excellent, e.g. the covering epithelium (both external and internal), the bone marrow cells and the lymphoid cells.

2. *Stable cells* — although normally the replacement requirements are minimal, they have not lost the capacity to proliferate in response to damage. Chances of regeneration are good, e.g. liver, endocrine glands, renal tubular epithelium.

3. *Permanent cells* — normally are unable to multiply after the growth phase early in life. Such cells cannot regenerate and healing is by granulation tissue with permanent loss of function, e.g. nerve cells.

The process of regeneration can be divided into two main components:

1. *Movement* of surviving cells into the vacant space made available by loss due to wounding or necrosis.
2. *Proliferation* of surviving cells to replace the loss.

The factors which control both regeneration and repair are extremely complex and their roles somewhat speculative.

Possible mechanisms are:

    1. Removal of contact inhibition allows movement of cells.
    2. Cell proliferation and formation of new capillaries stimulated as follows:

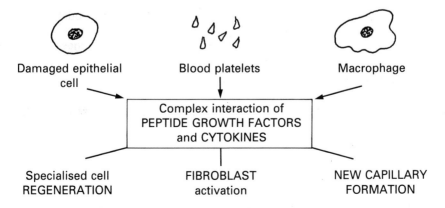

    3. The inhibitory mechanisms involved remain speculative.

HEALING – SPECIAL SITUATIONS

INTERNAL SURFACES

The regeneration of the covering epithelium is very similar to that of the skin, as seen for example in the alimentary tract.

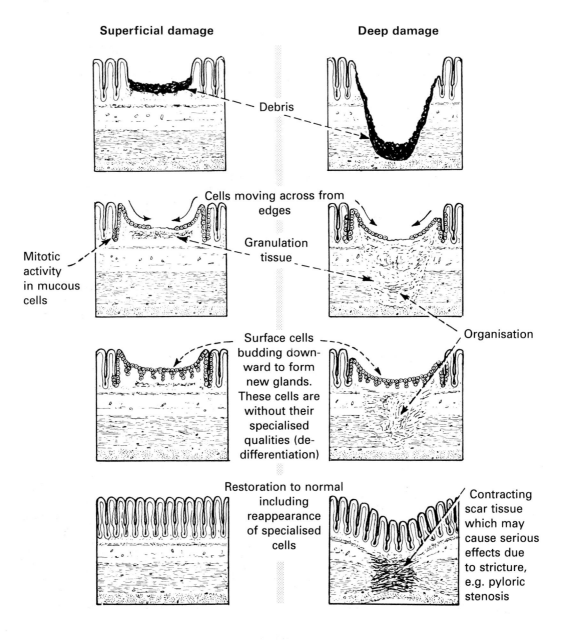

Superficial damage   **Deep damage**

Debris

Cells moving across from edges

Mitotic activity in mucous cells

Granulation tissue

Surface cells budding down-ward to form new glands. These cells are without their specialised qualities (de-differentiation)

Organisation

Restoration to normal including reappearance of specialised cells

Contracting scar tissue which may cause serious effects due to stricture, e.g. pyloric stenosis

HEALING – SPECIAL SITUATIONS

SOLID EPITHELIAL ORGANS

1. **Following gross tissue damage — including supporting tissue.**

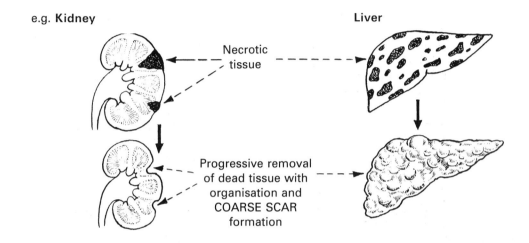

e.g. **Kidney**

Liver

Necrotic tissue

Progressive removal of dead tissue with organisation and COARSE SCAR formation

2. **Following cell damage with survival of the supporting (reticular) tissues**

e.g. **Tubular necrosis in kidney**

Perivenular hepatic cell necrosis

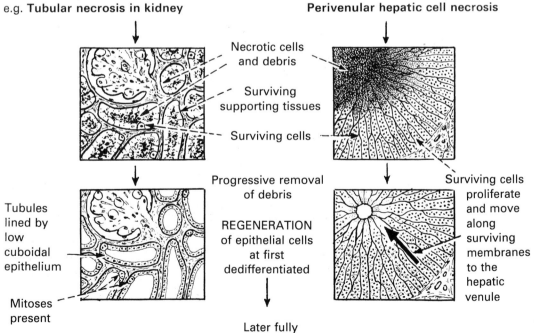

Necrotic cells and debris

Surviving supporting tissues

Surviving cells

Tubules lined by low cuboidal epithelium

Mitoses present

Progressive removal of debris

REGENERATION of epithelial cells at first dedifferentiated

Surviving cells proliferate and move along surviving membranes to the hepatic venule

Later fully RESTORED TO NORMAL

HEALING – SPECIAL SITUATIONS

MUSCLE

Muscle fibres of all 3 types — skeletal, cardiac and visceral — have only limited capacity to regenerate.

When a MASS of muscle tissue is damaged, repair by SCARRING occurs. This is particularly important in the HEART after infarction.

If the damage affects individual muscle fibres diffusely and with varying severity, then regeneration of the specialised fibres is possible (e.g. the myocardium may recover completely from the effects of diphtheria toxin and virus infection).

NERVOUS TISSUE

Central nervous system

Regeneration does not occur

In cases of acute damage, the initial functional loss often exceeds the loss of actual nerve tissue because of the reactive changes in the surrounding tissue. As these changes diminish, functional restoration commences.

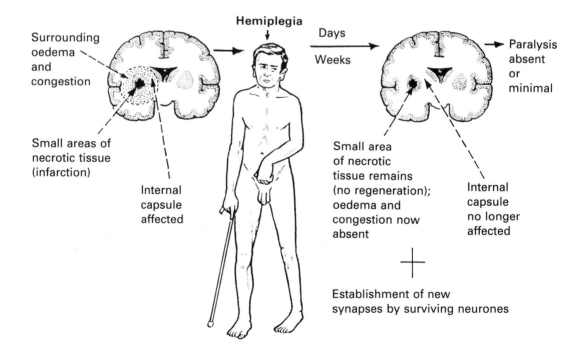

Surrounding oedema and congestion

Small areas of necrotic tissue (infarction)

Internal capsule affected

Hemiplegia

Days

Weeks

Small area of necrotic tissue remains (no regeneration); oedema and congestion now absent

Internal capsule no longer affected

Paralysis absent or minimal

Establishment of new synapses by surviving neurones

HEALING – SPECIAL SITUATIONS

NERVOUS TISSUE (continued)

Peripheral Nerves

When a peripheral nerve is damaged, the axon and its myelin sheath rapidly degenerate distally. The supporting tissues of the nerve (neurilemma) degenerate slowly.

Regeneration can occur because the central neurone of which the axon is a peripheral extension is remote from the site of damage.

A spinal motor nerve is taken as an example.

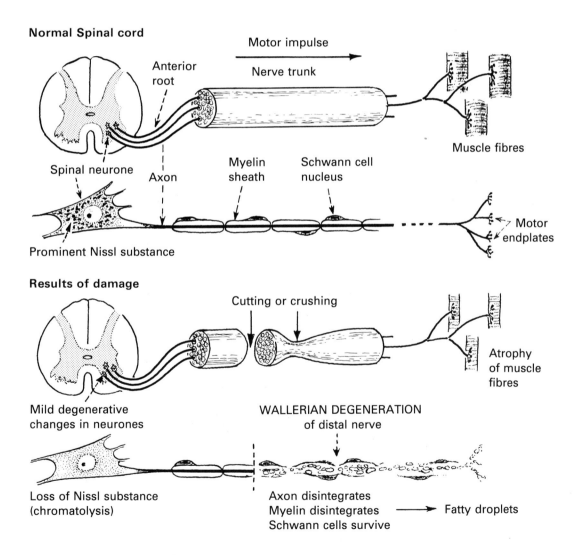

Normal Spinal cord

Motor impulse

Anterior root

Nerve trunk

Muscle fibres

Spinal neurone

Axon

Myelin sheath

Schwann cell nucleus

Motor endplates

Prominent Nissl substance

Results of damage

Cutting or crushing

Atrophy of muscle fibres

Mild degenerative changes in neurones

WALLERIAN DEGENERATION of distal nerve

Loss of Nissl substance (chromatolysis)

Axon disintegrates
Myelin disintegrates ⟶ Fatty droplets
Schwann cells survive

HEALING – SPECIAL SITUATIONS

PERIPHERAL NERVES (continued)

Regeneration takes the form of a sprouting of the cut ends of the axons.

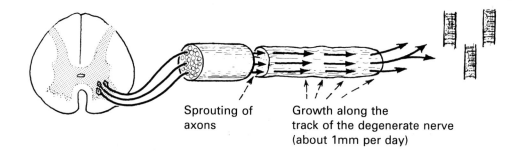

Sprouting of axons

Growth along the track of the degenerate nerve (about 1mm per day)

The results depend on the apposition of the distal remnant with the sprouting axons.

Good apposition

Good restoration

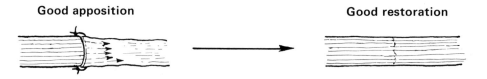

The best results are seen in crushing injuries where the sheaths remain in continuity.

Poor apposition

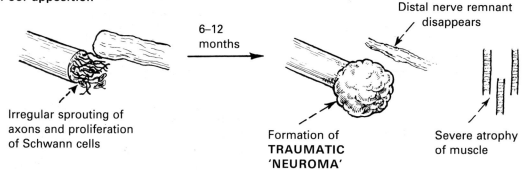

Distal nerve remnant disappears

6–12 months

Irregular sprouting of axons and proliferation of Schwann cells

Formation of **TRAUMATIC 'NEUROMA'**

Severe atrophy of muscle

HEALING – SPECIAL SITUATIONS

BONE

A fracture is usually accompanied by damage to or haemorrhage into adjacent soft tissues which are repaired by the process of organisation already described, while the bone fragments are reunited by regeneration.

Events following a fracture

(1) *Immediate effects*

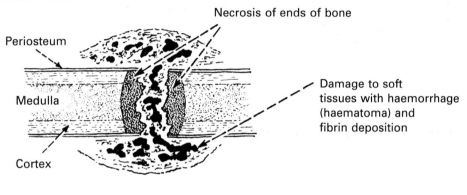

Periosteum

Necrosis of ends of bone

Medulla

Damage to soft tissues with haemorrhage (haematoma) and fibrin deposition

Cortex

(2) *Early reaction — inflammatory*
   First 4–5 days

(3) *Early bone regeneration*
   After 1st week,

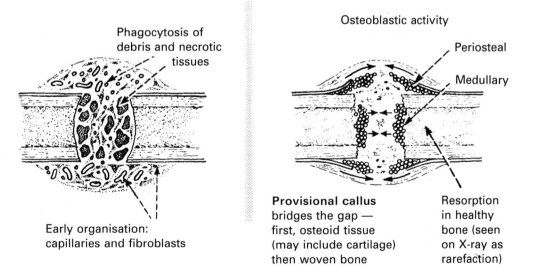

Phagocytosis of debris and necrotic tissues

Early organisation: capillaries and fibroblasts

Osteoblastic activity

Periosteal

Medullary

Provisional callus bridges the gap — first, osteoid tissue (may include cartilage) then woven bone

Resorption in healthy bone (seen on X-ray as rarefaction)

HEALING – SPECIAL SITUATIONS

Events following a fracture (continued)

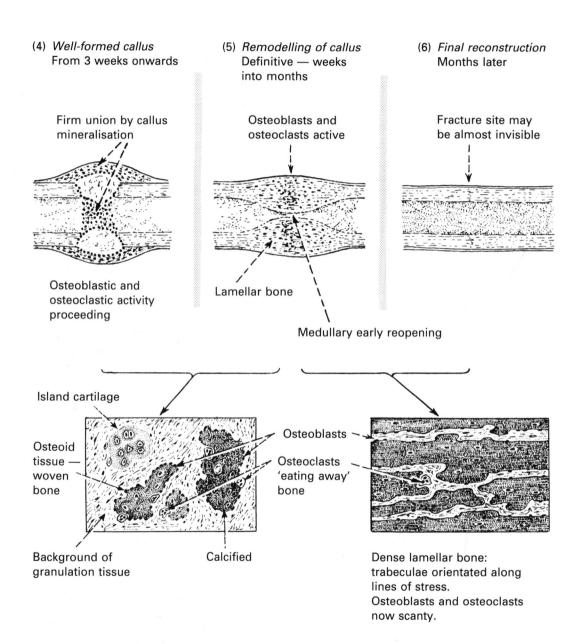

(4) *Well-formed callus*
From 3 weeks onwards

Firm union by callus
mineralisation

Osteoblastic and
osteoclastic activity
proceeding

(5) *Remodelling of callus*
Definitive — weeks
into months

Osteoblasts and
osteoclasts active

Lamellar bone

Medullary early reopening

(6) *Final reconstruction*
Months later

Fracture site may
be almost invisible

Island cartilage

Osteoid
tissue —
woven
bone

Background of
granulation tissue

Calcified

Osteoblasts

Osteoclasts
'eating away'
bone

Dense lamellar bone:
trabeculae orientated along
lines of stress.
Osteoblasts and osteoclasts
now scanty.

HEALING – SPECIAL SITUATIONS

EVENTS FOLLOWING A FRACTURE (continued)

Complications

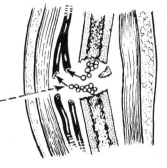

1. *Fat embolism* may occur in fracture of long bones due to entry of fat from the marrow cavity into the torn ends of veins.

2. *Infection*
   If the overlying skin is breached in any way, i.e. the fracture is 'compound', the risk of infection is greatly increased; this is an important adverse factor in the healing process.

   E.g.

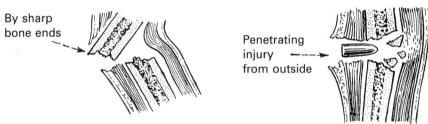

By sharp bone ends

Penetrating injury from outside

PATHOLOGICAL FRACTURE

When the break occurs at the site of pre-existing disease of the bone, the term 'pathological fracture' is applied.

A common condition is a secondary tumour growing in and destroying the bone

Mixture of tumour and haematoma — healing inhibited

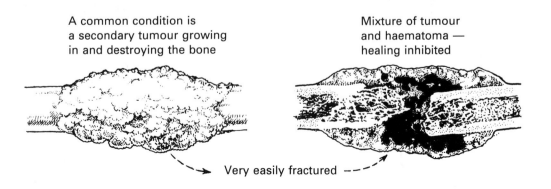

Very easily fractured

HEALING – SPECIAL SITUATIONS

FACTORS INFLUENCING HEALING OF FRACTURES

ADVERSE	FAVOURABLE

1. Local factors

(a) *Infection* ⎫ See previous
(b) *Pathological fracture* ⎬ page

(c) *Poor apposition and alignment* .... *Good apposition*

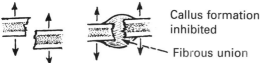

There may be interposition of soft tissue, *e.g.* muscle
Large irregular callus: slow repair, permanent deformity of bone

Small callus, quick repair

(d) *Continuing movement of bone ends* .... *Good immobilisation*

Callus formation inhibited

Fibrous union

In extreme cases, a rudimentary joint (pseudoarthrosis) may form

Small callus, good bone formation

(e) *Poor blood supply*.. *Good blood supply*

This is largely influenced by the anatomical site of the fracture, for example:
(a) Nutrient artery entering remote from the fracture or damaged by fracture (*e.g.* scaphoid, femoral head)
(b) Fracture through area devoid of periosteum (*e.g.* neck of femur)
(c) Minimal adjacent soft tissue (*e.g.* tibia).

In favourable conditions blood supply is derived from:
(a) periosteal arteries
(b) nutrient artery
(c) adjacent soft tissues.

2. General factors

(a) *Old age*... *Youth*
(b) *Poor nutrition* — e.g. famine conditions,............................ *Good nutrition* — especially
malabsorption lead to lack of protein, calcium, vit D and vit C.
protein, calcium, vit D and vit C.

CHAPTER 4

INFECTION

INFECTION

Most microorganisms are harmless; a few are **pathogenic**, i.e. have the potential to produce infectious disease.

BACTERIA and VIRUSES are the most common and most important groups of pathogenic organisms in man. Fungi and other groups (e.g. Chlamydia) less commonly cause disease.

COLONISATION AND COMMENSAL GROWTH

Vast numbers of bacteria normally colonise the external body surfaces (skin, alimentary and upper respiratory tracts). Most are of low pathogenicity and some may actually be beneficial to the host, for example:

1. By producing nutrient chemicals, e.g. vit B_{12}
2. By competing with and excluding pathogens.

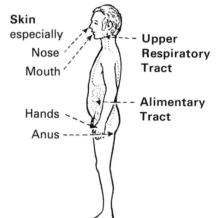

Common Sites of Contamination

Skin especially
Nose
Mouth
Hands
Anus

Upper Respiratory Tract

Alimentary Tract

INFECTION AND INFECTIOUS DISEASE

INFECTION occurs when microorganisms invade the sterile internal body tissues. (Multiplication usually follows invasion.)

An INFECTIOUS DISEASE occurs when infection is associated with clinically manifest tissue damage.

Routes of entry of infecting organisms

1. Through the *skin* or *mucous membranes*
   (a) By direct close contact, e.g. venereal disease.
   (b) By contamination of abrasions and wounds, e.g. wound infections, rabies.
   (c) By inoculation, e.g. insect bite — yellow fever, syringe — serum hepatitis, AIDS.

2. By *ingestion*
   Contaminated food and water, e.g. enteric fever, infective hepatitis (A), poliomyelitis, cholera.

3. By *inhalation*
   Dust and droplets, e.g. influenza.

INFECTION

Factors influencing the establishment of infection

1. *In the HOST*

In addition to a good state of general health and nutrition, the following mechanisms operate in preventing and limiting infection.

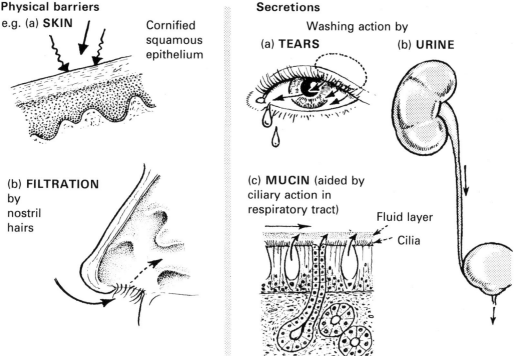

Physical barriers

e.g. (a) **SKIN** — Cornified squamous epithelium

(b) **FILTRATION** by nostril hairs

Secretions

Washing action by

(a) **TEARS**

(b) **URINE**

(c) **MUCIN** (aided by ciliary action in respiratory tract)

Fluid layer

Cilia

Chemical action

(1) Acid secretion in stomach and urinary tract.

(2) Lysozymes — enzymes capable of dissolving bacterial capsules, e.g. in tears and saliva.

(3) Immunoglobulin A (IgA) — a specialised immunoglobulin (see p. 105), — tears: intestinal secretions.

(4) Non-specific inhibitory substances — urine, sweat, sebum.

2. *In the MICRO-ORGANISM*

Factors potentiating invasive capacity include:

(1) **Quantity of dose** — the larger the dose the more likely that the defences are penetrated.

(2) **Virulence** — a variable factor, and often poorly defined, includes:

    (a) Capacity to resist phagocytosis and enzyme attack,

    (b) Adhesive properties,

    (c) Production of exoenzymes which act on host tissues, *e.g.* hyaluronidase (streptococci), coagulase (staphylococci) and of toxins, e.g. leucocidins, enterotoxins.

INFECTION

Factors influencing the course of infection

Once infection has occurred, important defence mechanisms operate:

1. **Inflammation** in the **acute** local reaction (see p.35) tends to limit the spread of organisms. In some important diseases, there is no acute local inflammatory response at the site of entry, e.g. Brucellosis (undulant fever) and many virus infections.
   In the **chronic** inflammatory reaction (see p.43), the formation of fibrous tissue also helps to localise infection.

2. **Phagocytosis** (see p.38) *NB* some organisms may survive or multiply within phagocytes — usually associated with chronic infection. Good examples are tuberculosis, brucellosis, leprosy.

3. **The Immune response**. (a) Humoral antibody reactions, e.g. agglutination, opsonisation, lysis via complement; (b) Cell-mediated reactions.

4. **Interferon production** (see p.90). In virus infection, interferon, a non-specific anti-viral agent produced by infected host cells, is important.

Examples of failure of protective and defence mechanisms

1. **In skin** — direct breach by wounding and burns; softening of the surface by exposure to water and sweat or due to skin disorders.

2. **In the respiratory tract** — inhibition of ciliary movement by nicotine in smokers potentiates infection.

3. **In the stomach** — in achlorhydria (no hydrochloric acid) organisms flourish in the stomach.

4. **When secretions are prevented from flowing freely** by narrowing of natural passages, bacterial growth in the 'stagnant' fluid is potentiated (e.g. enlarged prostate urethral obstruction, urinary infection).

5. **When commensal growth is impaired** by antibiotic treatment, pathogenic bacteria may colonise the 'vacant site'.

6. **Deficiency of the immunological system**:
   (a) natural deficiency due to hereditary defect,
   (b) acquired due to administration of drugs in treatment of disease, e.g. steroids, cytotoxic drugs; specific virus infection, e.g. Human Immunodeficiency Virus (HIV) causing Acquired Immune Deficiency Syndrome (AIDS).

7. **Deficiency of phagocytosis** — especially polymorphs.

8. **In debilitating diseases** such as diabetes, chronic renal failure and nutritional deficiency.

9. **Genetic susceptibility** — an important factor in some infections, e.g. the increased prevalence of several bacterial and fungal diseases in NON-SECRETORS of ABH blood group antigens (H = blood group O antigen). The mechanism remains obscure.

INFECTION

Mechanisms by which disease is produced

The local reaction to infections is usually INFLAMMATORY and is evoked by cellular damage and death. The detailed mechanisms are different in bacteria and viruses.

BACTERIA

1. Production of toxins (poisons)

Exotoxins	Endotoxins
Secreted by living bacteria	Integral part of bacterial cell wall Release on death of organism (usually Gram-negative)
Simple proteins	Lipid-polysaccharide complexes
Neutralised by specific antibody (antitoxin)	Do not stimulate antitoxin production
Often have specific enzyme activity and may act on specific organs or tissues	Cause fever and ENDOTOXIC SHOCK. Act by damaging capillaries and disturbing the coagulation system as well as causing necrosis. Activate fibrinolytic and complement cascades: facilitate release of chemical mediators of acute inflammation.

2. Hypersensitivity reaction causing tissue injury

This is a form of the immune response in which reaction between the bacterial protein and sensitised lymphocytes initiates the inflammatory reaction (see p. 117).

3. Tissue invasion: lymphatic spread and invasion of blood stream

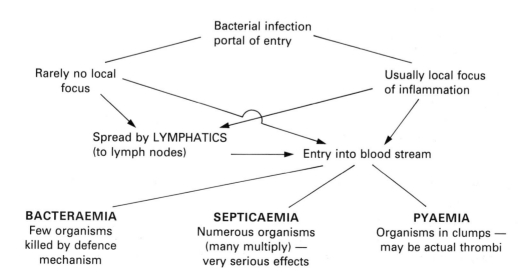

INFECTION

BACTERAEMIA
(a) Occurs commonly: usually of no serious significance
(b) An integral part of some infections, e.g. typhoid fever.

Important special cases

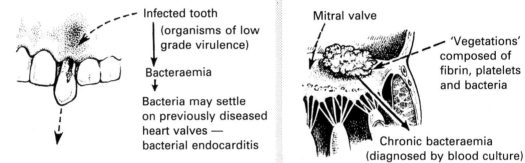

(1) *Dental extraction*

Infected tooth
(organisms of low
grade virulence)

↓

Bacteraemia

↓

Bacteria may settle
on previously diseased
heart valves —
bacterial endocarditis

(2) *Established bacterial endocarditis*

Mitral valve

'Vegetations'
composed of
fibrin, platelets
and bacteria

Chronic bacteraemia
(diagnosed by blood culture)

SEPTICAEMIA
Septicaemia is a very serious condition with severe toxaemia and shock. It may:

(a) be primary — usually caused by virulent organisms e.g. *meningococci, Streptococci pyogenes*
(b) complicate the shock syndrome initiated by other causes — especially when the alimentary tract is involved (coliform organisms)
(c) occur during medical treatment when immune mechanisms are disturbed (see opportunistic infections, p.91).

In septicaemia, unless antibiotic treatment is available, the infection is rapidly overwhelming and, at post-mortem, specific damage is difficult to detect. There may be massive adrenal haemorrhage and evidence of disseminated intravascular coagulation (see p.204).

PYAEMIA
Pyaemia is a serious condition with severe toxaemia — the organisms escape into the blood stream in the form of small aggregates — micro-emboli. This results in either (a) PYAEMIC ABSCESSES or (b) SEPTIC INFARCTION.

INFECTION

PYAEMIC ABSCESS

Septic focus — usually staphylococcal

↓

Thrombosis of venules incorporating bacteria

↓

Showers of very small (micro-) emboli

↓

Multiple, very small abscesses in various organs

Especially:

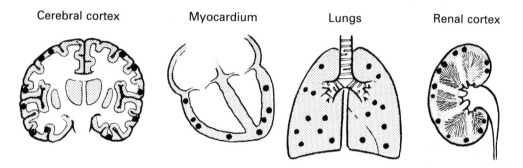

Cerebral cortex Myocardium Lungs Renal cortex

SEPTIC INFARCTION
The lesions are larger and less numerous than pyaemic abscesses.
They are associated with:

(a) Septic thrombosis of larger veins (b) Acute bacterial
  (suppurative thrombophlebitis)   endocarditis

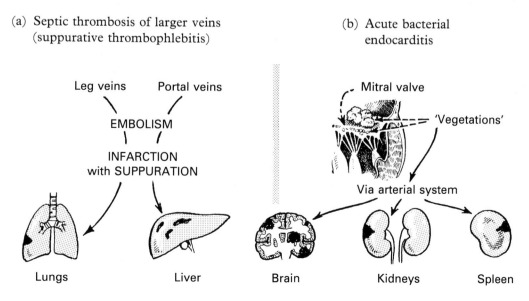

Leg veins Portal veins   Mitral valve

EMBOLISM   'Vegetations'

INFARCTION
with SUPPURATION   Via arterial system

Lungs Liver Brain Kidneys Spleen

ACUTE BACTERIAL INFECTION

PYOGENIC BACTERIA

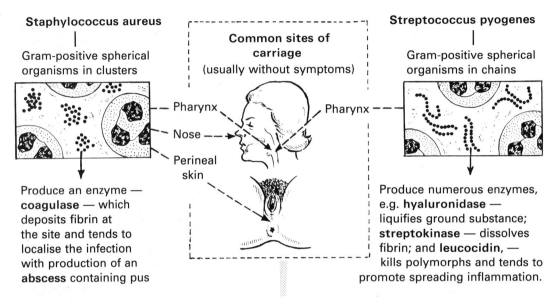

Staphylococcus aureus

Gram-positive spherical organisms in clusters

Common sites of carriage (usually without symptoms)

— Pharynx

— Nose

— Perineal skin

Pharynx

Streptococcus pyogenes

Gram-positive spherical organisms in chains

Produce an enzyme — **coagulase** — which deposits fibrin at the site and tends to localise the infection with production of an **abscess** containing pus

Produce numerous enzymes, e.g. **hyaluronidase** — liquifies ground substance; **streptokinase** — dissolves fibrin; and **leucocidin,** — kills polymorphs and tends to promote spreading inflammation.

Lesions produced

Skin infections — pustules, boils, carbuncles
Wound infection
Staphylococcal broncho-pneumonia may be a serious complication in epidemic influenza
Exotoxin production ➝ food poisoning

Skin infections — impetigo, erysipelas, cellulitis
Wound infection
TONSILLITIS and pharyngitis
Exotoxin production
↓
The skin rash of scarlet fever

GENERAL BLOOD SPREAD

PYAEMIA (and septicaemia)
OSTEOMYELITIS — acute inflammation of long bones — particularly in children

SEPTICAEMIA

NB Rheumatic fever and acute glomerulonephritis are complications of streptococcal infection in which the heart and kidneys are damaged. This is caused by disturbance in the immune mechanisms and is not due to the actual presence of streptococci in the heart and kidneys.

ACUTE BACTERIAL INFECTION

PYOGENIC BACTERIA (continued)

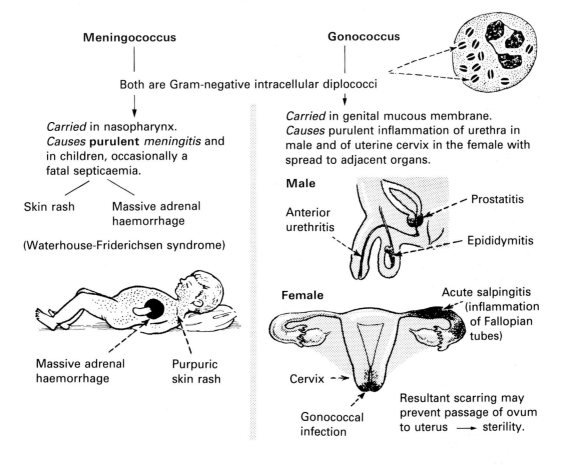

Meningococcus

Gonococcus

Both are Gram-negative intracellular diplococci

Carried in nasopharynx.
Causes **purulent** *meningitis* and in children, occasionally a fatal septicaemia.

Skin rash   Massive adrenal haemorrhage

(Waterhouse-Friderichsen syndrome)

Massive adrenal haemorrhage   Purpuric skin rash

Carried in genital mucous membrane.
Causes purulent inflammation of urethra in male and of uterine cervix in the female with spread to adjacent organs.

Male

Anterior urethritis

Prostatitis

Epididymitis

Female

Acute salpingitis (inflammation of Fallopian tubes)

Cervix

Gonococcal infection

Resultant scarring may prevent passage of ovum to uterus ⟶ sterility.

Gram-negative bacilli

These are usually commensals in the alimentary tract and include the broad group of aerobic 'coliform' organisms (*E. coli*, *B. proteus*, *Klebsiella*) as well as the anaerobic bacteroides.

They are of low grade virulence but can cause local inflammations in the alimentary tract, the urinary tract and wound infections.
The production of endotoxins is an important cause of shock.

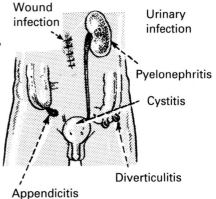

Wound infection

Urinary infection

Pyelonephritis

Cystitis

Diverticulitis

Appendicitis

ACUTE BACTERIAL INFECTION

GANGRENE

Gangrene is a form of NECROSIS in which a special type of bacterial activity is superimposed.

The bacteria proliferate in and digest the dead tissues often with the production of gases. There are two main types: PRIMARY and SECONDARY.

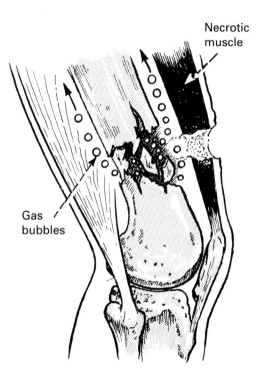

Necrotic muscle

Gas bubbles

Primary (gas gangrene)

This occurs only occasionally in civilian practice but is a serious complication of war wounds. It is due to infection of deep contaminated wounds (in which there is considerable muscle damage) by bacteria of the *CLOSTRIDIA* group — anaerobic sporulating Gram-positive bacilli which produce saccharolytic and proteolytic enzymes resulting in digestion of muscle tissue with gas formation. The infection rapidly spreads and there is associated severe toxaemia (spread of poisons in the blood).

Secondary

This is due to invasion of necrotic tissue usually by a mixed bacterial flora including putrefactive organisms. It occurs in two forms: WET and DRY.

Wet gangrene. The tissues are moist at the start of the process either due to oedema or venous congestion. Examples are in strangulation of viscera and occlusion of leg arteries in obese diabetic patients.

Dry gangrene. Occurs especially in the toes and feet of elderly people suffering from gradual arterial occlusion. The putrefactive process is very slow and only small numbers of putrefactive organisms are present.

ACUTE BACTERIAL INFECTION

TETANUS

This is a toxigenic disease — the organism itself does not cause local tissue damage. The effects are due to a powerful EXOTOXIN secreted by the organism. This is in contrast to the usual bacterial diseases where tissue damage is important and is due to the local bacterial action.

The infecting organism, *Clostridium tetani*, a STRICT ANAEROBE, is a Gram-positive rod. Often the presence of a terminal spore gives a characteristic drumstick appearance. The highly resistant spores are widespread in the environment due to contamination by animal faeces.

Method of Infection

Contamination of wounds in which there are anaerobic conditions, e.g. deep-penetrating wounds and wounds with severe soft tissue damage (road traffic accidents and battle casualties); only very occasionally trivial thorn punctures.

In primitive communities the umbilical stump of the newborn may be infected by faecal material.

Effects:

The exotoxin is highly potent and causes paroxysmal muscular spasm which becomes progressively more severe and is fatal in many cases.

Course

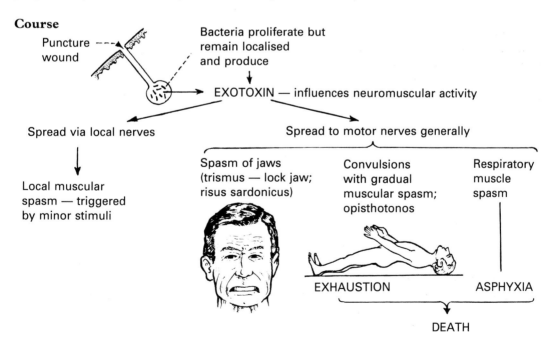

Immunity

● Active immunisation by **TOXOID** — prophylactic.
● Passive immunisation by **ANTITOXIN** — therapeutic
(only effective before toxin is fixed to nerve tissues).

77

CHRONIC BACTERIAL INFECTION (GRANULOMAS)

In these infections chronic inflammation is the basic mechanism (see p.47). The detailed evolution of the inflammatory reaction is modified by several factors of which the immune response of the host is important (see p.97).

TUBERCULOSIS

Tuberculosis is caused by the *Mycobacterium tuberculosis* (tubercle bacillus: TB) an organism which has a resistant waxy component in its structure and is acid and alcohol-fast (i.e. resists bleaching with strong acid and alcohol after being stained red with fuchsin).

The disease has rapidly declined in Western Europe and North America since World War II due to: (a) improved nutrition and hygiene, (b) chemotherapy and (c) BCG immunisation. Cases are occurring now in association with AIDS. It remains prevalent in developing countries, affecting both children and adults.

The tuberculous follicle (tubercle)

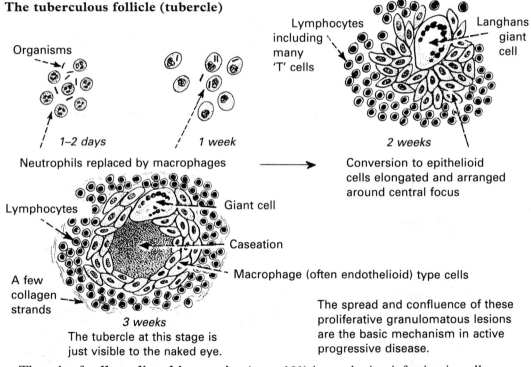

Organisms

1–2 days   *1 week*   *2 weeks*

Lymphocytes including many 'T' cells

Langhans giant cell

Neutrophils replaced by macrophages ⟶ Conversion to epithelioid cells elongated and arranged around central focus

Lymphocytes

Giant cell

Caseation

Macrophage (often endothelioid) type cells

A few collagen strands

3 weeks
The tubercle at this stage is just visible to the naked eye.

The spread and confluence of these proliferative granulomatous lesions are the basic mechanism in active progressive disease.

The role of **cell-mediated immunity** (see p.101) in combating infection is well seen in the evolution of the tuberculous follicle.

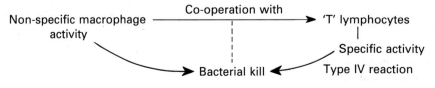

Non-specific macrophage activity ⟶ Co-operation with ⟶ 'T' lymphocytes

Specific activity

Bacterial kill ← Type IV reaction

The caseation is the result of the combined effects of (a) the Type IV hypersensitivity reaction, (b) bacterial activity and (c) ischaemia.

CHRONIC BACTERIAL INFECTION (GRANULOMAS)

TUBERCULOSIS (continued)

Primary infection

Usually seen in non-immune children in first contact with tuberculosis. A few bacilli infect the PRIMARY SITE — usually at the periphery of the lung but also occasionally in the pharynx (tonsil) or small intestine.

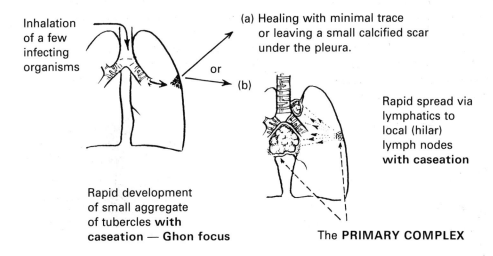

Inhalation of a few infecting organisms

(a) Healing with minimal trace or leaving a small calcified scar under the pleura.

or

(b)

Rapid spread via lymphatics to local (hilar) lymph nodes **with caseation**

Rapid development of small aggregate of tubercles **with caseation — Ghon focus**

The **PRIMARY COMPLEX**

Healing can occur at this stage, leaving calcified lymph nodes, or occasionally the disease spreads via blood stream (a) generally or (b) to individual organs.

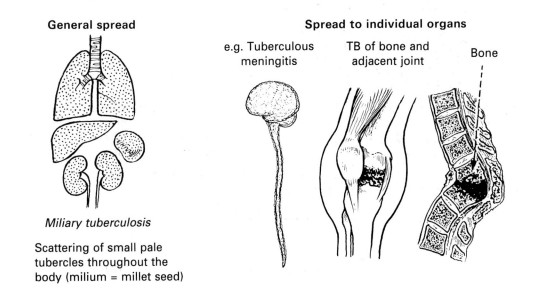

General spread

Spread to individual organs

e.g. Tuberculous meningitis

TB of bone and adjacent joint

Bone

Miliary tuberculosis

Scattering of small pale tubercles throughout the body (milium = millet seed)

CHRONIC BACTERIAL INFECTION (GRANULOMAS)

TUBERCULOSIS (continued)

Re-infection tuberculosis

This occurs in older children and adults who have had a primary infection or have received BCG vaccination by which a variable degree of immunity to the tubercle bacillus has been established.

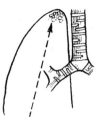

The evolution of the disease is much slower than in the primary infection and fibrosis tends to limit the spread, but in untreated cases gradual extension with destruction and scarring of tissues is usual.

The usual site of re-infection is the lung apex

Gradually progressive disease destroying lung tissue: CAVITATION is common.

If the individual's immunity is impaired for any reason, the disease may spread locally more rapidly with increased caseation or in the miliary form.

NB In apparently well-healed tuberculosis, the tubercle bacilli can survive for many years in scarred and calcified tissues and are able to re-establish active disease — REACTIVATION of tuberculosis. This is the commonest form nowadays in Western countries, occurring in late middle and old age among people who were originally infected when tuberculosis was common.

Variations in the basic mechanism

1. *Exudative* inflammation occurs particularly in serous cavities.

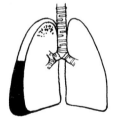

e.g. Pleurisy with effusion

Ascites in abdominal tuberculosis — with adherence of viscera

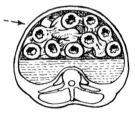

2. *Cold abscess* — where caseation is marked, the tuberculous pus may track to a surface as a 'cold' abscess and sinus.

3. *Fibrotic tuberculosis* — in this condition the body's reparative mechanism is dominant but not sufficient to ensure complete healing; a slow progressive fibrosis with scarring results. This is seen particularly in lung infections.

4. *Acute caseating 'non-reactive' tuberculosis* is seen when the individual's immunity is seriously impaired; massive caseation with little cellular reaction occurs.

CHRONIC BACTERIAL INFECTION (GRANULOMAS)

ACTINOMYCOSIS

Actinomycosis is a localised but gradually spreading chronic suppuration affecting the lower jaw particularly; the ileocaecal region of the bowel and occasionally the lung.

The organism — *Actinomyces* — widespread in nature, is a Gram-positive branching, filamentous anaerobe found around the teeth and in the pharyngeal crypts (the human variety is *Actinomyces israeli*). In the tissues, it forms yellow, densely felted together spherical colonies just visible to the naked eye: the pus is seen to contain 'sulphur granules'.

Sites of infection

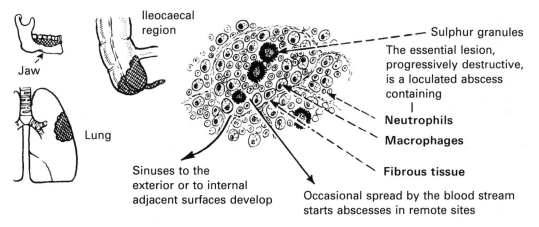

Ileocaecal region

Jaw

Lung

— Sulphur granules

The essential lesion, progressively destructive, is a loculated abscess containing
|
Neutrophils

Macrophages

Fibrous tissue

Sinuses to the exterior or to internal adjacent surfaces develop

Occasional spread by the blood stream starts abscesses in remote sites

LEPROSY

This slowly progressive disease which causes serious effects by damage to peripheral nerves is still widespread in the tropics and subtropics. The infection is acquired by close, prolonged contact and is due to a slender acid and alcohol-fast bacillus. The disease presents in two contrasting extreme forms and with cases of intermediate type.

1. **Lepromatous leprosy**	2. **Tuberculoid leprosy**
• Disfiguring nodularity of the skin — 'leonine facies'.	• Focal areas of skin pallor and anaesthesia due to early involvement of nerves.
• Peripheral nerves affected late.	
• The lesions contain lymphocytes, plasma cells and macrophages — filled with organisms.	• Basic lesion is a follicular granuloma (tubercle) not unlike the true tubercle follicle.
• Organisms + + + in tissues.	• Organisms are scanty.

These differences are due in the main to differences in the immune reaction of the host.

• Cell-mediated immunity is markedly diminished.	• Cell-mediated immunity is well developed.

81

CHRONIC BACTERIAL INFECTION (GRANULOMAS)

SYPHILIS

Syphilis is a venereal infection; the usual sites of entry of the infection are the penis and the vulva or vagina. Extra-genital infection is uncommon.

The organism is a spirochaete (*Treponema pallidum*) with a close set, regular spiral, demonstrated by dark ground illumination, silver staining or immuno-fluorescence. Although it very rapidly dies outside the body it has a highly invasive capacity on contact with mucous membranes.

10μ

PRIMARY SYPHILIS

During the first three weeks after infection, the spirochaetes spread in the blood throughout the body without any noticeable effects. Then the primary lesion — **hard chancre** — appears at the original site of entry.

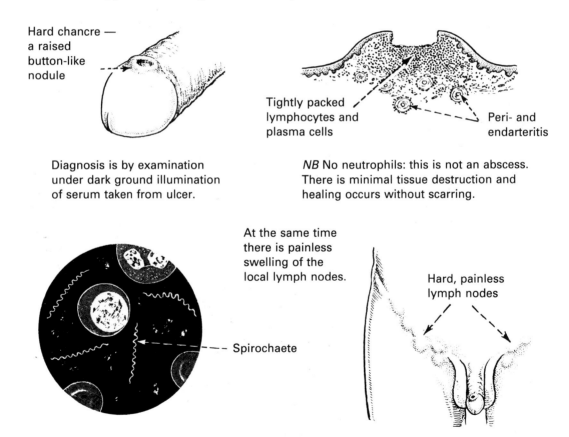

Hard chancre — a raised button-like nodule

Tightly packed lymphocytes and plasma cells

Peri- and endarteritis

Diagnosis is by examination under dark ground illumination of serum taken from ulcer.

NB No neutrophils: this is not an abscess. There is minimal tissue destruction and healing occurs without scarring.

At the same time there is painless swelling of the local lymph nodes.

Hard, painless lymph nodes

Spirochaete

In the course of the next two or three months, the effects of organisms which have spread throughout the body before and during the local reaction present as the SECONDARY STAGE of the disease.

CHRONIC BACTERIAL INFECTION (GRANULOMAS)

SECONDARY SYPHILIS

Secondary syphilis presents as a widespread skin rash (pox) of varying appearance, ulceration of mucous membranes, generalised lymphadenopathy, damage to various individual organs and tissues. There are constitutional effects — particularly fever and anaemia.

The essential pathology is the presence of very numerous spirochaetes accompanied by focal infiltration of lymphocytes, plasma cells and macrophages with mild arteritis. Infectivity is very high. Tissue destruction is minimal and healing occurs without scarring. A latent stage of long duration is followed in 35% of cases by tertiary syphilis.

TERTIARY (Late) SYPHILIS

The lesions which may occur at any time for many years after the healing of the secondary phase offer striking contrasts. This stage is characterised mainly by local destructive lesions, the result of cell-mediated immune reactions (T cells) causing necrosis of tissue. The main forms are:

1. **Gumma**

   This is a localised area of necrosis which may affect large parts of any organ or tissue but particularly bones, testis and liver.

2. **Syphilitic aortitis**

   The aorta (arch and thoracic portion) is affected by an infiltration of lymphocytes and plasma cells beginning around the vasa vasorum and extending into the media, causing weakening due to focal destruction ('windowing') of the specialised elastic tissues. There is compensatory irregular thickening of the intima (tree-bark appearance), but the important effect is expanding ANEURYSM formation.

Normal

Serious local pressure effects or rupture

Tree-bark thickening

Expanding aneurism formation

Periarteritis and endarteritis

'Windowing'

CHRONIC BACTERIAL INFECTION (GRANULOMAS)

TERTIARY SYPHILIS (continued)

3. Neurological syphilis
  (a) **Meningovascular** — mainly affects the meningeal blood vessels and causes neurological impairment secondarily.

  (b) **Parenchymatous** —

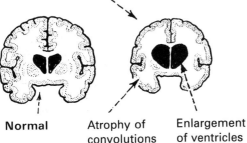

(a) General paralysis of the insane — severe destruction of cerebral tissue

Normal Atrophy of convolutions Enlargement of ventricles

(b) Tabes dorsalis — the damage specifically affecting the posterior roots and columns of spinal cord — is associated with characteristic clinical symptoms due to loss of proprioceptive sensation in the legs

CONGENITAL SYPHILIS

Transplacental infection of the fetus occurs with the following possible consequences:
  (a) abortion or stillbirth — many organs damaged
  (b) birth of marasmic infant — organ and tissue damage at birth and in later childhood.

IMMUNITY IN SYPHILIS

Antibody production and diagnostic tests
1. *Screening tests*
  Antibodies of uncertain origin which bind to a phospholipid (cardiolipin): these are detected in Wasserman and VDRL (Venereal Diseases Reference Laboratory) tests.
2. *Specific diagnostic tests*
  Specific anti-treponemal antibodies: these are detected in Treponema immobilisation, haemagglutination and fluorescent antibody tests.

Cell-mediated delayed hypersensitivity also develops.
  Sensitivity reactions are important in the mechanism of syphilitic damage to tissues.

VIRUS INFECTIONS

Viruses, the smallest microorganisms in nature (measured in nm), are not visible by light microscopy but can be studied using the electron microscope (EM). The virus particle (*virion*: elementary body) consists of a central core of genetic material, either ribonucleic acid (RNA) or deoxyribonucleic acid (DNA) surrounded by a protein coat (capsid). The virus particle in itself does not contain the biochemical mechanism for replication; it is wholly dependent on the resources of the infected cell.

The diagram shows how, by taking control of and utilising the nucleic acid of the invaded cell, replication is accomplished.

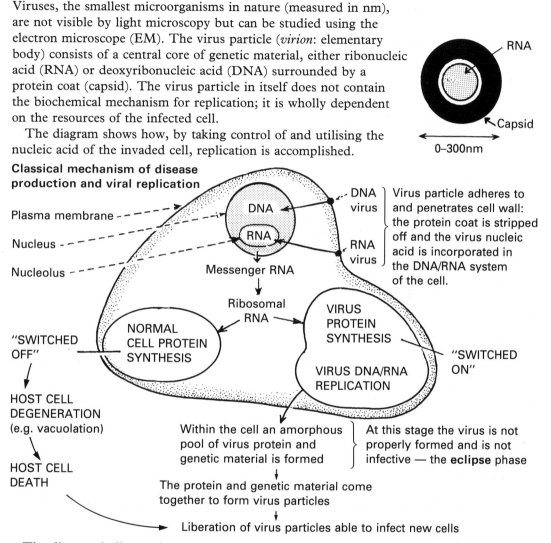

The diagram indicates the direct cytopathic effects of the virus. An alternative and important cause of damage to the host cell is the side effects associated with antibody and cell-mediated immune reactions.

RETROVIRUSES

An important variation occurs in a small group of RNA viruses. These contain an enzyme — **reverse transcriptase** — which, within the cell cytoplasm, is able (using the virus RNA as the template) to synthesise virus DNA which is then incorporated into the nuclear genetic material (note that messenger RNA is not required).

The virus DNA may remain there inactive for long periods. When activity is resumed, replication and cytopathic changes are effected as indicated in diagram.

Retroviruses are important agents in carcinogenesis and AIDS (see p. 115).

85

VIRUS INFECTIONS

ACUTE VIRUS INFECTION

The evolution of a typical acute virus infection can be understood in terms of virus replication, release and spread within the body, and of the host's reaction.

Typical evolution

Incubation period

Penetration of cells at site of infection
↓
Replication of VIRUS within
CELLS LOCALLY
↓
CELL DEATH
liberation of virus
↓
VIRUS spread to
LOCAL LYMPH NODES
↓
Further replication of virus
Cell death

Local lesion

Local symptoms.
The common cold,
Influenza,
Enteritis (due to
enterovirus)
illustrate diseases
of this type

— —

Overt disease

Primary viraemia

Liberation of virus into blood stream
↓
VIRUS spread by blood to
LYMPHOID TISSUES GENERALLY
↓
Further replication of virus

General malaise and
fever with lymph
node enlargement.

Secondary viraemia

CELL DEATH
Liberation of virus into blood stream
↓
Virus spread, GENERALLY
throughout the body with
effects seen particularly
in organs and tissues which
possess specific receptors
for particular viruses

Specific symptoms
referable to organ
or tissue damage,
e.g. poliomyelitis —
nerve cells, infective
hepatitis — liver cells,
small pox — skin cells.

This typical evolution is produced by successive waves of virus. However, the great majority of virus infections are clinically latent or mild because virus replication and spread are prevented by the body's defence mechanisms. Severe overt disease occurs when there is a specially virulent virus or when the body's resistance is inadequate, especially in a primary infection.

Not all virus infections cause disease in this way. 3 important variations are:

(1) LATENT   (2) ONCOGENIC   (3) SLOW

VIRUS INFECTIONS

LATENT VIRUS INFECTION

A good example is the common 'cold sores' of the lips and face caused by the virus **Herpes simplex** (an enveloped DNA virus).

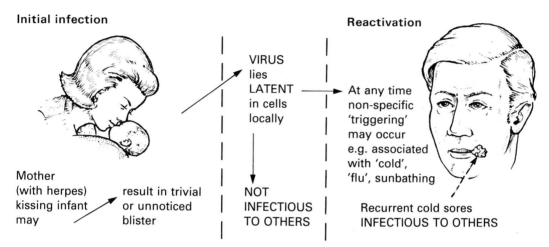

Initial infection

Reactivation

VIRUS lies LATENT in cells locally

At any time non-specific 'triggering' may occur e.g. associated with 'cold', 'flu', sunbathing

Mother (with herpes) kissing infant may → result in trivial or unnoticed blister

NOT INFECTIOUS TO OTHERS

Recurrent cold sores INFECTIOUS TO OTHERS

Another example is **herpes zoster (shingles)**.

This is a painful affection of segmental sensory nerves and root ganglia due to infection by CHICKEN POX VIRUS **Varicella**.

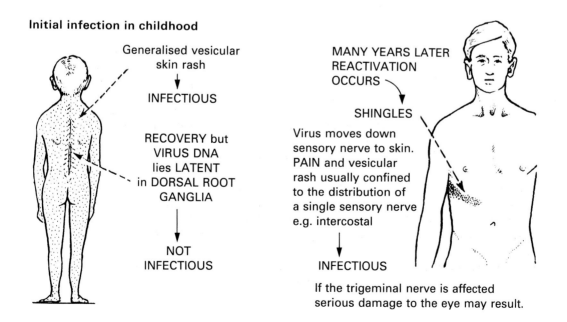

Initial infection in childhood

Generalised vesicular skin rash

↓

INFECTIOUS

RECOVERY but VIRUS DNA lies LATENT in DORSAL ROOT GANGLIA

↓

NOT INFECTIOUS

MANY YEARS LATER REACTIVATION OCCURS

SHINGLES

Virus moves down sensory nerve to skin. PAIN and vesicular rash usually confined to the distribution of a single sensory nerve e.g. intercostal

↓

INFECTIOUS

If the trigeminal nerve is affected serious damage to the eye may result.

VIRUS INFECTIONS

ONCOGENIC VIRUS INFECTION

In animals, viruses have been clearly proved to cause malignant tumours, and there is good evidence that some tumours in man are caused by viruses (see also p.160).

Examples include the following:

(a) **The common wart** *verruca vulgaris* is due to infection by human papilloma viruses (HPV) and there is a close association of these viruses with **cervical carcinoma**.

(b) **The Epstein-Barr virus** (a member of the herpes group) causes glandular fever (infectious mononucleosis — a non-malignant condition) in young adults in Western societies. This virus is also closely associated with Burkitt's lymphoma (a malignant tumour) found in young Africans living in malarial areas. Virus genetic material is present in the tumour cells.

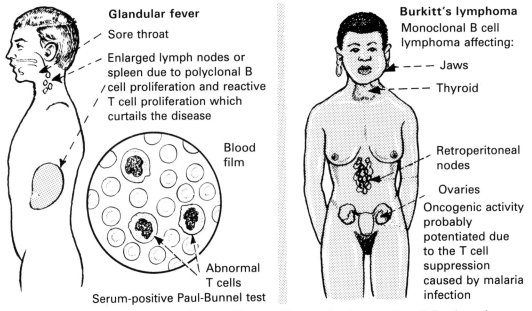

Glandular fever
- Sore throat
- Enlarged lymph nodes or spleen due to polyclonal B cell proliferation and reactive T cell proliferation which curtails the disease

Blood film

Abnormal T cells

Serum-positive Paul-Bunnel test

Burkitt's lymphoma
Monoclonal B cell lymphoma affecting:
- Jaws
- Thyroid

Retroperitoneal nodes

Ovaries
Oncogenic activity probably potentiated due to the T cell suppression caused by malaria infection

(c) *T cell leukaemias* are caused by specific retroviruses, i.e. human T cell Leukaemia-Lymphoma Virus (HTLV)

The mechanisms by which viruses cause tumours are illustrated on page 160.

SLOW VIRUS INFECTION

PRION DISEASE   SCRAPIE in sheep and SPONGIFORM ENCEPHALOPATHY in cattle ('mad cow disease') after long incubation periods cause severe damage to the brain. KURU and CREUTZFELDT-JAKOB disease are the human equivalents.

The essential pathological changes consist of microscopic cerebral cystic degeneration.

The infective agents are very resistant to the usual sterilizing methods and, although they replicate, do not conform completely to the definition of a virus.

The name PRION has been given to agents of this type.

LENTIVIRUSES   The progress of disease caused by LENTIVIRUSES (a type of retrovirus) is usually very slow. AIDS due to HIV infection is the prime example (see p.115).

HOST/VIRUS INTERACTION

The reactions occurring in the host are important.

1. Changes in the infected cells

(a) Cell degeneration
(with loss of function)
leading to cell death.

Vacuolation

Rapid degeneration
and lysis

Nuclear and cytoplasmic
condensation

Slow lysis

(b) Fusion of adjacent infected
cells — giant cell formation,
e.g. the Warthin-Winkeldy
cell of measles,

Lymphocytes

(c) Cell proliferation.

Proliferation of skin
epithelial cells
causing a warty growth

(d) Formation of 'inclusion'
bodies within cytoplasm
or nucleus: they consist
of aggregates of virus
and/or products of cell
degeneration.

Diagnostic eosinophilic
intracytoplasmic
Negri bodies in nerve
cells of the hippocampus
in **RABIES**

Nuclear and
cytoplasmic
inclusion in
cytomegalic
virus infection
of salivary ducts

(e) No apparent change in cell but virus remains latent — reactivation later with
continuous and slow release associated with gradually progressive disease.

(f) No apparent change but later malignant proliferation occurs, i.e. oncogenic infection.

HOST/VIRUS INTERACTION

REACTIONS IN HOST (continued)

2. **Interferon production** by the infected cells and specifically activated T lymphocytes. Interferon is a protein but not an antibody. It represents the first and very important line of defence by interfering with the synthesis of viral protein and thus protects healthy cells.

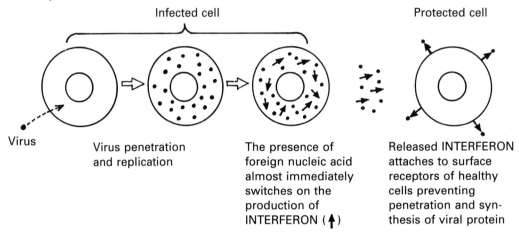

Infected cell   Protected cell

Virus

| Virus penetration and replication | The presence of foreign nucleic acid almost immediately switches on the production of INTERFERON ($\uparrow$) | Released INTERFERON attaches to surface receptors of healthy cells preventing penetration and synthesis of viral protein |

3. **The immune response** (see p.95) begins 4–7 days after initial infection.

 (a) Antibodies to virus   }   limit initial infection but are very
 (b) Cell-mediated immunity }   important in protecting against RE-INFECTION.
 (c) Occasionally virus antibody complexes cause special types of reaction in the host, e.g. inflammatory necrosis of arteries (arteritis), some forms of kidney damage, and the skin rashes of childhood viral infections.

4. **The inflammatory response**

The vascular and exudative elements follow the usual pattern; neutrophils are not a feature unless there is considerable tissue necrosis or secondary bacterial infection. However, macrophage phagocytic activity is important in the defence against viral infection. There is often a relative lymphocytosis.

OPPORTUNISTIC INFECTIONS

This term is used for infections caused by organisms which are often nonpathogenic or of low grade virulence, occurring in individuals whose resistance to infection is impaired. They are occurring more frequently in modern medical practice because of the increasing use of powerful immunosuppressive drugs.

CAUSES OF LOWERED RESISTANCE

1. Congenital immunological deficiencies (rare).
2. Acquired
   (a) *the result of disease*: HIV infection (AIDS);
           uraemia; liver disease; malignant tumours,
           particularly Hodgkin's disease and leukaemias;
   (b) *the result of therapy*: e.g.
           immunosuppression in transplant surgery;
           immunosuppression — a side effect of tumour therapy;
           antibiotics — changing commensal populations;
           introduction of foreign material, e.g. heart valve prostheses;
           I.V. long lines in intensive care; tracheostomy.

Examples of infecting organisms

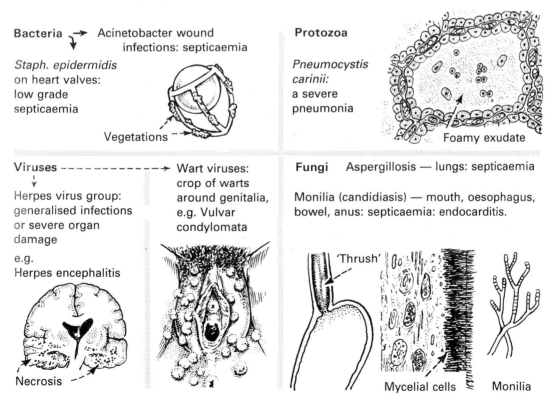

Bacteria → Acinetobacter wound infections: septicaemia

Staph. epidermidis on heart valves: low grade septicaemia

Vegetations

Protozoa

Pneumocystis carinii: a severe pneumonia

Foamy exudate

Viruses → Wart viruses: crop of warts around genitalia, e.g. Vulvar condylomata

Herpes virus group: generalised infections or severe organ damage

e.g. Herpes encephalitis

Necrosis

Fungi Aspergillosis — lungs: septicaemia

Monilia (candidiasis) — mouth, oesophagus, bowel, anus: septicaemia: endocarditis.

'Thrush'

Mycelial cells   Monilia

INFECTION – GENERAL EFFECTS

The more general body reactions in infection are: FEVER and CHANGES IN METABOLISM.

FEVER (PYREXIA)

The body temperature rises above normal initially due partly to an imbalance between heat production and loss, but mainly due to a resetting at a higher level of the 'thermostat' mechanism in the hypothalamus. This results in:

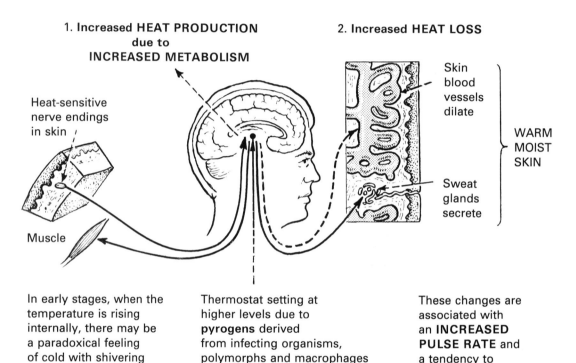

1. Increased HEAT PRODUCTION due to INCREASED METABOLISM

Heat-sensitive nerve endings in skin

Muscle

2. Increased HEAT LOSS

Skin blood vessels dilate

Sweat glands secrete

WARM MOIST SKIN

In early stages, when the temperature is rising internally, there may be a paradoxical feeling of cold with shivering (rigor).

Thermostat setting at higher levels due to **pyrogens** derived from infecting organisms, polymorphs and macrophages mediated by prostaglandin E.

These changes are associated with an **INCREASED PULSE RATE** and a tendency to **DEHYDRATION**.

Pyrexia also occurs when there is:

(a) Considerable tissue necrosis, e.g. infarction and tumours

(b) Cerebral disease — especially in the region of the pons

(c) Heat-stroke — where the environmental temperature and humidity are high and there is excessive water and salt loss.

Hyperpyrexia [when the temperature exceeds 41°C (106°F)] is extremely dangerous because of damage to the nerve cells in the brain.

INFECTION – GENERAL EFFECTS

CHANGES in METABOLISM

Tissue breakdown is greatly increased, and in some infectious fevers there is a marked loss of body weight.

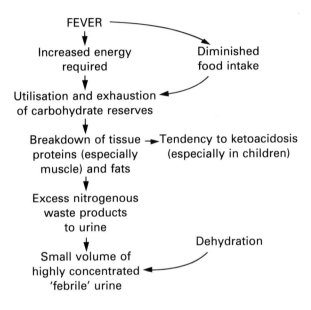

CHANGES in the BLOOD

Plasma proteins

In many chronic bacterial infections subtle changes in the blood protein content are reflected in a **rise in the ESR** (Erythrocyte Sedimentation Rate). In a few chronic infections an increase in immunoglobulins results in **hyperglobulinaemia**. Serum amyloid A proteins (SAA) are raised and, in very long-standing chronic inflammatory processes, potentiate amyloidosis (see p.24).

In many acute bacterial infections there is a neutrophil leucocytosis (see p.357): in contrast, in virus infections a relative or absolute lymphocytosis is common.

Leucopenia occurs in typhoid fever and chronic debilitating infections.

IMMUNITY

IMMUNITY

It has been known from historical times that a person who has recovered from an infectious disease, e.g. smallpox, is most unlikely to suffer from it again — even when exposed maximally — although he would remain susceptible to other infections.

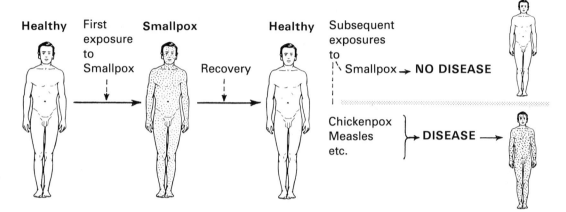

That is, during the recovery period he has ACQUIRED SPECIFIC IMMUNITY to smallpox but not to other infections.

Of course, in its literal meaning, immunity — the inability to be infected — includes NON-SPECIFIC mechanisms, some of which have been mentioned previously.

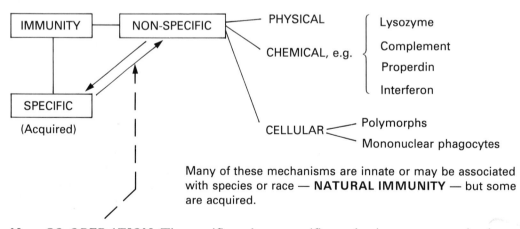

Many of these mechanisms are innate or may be associated with species or race — **NATURAL IMMUNITY** — but some are acquired.

Note: *CO-OPERATION*. The specific and non-specific mechanisms are conveniently separated but they have important influences on each other.

The modern science of IMMUNOLOGY is engaged mainly in the study of the mechanisms involved in the establishment of specific immunity, i.e. the IMMUNE RESPONSE and its CONSEQUENCES.

THE SPECIFIC IMMUNE RESPONSE

The sequence of events in an infection is as follows:

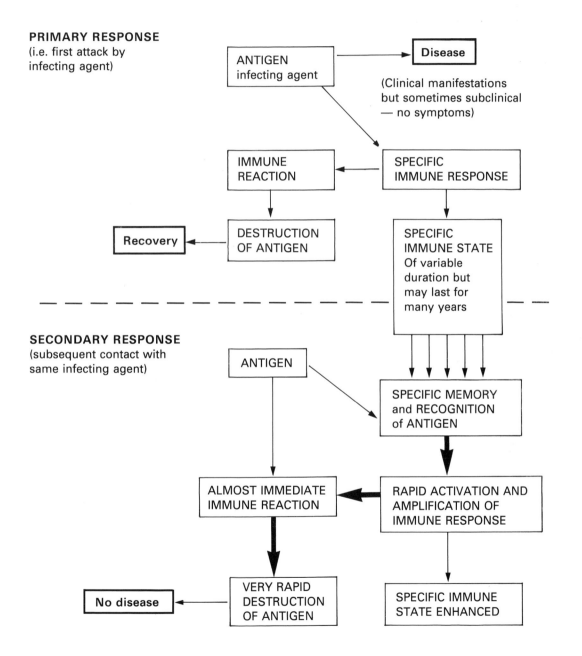

PRIMARY RESPONSE
(i.e. first attack by
infecting agent)

ANTIGEN
infecting agent

Disease

(Clinical manifestations
but sometimes subclinical
— no symptoms)

IMMUNE
REACTION

SPECIFIC
IMMUNE RESPONSE

DESTRUCTION
OF ANTIGEN

Recovery

SPECIFIC
IMMUNE STATE
Of variable
duration but
may last for
many years

SECONDARY RESPONSE
(subsequent contact with
same infecting agent)

ANTIGEN

SPECIFIC MEMORY
and RECOGNITION
of ANTIGEN

ALMOST IMMEDIATE
IMMUNE REACTION

RAPID ACTIVATION AND
AMPLIFICATION OF
IMMUNE RESPONSE

VERY RAPID
DESTRUCTION
OF ANTIGEN

No disease

SPECIFIC IMMUNE
STATE ENHANCED

ANTIGEN

The most familiar antigens are infectious agents such as bacteria and some viruses, but other substances foreign to the human body will stimulate the immune process. Most of them are of protein nature, but complex chemical substances such as some large carbohydrate molecules, lipoproteins and lipopolysaccharides will induce antibody formation. At the other end of the scale, immune reactions are provoked by fungi, protozoa such as malarial parasites, and helminths.

Antigens can be chemically split into two fractions. One of these binds the antigen to the antibody — the HAPTEN FACTOR — but is itself unable to induce the formation of antibodies. Only the complete antigen will do this. Many simpler chemicals can act as haptens. Their importance is twofold. By combining with antibody they can block the antibody antigen Ab/Ag reaction. Secondly, if they become attached to a protein they become strongly antigenic.

The union of antigen with antibody is a physicochemical reaction and takes place at specific sites on the antigen molecule — called DETERMINANTS. Their number influences the strength of the Ab/Ag binding.

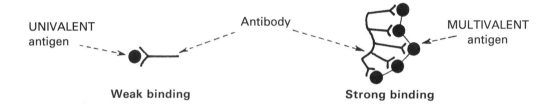

UNIVALENT antigen — Antibody — MULTIVALENT antigen

Weak binding   **Strong binding**

Cross-reactions

Complex antigens may have common determinant sites; this explains why the specific antibody to one may cross-react with other antigens. It may lead to confusion when immunological diagnostic tests are used in the laboratory.

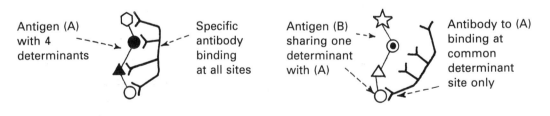

Antigen (A) with 4 determinants — Specific antibody binding at all sites — Antigen (B) sharing one determinant with (A) — Antibody to (A) binding at common determinant site only

Strong specific binding   **Weak cross-reaction**

Antigens evoke the strongest response when they are introduced to the tissues parenterally, because the protein molecule is presented to the lymphoid tissues (site of immune response) unaltered by the digestive processes. But some diseases are caused by surface absorption of antigen, e.g. gluten enteropathy (coeliac disease) and hay fever.

THE SPECIFIC IMMUNE RESPONSE

The process is essentially an activity of the small lymphocytes of which there are two main types. They are indistinguishable by light microscopy using conventional stains but show clear differences, under the electron microscope, in their surface properties and in their function.

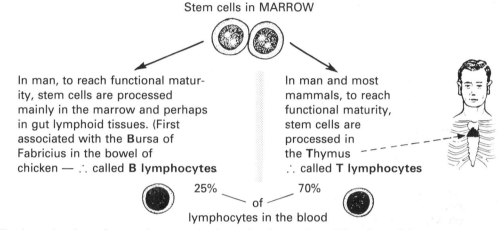

Stem cells in MARROW

In man, to reach functional maturity, stem cells are processed mainly in the marrow and perhaps in gut lymphoid tissues. (First associated with the **B**ursa of Fabricius in the bowel of chicken — ∴ called **B lymphocytes**

In man and most mammals, to reach functional maturity, stem cells are processed in the **T**hymus ∴ called **T lymphocytes**

25% — of — 70%
lymphocytes in the blood

The introduction of an antigen results in activation and proliferation of these two lymphocyte populations. This activity takes place in the lymphoid tissues (see p.558 et seq.).

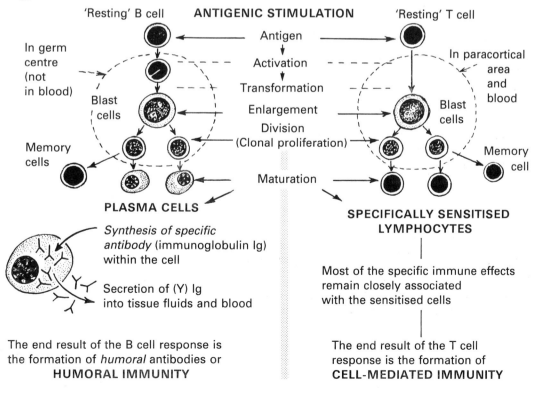

'Resting' B cell   **ANTIGENIC STIMULATION**   'Resting' T cell

In germ centre (not in blood)

Antigen

Activation

Transformation

In paracortical area and blood

Blast cells

Enlargement

Division (Clonal proliferation)

Blast cells

Memory cells

Memory cell

Maturation

PLASMA CELLS

SPECIFICALLY SENSITISED LYMPHOCYTES

Synthesis of specific antibody (immunoglobulin Ig) within the cell

Secretion of (Y) Ig into tissue fluids and blood

Most of the specific immune effects remain closely associated with the sensitised cells

The end result of the B cell response is the formation of *humoral* antibodies or **HUMORAL IMMUNITY**

The end result of the T cell response is the formation of **CELL-MEDIATED IMMUNITY**

99

GENETIC INFLUENCES ON THE IMMUNE RESPONSE

The immune response is effected at molecular level on cell surfaces, within cells and in the tissue fluids. Minor genetic variations explain the differences between individuals in the quality and quantity of the immune response.

The HUMAN LEUCOCYTIC ASSOCIATED ANTIGEN (HLA) system [alternative name: the MAJOR HISTOCOMPATIBILITY COMPLEX (MHC)] illustrates one aspect:

The complex is a group of genes on chromosome 6 encoding for cell membrane glycoproteins which play important roles in the immune response.

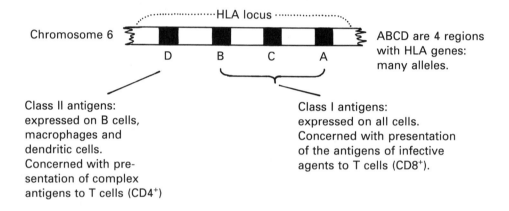

The important roles in medicine are:

(1) Association with disease processes — particularly AUTO-IMMUNE disorders (see p.117 et seq.).

   The most striking association is ANKYLOSING SPONDYLITIS where 90% are HLA B27.

   Most other auto-immune disorders associate with the D group HLA locus.

(2) (a) Combating infection (see above).

   (b) Effecting graft rejection in incompatible hosts (the better the HLA match the better the chances of graft survival).

CELL-MEDIATED IMMUNITY

To ensure maximal specific T cell response the antigen is linked to molecular components of the HLA system (by B cells, dendritic cells and macrophages) and presented to the T cell.

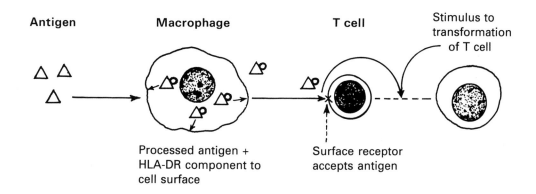

| Antigen | Macrophage | T cell | Stimulus to transformation of T cell |

Processed antigen + HLA-DR component to cell surface

Surface receptor accepts antigen

The transformed blast cell undergoes progressive mitotic division and each cell of the resulting clone has the same specific immune potential.

The subsequent T cell activities tend to remain local at the site of the antigen concentration and this cell-mediated immunity (CMI) is delayed, i.e. at least 24 hours are required for a significant local concentration of sensitised T cells.

T cell functions and mechanisms

1. *Overall regulation of the immune response and reactions.* This is effected by **HELPER T cells** which promote, and **SUPPRESSOR T cells** which inhibit immune reactions. In the peripheral blood, 2/3 of the T lymphocytes are helper and 1/3 suppressor. Using monoclonal antibodies, helper cells carry the T_4 surface antigen and suppressor cells the T_8.

2. *T cell effector mechanisms:*
   (a) Cytotoxic T cells cause antigen-specific lysis by direct cell to cell contact.
   (b) Natural killer cells, again cause lysis by direct cell to cell contact but usually the killing action is non-specific.
   (c) Delayed hypersensitivity reactions are mediated by the release of LYMPHOKINES from the specifically activated T cells. They promote a wide range of cellular activity associated with the promotion and control of the immune response and the inflammatory reaction.

The diagrams on the following pages indicate in summary the complex T cell activities.

T-CELL ACTIVITIES

1. Influence on B cells

2. Lymphokines controlling cell proliferation

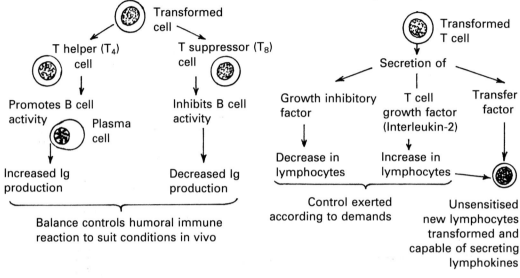

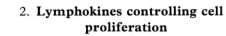

3. Action on neutrophils and macrophages

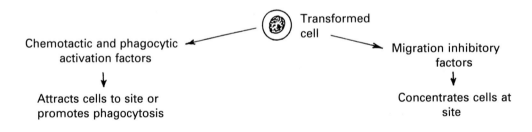

Practical tests for the detection of specific sensitised T lymphocytes in the blood are:

(a) **The lymphocyte transformation test:** During incubation with a specific antigen, the rate of transformation, as indicated by DNA synthesis or mitotic activity, is measured.

(b) **The macrophage migration inhibition test:** The migration of macrophages in the presence of specific antigen is measured and the amount of inhibition is an indicator of the specific T lymphocyte activity.

(c) **The Tuberculin test:** This is a good example of the use of cell mediated immunity in diagnosis in clinical practice. In individuals who are or have been infected by mycobacterium tuberculi or BCG, sensitised T cells are present in the blood. Intradermal injection of a small quantity of tuberculoprotein results in an inflammatory reaction (papule) appearing after 24 hours and lasting for several days.

HUMORAL ANTIBODIES – IMMUNOGLOBINS (Ig)

The basic immunoglobulin is a protein molecule consisting of 2 pairs of polypeptide chains arranged in a particular way.

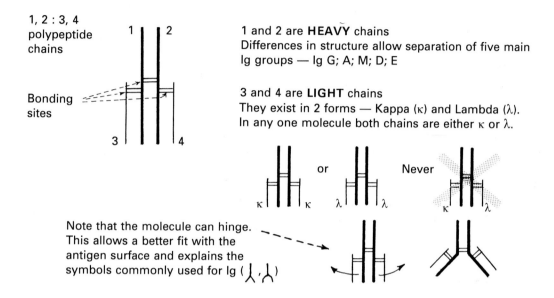

1, 2 : 3, 4 polypeptide chains

1 and 2 are **HEAVY** chains
Differences in structure allow separation of five main Ig groups — Ig G; A; M; D; E

Bonding sites

3 and 4 are **LIGHT** chains
They exist in 2 forms — Kappa (κ) and Lambda (λ).
In any one molecule both chains are either κ or λ.

Note that the molecule can hinge. This allows a better fit with the antigen surface and explains the symbols commonly used for Ig (⅄ , ⅄)

Enzymatic digestion (papain) splits the molecule into named fragments.

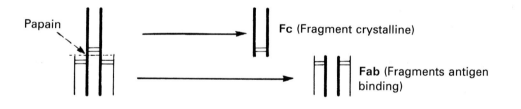

Papain

Fc (Fragment crystalline)

Fab (Fragments antigen binding)

Fc is the *constant* part of the molecule and does not participate in antigen binding.
However, the Fc fragment is associated with secondary effects after binding has occurred, e.g. complement activation; attraction of lymphocytes and particularly the facilitation of phagocytosis by macrophages which carry Fc receptors (see p.99).

Antigen
Fc
Fab
Fab

Fab are the *variable* parts of the molecule and are the site of antigen binding, the variation in amino acid content allowing a wide range of specific activity.

IMMUNOGLOBULINS

MAIN GROUPS

These groups are named according to the composition of the heavy chains.

IgM

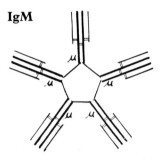

IgM (heavy chain = μ) is a polymer of five identical basic molecules, therefore called macroglobulin. Although in low concentration in the blood, 0.5–2 mg/ml, it is the main Ig on the surface of B lymphocytes (before conversion to plasma cells) and is active in the early phase of the immune response. It neutralises viruses. In combination with complement, it is actively bactericidal and is especially effective in bacteraemia.

Note: The numerous (10) antigen-binding sites increase its efficiency.

The natural blood group antibodies, anti-A and anti-B are M globulins.

IgG

IgG (heavy chain = γ) is a single molecule with two antigen binding sites.

It is produced mainly in **secondary response**.

IgG has the highest concentration of all immunoglobulins in the blood — within a range of 8–16 mg/ml dependent on antigenic stimulation at the time. Of its several activities, the important ones take place in the blood and tissue fluids and are:

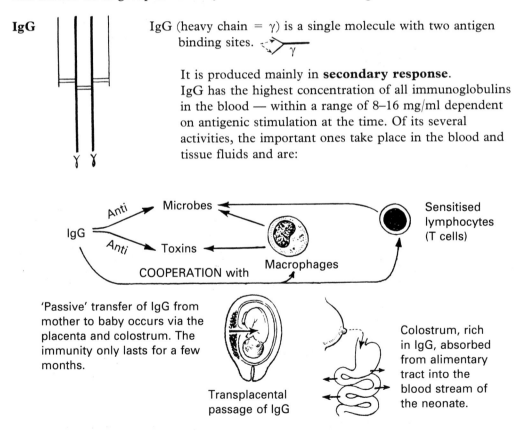

'Passive' transfer of IgG from mother to baby occurs via the placenta and colostrum. The immunity only lasts for a few months.

Transplacental passage of IgG

Colostrum, rich in IgG, absorbed from alimentary tract into the blood stream of the neonate.

IMMUNOGLOBULINS

IgA

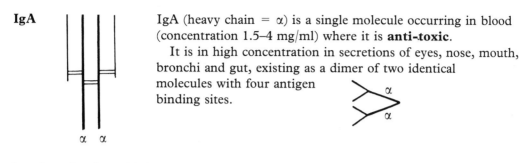

IgA (heavy chain = α) is a single molecule occurring in blood (concentration 1.5–4 mg/ml) where it is **anti-toxic**.

It is in high concentration in secretions of eyes, nose, mouth, bronchi and gut, existing as a dimer of two identical molecules with four antigen binding sites.

Local production of IgA e.g. in alimentary tract

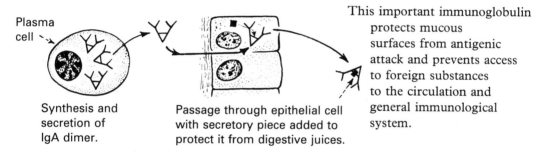

Plasma cell

Synthesis and secretion of IgA dimer.

Passage through epithelial cell with secretory piece added to protect it from digestive juices.

This important immunoglobulin protects mucous surfaces from antigenic attack and prevents access to foreign substances to the circulation and general immunological system.

IgD (heavy chain △) of uncertain function: concentration in blood very low. Like IgM it is present on the surface of lymphocytes prior to transformation.

IgE (heavy chain ε) — a single molecule similar to IgG and IgA.

It is sometimes called REAGIN: concentration in blood is low (20–500 ng/ml).

The serum level is raised in worm infestation and is probably protective.

Its main activity is mediated by MAST CELLS (or BASOPHILS).

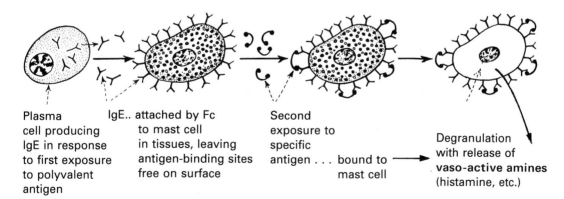

Plasma cell producing IgE in response to first exposure to polyvalent antigen

IgE.. attached by Fc to mast cell in tissues, leaving antigen-binding sites free on surface

Second exposure to specific antigen . . . bound to mast cell

Degranulation with release of **vaso-active amines** (histamine, etc.)

The range of antigens is immense and B cells produce an infinite number of specific antibodies by interchanging and rearranging the shape of the terminal amino acids of the FAB fraction to suit the antigen determinants.

IMMUNE REACTIONS

The basic reaction is the combination of antigen (Ag) and antibody (Ab) to form an Ag/Ab complex.

This reaction is reversible in varying degree (Ag + Ab $\rightleftharpoons$ Ag/Ab).

IMMEDIATE AND DELAYED REACTIONS

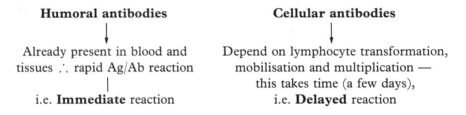

Humoral antibodies

Already present in blood and tissues ∴ rapid Ag/Ab reaction

i.e. **Immediate** reaction

Cellular antibodies

Depend on lymphocyte transformation, mobilisation and multiplication — this takes time (a few days), i.e. **Delayed** reaction

The forces binding the antigen and antibody are essentially non-specific and are the same as those operating in most situations where protein molecules are in proximity.

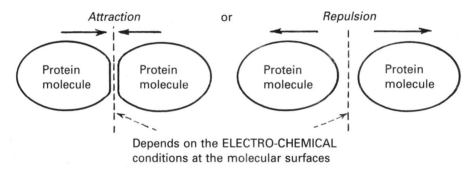

Attraction   or   *Repulsion*

Protein molecule | Protein molecule | Protein molecule | Protein molecule

Depends on the ELECTRO-CHEMICAL conditions at the molecular surfaces

In antigen/antibody binding, these forces of attraction are boosted by the shape and flexibility of the Ig molecule ensuring a good 'fit' with determinants on the antigen surface.

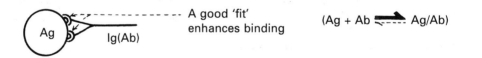

Ag Ig(Ab) A good 'fit' enhances binding   (Ag + Ab $\rightleftharpoons$ Ag/Ab)

There are several consequences of the basic Ag/Ab combination which have been extensively studied *in vitro*.

1. PRECIPITATION
2. AGGLUTINATION
3. ANTI-TOXIC effect
4. ENHANCEMENT of the natural non-specific defence mechanisms

IMMUNE REACTIONS

1. PRECIPITATION

A soluble antigen is rendered insoluble by aggregation of the Ag/Ab complexes into a lattice.

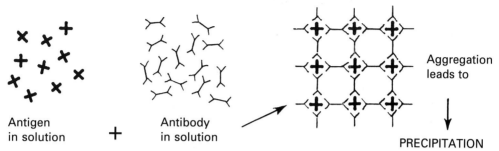

Antigen in solution + Antibody in solution → Aggregation leads to PRECIPITATION

2. AGGLUTINATION

Particulate antigen, e.g. bacteria and red blood cells, are aggregated in the same way as in the precipitation reaction and the process is called AGGLUTINATION.

3. ANTI-TOXIC Effect

The Ag/Ab combination neutralises the toxic activity.

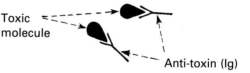

Toxic molecule

Anti-toxin (Ig)

4. ENHANCEMENT of the natural non-specific defence mechanisms

(a) Phagocytic activity

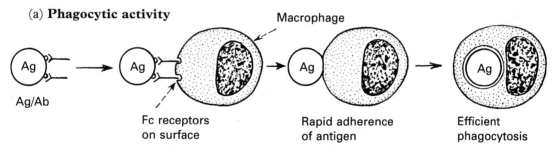

Macrophage

Ag/Ab

Fc receptors on surface

Rapid adherence of antigen

Efficient phagocytosis

Antibodies with this property are called **opsonins**.

(b) Complement activation

Humoral immune reactions frequently involve activation of the complement system. Complement consists of nine main protein components circulating in inactive form in the blood. Activation is affected by Ag/Ab complexes. The complex attaches itself to complement via the Fc part of the Ab (IgG or IgM). When the first protein (C1) is activated it acts as an enzyme, splitting the second protein (C2) into two parts, one an effector and the other an enzyme which splits the third protein (C3) into two parts, an effector and an enzyme and so on down the cascade.

The ultimate objective is to enhance the immune reaction particularly by killing micro-organisms, by improving phagocytosis and mediating the inflammatory response (see p.38 et seq.).

107

IMMUNE REACTIONS

COMPLEMENT SYSTEM

The sequence of the reactions and the substances produced are as follows:

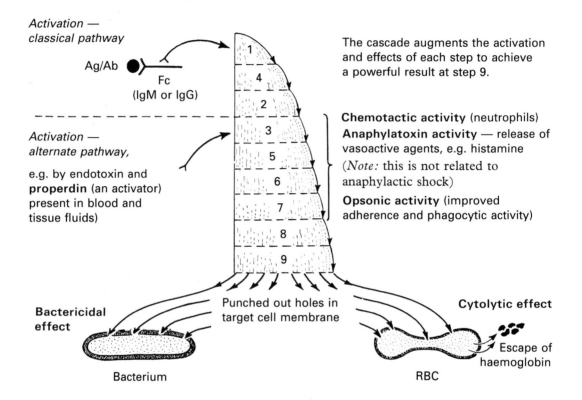

*Activation —
classical pathway*

Ag/Ab

Fc
(IgM or IgG)

The cascade augments the activation
and effects of each step to achieve
a powerful result at step 9.

*Activation —
alternate pathway,*

e.g. by endotoxin and
properdin (an activator)
present in blood and
tissue fluids)

Chemotactic activity (neutrophils)
Anaphylatoxin activity — release of
vasoactive agents, e.g. histamine
(*Note:* this is not related to
anaphylactic shock)
Opsonic activity (improved
adherence and phagocytic activity)

**Bactericidal
effect**

Punched out holes in
target cell membrane

Cytolytic effect

Escape of
haemoglobin

Bacterium

RBC

B lymphocytes, neutrophils, monocytes, macrophages and red cells have receptors for complement and thus concentrate the released kinins at the reaction site.

Activation of C by Ag/Ab complex is called **fixation of complement**. Antibodies with this property are termed **amboceptors**. Using red cells as markers, this fixation can detect the presence of antigen or antibody in serum.

E.g. Test serum + antigen + C.
    If serum contains antibody, C is fixed, otherwise it remains free.
    Add sensitised RBC (coated with Ab).
    Lysis of RBC ≡ complement still free ∴ no Ab in original serum.
    No lysis = C was fixed by Ab in test serum.

MONONUCLEAR PHAGOCYTE SYSTEM

The cells of this system have important roles in many disease processes and appear throughout the book. Although their main functions are essentially *non-specific*, they have important roles in the immune response, particularly in cooperation with T lymphocytes. Found at many sites throughout the body, they are derived from **STEM CELLS** in the bone marrow.

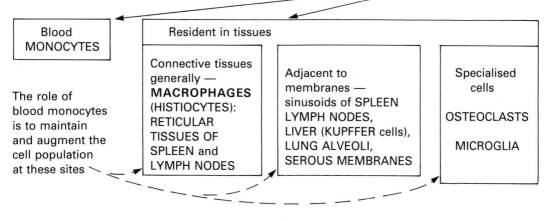

Historically, cells with varying degrees of phagocytic activity recognised at many of these sites were grouped into the **RETICULOENDOTHELIAL** system, but since reticulum cells are still ill-defined and endothelial cells have little phagocytic function the term is inappropriate and (although still used by some) has become obsolete.

Main functions

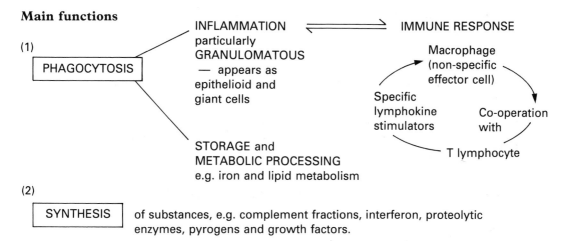

The System in Disease

Primary disorders of the system are rare. Participation in many disease processes is well recognised and detailed mechanisms are being elucidated.

TOLERANCE

Humoral and cell-mediated immunity are specific responses with a protective function.

In certain circumstances an antigen does not evoke these specific responses. This is not a failure of immunologically competent lymphocytes but is a third type of specific activity — TOLERANCE.

Natural tolerance   **Acquired tolerance**

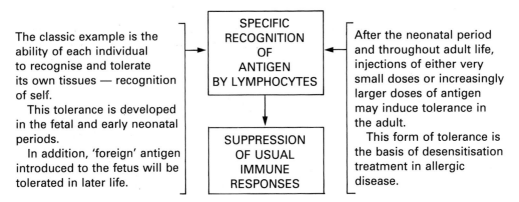

The classic example is the ability of each individual to recognise and tolerate its own tissues — recognition of self.

This tolerance is developed in the fetal and early neonatal periods.

In addition, 'foreign' antigen introduced to the fetus will be tolerated in later life.

SPECIFIC RECOGNITION OF ANTIGEN BY LYMPHOCYTES

SUPPRESSION OF USUAL IMMUNE RESPONSES

After the neonatal period and throughout adult life, injections of either very small doses or increasingly larger doses of antigen may induce tolerance in the adult.

This form of tolerance is the basis of desensitisation treatment in allergic disease.

The mechanisms of inducing tolerance are not yet completely understood. There are three possibilities:

1. Burnet's 'forbidden clone theory' (clonal selection theory) — in fetal life all lymphoid cells which could respond immunologically to 'self' antigens are eliminated.

2. In adults, acquired tolerance is associated primarily with specific SUPPRESSOR T cell activity which inhibits the response to both helper T cells and B cells.

3. Modification of antigen structure and the form of presentation to lymphoid cells — the effect may be a functional blocking of the immune reaction (anergy of T and/or B cells).

PERSISTING TOLERANCE IS A FUNCTION OF T CELLS. B cell activity is of short term significance (e.g. infections) but where the antigen is persistent i.e. exists as a reservoir in the body or is repeatedly introduced, T cells are involved and long-lasting tolerance can be induced, e.g. a tissue graft with foreign cell clones.

Tolerance is an important protective mechanism. When it breaks down, the serious effects give rise to autoimmune disease (see p.117).

IMMUNOPATH

The complicated and delicately balanced immune mechanisms clearly have been developed to protect against antigens, particularly infections. When these immune reactions are upset, the protective mechanism can itself be a source of disease states.

There are three main categories: (1) hypersensitivity states, (2) immune deficiency states and (3) autoimmune diseases.

HYPERSENSITIVITY REACTIONS

Basically these consist of an exaggerated response by an individual to an antigen, following a previous exposure. The resulting Ag/Ab reaction induces the release of large quantities of chemicals, enzymes and cell stimulators. Depending on the main type of immune response concerned these are classified as follows:

(a) Those associated with
   HUMORAL ANTIBODIES
   ∴ immediate — types I, II, III

(b) Those associated with
   CELL-MEDIATED IMMUNITY
   ∴ delayed (24–72 hours) — type IV.

As previously stated this classification is to some extent artificial. Hypersensitivity may start as an immediate humoral reaction but end in a mixed state with both humoral and cell-mediated activities.

Type 1 Anaphylaxis, atopy, allergy

All three terms have been used for this reaction. The basic mechanism is as follows:

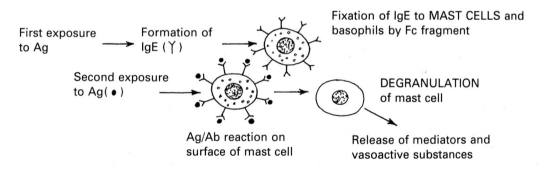

First exposure to Ag → Formation of IgE (Y) → Fixation of IgE to MAST CELLS and basophils by Fc fragment

Second exposure to Ag(•) →

Ag/Ab reaction on surface of mast cell

DEGRANULATION of mast cell

Release of mediators and vasoactive substances

Antigens and 'allergens'

The most potent antigens are usually very large molecules with molecular weights up to 40,000. Examples of common 'allergens' are: anti-tetanic serum, penicillin, bee venom, pollen, house mite dust, food, drugs, etc.

Antibody

This is IgE. Plasma cells forming IgE are found extensively in the internal secretory surfaces of the body — tonsils, adenoids, bronchi, gastrointestinal tract and urinary bladder.

HYPERSENSITIVITY STATES

Mast cells

These have a wide distribution but are prominent in the same areas as the IgE-producing plasma cells, plus skin, uterus and synovial membranes. This explains the frequently used term 'target organs' when discussing hypersensitivity.

Clinical examples of Type I reaction

ANAPHYLACTIC SHOCK

1st injection of e.g. horse serum (e.g. antitetanic serum, ATS) penicillin or a bee sting → General sensitisation

– – – – – – – – – – – – – – – –

2nd injection of above → Acute collapse: bronchial constriction; vomiting; diarrhoea; perhaps a skin rash. May be fatal. Note that the antigens are injected — enter blood stream → basophils affected → widespread reaction

HAY FEVER

1st contact with grass pollen → Local sensitisation of conjunctiva and nasal passages

– – – – – – – – – – – – – –

2nd contact with above → Irritation or swelling of conjunctiva with excessive watery secretion

ASTHMA

1st contact with house mite dust or animal dander → Local sensitisation of bronchi

– – – – – – – – – – – – –

2nd contact with above → Bronchial constriction and secretion of thick mucus cause dyspnoea (difficult breathing)

Chronic asthma may involve cell-mediated immunity with tissue destruction.

Allergic conditions are often familial with a genetic basis. If both parents are allergic = 75% chance of allergic offspring; one parent = 50%.

Type II — Cytotoxic type

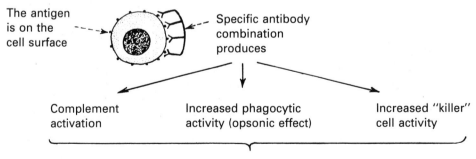

The antigen is on the cell surface – – → Specific antibody combination produces

Complement activation → Increased phagocytic activity (opsonic effect) → Increased "killer" cell activity

DESTRUCTION OF CELL

This cytotoxic reaction causes some forms of haemolytic anaemia and some blood transfusion reactions.

In some auto-immune disorders antibodies of this type are directed against specialised cell surface receptors, e.g. Graves' disease or myasthenia gravis (see p.119).

HYPERSENSITIVITY STATES

Type III — Immune complex (Arthus) type

The reaction is due to the consequences of specific direct antigen/antibody combination — particularly complement activation (p.108) and platelet aggregation. The antibodies involved are commonly IgG or IgM.

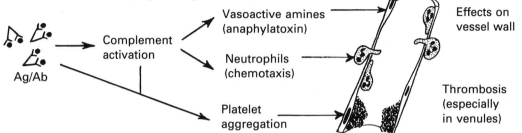

In most cases where there is Ag/Ab reaction, hypersensitivity does not develop. Where it does so, the Ag/Ab complexes tend to aggregate in small vessels and, with complement, cause tissue destruction, e.g. renal glomeruli. Serum sickness is acute short term disease of this type.

Type IV — Cell-mediated (delayed) type

This reaction is usually local and is due to the activities of specifically sensitised T cells.

The classical example of this type of reaction is the tubercle follicle; it is concerned also in other granulomatous disease processes, the rashes of virus infections and the rejection of grafts.

The skin reaction to chemicals — **contact dermatitis** — is illustrative. This condition is now common due to the increasing use of chemicals in industry and for topical application. The chemical — often of a simple nature, e.g. nickel — acts as a hapten, evoking an immune response.

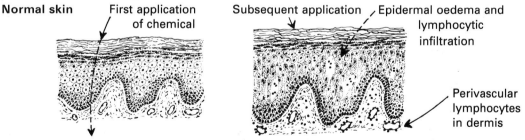

Chemical + tissue protein = 'foreign' antigen → cell-mediated immunity → inflammation

Another interesting common illustration of this type of reaction is the recurrent activity at the site of an insect bite often for several days after — possibly explained by the intermittent arrival of sensitised lymphocytes.

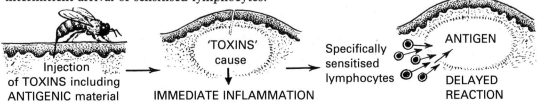

113

IMMUNE DEFICIENCY STATES

The systems involved are:

(1) **THE SPECIFIC SYSTEM** — humoral
cell-mediated

(2) **THE NON-SPECIFIC SYSTEM** — phagocytes
complement

Failure in any one alters the immune response. The deficiencies may be of a primary nature, commonly genetic in origin, or secondary to some other disease or circumstance. Equally, the alteration in any system may be quantitative or qualitative. In many of these deficiencies there is a failure in more than one system.

Primary (inherited) deficiencies of the specific system are rare. They include B cell, T cell and combined B and T cell deficits and are associated with recurring infections, particularly of the respiratory and alimentary tracts.

Secondary deficiencies of the specific system are common. Usually T cell activity is affected, resulting in deficient cell-mediated immunity and, later, B cell deficit occurs.

Currently the acquired immune deficiency syndrome (AIDS) is causing great concern. However more common predisposing conditions and diseases are:

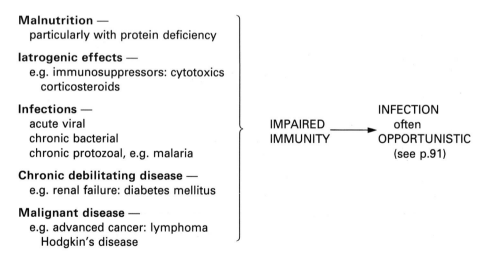

Malnutrition —
    particularly with protein deficiency

Iatrogenic effects —
    e.g. immunosuppressors: cytotoxics
        corticosteroids

Infections —
    acute viral
    chronic bacterial
    chronic protozoal, e.g. malaria

Chronic debilitating disease —
    e.g. renal failure: diabetes mellitus

Malignant disease —
    e.g. advanced cancer: lymphoma
        Hodgkin's disease

IMPAIRED IMMUNITY ⟶ INFECTION often OPPORTUNISTIC (see p.91)

Deficiencies of the non-specific system are rare. The disorders of neutrophil function are described on page 538.

IMMUNE DEFICIENCY STATES — AIDS

The Acquired Immune Deficiency Syndrome (AIDS) is now distributed worldwide, but has assumed epidemic status in many parts of the world — particularly CENTRAL AFRICA and WESTERN HOMOSEXUAL COMMUNITIES.

It is due to infection by a lentiretrovirus — human immunodeficiency virus (HIV).

The disease is slowly progressive and is usually fatal.

Infection	Latent and prodromal stages	Stages of opportunistic
	[AIDS-related complex (ARC)] (months up to several years)	infection and tumours (1–2 years)
No initial symptoms	Virus present in lymphocytes — at first, no signs, — later, may be persistent lymph node enlargement and fever.	Infection ⟨ opportunistic / others
T_4 (helper) lymphocytes > 500/mm^3	T_4 cells < 200/mm^3	Malignant tumours ⟨ Kaposi's sarcoma / lymphomas T_4 cells < 200/mm^3

The whole range of opportunistic infection (see p.91), including disseminated virus infection (e.g. herpes simplex and cytomegalovirus), occurs.

The diagram shows the more common AIDS-associated diseases and sites:

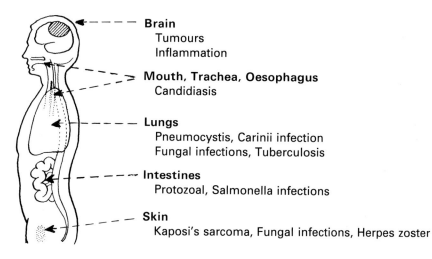

Brain
Tumours
Inflammation

Mouth, Trachea, Oesophagus
Candidiasis

Lungs
Pneumocystis, Carinii infection
Fungal infections, Tuberculosis

Intestines
Protozoal, Salmonella infections

Skin
Kaposi's sarcoma, Fungal infections, Herpes zoster

Blood changes

Antibodies — after infection, up to 6 months may elapse before anti-HIV antibodies appear; in the later stages the titre may drop greatly.

Immunoglobulins are usually elevated in the early stages.

T4 (helper) lymphocytes are severely reduced, producing a lymphopaenia. T4/T8 ratio reversed.

115

IMMUNE DEFICIENCY STATES — AIDS

EPIDEMIOLOGY AND TRANSMISSION

Although the virus may be present in many body fluids and secretions, transmission is by the parenteral route, usually by (1) **sexual contact** or (2) **injection of blood** or **blood products**.

Transmission does not occur with normal social contact and there is no risk to medical or nursing personnel using normal procedures.

1. *Sexual transmission*

(a) MALE HOMOSEXUAL PRACTICE: HIV in seminal fluid → via anorectal abrasion to passive partner.

(b) HETEROSEXUAL TRANSMISSION is less common except where there is a high prevalence in prostitutes.

> Female to male — infectious genital secretions and blood → via penis to male (risk increased in uncircumcised).
>
> Male to female — infectious seminal fluid and blood → to female cervix uteri and vagina.

In both sexes the risks are very considerably increased where there is genital ulceration or abrasion.

2. *Transmission by blood*

- The risk from blood transfusion and blood products has now been virtually eliminated by screening and sterilisation procedures.
- The communal use of contaminated syringes and needles continues to be important among drug addicts.

Cellular mechanisms

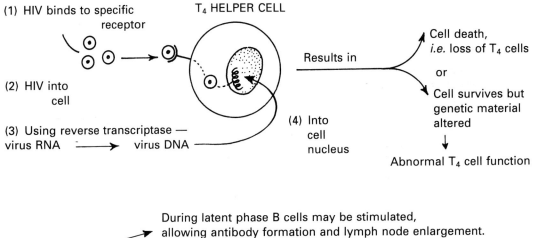

(1) HIV binds to specific receptor

T₄ HELPER CELL

(2) HIV into cell

(3) Using reverse transcriptase — virus RNA ⇢ virus DNA

(4) Into cell nucleus

Results in

Cell death, i.e. loss of T₄ cells

or

Cell survives but genetic material altered

↓

Abnormal T₄ cell function

T₄ cell deficiency

During latent phase B cells may be stimulated, allowing antibody formation and lymph node enlargement.

Gradual failure of immune effector mechanisms.

AUTOIMMUNE DISEASES

Autoimmune diseases result from, or are associated with, an immune response against the individual's own cells, or in some cases cell products. The phrase 'associated with' is used advisedly since the autoimmune response is often a phase or feature, generally of late onset, in an ongoing disease state and is not a primary cause. It involves changes in humoral, cell-mediated immunity and in tolerance.

Aetiology

The aetiology of autoimmune diseases is not established, but clues to their genesis are available.

An increased FAMILIAL incidence of autoimmune diseases in general and of particular individual diseases	The overlapping of the incidence of antibodies and of the types of damage produced	An increased incidence of malignant tumours among affected individuals

Suggest
an INBORN INSTABILITY OF IMMUNE TOLERANCE
particularly associated with inheritance of specific HLA-D antigens.

The possible changes in the immune mechanism are complex and involve several factors of which the two most important are (1) antigenic abnormality and (2) abnormality of the effector response (particularly T cell activity).

(1) Antigenic abnormality

   (a) cell surface antigens modified by drugs or chemicals.
   (b) cell antigens modified by proteolysis associated with disease processes, particularly inflammation when 'new' antigens are formed.
   (c) microbial cross-reacting antigens.

(2) Abnormality of effector response

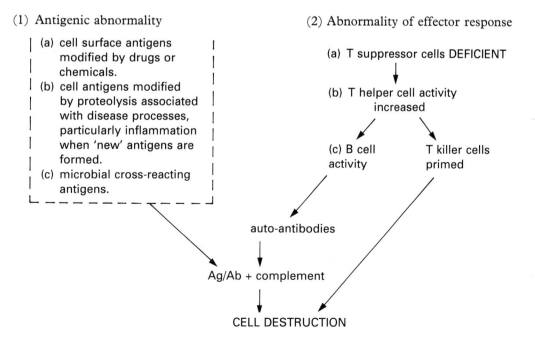

(a) T suppressor cells DEFICIENT

(b) T helper cell activity increased

(c) B cell activity   T killer cells primed

auto-antibodies

Ag/Ab + complement

CELL DESTRUCTION

117

AUTOIMMUNE DISEASES

	Antibody to	Target Organ	Associated Diseases
ORGAN-SPECIFIC	(a) Thyroid cells and hormones, or (b) TSH receptor	Thyroid	Primary myxoedema Hashimoto's disease (auto-immune thyroiditis) Thyrotoxicosis (Graves' disease)
	Parietal cells Intrinsic factor Intrinsic factor/B12 complex	Stomach	Pernicious anaemia
	Red blood cells	Red blood cells	Haemolytic anaemia
	Pancreatic islet beta cells	Pancreas	Type 1 diabetes
	Adrenal cortical cells ACTH receptor	Adrenal	Addison's disease
	Parathyroid cells	Parathyroid	Primary hypoparathyroidism
	Acetylcholine receptor	Voluntary muscle	Myasthenia gravis

	Antibody to	Target Organ	Associated Diseases
NON-ORGAN-SPECIFIC	Mitochondria	Liver	Primary biliary cirrhosis
	Smooth muscle	Liver	Chronic active hepatitis
	Nuclear constituents	Skin and muscles	The connective tissue diseases Dermatomyositis
	IgG	Skin, kidney endocardium, blood vessels, joints	Rheumatoid arthritis Systemic lupus erythematosus (SLE)
	Many other body proteins		Progressive systemic sclerosis

AUTOIMMUNE DISEASES

Primary thyrotoxicosis (Graves' disease) and myasthenia gravis are of particular interest. The activity of the auto-antibodies is a modification of the Type II reaction in that the specific antibody combines with antigen on the cell surface and either stimulates or blocks the action of the physiological agent which would normally turn on the activity of the cell.

Stimulatory effect
In Graves' disease, excessive amounts of thyroid hormone are produced. LATS (long acting thyroid stimulator), an IgG auto-antibody, combines with antigen on the thyroid cell surface and produces changes mimicking those produced by TSH (thyroid stimulating hormone) — physiologically manufactured by the pituitary.

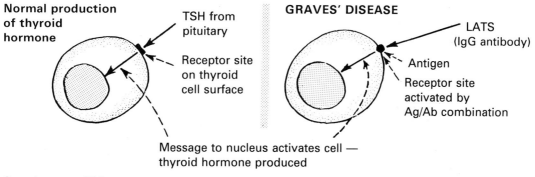

See also page 816

Blocking effect
In myasthenia gravis, the acetylcholine formed at the motor nerve endings is prevented from stimulating the muscle motor end plate due to the antibody blocking the specific acetylcholine receptors. The end plate is also damaged (Ag/Ab + complement).

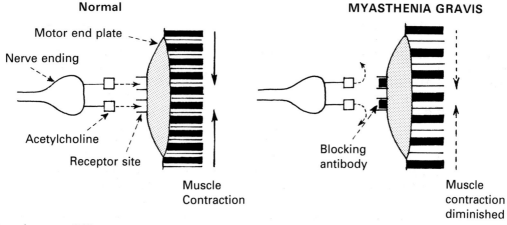

See also page 768

119

APPLIED IMMUNOLOGY

Immunohistochemical identification

Immunohistochemical techniques are developing rapidly. They allow the clear identification of specific substances in histological sections.

Example:

Microscopic result

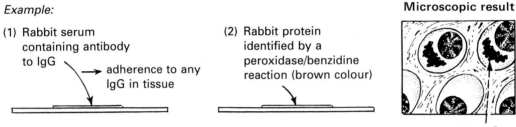

(1) Rabbit serum containing antibody to IgG → adherence to any IgG in tissue

Histological slide containing plasma cell infiltrate

(2) Rabbit protein identified by a peroxidase/benzidine reaction (brown colour)

Only plasma cells containing IGg are coloured brown

This or similar techniques may be used to identify a wide range of substances.

Prophylaxis and treatment of infections

1. **Passive immunisation** is the term used when antibody formed in one individual is given to another individual who is at risk of infection — the protection is temporary. Examples include:
   - Pooled human γ-globulin → general protection — particularly useful in cases of immune deficiency.
   - Horse serum containing antibodies to **tetanus** or **diphtheria** → specific protection. *NB* the foreign horse protein may itself cause immunological reactions, e.g. serum sickness or anaphylactic shock.

2. **Active immunisation** is the term used when the infective agent is modified in some way to eliminate its harmful effects without loss of antigenicity. The subject's own immune response is activated. Examples include:

   TOXOID — e.g. tetanus toxin modified chemically
   KILLED ORGANISMS — e.g. TAB (typhoid, paratyphoid A and B) vaccine
   ATTENUATED ORGANISMS — e.g. viruses; cowpox, polio, measles.

Diagnosis of disease

Diagnosis is confirmed by the detection in serum of specific antibodies using known antigens. The immune reactions, such as agglutination and specific complement fixation, are indicators.

Infections and autoimmune disease are investigated by these means. The specificity of such tests has been greatly improved by the use of **monoclonal antibodies**.

APPLIED IMMUNOLOGY — TISSUE TRANSPLANTATION

In the past, allografting (transplanting of tissues or organs from one individual to another of the same species) inevitably led to rejection of the graft by the host. Understanding of the mechanisms has allowed intervention so that nowadays successful survival of grafts is usual (e.g. 90% survival of renal transplants after 1 year).

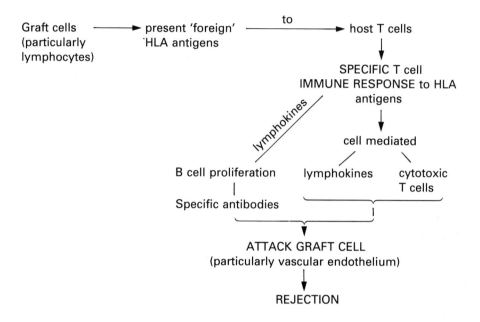

Rejection may occur very rapidly if pre-existing antibodies are present (e.g. due to previous incompatible blood transfusion).

Usually rejection takes 2–4 weeks while the immune response is building up.

The remarkable improvement in transplant prognosis is due to:

    (a) careful matching of HLA compatibility,
    (b) use of immuno-suppressive agents (particularly cyclosporin A),
    (c) screening for the presence of pre–existing HLA and cytotoxic antibodies.

Paradoxically the pre-transplant transfusion of compatible blood improves the chances of graft survival.

GRAFT versus HOST (GVH) DISEASE

In a minority of cases, particularly when the recipient is immuno-suppressed, the lymphocytes of the donor (graft) proliferate in the recipient (host) and establish an immune response against the host tissues: the main target organs are the skin, the liver and the alimentary tract.

CHAPTER 6

NEOPLASIA

NON-NEOPLASTIC PROLIFERATION

Enlargement of an organ due to increase in the parenchymal cell mass may be due to:

(1) an increase in the size and functional capacity of the individual cells — **hypertrophy**
or (2) an increase in the number of cells — **hyperplasia**
or (3) commonly a combination of (1) and (2)

The stimuli responsible are:
   (a) increase in functional demand
   (b) increased trophic hormonal activity.

Physiological enlargement of organs is common and well illustrated by the increase in muscle bulk consequent upon training and the enlargement of uterus and breasts in pregnancy.
Pathological enlargement is the result of disease processes.

HYPERTROPHY (pathological)

Enlargement of the heart as a result of hypertension is a good example of pure hypertrophy: the result of the increased functional demands to maintain the high blood pressure is an increase in the size of the myocardial cells.

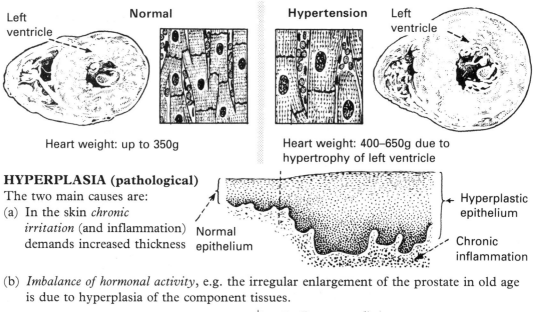

Left ventricle   **Normal**   **Hypertension**   Left ventricle

Heart weight: up to 350g   Heart weight: 400–650g due to hypertrophy of left ventricle

HYPERPLASIA (pathological)

The two main causes are:

(a) In the skin *chronic irritation* (and inflammation) demands increased thickness

Normal epithelium

Hyperplastic epithelium

Chronic inflammation

(b) *Imbalance of hormonal activity*, e.g. the irregular enlargement of the prostate in old age is due to hyperplasia of the component tissues.

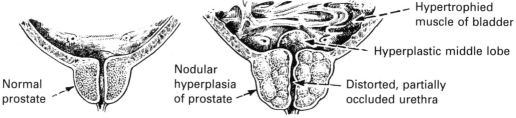

Hypertrophied muscle of bladder

Hyperplastic middle lobe

Normal prostate

Nodular hyperplasia of prostate

Distorted, partially occluded urethra

Note: If the abnormal stimulus is removed, the affected organ can return to normal.

NON-NEOPLASTIC PROLIFERATION

METAPLASIA

This is a change from one type of differentiated tissue to another, usually of the same broad class but often less well specialised. The change is commonly seen in lining epithelia but occurs also in connective tissues and lining of serous cavities. There is frequently an associated hyperplasia.

e.g. (a) Change from mucus-secreting epithelium to stratified squamous epithelium as in the bronchial irritation associated with smoking.

(b) Formation of bone in fibrous tissue — sometimes in healing process, e.g. prostatectomy scars.

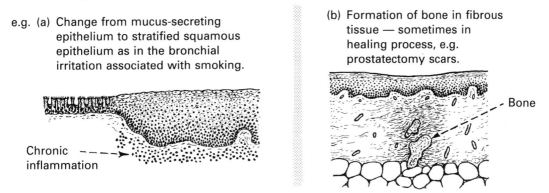

Chronic inflammation

Bone

In some cases metaplasia is associated with chronic irritation, but the intimate causes are unknown in most instances. Lack of vitamin A however results in widespread squamous metaplasia of respiratory and salivary epithelium.

DYSPLASIA

This means disordered development, as observed in histological sections.

The changes consist of increased mitosis, the production of abnormal cells in varying numbers and a tendency to disorder in their arrangement (cellular ATYPIA). Some cases of dysplasia progress to malignancy.

The diagram illustrates changes which are common in the uterine cervix (see also p.660).

| Mucus-secreting epithelium | Squamous metaplasia | Dysplastic epithelium |

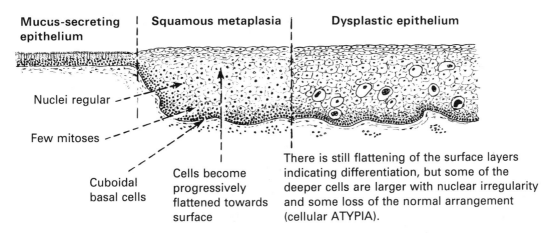

Nuclei regular

Few mitoses

Cuboidal basal cells

Cells become progressively flattened towards surface

There is still flattening of the surface layers indicating differentiation, but some of the deeper cells are larger with nuclear irregularity and some loss of the normal arrangement (cellular ATYPIA).

Note: Both metaplasia and dysplasia may be reversible, but many of the characteristics of dysplastic cells are common to malignant cells (see p.136).

NEOPLASTIC PROLIFERATION

A tumour is a proliferation of cells which is:

1. **Progressive**

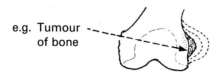

e.g. Tumour
of bone

2. **Purposeless** e.g. Tumour of fibrous tissue

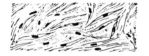   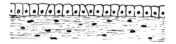

The fibres of a tumour of fibrous
tissue have no regular arrangement
and serve no useful purpose.

In normal fibrous tissue, the strands
have a definite arrangement, supporting
some structure such as an
epithelial surface.

NB Individual cells of a tumour may exhibit function — the fibrocytes form collagen —
but it has no purpose.

3. **Regardless of surrounding tissue,**

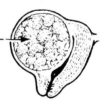

e.g. Smooth muscle tumour of uterus — — — — —
compresses normal tissues and distorts
uterine cavity

4. **Not related to needs of the body,**

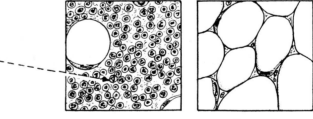

e.g. Certain tumours of
bone-marrow cells
produce, needlessly,
enormous numbers
of leucocytes which
enter the blood stream

Normal

5. **Parasitic**
The tumour draws its nourishment from the body while contributing nothing to its
function. It induces the body to provide a blood supply and, in the case of epithelial
tumours, a supporting stroma.

Since the development of a neoplasm is independent of the normal processes in the body
it is *autonomous* although its growth may to some extent be influenced by these processes.

NEOPLASMS — CLASSIFICATION

Tumours may be classified in two ways: (1) clinical and (2) histological origin.

1. CLINICAL

The tumour is classified according to its morbid anatomy and behaviour. Two main groups are recognised — *benign* (simple) and *malignant*. The contrast between these two groups is as follows:-

	BENIGN	MALIGNANT
Spread (the most important feature)	Remains localised	Cells transferred via lymphatics, blood vessels, tissue planes and serous cavities to set up satellite tumours (metastases)
Rate of Growth	Usually slow	Usually rapid
Boundaries	Circumscribed, often encapsulated	Irregular, ill-defined and non-encapsulated
Relationship to surrounding tissues	Merely compresses normal tissue	Invades and destroys normal tissues
Effects	Produced by pressure on vessels, tubes, nerves, organs etc. Removal will alleviate.	Destroys structures and removal of tumour will not restore function

In practice, there is a spectrum of malignancy. Some tumours may grow locally and destroy normal tissues but never produce metastases. Others will produce metastases only after a very considerable time while, at the other end of the spectrum, there are tumours which metastasise very early in their development.

2. HISTOLOGICAL ORIGIN

Although tumours may arise from any tissue in the body, they can be conveniently accommodated in six groups.

1. Mesodermic connective tissues including muscle, bone and cartilage
2. Epethelia
3. Neuroectoderm
4. Haemopoietic tissues
5. Blood and lymph vessels
6. Cells originating from developmental abnormalities

In practice, tumours most often take origin from tissues which normally have a rapid turnover of cells and are active in repair — epithelia of skin and mucous membranes, breast and female reproductive organs, connective tissue, bone and haemopoietic cells.

CYTOLOGICAL DIFFERENTIATION

Tumour cells may be broadly divided into two types:
(1) Differentiated and (2) Undifferentiated.

The degree of differentiation roughly corresponds to the character of the neoplasm. Cells of simple tumours are well differentiated; those of malignant tumours tend to remain undifferentiated, and the more primitive the cells the greater the malignancy.

DIFFERENTIATED CELLS (BENIGN TUMOURS)

1. **Mimic the structure of their parent organ.**

e.g. In an adenoma (simple gland-forming tumour) of colon the cells arrange themselves in acini. – – – –

In a skin papilloma (wart) the squamous epithelium still forms a covering for underlying connective tissue

2. **Resemble their cells of origin.**

e.g. The cells of a skin papilloma are squamous

The cells of a myoma are muscle cells

The cells of a chondroma are recognisable cartilage cells

3. As in normal tissue, **show a remarkable uniformity in size, shape and nuclear configuration**. – – – – – – – →

4. **Show evidence of normal function even if useless.**

– – Mucous secretion in acinus of an adenoma

5. **Have relatively infrequent mitotic figures:** these are of normal type.

Division into two identical daughter cells.

Equatorial chromosomes

CYTOLOGICAL DIFFERENTIATION

UNDIFFERENTIATED CELLS (MALIGNANT TUMOURS):

1. **Generally show a haphazard arrangement.**   →   e.g. Carcinoma of breast

2. **Bear little resemblance to the cells of origin.**

3. **Tend to vary widely in size, shape and nuclear configuration.** → e.g. Pleomorphic sarcoma

4. **Provide little evidence of normal function.** → e.g. Adeno carcinoma of bowel (Secretory activity very limited)

5. **Show frequent mitoses often of abnormal type.**   Three daughter cells

Lack of differentiation is often termed anaplasia, and anaplastic tumours are highly malignant. There is a spectrum of change in neoplasms from the very slowly growing, highly differentiated simple types to the rapidly growing, undifferentiated malignant examples.

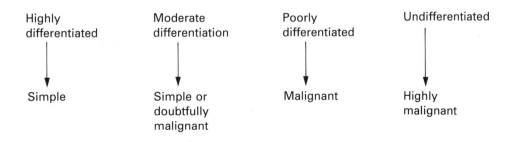

Highly differentiated	Moderate differentiation	Poorly differentiated	Undifferentiated
↓	↓	↓	↓
Simple	Simple or doubtfully malignant	Malignant	Highly malignant

SIMPLE CONNECTIVE TISSUE TUMOURS

These tumours are composed of differentiated connective tissues of the body — fibrous tissue, cartilage, bone, muscle, fatty tissue. They all tend to be rounded or lobulated, well-encapsulated and merely compress the surrounding tissues.

TUMOURS OF FIBROUS TISSUE

So-called FIBROMAS are extremely rare in the soft tissues. They occur in the ovary and kidney as firm nodules.

Neurofibroma and Schwannoma

These are derived from the connective tissues of the peripheral nerves. They may be single or multiple and cause compression effects (see p.756).

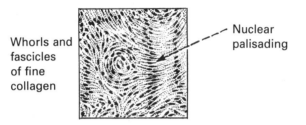

Whorls and fascicles of fine collagen

Nuclear palisading

TUMOUR-LIKE GROWTHS of fibrous tissue also occur. Examples are:

Keloid is an overgrowth of fibrous tissue in scars. It follows radiation burns but may complicate operation scars (see p.55).

Palmar fibromatosis, at first nodular, causes flexion deformities of fingers (Dupuytren's contracture) due to contraction of fibrous tissue within the palmar fascia. A similar condition may affect the plantar fascia.

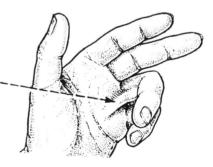

Juvenile aponeurotic fibroma — of palms and soles in children.

Nodular fasciitis — of the subcutaneous tissues of adults.
Both of the above appear malignant in that they invade adjacent structures, but they are self-limiting and yield to local excision.

Musculoaponeurotic fibromatosis (desmoid fibromatosis) is a similar lesion but recurs frequently after excision. It grows progressively infiltrating surrounding structures.

SIMPLE CONNECTIVE TISSUE TUMOURS

LIPOMA

Circumscribed masses of fat cells are commonly found in the subcutaneous tissue of the arms, shoulders and buttocks. They may also be found in the peritoneal cavity in relation to the kidney, omentum or mesentery, but very rarely in solid organs.

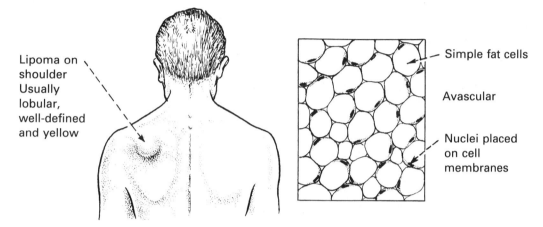

Lipoma on shoulder Usually lobular, well-defined and yellow

Simple fat cells

Avascular

Nuclei placed on cell membranes

Sometimes lipomas may have projections into the surrounding tissues which make complete removal difficult.

CHONDROMA

Two types are sometimes described:

1. **Solitary enchondroma**. This type is found in the tubular bones of the hands and feet and also in the long bones. It forms in the substance or at the surface of the bone and causes destruction of the bone by expansion and pressure.

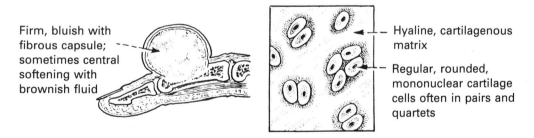

Firm, bluish with fibrous capsule; sometimes central softening with brownish fluid

Hyaline, cartilagenous matrix

Regular, rounded, mononuclear cartilage cells often in pairs and quartets

Growth occurs by the proliferation and metaplastic transformation of the capsular fibrocytes.

2. **Multiple enchondromatosis**. These are cartilagenous masses which appear in children, in the hands and feet but also importantly in the long bones where deformities may result. They usually cease to grow when adulthood is reached and ossify or regress; therefore they are probably in the nature of developmental abnormalities rather than true neoplasms. Occasionally they may continue to grow, and may even become malignant.

131

SIMPLE CONNECTIVE TISSUE TUMOURS

OSTEOMA

As with chondromas, two types are described:

1. **Ivory osteoma**. This is a true tumour and is mainly found in the long bones of the skull, although it may occur in the long bones. Osteomas are usually relatively small but may produce severe symptoms because of their situation.

2. **Cancellous bony growths**. These are found at the end of long bones and are the ossified remains of cartilagenous exostoses. They are formed from developmentally displaced epiphyseal cartilage.

   Growth continues until epiphyses unite. A cap of cartilage covers the mass and growth takes place by proliferation of the cartilage and transformation into bone.

Osteoma on floor of orbit causing protrusion of eyeball

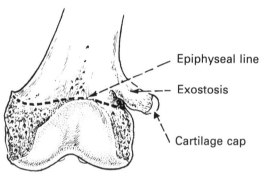

Epiphyseal line

Exostosis

Cartilage cap

LEIOMYOMA

Simple tumours of muscle are derived from smooth muscle (leiomyoma), and the majority occur in the uterus where they are extremely common. They are firm, rounded masses which usually begin in the myometrium. Subsequently, they may move inward to the uterine cavity forming polypi, or towards the serous surface.

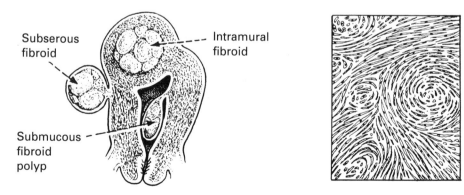

Subserous fibroid

Intramural fibroid

Submucous fibroid polyp

Fibres in parallel bundles which in turn are whorled

Occasionally, similar tumours may be found in the gastrointestinal tract, ovaries, prostate and bladder. Degenerative changes are common in myomas. **Many have a large fibrous component and, in the uterus, are termed fibroids**.

SIMPLE EPITHELIAL TUMOURS

Simple epithelial tumours are essentially of two types: (1) papillomas and (2) adenomas.

PAPILLOMA
Papillomas take origin from an epithelial surface. As the epithelium proliferates it is thrown into folds which become increasingly complex.

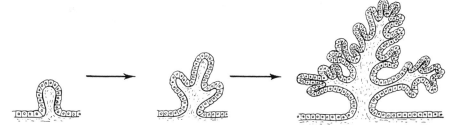

The epithelial proliferation is accompanied by a corresponding growth of supporting connective tissue and blood vessels.

Typical examples are found in the skin, e.g. the common wart.

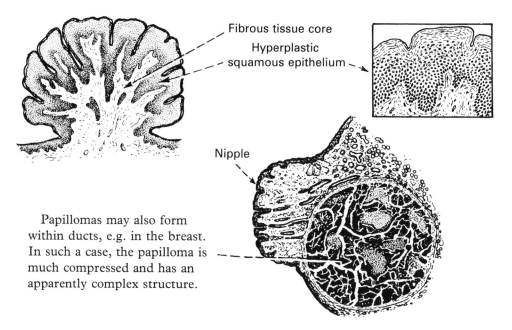

Fibrous tissue core

Hyperplastic squamous epithelium

Nipple

Papillomas may also form within ducts, e.g. in the breast. In such a case, the papilloma is much compressed and has an apparently complex structure.

In these simple tumours:

(a) The normal arrangement of epithelial cells is maintained, e.g. in skin papillomas the surface cells are squamous and proliferation is confined to the deepest layers.
(b) The relationship of epithelium to connective tissue is normal.
(c) Blood vessels are well formed.

SIMPLE EPITHELIAL TUMOURS

ADENOMA

Adenomas are derived from the ducts and acini of glands, although the name is also used to cover simple tumours arising in solid epithelial organs.

Again the proliferation of epithelium of a gland causes the formation of tubules which ramify and become increasingly compound. The original communication with the parent gland duct or acinus tends to become lost. — —

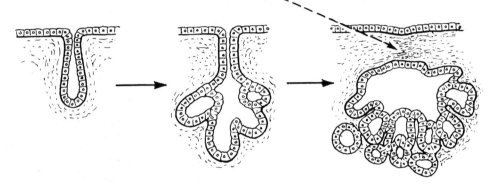

In the case of a hollow viscus, such as the intestine or gall bladder, the adenomatous proliferation, instead of growing down into the subjacent connective tissue, is usually pushed upwards into the lumen of the viscus. — — —

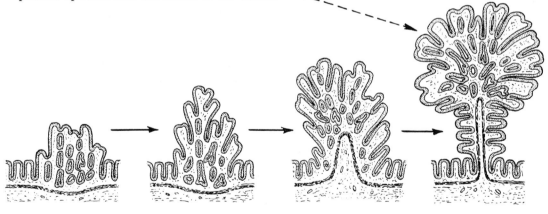

The growth therefore combines the features of a papilloma and an adenoma. The term adenomatous polyp is often applied in such a case.

SIMPLE EPITHELIAL TUMOURS

ADENOMA (continued)

In the type which grows into the subjacent connective tissue, the constant budding of the epithelium results in new acini which become nipped off from the parent acini.

In cases in which retention of secretion is marked, a cyst forms and the tumour is then called a cystadenoma which may reach an enormous size, e.g. some cystadenomas of the ovary may be 30–40 cm in diameter, particularly those which secrete mucus.

Normal ovary — Cystadenoma — Cut surface — Tall mucus-secreting cells

As in a hollow viscus, the proliferating epithelium may be heaped to form papillomas and the tumour then becomes a papillary cystadenoma. These are also common in the ovary (see p. 673).

In some organs the supporting connective tissue of the adenoma is a prominent component of the tumour. This is commonly seen in the BREAST, and the name FIBROADENOMA is used. Depending on the distribution of the fibrous tissue the histological appearances are variable.

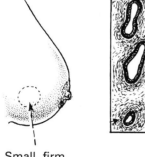

Small, firm, palpable mobile lump

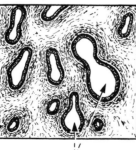

Well formed acini

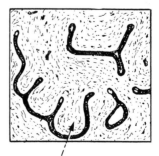

Slit-like acini compressed by fibrous tissue

CARCINOMA IN SITU (INTRAEPITHELIAL NEOPLASIA)

This represents an intermediate stage in the production of a cancer. All the cytological features of malignancy are present, but the cells have not invaded the surrounding tissues. It is frequently found in the cervix uteri at the junction of ecto and endocervix.

Normal cervix

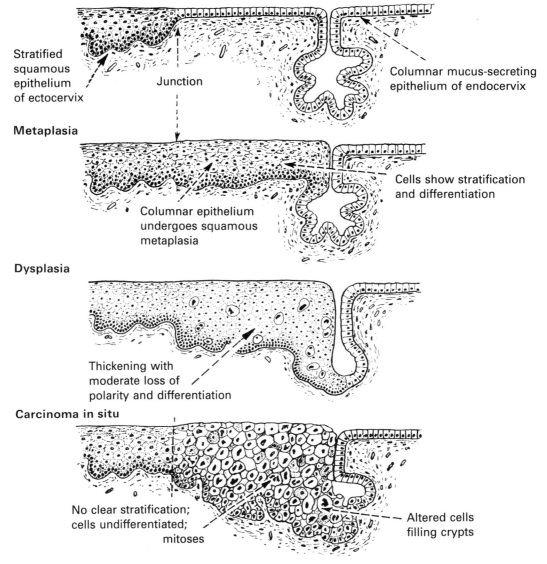

Stratified squamous epithelium of ectocervix

Junction

Columnar mucus-secreting epithelium of endocervix

Metaplasia

Columnar epithelium undergoes squamous metaplasia

Cells show stratification and differentiation

Dysplasia

Thickening with moderate loss of polarity and differentiation

Carcinoma in situ

No clear stratification; cells undifferentiated; mitoses

Altered cells filling crypts

Intraduct carcinoma of the breast is another example.

These premalignant conditions may revert to normal, but most commonly they become truly malignant and invade the surrounding tissues. The determining factors are unknown.

The concept of progressive premalignant proliferation applies equally in other organs (e.g. stomach, bowel, bronchus, etc.).

MALIGNANT EPITHELIAL TUMOURS

The generic term for a malignant epithelial tumour is
CARCINOMA (Greek: *Karkinos*, a crab). This
refers to the irregular jagged shape often assumed. It
is due to the local spread of carcinoma.

The proliferating cells break
through normal barriers.

Further growth is by permeation of
the tissue spaces.

Malignant
epithelium
breaks through basement membrane
and subjacent connective tissue

Malignant
cells
permeating
spaces

An important principle is that these permeating tumour cells take the line of least
physical resistance.

Growth of malignant cells may
stimulate the production of new
collagen fibres which are
sometimes converted into dense
fibrous tissue → contracts and fixes
the growth to surrounding
structures

e.g. Carcinoma of breast.

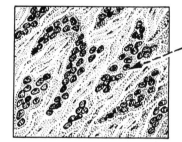

Retracted
nipple

Carcinoma
fixed to
underlying
muscle

Fibrous
tissue

The following diagram illustrates the basic mechanisms of cancer cell invasion.

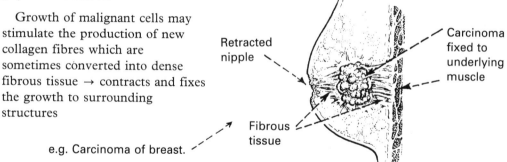

(1) Cancer cells

Ability to secrete
lytic enzymes,
e.g. collagenases

Basement
membrane
breached

(2)

Cells are less
adhesive
than normal

(3)

Spread
and subsequent
replication

Increased amoeboid
movements — penetration
and spread

137

SPREAD OF CARCINOMA

By definition, all carcinomas spread primarily into the adjacent tissues, and after a varying period, metastasis to more distant structures occurs in the following ways:

LYMPHATIC SPREAD

This is the commonest mode of spread. The carcinoma cells easily invade lymphatic channels from the tissue spaces.

Groups of cells form *emboli* in the lymph stream and are carried to the nearest node.

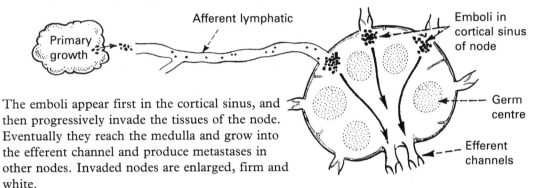

The emboli appear first in the cortical sinus, and then progressively invade the tissues of the node. Eventually they reach the medulla and grow into the efferent channel and produce metastases in other nodes. Invaded nodes are enlarged, firm and white.

These emboli are microscopic and can escape notice at operation. They account for recurrence of growth in many cases.

Growth of carcinoma cells in a node results in occlusion of afferent and efferent channels. Lymph flow is thus diverted and this has two effects:

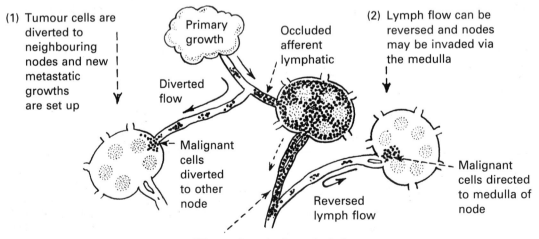

This accounts for the spread of carcinoma in a diverse and often irregular manner.

SPREAD OF CARCINOMA

LYMPHATIC SPREAD (continued)

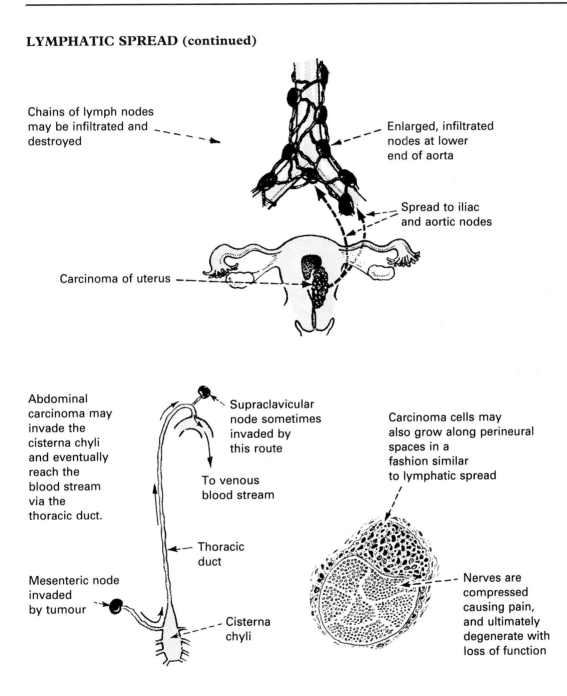

Chains of lymph nodes may be infiltrated and destroyed

Enlarged, infiltrated nodes at lower end of aorta

Spread to iliac and aortic nodes

Carcinoma of uterus

Abdominal carcinoma may invade the cisterna chyli and eventually reach the blood stream via the thoracic duct.

Supraclavicular node sometimes invaded by this route

To venous blood stream

Thoracic duct

Mesenteric node invaded by tumour

Cisterna chyli

Carcinoma cells may also grow along perineural spaces in a fashion similar to lymphatic spread

Nerves are compressed causing pain, and ultimately degenerate with loss of function

Although lymphatic embolism is of major practical importance, tumour cells may also grow along lymphatic channels in continuous solid columns — lymphatic permeation.

SPREAD OF CARCINOMA

BLOOD SPREAD (VENOUS)
VIA VENULES

The entry of malignant cells into the blood is via invasion of VENULES and by lymphatic embolism through the thoracic duct into the subclavian vein.

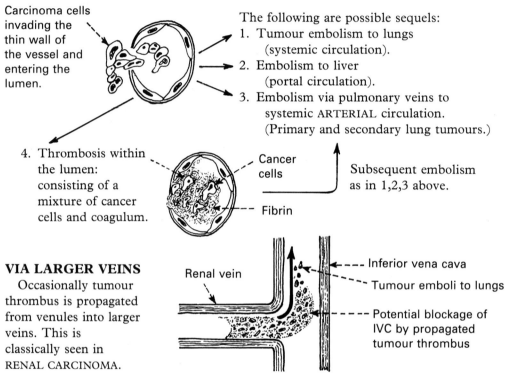

Carcinoma cells invading the thin wall of the vessel and entering the lumen.

The following are possible sequels:
1. Tumour embolism to lungs (systemic circulation).
2. Embolism to liver (portal circulation).
3. Embolism via pulmonary veins to systemic ARTERIAL circulation. (Primary and secondary lung tumours.)

4. Thrombosis within the lumen: consisting of a mixture of cancer cells and coagulum.

Cancer cells

Fibrin

Subsequent embolism as in 1,2,3 above.

VIA LARGER VEINS

Occasionally tumour thrombus is propagated from venules into larger veins. This is classically seen in RENAL CARCINOMA.

Renal vein

Inferior vena cava

Tumour emboli to lungs

Potential blockage of IVC by propagated tumour thrombus

Larger veins may suffer compression effects in 2 ways:

(1) Compression by tumour: vein may ultimately be obliterated.

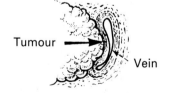

Tumour

Vein

(2) Lumen reduced by growth of fibrous tissue stimulated by the neoplasm.

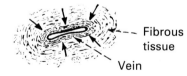

Fibrous tissue

Vein

Rarely, a malignant process may be complicated by thrombosis of distant veins (thrombophlebitis migrans). This is not due to malignant invasion of the veins but is caused by the action of circulating thromboplastins formed by the tumour, or as a result of tissue degeneration.

ARTERIAL SYSTEM

Direct invasion of arteries and arteriolar lumens is very rare because of the physical barrier provided by the thick muscular and elastic walls.

SPREAD OF CARCINOMA

DESTINATION of EMBOLI
This depends on the vessel invaded.

(1) Portal venous system
— emboli pass to liver

(2) Systemic venous system — emboli pass to lungs. There are exceptions (see 'Retrograde Spread' below).

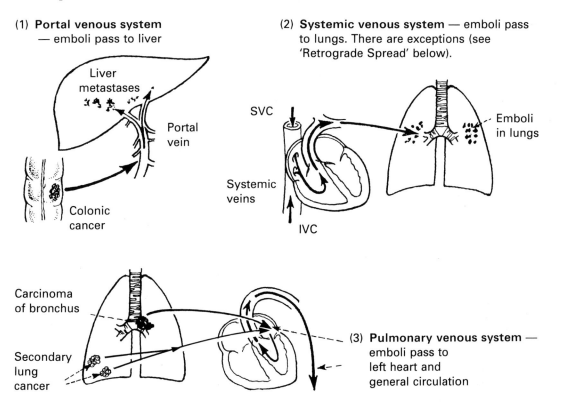

(3) Pulmonary venous system — emboli pass to left heart and general circulation

RETROGRADE VENOUS SPREAD
As in lymphatics, growth of tumour within a vein may cause reversal of blood flow. In addition, reversal of flow is apt to happen in certain areas of the body where veins form a rich plexus and are deficient in valves, e.g. in the pelvis and around vertebrae. Changes in intra-abdominal and intrathoracic pressures easily induce changes in blood flow in these channels. It is for this reason that secondary tumours are relatively common in vertebral bodies.

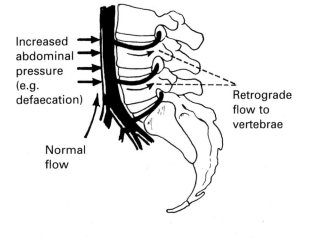

141

SPREAD OF CARCINOMA

FATE of CARCINOMATOUS EMBOLI

SEED and SOIL ANALOGY

The distribution of carcinomatous emboli is determined in part by anatomy, but many complex factors both in the 'seed' (the cancer cell) and the 'soil' (the potential metastatic site) are at play in the establishment of metastases at particular sites. They include surface properties and secretory products of the cancer cells and receptors present in the cells and matrix at the metastatic site. Variation in the host IMMUNE RESPONSE is also important.

The following facts emerge:

1. **Size of embolus**
   Most malignant emboli are tiny and contain few cancer cells. On impaction, the cells commonly die and only an extremely small percentage survive to produce metastases.
2. **Changes at site of embolic impaction**
   The malignant embolus produces the same changes as any embolus and is treated by the tissues in the same way. Thrombus is deposited on the embolus and platelet and leucocyte functions are stimulated.
3. **The organ affected**
   Metastatic tumours are **common** in:
   (a) *Lungs*. This is due to the large number of emboli reaching them in cases of malignancy. Most of the emboli are destroyed but some are bound to survive.
   (b) *Liver*. Malignant emboli seem to find this organ particularly favourable for further growth, possibly due to the high concentration of nutrient material in the portal blood.
   Metastases are **uncommon** in:
   (a) *Spleen*.
   (b) *Actively moving tissues*: muscle, tendon.
4. Cancer cells may remain latent at remote sites (e.g. breast cancer cells in vertebral bone marrow) and commence aggressive growth after months or years.

GRADING AND STAGING OF CANCER

Two important factors in assessing the prognosis in an individual case of cancer are:
   1. The histological appearance indicating the grade of malignancy.
   2. The size and extent of spread of tumour.
Grading and staging are attempts to quantify these factors.

Pathological grading

Because this assessment is subjective, it is usual to assign no more than 3 histological grades: well (Grade I), moderately (Grade II) and poorly differentiated (Grade III).

Clinico-Pathological staging

This is well exemplified in Hodgkin's disease where numerical staging has proved very useful (see p.583).

TNM staging is widely used: T 0–3 indicates local tumour spread, N 0–1 indicates lymph node metastases and M 0–1 distant metastases.

SPREAD OF CARCINOMA

VIA SEROUS SACS

This is an important and frequent route of spread in the peritoneal and pleural cavities. It also takes place in the pericardial sac.

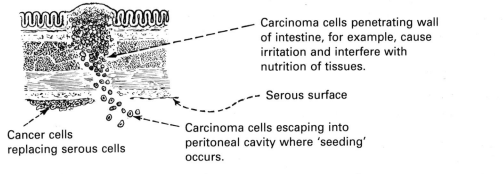

Carcinoma cells penetrating wall of intestine, for example, cause irritation and interfere with nutrition of tissues.

Serous surface

Cancer cells replacing serous cells

Carcinoma cells escaping into peritoneal cavity where 'seeding' occurs.

As malignant cells sink in peritoneal cavity, they will settle in various sites. They cause an inflammatory reaction with fibrin formation. This anchors the cells and also causes adhesions between organs, providing routes for further spread.

An inflammatory reaction can obscure the presence of carcinoma and make diagnosis difficult.

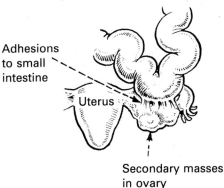

Adhesions to small intestine

Uterus

Secondary masses in ovary

INTRA-EPITHELIAL SPREAD

This form of spread may occur where carcinoma develops in a gland or its duct, e.g. in the breast. Carcinoma cells spread in the areolar skin. (Paget's disease of the nipple.)

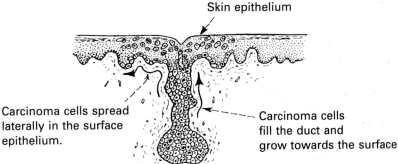

Skin epithelium

Carcinoma cells spread laterally in the surface epithelium.

Carcinoma cells fill the duct and grow towards the surface

143

TYPES OF CARCINOMA

SQUAMOUS CELL CARCINOMA

This is commonly found on the skin, especially exposed surfaces, but also develops in other sites covered by stratified squamous epithelium, *e.g.* lips, tongue, pharynx, oesophagus and vagina. In addition, it may occur on surfaces covered by glandular type epithelium through metaplastic transformation as in the bronchus, gall bladder and uterine cervix.

(1) It starts as a small papular mass

(2) The surface breaks down and a characteristic irregular ulcer is produced.

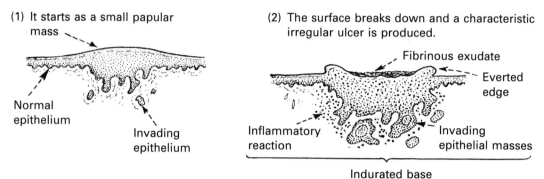

Histologically, it is composed of irregular strands and columns of invading epithelium which infiltrate the subjacent connective tissue. If well differentiated, the central cells of the invading masses show conversion into eosinophilic keratinised squames, while the outer layer consists of young basophilic cells. In cross-section, the appearance is typical.

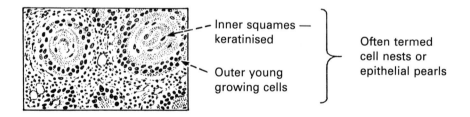

The usual features of malignancy — variation in size and shape of cell accompanied by frequent mitotic activity — are present.

Squamous cell carcinoma of skin is usually cornified and slowly growing. Metastasis to the local lymph nodes tends to occur relatively late.

In tumours arising in mucous membranes, growth is more rapid, cornification is inconspicuous and, due to the rich lymphatic drainage, metastasis to lymph nodes occurs early.

TYPES OF CARCINOMA

BASAL CELL CARCINOMA (Rodent ulcer)

This tumour may arise in any part of the skin but is most common in the face, near the eyes and nose.

First stage
It starts as a flattened papilloma which slowly enlarges over months or perhaps a year or two.

Second stage
The surface breaks down and a shallow, ragged ulcer with pearly edges is formed.

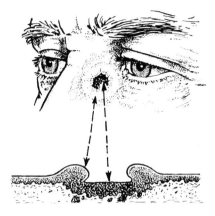

Usually the malignant tissue spreads slowly but progressively, mainly in a lateral direction. It is composed of cells resembling those of the basal layer of the skin from which it takes origin and has a characteristic histological appearance.

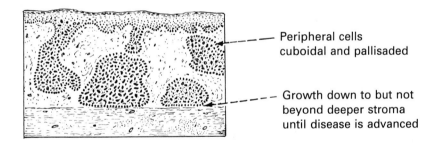

Peripheral cells cuboidal and pallisaded

Growth down to but not beyond deeper stroma until disease is advanced

Sometimes it takes origin from basal cells of skin appendages and may show pseudoglandular structures: melanin deposition occurs in some tumours.

It is a locally invasive growth which almost never metastasises, but nevertheless may be very destructive.

TYPES OF CARCINOMA

CARCINOMA of GLANDULAR ORGANS

These may take origin from gland acini, ducts or the glandular epithelium of mucous surfaces. The anatomical structure varies.

(A) On mucous surfaces they may start as a polypoid growth or as a thick plaque. e.g. Carcinoma of colon

Ulceration with the formation of an irregular crater follows.

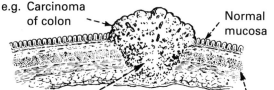
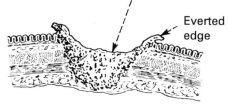

Normal mucosa

Everted edge

Invading carcinoma   Muscular coats

(B) In compound glands, e.g. the breast, the cancer forms an irregular penetrating mass — the typical crab-like appearance.

(C) Some malignant tumours are cystic. Quite commonly the malignant growth originates in a pre-existing benign cyst. This is more likely to occur when there are papillomatous structures within the cyst.

Histologically, carcinomas of glandular tissue have three basic forms.

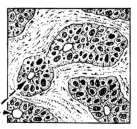

(1) Adenocarcinoma. In this form the growth shows a varying degree of differentiation with attempts at acinus formation.

(2) The carcinoma may be undifferentiated and take the form of solid masses or columns of pleomorphic cells.

(3) Occasionally a carcinoma will produce large quantities of mucus and merit the term mucoid carcinoma. The tumour alveoli may be filled with mucus in which only a few carcinoma cells persist, the cells appearing to dissolve in the mucus. They are commonest in organs normally containing large numbers of mucus-secreting cells, e.g. large intestine, stomach, etc.

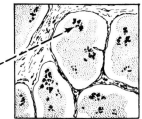

MALIGNANT CONNECTIVE TISSUE TUMOURS

These tumours are grouped under the descriptive term **SARCOMA**, from the Greek *sarkoma* meaning 'flesh'.

Sarcomas are less common than carcinomas. Next to leukaemia, they are the most common malignant tumours in children and young adults. In older age groups, 90% of malignant tumours are carcinomas.

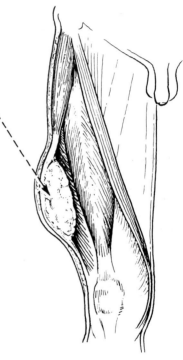

Unlike the sinuous infiltrating carcinoma, sarcomas are large fleshy tumours. Arising from and within connective tissues means that infiltration between normal cells is not a feature. The malignant cells advance on a broad front destroying and replacing normal cells. The result is a rounded growth with fairly definite margins.

On naked eye assessment these appearances give a false impression and surgical 'shelling out' procedures are almost inevitably followed by local recurrence due to microscopic aggregates of malignant cells remaining in the tumour bed.

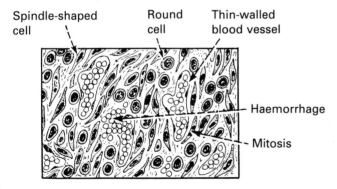

The neoplastic process is associated with the formation of many large, new, thin-walled blood vessels. As a result, haemorrhage and necrosis are frequent in sarcomas.

Metastatic spread

Sarcoma cells, like all connective tissue cells, are strongly motile. They easily invade the venules and early lung metastases are common.

MALIGNANT CONNECTIVE TISSUE TUMOURS

FIBROSARCOMAS

These arise most commonly from fascia, intermuscular septa, subcutaneous tissue and sometimes periosteum. As usual, cellular differentiation varies with the degree of malignancy.

Malignant Fibrous Histiocytoma (MFH) is the most common soft tissue sarcoma: it occurs in the limbs and retroperitoneal tissues. It is a rapidly growing aggressive tumour with a poor prognosis.

The histological appearances are variable and include:

Large multinucleated tumour cells ------

Spindle cells ------

Foamy histiocytes (reactive) ------

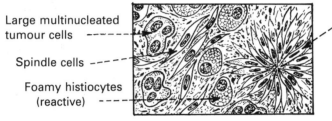

A 'storiform' arrangement of spindle cells — mimicking the spokes of a wheel — is an important diagnostic feature.

Spindle cell sarcoma

The cells are fairly uniform and resemble fibroblasts. Intercellular matrix varies in quantity. Considerable collagen may be formed and the term fibrosarcoma may be applied.

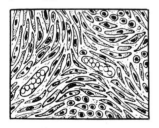

Pleomorphic or anaplastic sarcoma

Such tumours bear little resemblance to connective tissue. They are highly malignant. The commonest sites are the bones and perimysial connective tissue.

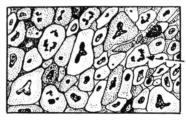

Bizarre cells ← --- and nuclei

Irregular mitotic figures

Absence of matrix

These are convenient morphological compartments which are further delineated by special marking techniques which indicate the possible line of differentiation or type cell of origin.

SARCOMAS arising from or differentiating towards specialised connective tissues.

These are malignant counterparts of benign mesenchymal tumours and produce a few of the features of the tissues from which they have arisen. Generally this is patchy and incomplete and is little indication of the malignancy of the growth.

MALIGNANT CONNECTIVE TISSUE TUMOURS

OSTEOGENIC SARCOMAS

Most of these tumours occur in patients between 10 and 25 years of age. Occasionally it may complicate Paget's disease in the elderly.

They affect the metaphysial ends of long bones, especially the upper end of the tibia, lower end of the femur and upper end of the humerus.

The tumour may be endosteal in origin when it is usually solid and relatively hard. In other cases, it may arise from the periosteum and frequently presents a characteristic fir-tree appearance on X-ray due to spicules of bone radiating at right angles from the shaft.

It is a highly malignant tumour producing metastases at a relatively early stage.

Histologically they show irregular spicules of calcified bone and osteoid tissue among masses of pleomorphic cells.

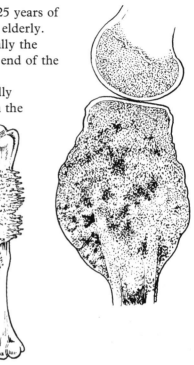

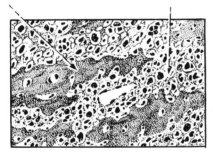

Many tumours show several forms of matrix — fibrous, cartilagenous, osseous and myxomatous.

GIANT CELL TUMOUR OF BONE (Osteoclastoma)

This is a tumour found at the extremities of long bones. It consists of multinucleated osteoclasts and spindle cells.

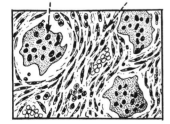

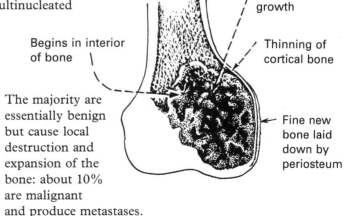

Haemorrhagic growth

Begins in interior of bone

Thinning of cortical bone

The majority are essentially benign but cause local destruction and expansion of the bone: about 10% are malignant and produce metastases.

Fine new bone laid down by periosteum

149

MALIGNANT CONNECTIVE TISSUE TUMOURS

CHONDROSARCOMA

This tumour occurs in older age groups arising usually at the proximal ends of long bones of the pelvis. The majority are slowly growing and of low-grade malignancy: they cause difficulty in histological assessment. The diagram shows a high-grade tumour where the malignant cellular characteristics are obvious.

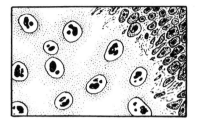

LIPOSARCOMA

This is an uncommon tumour. It may arise in connection with simple lipoma. Like ordinary adipose tissue, it is lobulated.

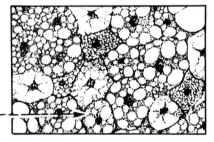

Pleomorphic cells with — — coarse emulsion of lipid

MYOSARCOMA

There are two varieties:

1. **Leiomyosarcoma**
   These rare tumours arise in the skin, deep soft tissues, the stomach and particularly in the uterus from pre-existing myomas.

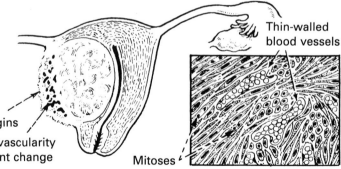

Thin-walled blood vessels

Indefinite margins

Increased vascularity at malignant change

Mitoses

2. **Rhabdomyosarcoma**
   This is a rare tumour occurring mainly in children. They occur very rarely in skeletal muscles. More common but still rare are polypoid tumours in the bladder, uterus and vagina, sometimes called sarcoma — — — — > botryoides.

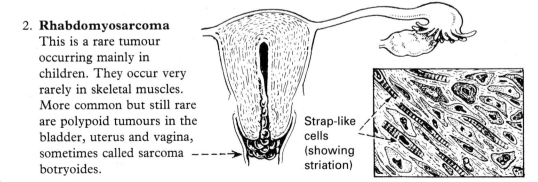

Strap-like cells (showing striation)

SPECIAL TUMOURS

MIXED TUMOURS

These are tumours which appear to be composed of both epithelial and connective tissue cells. The commonest example is the mixed parotid tumour.

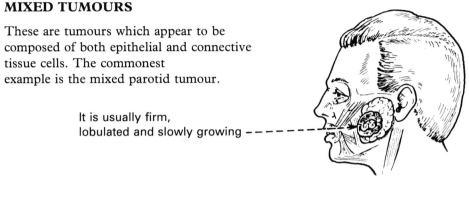

It is usually firm, lobulated and slowly growing – – – – – – –

The histology is complex and variable.

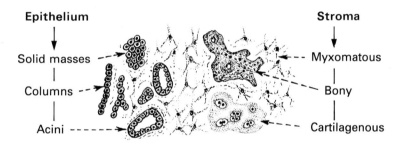

Epithelium

Solid masses

Columns

Acini

Stroma

Myxomatous

Bony

Cartilagenous

It is now considered that both stroma and epithelium are derived from a single cell type, the stroma being a manifestation of metaplasia.

Malignant tumours also occur which appear to be a combination of carcinoma and sarcoma. In almost all cases, the sarcomatous element is merely a very anaplastic area of the carcinoma.

TERATOMA

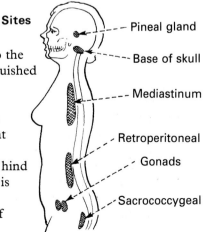

Sites
— Pineal gland
— Base of skull
— Mediastinum
— Retroperitoneal
— Gonads
— Sacrococcygeal

This is a tumour composed of multiple tissues foreign to the site of growth. It is a true neoplasm and must be distinguished from developmental anomalies in which tissues may be displaced.

Teratomas arise in the gonads or in the midline of the body. It is now considered that they arise from totipotent germ cells. In the embryo, these appear in the mid-line beneath the coelomic epithelium, in association with the hind gut. Normally they migrate to the gonadal ridges, but it is thought that some fail to reach the gonads and remain distributed along the mid-line. The most common site of teratoma is in the ovaries.

151

SPECIAL TUMOURS

TERATOMA (continued)
Two main types are described: benign cystic and solid teratoma.

1. Benign cystic teratoma
This consist mainly of ectodermal structures such as skin and its appendages and neural tissue. Frequently respiratory epithelium, intestinal epithelium, bone and cartilage are present.

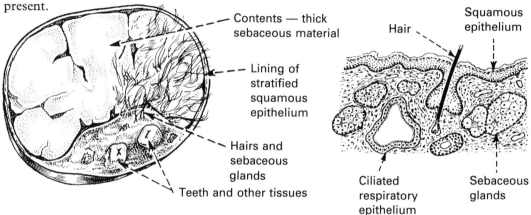

Contents — thick sebaceous material

Lining of stratified squamous epithelium

Hairs and sebaceous glands

Teeth and other tissues

Hair

Squamous epithelium

Ciliated respiratory epithelium

Sebaceous glands

2. Solid teratoma
This tumour is most commonly found in children and is frequently highly malignant. Embryonic, fetal and adult tissues of all types may be found. The malignant tumour may consist of a mixture of immature tissues, but one particular tissue may undergo malignant change and over-run the others.

HAMARTOMA
A hamartoma is a tumour-like but non-neoplastic malformation consisting of a mixture of tissues normally found at the particular site.

The commonest forms of hamartoma are those composed of blood vessels and those involving pigment cells of the skin.

HAEMANGIOMA
Two main varieties exist:

1. Capillary angioma
These are common in the skin as 'birth-marks' which vary in size. Occasionally they may be found in internal organs. They are well defined, deep red or purple. A single artery provides a supply separate from the surrounding tissue.

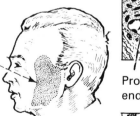

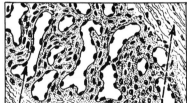

Prominent endothelial cells

Well formed collagen

2. Cavernous angioma
This type is confined to internal organs and quite often found in the liver. Like the capillary variety they are well defined and deep purple. Similar tumours are found involving the lymphatic system but less commonly.

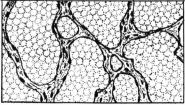

SPECIAL TUMOURS

BENIGN PIGMENTED NAEVUS or LENTIGO (Melanotic naevus or mole)

This is a common congenital lesion, hence the term 'naevus', meaning a 'birth mark'.

During fetal life melanin-pigment-forming neuroectodermal cells migrate to the skin and are found in small numbers in the basal layer of the skin.

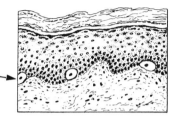

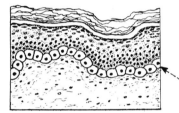

The common congenital pigmented mole or lentigo is the result of an abnormality in migration, proliferation and maturation of these neuroectodermal cells. A continuous layer of pigmented cells is found adjacent to the basal epidermal cells.

The resulting naevi vary in size and appearance, varying from small flat macular brown areas or smooth papular lesions to warty hairy excrescences. Pigmentation is variable.

Sometimes proliferation of the 'naevus' cells is a striking feature and this varies in degree and extent:

Junctional naevus
In this case proliferation is local and confined to the dermoepidermal junction

Compound naevus
Proliferation is found in the dermis as well as the junctional area.

Intradermal naevus
Proliferation is wholly in the dermis.

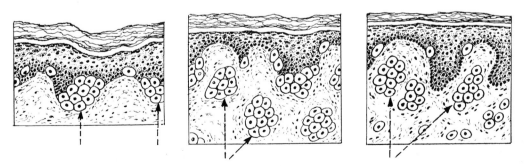

SPECIAL TUMOURS

BENIGN PIGMENTED NAEVUS (continued)

Another variation is the 'blue' naevus. Melanocytes are arrested in migration in the dermis.

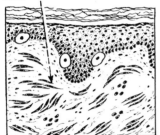

Active proliferative activity may extend into adult life, but the great majority of these lesions undergo a degree of involution. One feature which differentiates them from the malignant change is that the deeper the cells penetrate the dermis the smaller they become and the less active.

Continuing active junctional change is said to potentiate malignant change, but this transformation is very rare.

Hamartomas are also found involving the peripheral nerves — neurofibromatosis and its variants — the intestinal tract, congenital polypi, and in many other organs. Tuberous sclerosis is a condition in which hamartomas are found in many of the organs. Osteomas, enchondromas and lipomas are considered by many as hamartomas.

Although hamartomas are not neoplastic, true tumour growth may develop from a hamartoma.

Hamartoma	True neoplasm
Developmental abnormality.	New growth.
Present and often visible at birth.	Most occur in adults.
Enlargement continues until physiological growth ceases (i.e. on reaching adulthood).	Growth is progressive, autonomous and not related to stages of body development.
Condition is essentially benign.	May be malignant.

It will be appreciated that the borderline between hamartoma and some types of benign neoplasm is ill-defined and the distinction is often not of practical importance.

SPECIAL TUMOURS

MALIGNANT MELANOMA

Malignant proliferation of melanocytes usually arises de novo. The aetiology is unknown, but excessive exposure of white skin to sunlight is important. The exposure may be:

1. *Chronic* — over many years — especially relevant in the elderly.
2. *Acute* — causing burning. This may be important in the young.

Sites

1. Skin of (a) face, soles of feet, palms of hands, nail beds,
       (b) legs (women) and (c) trunk (in men).
2. Mucous membranes of mouth, arms and genitalia — rare.
3. Eye and meninges — rare.

Some growths are amelanotic (non-pigmented). The rate of growth is variable.

Four types of growth may occur:

1. *Lentigo maligna* — an 'in situ' lesion occurring on the face of the elderly. It may spread at one angle and regress at another.

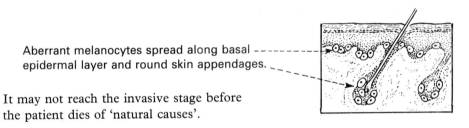

Aberrant melanocytes spread along basal epidermal layer and round skin appendages.

It may not reach the invasive stage before the patient dies of 'natural causes'.

2. *Superficial spreading melanoma* — occurs on female leg, male trunk. It accounts for 50% of all skin melanomas in northern countries.
3. *Acral lentiginous melanoma* — found on palms of hands, soles of feet and mucous membranes.
4. *Nodular malignant melanoma* — usually on trunk. It invades early and ulceration is common.

Types 2, 3 and 4 occur in younger adults, and both 2 and 3 have an in situ stage.

The essential features of malignant melanoma are:

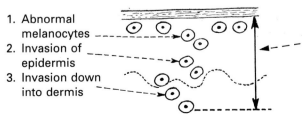

1. Abnormal melanocytes
2. Invasion of epidermis
3. Invasion down into dermis

Two-thirds are cured by excision.

The prognosis depends on depth of invasion, measured as follows:

1.5 mm or less — good prognosis
1.5–3 mm — fair prognosis
3 mm — poor prognosis.

155

CARCINOGENESIS

The ultimate mechanisms which cause cancer, i.e. allow cells to proliferate continuously, break through normal bounds and invade other tissues remain unknown.

There are, however, three classes of agent which will induce cell proliferation and are associated with tumour formation: 1. **Chemical carcinogens**, 2. **Radiant energy** and 3. **Viruses**.

Many of the changes within the cell prior to complete malignant transformation are known.

The first changes are mutations in the nuclear DNA (see p.158 et seq.) of proliferating cells followed by progressive multiple disturbances of the effector and suppressor mechanisms controlling cell proliferation, adhesion and mobility.

CHEMICAL CARCINOGENS

Historically, chemical agents were the first to be associated with cancer; nowadays many chemical carcinogens are known and their number is continuously increasing associated with (a) industrial process and changes in (b) diet and (c) social habits.

Industry	Tumour	Chemical responsible
Aniline Dyes	Bladder cancer	Naphthylamine
Mineral Oil and tar	Skin cancers	Benzpyrene and other hydrocarbons
Plastics	Angiosarcoma of Liver	Vinyl chloride monomer
Insulation	Mesothelioma	Asbestos (carcinogenic activity depends on the **physical** configuration of the fibres)

Diet

It is possible that chemicals in food are carcinogenic. Nitrosamines and aflotoxins are examples; some modern synthetic additives and flavourings are potential carcinogens.

Social habits

The increasing urban concentration of population increases exposure to the combustion products of organic compounds, some of which are carcinogenic, and smoking and chewing of tobacco are associated with cancers of the lung and mouth.

Note: Chemical carcinogens may act in two ways:
1. Directly at the site of application or portal of entry, e.g. skin and lung cancers
2. Through degradation products either at the sites of metabolism or excretion, e.g. liver and urinary tract tumours.

CARCINOGENESIS

CHEMICAL CARCINOGENESIS (continued)

This is a multistep process of long duration.

The stages of **initiation** and **promotion** are important and are exemplified in experimental skin carcinogenesis.

(1) **Normal skin**

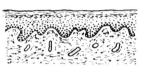

Application
of
Benzpyrene
(carcinogen) ⟶

(2) **INITIATION**
Skin appears normal
but important changes
have occurred in the
cell nuclear DNA

(3) **PROMOTION** — initiated by e.g. croton oil, turpentine (co-carcinogens).

Visible surface and histological changes are seen.

(a) Keratosis and papilloma
    formation

(b) Dysplasia

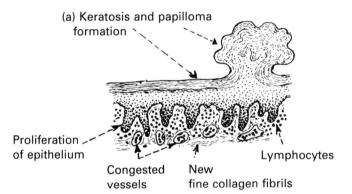

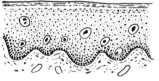

Proliferation
of epithelium

Congested
vessels

New
fine collagen fibrils

Lymphocytes

These stages are reversible

(4) **Appearance of MALIGNANT TUMOUR** — [An irreversible change]

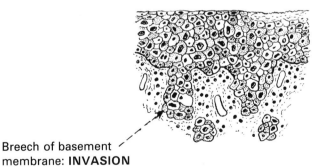

Breech of basement
membrane: **INVASION**

In rodents these changes take months; in humans the time scale is years and is exemplified in the skin, cervix uteri, bronchus, urinary bladder, colon and breast.

CARCINOGENESIS

RADIANT ENERGY
The dangers from this source have increased greatly in recent years.

Source of radiation	Possible tumours	Type of radiant energy
X-ray workers	Skin cancer, leukaemia	X-rays (ionising)
Administration of radioisotopes (therapeutic)	Various, e.g. thyroid carcinoma due to radioactive iodine	Atomic rays (ionising)
Industrial processes involving radioactive substances	Various	Atomic rays (ionising)
Atomic explosions	Skin cancer, leukaemia, bone cancer	Atomic rays (ionising)
Mining of radioactive substances	Lung cancer	Atomic rays (ionising)
Exposure to sunlight	Skin cancer	Ultraviolet rays (non-ionising)

Effects of radiations on cells

The ionising activity of X-rays and atomic radiations produce many changes in the nuclear DNA ranging from single gene mutation to gross chromosomal damage.

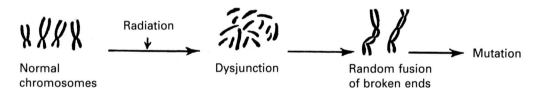

Normal chromosomes — Radiation → Dysjunction → Random fusion of broken ends → Mutation

Proliferating cells are particularly vulnerable.
New clones of mutant cells arise which may produce tumour growth.

ONCOGENIC VIRUSES
Viruses have long been known to cause cancer in animals, and for several years a few human malignancies have been associated with specific viruses.

Recently the role of retroviruses in carcinogenesis has revealed new important intracellular mechanisms leading to malignant transformation.

In addition, vaccines have been manufactured against these viruses and have proved successful in the prevention of leukaemia in ANIMALS.

CARCINOGENESIS — VIRUSES

In *animals*: Examples of viruses associated with tumours are:

Virus	Type	Host	Tumour
Shope papilloma V.	DNA	Rabbits	Skin papilloma
Polyoma V.	DNA	Rodents Hamsters	Sarcoma
Rous sarcoma V.	RNA (acute)	Chickens	Sarcoma
Onco-retroviruses	RNA (slow)	Cats Chickens, etc.	Leukaemias and lymphomas

The **mouse mammary tumour virus** (Bittner milk factor) — an onco-RNA virus — is of interest; it is transmitted to offspring during suckling and results in breast cancer

Effect of Suckling

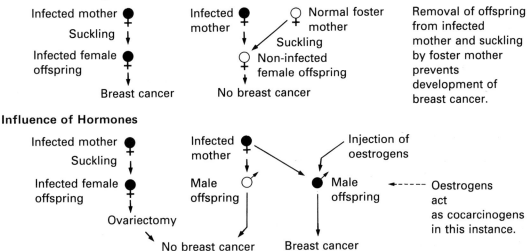

Influence of Hormones

Comment: The development of breast cancer has been shown to be the result of the passage of the virus from the mother to the offspring. However, in addition to hormone status (illustrated above), age and the strain of mouse are other important co-factors determining the development of breast cancer.

N.B. There is no clear evidence linking a milk factor with human breast cancer.

In *humans*:

Human papilloma virus (HPV)	DNA	Human	Skin papilloma Cervical cancer
Herpes group Epstein-Barr v (EBV)	DNA	Human	Burkitt's lymphoma Naso-pharyngeal Ca.
Hepatitis B	DNA	Human	Liver cancer
Onco-retrovirus group Human T cell leukaemia virus (HTLV)	RNA (slow)	Human	Leukaemia and lymphoma

CARCINOGENESIS — VIRUSES

Mode of action on oncogenic viruses

The essential feature is addition of new DNA to the nucleus of host cells resulting in mutants, but the way in which this is achieved differs in the two types of virus.

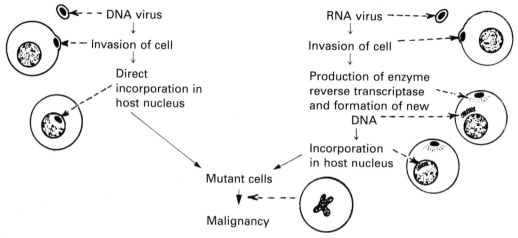

Oncogenes

The normal human cell nucleus contains genes — proto-oncogenes or cell oncogenes (c-onc) — which code for several important cellular activities. The oncogenic retroviruses contain genes (v-onc) which are homologous to the proto-oncogenes.

Oncogenic viruses either replace or alter the human cell oncogenes in such a way that they code for malignant transformation. Examples are:

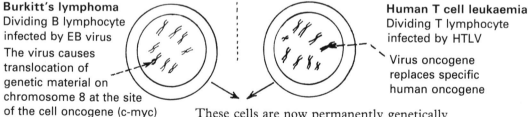

Burkitt's lymphoma
Dividing B lymphocyte infected by EB virus
The virus causes translocation of genetic material on chromosome 8 at the site of the cell oncogene (c-myc) which is altered.

Human T cell leukaemia
Dividing T lymphocyte infected by HTLV

Virus oncogene replaces specific human oncogene

These cells are now permanently genetically altered and programmed for malignancy

Several important cellular activities normally controlled by proto-oncogenes may become seriously abnormal: (1) DNA replication, (2) control of gene expression, (3) the production of growth factors, (4) production of enzymes, particularly phosphorylases.

The resulting in-coordination and deregulation cause marked disturbance of cell metabolism.

There is a progressive build up of intracellular abnormalities until malignant transformation occurs in one cell.

Anti-oncogenes (tumour suppressor genes)

Another factor is the loss or defective functioning of these genes which are involved in normal cellular differentiation and inhibit the 'proliferative' activities of the proto-oncogenes. Disorder of the anti-oncogene p53 is present in at least half of all human cancers.

CARCINOGENESIS

CO-FACTORS in CARCINOGENESIS

Heredity.   The genetic influence is now widely recognised.

(1) However, in only a few instances is there a strong or inevitable link between a hereditary genetic abnormality and the development of cancer.
Illustrative examples are:

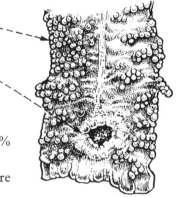

    (a) ***Polyposis coli***, an excellent example, is a familial condition in which numerous polypi appear in the large intestine about the age of 20 and inevitably lead to adenocarcinoma (abnormality of chromosome 5).

    (b) ***Xeroderma pigmentosum***, in which there is excessive sensitivity to sunlight, is another hereditary condition which leads to skin malignancy.

    (c) ***Neurofibromatosis*** (multiple tumours of nerves) (1% sarcomatous change: defect on chromosome 17).

    (d) ***Retinoblastoma*** (abnormality of chromosome 13) are conditions which have a familial incidence.

(2) In most tumours the genetic abnormality, either inherited or acquired, is only one of many factors conditioning a cell towards malignancy (see p.163).

Race.   The white races appear to be more susceptible to skin cancers due to lack of pigment which protects against ultra-violet radiations. Far Eastern, possibly mongol races, have an extremely high incidence of choriocarcinoma and lymphoepithelioma. Not all 'racial' incidences are genetically determined: local environmental factors are often operative.

Geography.   There is undoubtedly a variation in the incidence of various cancers in different parts of the world. This is mainly a result of human activities — industrial processes, pollution, diet and social habits. In a few instances it may be related to natural background radiation in the soil, or parasites.

Age.   Most cancers arise in later adult life. Throughout life, abnormal mutant cells are produced during cell proliferation and these are destroyed.

In later life, as control mechanisms break down, (a) the recognition and destruction of mutant cells is less active and (b) more mutant cells are produced and the chances of a malignant mutant arising are much increased.

Hormones.   In the female, the rate of growth of cancer of the breast and cancer of the uterine endometrium often appears to be dependent upon hormone secretion, usually oestrogen. Similarly in the male prostate, cancer is stimulated by testosterone and depressed by oestrogen. There is however no real evidence that hormones of themselves cause cancer.

Chronic irritation.   This is rarely involved per se in carcinogenesis. Its role as a co-factor probably depends on the increased replication rate of damaged tissues being associated with an increased prevalence of random mutations.

Trauma.   Malignant tumours are sometimes discovered after trauma but it is likely that trauma merely draws attention to a pre-existing malignant condition.

CARCINOGENESIS

CLONES and MALIGNANCY

A clone is a cell line derived from a single cell whose unique identifying characteristics are, by definition, passed to the daughter cells.

Monoclonal tumours

Certain tumours are composed of cells remarkably uniform in form and behaviour. In a few it can be shown by special methods that all of the cells are identical. A good example is plasma cell myeloma which produces multiple tumours of bone marrow.
Plasma cells produce immunoglobulins, each cell producing one type of immunoglobulin.
Using light chain markers it can be shown that a plasma cell myeloma is derived from a single cell — a monoclonal tumour.

Plasma Cell Myeloma

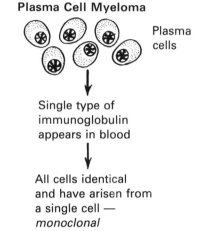

Plasma cells

Single type of immunoglobulin appears in blood

All cells identical and have arisen from a single cell — *monoclonal*

Monoclonal/multiple clone tumours

Although most tumours show a variation in cell type, and the more malignant the tumour the greater the variation is likely to be, there is very strong evidence that they always arise from the proliferation of a single transformed cell, i.e. they are monoclonal in origin. During subsequent tumour growth mutations account for the cellular heterogeneity. This explains why most cancers arise as a single focal lesion.

Evolution of cancer

(1) Precancerous state
   e.g. dysplasia

(2)

(3) Carcinoma

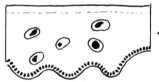 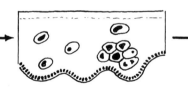 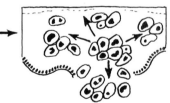

Several cells show abnormality

One cell undergoes malignant transformation
i.e. monoclonal proliferation.

Non-malignant neighbouring cells replaced.
Further mutation
↓
Cells heterogeneous, malignant properties enhanced.

Field change
In a tissue or organ such as the skin and breast, precancerous cells may be present over a wide area. The chances of subsequent single cell transformation to malignancy are increased with the formation of separate tumour(s). Such a concept is important in surgical practice where the limits of excision should be wider than the field change.

CARCINOGENESIS — SUMMARY

A multitude of factors determine whether a proliferative lesion will progress to frank malignancy. Malignant change can be viewed as taking place by a series of steps — the *'multi-step theory of carcinogenesis'*. At each step, according to circumstances, the process can halt and may revert to normal or it may progress.

Four stages can be recognised:

1. Stage of INITIATION

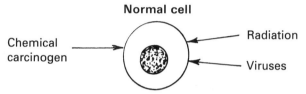

Two changes are involved at this stage.

(a) *Biochemical*

The 'carcinogenic' stimuli are converted into biochemically active substances.

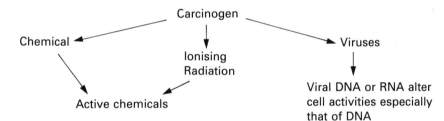

(b) *Interaction with cell components especially DNA*

The activated substances are positively charged molecules reacting vigorously with electrons, especially those in DNA. A variety of products are produced — altered forms of DNA. Some of these will revert to normal, but if others persist, they will be handed on to daughter cells thus forming new clones of cells with new potentialities. Viral genes are incorporated in the nuclei of cells.

An important mechanism by which these various nuclear changes may be unified is the production of abnormal oncogenic activity or the suppression of anti-oncogenes. The proliferative and control mechanisms within the cell are progressively seriously disturbed.

2. LATENT stage

These initiated cells are not yet autonomous and are still subject to normal controls. This accounts for the varying period between exposure to a carcinogen and neoplastic activity.

163

CARCINOGENESIS — SUMMARY

3. Stage of PROMOTION

The initiated cells may be 'promoted' by many substances. Promoters (co-carcinogens) exert a selective stimulation on initiated cells.

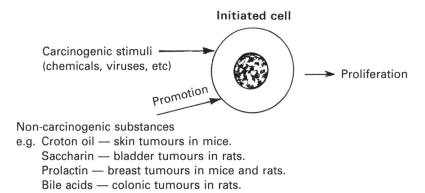

Non-carcinogenic substances
e.g. Croton oil — skin tumours in mice.
Saccharin — bladder tumours in rats.
Prolactin — breast tumours in mice and rats.
Bile acids — colonic tumours in rats.

In this phase there are often multiple areas of proliferation in a tissue or organ, but these lesions are focal and not yet malignant.

4. MALIGNANT CHANGES

Two possibilities exist at this point.

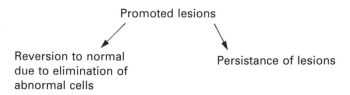

The vast majority of such lesions disappear due to defence mechanisms, particularly within the cells and also an immune response.

In some of the lesions which persist, foci of morphologically altered cells ultimately appear. The changes are described in terms such as a typical hyperplasia, dysplasia and carcinoma-in-situ and are due to progressive nuclear disturbance. Reversal to normal is still possible, presumably by the elimination of the abnormal cells.

Other factors are involved in the final step — the conversion of a single cell to the malignant state.

Note: (a) During carcinogenesis many abnormal cells are eliminated by the very efficient normal control mechanisms.
(b) It is not known exactly what changes are required to complete malignant transformation.

IMMUNOLOGY AND CANCER

It has been thought for a very long time that cancers stimulate immunological reactions. This is suggested by the following clinical observations:

(a) Some cancers do regress

(b) Secondary tumours are relatively rare in the spleen, presumably due to the ability of the spleen to destroy abnormal cells in the circulation

(c) In some tumours a lymphocyte response in the malignant tissue may be associated with a more favourable prognosis,

e.g. some cases of carcinoma of breast.

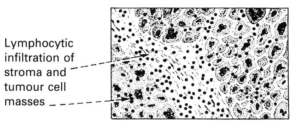

Lymphocytic infiltration of stroma and tumour cell masses

Experimental investigations

Immunity to cancers can be induced in animals by the same methods as those used to immunise against infection. These methods include:

1. Injection of very small doses of tumour cells — too small to cause the development of neoplasm

2. Injection of tumour cells made inactive by irradiation or chemotherapy

3. Injection of parts of malignant cells especially cell membranes.

These are all forms of vaccination, but they only tend to be effective if given prior to implanting the tumour as a graft.

In the case of tumours induced by viruses, however, a vaccine of the virus can sometimes protect the animal, e.g. feline leukaemia.

IMMUNOLOGY AND CANCER

Both humoral and cell-mediated immunity can be demonstrated in ANIMALS bearing tumours. Three features are of interest:

1. Antibodies have a protective role only when the tumour cells are in a fluid medium, e.g. leukaemic cells in the blood or tumour cells in body cavities.
2. In solid cancers, only cell-mediated (lymphocytes) immunity is effective.
3. Reaction is strongest in small tumours and disappears when they enlarge.

An interesting feature has been noted in experimental carcinogenesis: a virus may produce several different types of tumour, and vaccine of the cells of one tumour will induce protection against all other tumours produced by the same virus.

A chemical carcinogen can also produce several different types of tumour but immunity to one does not confer protection against another. Each tumour has its own specific antigens.

Immunological studies in man

The circumstances in man have similarities to those in animals.

(1) Antibodies and specific cell-mediated immunity have been demonstrated in patients with cancer.
(2) There is a higher incidence of cancers in patients with immune deficiency status e.g. AIDS.
(3) Therapeutic implications:
   (a) Some forms of cancer therapy attempt to evoke or enhance immune reactions against the cancer cells.
   (b) Attempts are being made to kill cancer cells specifically by linking cell poisons to specific monoclonal antibodies to the cancer cells.

Antigens as tumour markers

(a) Alpha feto-protein. Serum concentrations are much increased in cases of hepatic cancer and certain germ cell tumours of the gonads.
(b) Carcinoembryonic antigen. This is found in cases of cancer of intestinal and urinary tracts.

Neither of these is truly specific: they are products of normal genes and are found in other tumours and in hepatitis, but the high concentration together with local signs may make them useful in diagnosis, and they are important in monitoring progress.

Histological markers

Monoclonal antibodies to a great variety of tumour cell membranes and products are used extensively in histo-pathology to improve the accuracy of cancer diagnosis.

Other serological markers

These are substances formed by tumours and can be used as diagnostic markers and treatment monitors, for example:

Acid phosphatase is secreted by prostatic cancers.
5-hydroxytryptamine is produced by carcinoids.
Catecholamines appear in the blood and urine in phaeochromocytoma.

CIRCULATORY DISTURBANCES

THROMBOSIS

A thrombus is a mass formed from the blood constituents within a vessel or the heart during life.

MECHANISM OF FORMATION

Platelets adhere to the endothelium and to each other, forming a projecting mass.

(1)

The liberation of **thromboplastin** initiates a "chemical cascade" leading to coagulation.

Release of thromboplastins

↓

Thrombin formation

+

Fibrinogen

↓

Fibrin strands

If the rate of flow is slow, as in a vein, red cells are entangled so that the lumen is occluded.

(2)

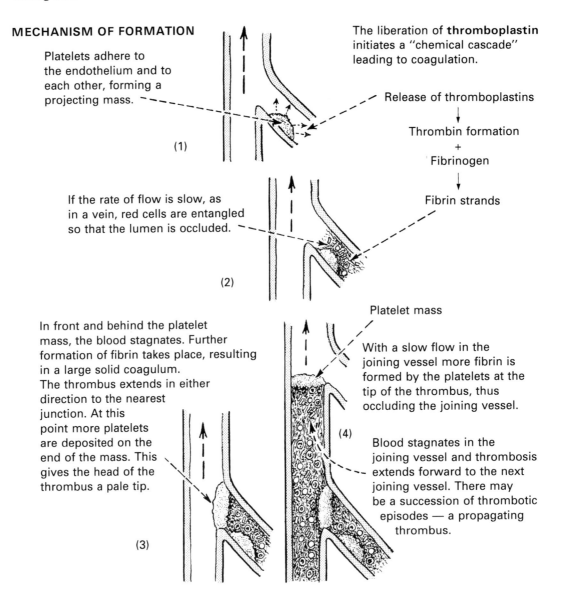

Platelet mass

In front and behind the platelet mass, the blood stagnates. Further formation of fibrin takes place, resulting in a large solid coagulum. The thrombus extends in either direction to the nearest junction. At this point more platelets are deposited on the end of the mass. This gives the head of the thrombus a pale tip.

(3)

With a slow flow in the joining vessel more fibrin is formed by the platelets at the tip of the thrombus, thus occluding the joining vessel.

(4)

Blood stagnates in the joining vessel and thrombosis extends forward to the next joining vessel. There may be a succession of thrombotic episodes — a propagating thrombus.

FACTORS LEADING TO THROMBOSIS

There are 3 MAIN factors leading to thrombosis: they are closely concerned with local changes in the coagulability of the blood (see pp. 548 et seq.).

1. ALTERATIONS OF BLOOD FLOW

The main effect is to bring platelets into contact with the vessel wall. This results from:
Slowing of blood flow, e.g. in cardiac failure or during bed rest. With slowing, the normal axial stream of blood cells is lost and white cells and platelets fall out of the main stream and accumulate in the peripheral plasma zone.

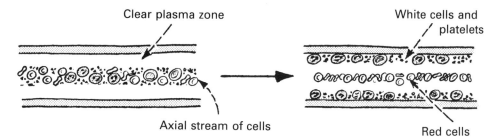

Clear plasma zone

White cells and platelets

Axial stream of cells

Red cells

Turbulence, e.g. by deformation of vessel wall or around venous valves.

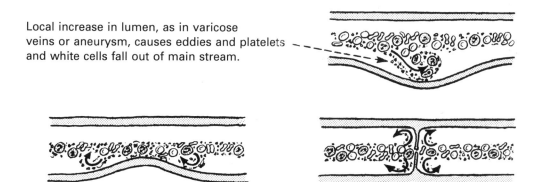

Local increase in lumen, as in varicose veins or aneurysm, causes eddies and platelets and white cells fall out of main stream.

Swelling or compression of vessel wall by disease. Eddies form in front and behind obstruction.

Eddies form around valves if flow slows.

FACTORS LEADING TO THROMBOSIS

2. DAMAGE TO ENDOTHELIUM OF VESSEL

This leads to platelet adhesion and aggregation. Common causes are:

(a) Disease in vessel wall e.g. atheroma.

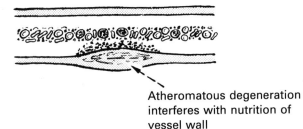

Atheromatous degeneration
interferes with nutrition of
vessel wall

(b) Toxins from nearby inflammatory processes.
(c) Local compression of vessels (e.g. during operation).

3. CHANGES IN THE COMPOSITION OF THE BLOOD

(a) **Increase in platelets, fibrinogen and prothrombin**, e.g. after operations and childbirth.

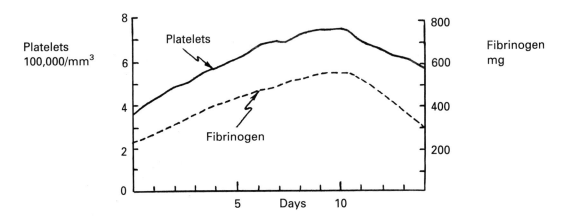

(b) **Change in platelet adhesiveness** — This increases after operations and childbirth and is most marked around the 10th day, at the same time as the other changes reach a peak.

MISCELLANEOUS AETIOLOGICAL FACTORS

These include smoking, oestrogen contraception, obesity and increased blood coagulability associated with some diseases e.g. certain cancers and systemic lupus erythematosus.

VARIETIES OF THROMBOSIS

The following types are recognised:

WHITE
Composed mainly of platelets, they occur chiefly
where the circulation is rapid, e.g. in arteries.
They tend to be non-occlusive (mural).

RED
In this case the thrombus, starting as a small
aggregate of platelets, produces fibrin strands
entangling the blood cells.

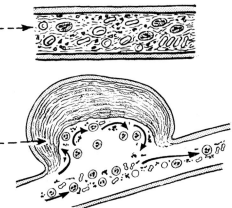

MIXED OR LAMINATED
This type of thrombus consists of alternate layers
of red and white thrombi. Commonly found in
aneurysms.

Red thrombi are the commonest type and have to be distinguished from postmortem
clots. The former are dry, granular, firm but friable. They are usually adherent to the
vessel wall at their point of origin and a network of fine white lines of fibrin (striae of
Zahn) can be seen on the surface. Postmortem clots are shiny in appearance and jelly-like
in consistency.

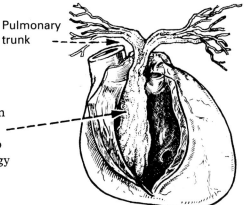

Pulmonary
trunk

AGONAL
These are formed in the last minutes of life when
death occurs slowly. They are composed mainly
of yellowish fibrin. Commonly found attached to
the apex of the right ventricle, they form a stringy
mass extending into pulmonary arteries.

171

COMMON SITES OF THROMBOSIS

ARTERIAL

Thrombi are common in the aorta due to disease, e.g. atheroma or arteriosclerosis. Due to high pressure and rapid flow, they are of platelet variety. An exception is the laminated thrombus in aneurysms.

In smaller arteries they may be of the more mixed type, for example:

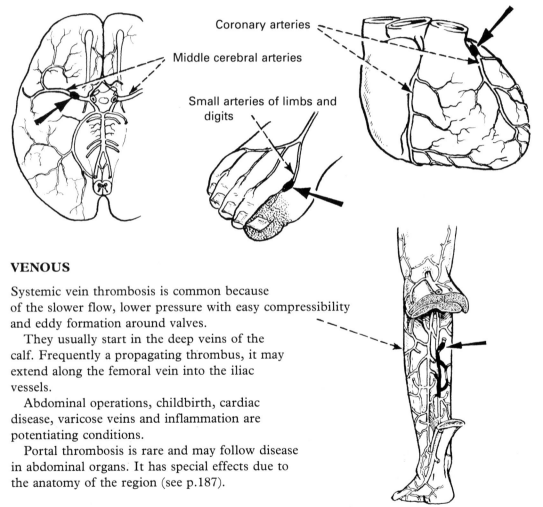

Coronary arteries

Middle cerebral arteries

Small arteries of limbs and digits

VENOUS

Systemic vein thrombosis is common because of the slower flow, lower pressure with easy compressibility and eddy formation around valves.

They usually start in the deep veins of the calf. Frequently a propagating thrombus, it may extend along the femoral vein into the iliac vessels.

Abdominal operations, childbirth, cardiac disease, varicose veins and inflammation are potentiating conditions.

Portal thrombosis is rare and may follow disease in abdominal organs. It has special effects due to the anatomy of the region (see p.187).

CAPILLARY

Thrombi, composed mainly of fused red cells, form when capillaries are damaged, usually in acute inflammatory processes.

Capillaries are occluded by fibrin thrombi in cases of disseminated intravascular coagulation (DIC — see p.553).

COMMON SITES OF THROMBOSIS

CARDIAC

Antemortem thrombi may be formed
in the auricles, ventricles or on the heart
valves. The auricular appendage may be
filled with red thrombus, or small pale
globular thrombi (cardiac polypi) may form
between the muscular columnae.

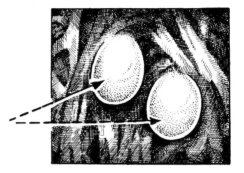

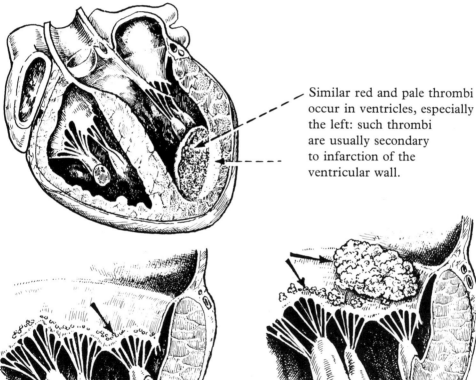

Similar red and pale thrombi
occur in ventricles, especially
the left: such thrombi
are usually secondary
to infarction of the
ventricular wall.

Thrombi of pale variety occur
on the heart valves in
rheumatic endocarditis.

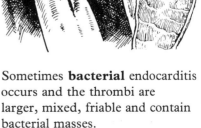

Sometimes **bacterial** endocarditis
occurs and the thrombi are
larger, mixed, friable and contain
bacterial masses.

173

FIBRINOLYSIS

Clotting of blood naturally occurs in vessels, even after trivial injury (see p.548). To control this process, another mechanism — the fibrinolytic system — exists which limits clot deposition by lysing fibrin (see p.557).

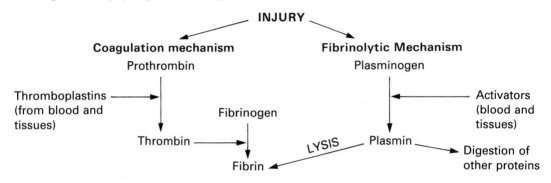

Normally these two mechanisms are activated at the same time and are in dynamic equilibrium. The lytic activity modifies the coagulation process, preventing excessive or continued clotting.

In trivial injury the two processes are activated and together they limit the results of injury and take part in the restoration of the tissues to normal. With very large thrombi, fibrinolysis limits the extension of the thrombotic process and aids the removal of the thrombus during the period of organisation.

Fibrinolysis is also activated during repair of wounds, helping to remove the fibrin scaffold when no longer required. A similar activity is seen during the removal of inflammatory fibrin exudates.

THROMBOXANE and PROSTACYCLIN (PROSTAGLANDINS)

Prostaglandins, substances first discovered in semen, have an important influence in coagulation. They are produced and act locally, THROMBOXANE from platelets and PROSTACYCLIN by ENDOTHELIAL CELLS.

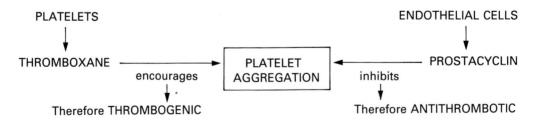

In health the mechanisms are in balance.

PROPHYLAXIS and THERAPY of thrombosis aims at:

1. Reducing coagulability utilising (a) anticoagulants aimed at specific sites in the coagulation cascade e.g. warfarin derivatives, heparin (see p.549) and (b) inhibiting specific prostaglandin synthesis e.g. aspirin.
2. Encouraging fibrinolysis, using fibrinolysins.

SEQUELS OF THROMBOSIS

ORGANISATION

Capillaries grow into the point of thrombus attachment within a day or two. Fibroblasts and phagocytic cells accompany the capillaries, and gradually the thrombus material is dissolved and replaced by a fibrovascular tissue. At the same time endothelium covers the ends of the thrombus, thus limiting the thrombotic process.

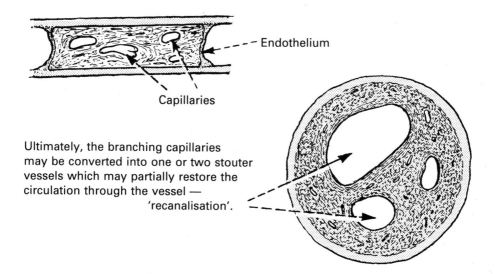

Endothelium

Capillaries

Ultimately, the branching capillaries may be converted into one or two stouter vessels which may partially restore the circulation through the vessel — 'recanalisation'.

CALCIFICATION

In diseased vessels, organisation may not take place. The thrombus shrinks, calcium salts are deposited and convert it into a phlebolith.

INCORPORATION

A mural thrombus, e.g. in a large artery, may be covered by endothelium and incorporated in the vessel wall. This process may be important in the formation of atheroma.

EMBOLISM

Part of the thrombus may be detached and carried along in the blood stream to impact in a distant vessel.

EMBOLISM

An embolus is any abnormal mass of matter carried in the blood stream and large enough to occlude some vessel. Emboli may be:

1. Generated within the vascular system, e.g. fragments of thrombus, or material from atheromatous plaques. Thromboembolism is the commonest.

2. Matter entering the vessels:
   (a) Solid e.g. tumour cells, bacterial clumps, parasites, foreign bodies
   (b) Gaseous — air
   (c) Liquid — amniotic fluid, fat.

Source and destination of emboli

Systemic veins ⟶ Pulmonary arteries

Left side of heart or } ⟶ { Systemic arteries, e.g. in brain, kidney,
large arteries   spleen, intestine, lower limbs

Gaseous and fluid emboli, being malleable, may traverse the lung and appear in the systemic arterial circulation causing occlusion at various sites.

Gas embolism occurs mainly in two forms:

1. *Single embolism*. Atmospheric air may enter the blood when a neck or intracranial vein is incised. Inspiration induces a suction effect by causing a negative pressure in the veins. As a result of frothing in the right ventricle cardiac action is seriously impaired.
2. *Multiple 'embolism'*, in 'Caisson disease'. This occurs in persons working in barometric pressures of several atmospheres, e.g. diving to great depths. The atmospheric gases go into solution in high concentration in the blood and tissues. If decompression occurs too quickly these gases 'boil' off and appear as bubbles in the circulation. The oxygen is taken up by the tissues but insoluble gases cause widespread 'embolism', especially in the nervous system.

Fluid embolism
1. *Fat embolism*. This may occur when a long bone is fractured. Fat globules enter the veins of the bones and pass to the lungs, obstruct the pulmonary blood flow and cause anoxaemia. Cerebral symptoms are common due to this and also to the actual arrival of fat particles which have passed through the lungs.

2. *Amniotic fluid embolism*. During parturition, amniotic fluid may enter a uterine vein, especially after manipulations or with certain obstetric treatments. Vernix, hairs and squames enter the circulation. In addition to embolic phenomena, there are also coagulation disorders.

RESULTS OF ARTERIAL OBSTRUCTION

Results of vascular obstruction vary with type of vessel and anatomy of the part.

1. ARTERIES WITH GOOD COLLATERAL ANASTOMOSIS

Three phases can be recognised.

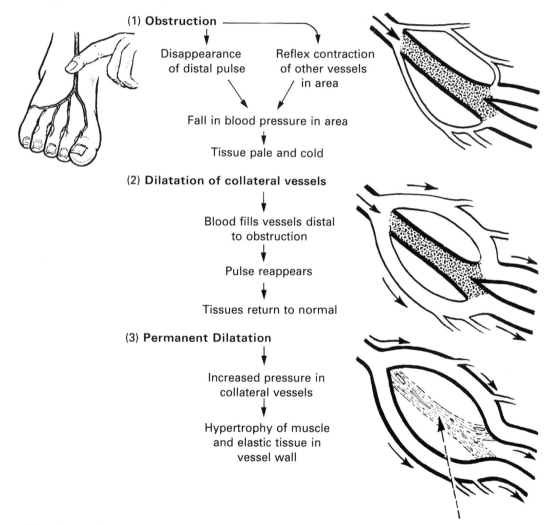

(1) Obstruction

Disappearance of distal pulse

Reflex contraction of other vessels in area

Fall in blood pressure in area

Tissue pale and cold

(2) Dilatation of collateral vessels

Blood fills vessels distal to obstruction

Pulse reappears

Tissues return to normal

(3) Permanent Dilatation

Increased pressure in collateral vessels

Hypertrophy of muscle and elastic tissue in vessel wall

The obstruction in the artery organises and the vessel is filled by vascular fibrous tissue. Very occasionally it may effectively recanalise.

RESULTS OF ARTERIAL OBSTRUCTION

2. END ARTERIES

These may have:

   (a) No collateral anastomosis e.g. splenic artery;

or (b) Capillary anastomosis, e.g. renal arteries, coronary arteries;

or (c) Arterial anastomosis, but too small to maintain circulation, e.g. superior mesenteric artery.

   Result: Obstruction of end artery

                ↓

             Dilatation of collateral vessels

                ↓

             Stagnation of blood

                ↓

             Anoxia of tissues

                ↓

             Congested necrotic area = INFARCTION (Latin, *infarctire* — to stuff in)

Infarction

An infarct is an area of necrosis due to ischaemia usually found at the periphery of an organ e.g. kidney.

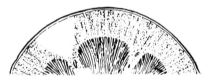

After 12 hours: Area is pale. Degenerative changes already seen with electron microscope or histochemical tests.

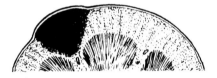

By 24 hours: Collateral vessels have dilated. Blood fills area, stagnates and causes red swelling.

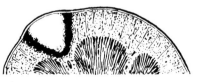

At 36 hours: Area shows coagulative necrosis. In solid organs, infarct may become pale. Breakdown of cell molecules
→increased number of small molecules
→rise in osmotic pressure→cells swell
→blood pressed out of area.

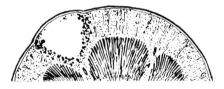

At 72 hours: Stagnant blood breaks down. Polymorphs and macrophages appear at periphery and break down dead tissue.

Healing

This takes place slowly. Capillaries and fibroblasts replace the necrotic tissue. Collagen is formed, contracts and results in a depressed scar.

IMPORTANT SITES OF INFARCTION

HEART

Infarction is almost always due to thrombosis.

Diseased coronary arteries

↓

Thrombosis

↓

Infarction of ventricle

Cardiac action is immediately upset, eddies form, the endocardium may be damaged and a thrombus form on the inner surface of the infarcted area. The damage may extend to the external surface causing pericarditis.

If the patient survives, the infarct heals by fibrosis.

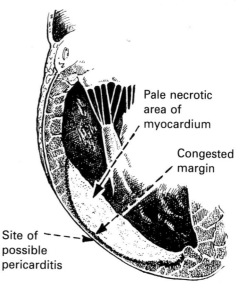

Pale necrotic area of myocardium

Congested margin

Site of possible pericarditis

BRAIN

Infarcts are commonly due to thrombosis of diseased vessels, e.g. MIDDLE CEREBRAL, posterior cerebral and basilar arteries.

The usual changes of infarction take place, but the necrosis is colliquative — cerebral softening.

Embolism is less common and may cause infarcts in almost any part of the brain.

Infarction may occur without arterial occlusion in severe, prolonged hypotension (shock).

Parts of the brain at the junction or arterial territories are affected (boundary zone or watershed infarcts) (see p.201).

Middle cerebral infarct

IMPORTANT SITES OF INFARCTION

LUNG

With a double blood supply — pulmonary and bronchial arteries — and a vast anastomosis, obstruction of a pulmonary artery branch does not necessarily cause infarction. When there is pre-existing circulatory stagnation within the lung, the arrival of an embolus in the pulmonary arterial tree will cause infarction.

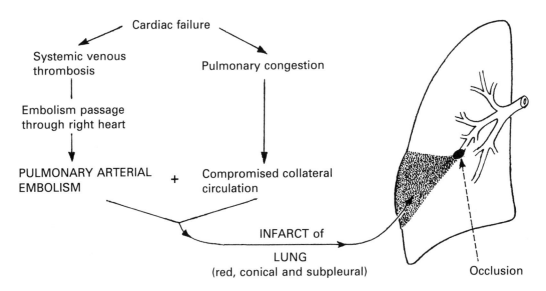

Cardiac failure

Systemic venous thrombosis

Pulmonary congestion

Embolism passage through right heart

PULMONARY ARTERIAL EMBOLISM   +   Compromised collateral circulation

INFARCT of

LUNG
(red, conical and subpleural)

Occlusion

KIDNEY

Embolism is usually a complication of thrombus formation in the left side of the heart (associated with atrial fibrillation or myocardial infarction) or severe atheroma of the aorta.

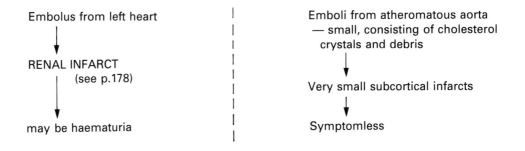

Embolus from left heart

RENAL INFARCT
(see p.178)

may be haematuria

Emboli from atheromatous aorta — small, consisting of cholesterol crystals and debris

Very small subcortical infarcts

Symptomless

IMPORTANT SITES OF INFARCTION

INTESTINE

Infarctions, which are relatively uncommon, are usually smaller than expected due to arterial anastomosis, and embolism is the usual cause. The sequence of changes seen in solid organs is altered in the terminal stages.

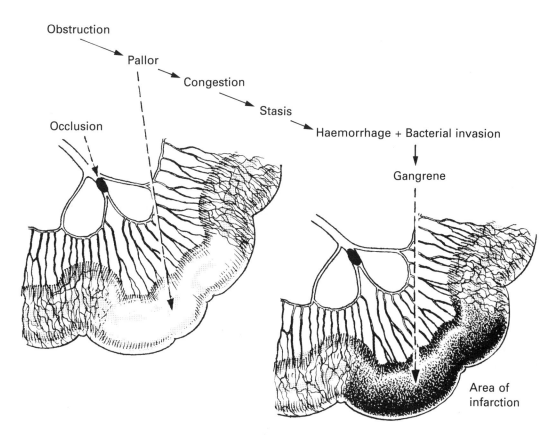

SPLEEN

Infarcts are common in arterial embolic conditions. Being true end arteries without collateral anastomosis, obstruction of splenic artery branches results in pale red infarcts becoming yellow as the stagnant blood breaks down.

PARTIAL OR SLOW ARTERIAL OCCLUSION/VENOUS OBSTRUCTION

This is common in old age and in chronic systemic arterial disease such as atheroma. Parenchymal cells atrophy and are replaced by fibrous tissue. Serious functional disturbance may result.

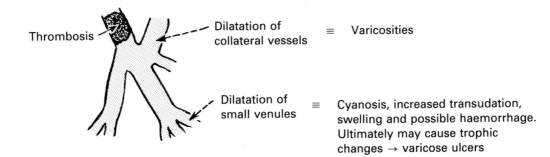

Renal artery stenosis	Coronary artery atheroma	Narrowing of lower limb arteries
↓	↓	↓
Ischaemia	Myocardial fibrosis	Anoxia of muscles
↓	↓	↓
HYPERTENSION	Cardiac failure	Intermittent claudication

VENOUS OBSTRUCTION

Acute obstruction is usually due to thrombosis but in certain sites may be caused by mechanical pressure, e.g. in strangulation of the bowel.

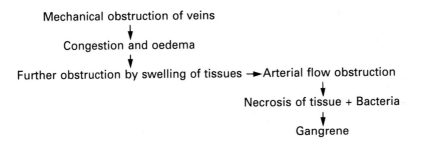

Thrombosis

Dilatation of collateral vessels ≡ Varicosities

Dilatation of small venules ≡ Cyanosis, increased transudation, swelling and possible haemorrhage. Ultimately may cause trophic changes → varicose ulcers

STRANGULATION OF BOWEL

This may follow hernia, volvulus or intussusception. The sequence of events is as follows:

Mechanical obstruction of veins
↓
Congestion and oedema
↓
Further obstruction by swelling of tissues → Arterial flow obstruction
↓
Necrosis of tissue + Bacteria
↓
Gangrene

CHRONIC VENOUS CONGESTION

General venous congestion is a condition where *all* the veins of the body are distended with blood. It is associated with disease of the heart or lungs since all the circulating blood must pass through them.

Chronic cardiac failure or lung disease which reduces the pulmonary vascular bed, e.g. fibrosis or emphysema, are the usual causes.

The basic mechanism is:

CHRONIC CARDIAC FAILURE

REDUCED left ventricular output
+ MITRAL valve incompetence

chronic **PULMONARY VENOUS CONGESTION**

+ increased pulmonary arterial pressure

LUNG DISEASE

increased pulmonary vascular resistance

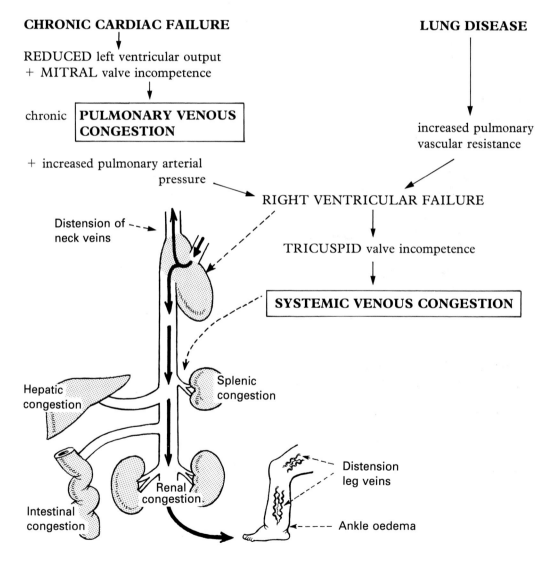

RIGHT VENTRICULAR FAILURE

Distension of neck veins

TRICUSPID valve incompetence

SYSTEMIC VENOUS CONGESTION

Hepatic congestion

Splenic congestion

Intestinal congestion

Renal congestion

Distension leg veins

Ankle oedema

CHRONIC VENOUS CONGESTION

GENERAL EFFECTS

1. **Increased blood volume**. This is related to the REDUCED OUTPUT from the LEFT VENTRICLE: the mechanism involves retention of sodium and water:

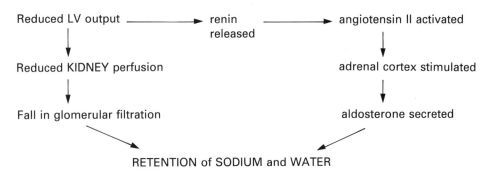

The increasing volume is accommodated in the venous side of the circulation.

2. **Hypoxia**. There are two types: anoxic and stagnant.
   (a) *Anoxic*. Whether the primary cause is cardiac or pulmonary, oxygenation of the blood is reduced because gaseous interchange in the lungs is made difficult.

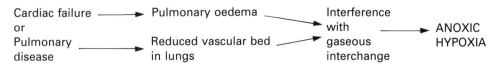

   Reduction in left heart output increases the effect of this on the organs.

   (b) *Stagnant*. The slow flow of venous blood results in excessive amounts of reduced haemoglobin in the circulation.

3. **Cyanosis**. Slow venous blood flow and the rise in the blood volume increase the amount of reduced haemoglobin in the distended venules, thus causing the general 'blue' colour. If the patient happens to be anaemic the amount of reduced haemoglobin may not be sufficient to alter coloration.

4. **Oedema**. Two mechanisms are mainly responsible:

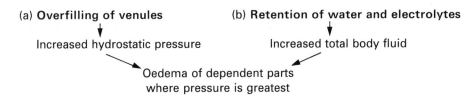

CHRONIC VENOUS CONGESTION

PATHOLOGICAL CHANGES IN ORGANS

Because of the increase in venous blood, the organs become swollen and purplish. With long continued over-distension, the walls of the venules show reactive thickening and there is mild interstitial fibrosis of the organs, giving them a very firm consistency. These changes are seen typically in the kidney and spleen.

Important additional changes are found in the lungs and liver.

LUNGS

The lungs are bulky, congested and brownish in colour.

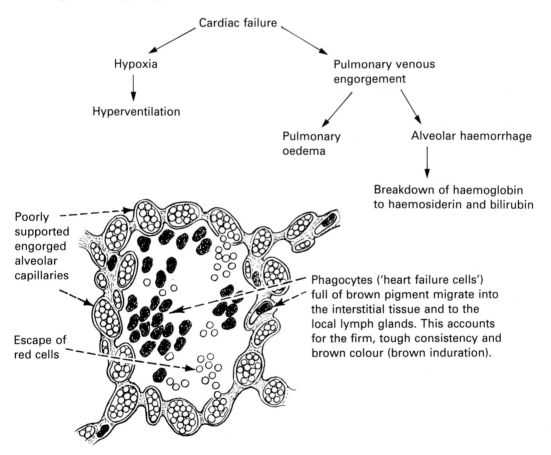

Cardiac failure

Hypoxia

Hyperventilation

Pulmonary venous engorgement

Pulmonary oedema

Alveolar haemorrhage

Breakdown of haemoglobin to haemosiderin and bilirubin

Poorly supported engorged alveolar capillaries

Escape of red cells

Phagocytes ('heart failure cells') full of brown pigment migrate into the interstitial tissue and to the local lymph glands. This accounts for the firm, tough consistency and brown colour (brown induration).

At post mortem, application of potassium ferrocyanide and hydrochloric acid to the lung results in a blue colour (Prussian blue reaction) indicating the presence of free iron.

185

CHRONIC VENOUS CONGESTION

PATHOLOGICAL CHANGES IN ORGANS (continued)

LIVER

Mechanical distension of the veins causes considerable enlargement of the liver so that it can be felt below the costal margin.

The parenchymal cells furthest from the arterial blood supply, i.e. around the hepatic venules (centrilobular), undergo degeneration with atrophy and ultimately disappear. Cells nearer the arteries show an accumulation of fat.

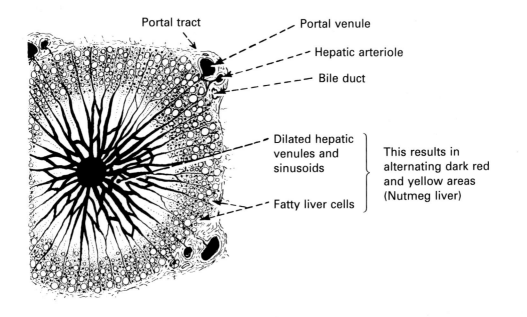

Portal tract

Portal venule

Hepatic arteriole

Bile duct

Dilated hepatic venules and sinusoids

Fatty liver cells

This results in alternating dark red and yellow areas (Nutmeg liver)

Much of the liver parenchyma may be destroyed. If the patient has periods of remission, the remaining liver cells may undergo compensatory hyperplasia. This results in small, irregular, pale nodules alternating with areas of fibrosis — so-called cardiac cirrhosis. It is not a true cirrhosis and does not cause hepatic failure.

PORTAL VENOUS CONGESTION

PORTAL VENOUS CONGESTION
This is the result of vascular obstruction in the liver since the whole of the portal circulation must pass through that organ. The usual cause is hepatic cirrhosis.

Congestion affects the spleen, the gastrointestinal tract and the peritoneum. Portal venous congestion is one of the main causes of ASCITES — accumulation of fluid in the peritoneal cavity (see p.190).

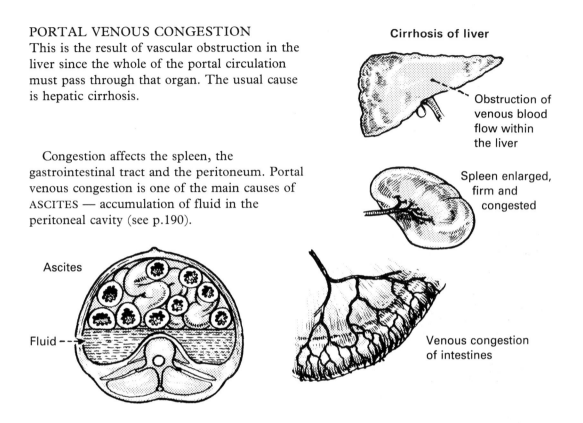

Cirrhosis of liver

Obstruction of venous blood flow within the liver

Spleen enlarged, firm and congested

Ascites

Fluid

Venous congestion of intestines

Certain collateral anastomotic connections do exist, and these dilate and become varicose. These include haemorrhoidal veins around the rectum and veins at the lower end of the oesophagus. Haemorrhage may occur from these sites.

Less important are vessels around the umbilicus and over the anterior abdominal wall.

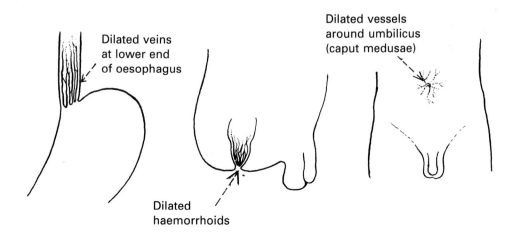

Dilated veins at lower end of oesophagus

Dilated vessels around umbilicus (caput medusae)

Dilated haemorrhoids

BODY WATER CONTROL

NORMAL TISSUE FLUID CIRCULATION

There is a continuous interchange of fluid between blood and tissues. Some fluid enters the lymphatics before eventually returning to the blood stream.

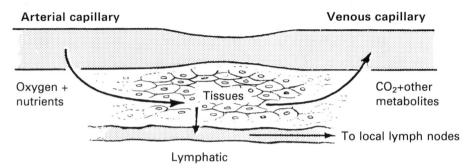

In order to maintain this normal circulation two main forces operate a pressure gradient which controls the rate and direction of fluid movement.

1. **Hydrostatic pressure**, i.e. capillary blood pressure (BP) encouraging the passage of fluid through the capillary wall, = 35 mm mercury.
2. **Protein osmotic pressure**, (OP), i.e. the plasma proteins encourage the retention of fluid in the capillaries to try and maintain osmotic equilibrium. This pressure is equivalent to 25 mm mercury.

At the arterial end the blood pressure is greater than the osmotic pressure and fluid is forced out of the capillary. The reverse is true at the venous end and fluid is attracted into the vessel.

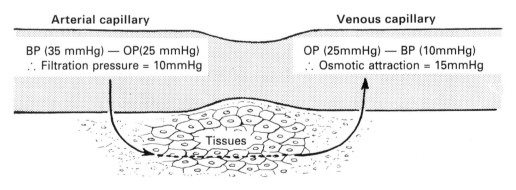

Some fluid enters lymphatics. This may be partly the result of tissue pressure and partly due to osmotic attraction of proteins in the lymphatic system.

BODY WATER CONTROL: OEDEMA

In addition to those forces operating at capillary level, there are other mechanisms which influence the movement of fluid within the body in a general manner.

1. **Fluid intake**
   Intake via the gut or parenterally may exceed the ability of the kidneys to eliminate water.

2. **Integrity of the kidneys**
   Damage to the renal parenchyma may diminish the elimination of fluid.

3. **Hormone activity**

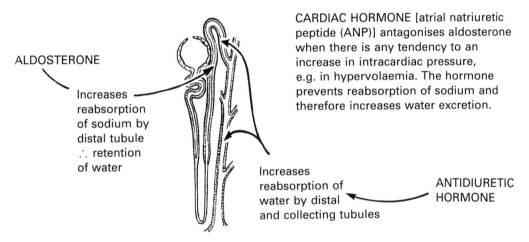

CARDIAC HORMONE [atrial natriuretic peptide (ANP)] antagonises aldosterone when there is any tendency to an increase in intracardiac pressure, e.g. in hypervolaemia. The hormone prevents reabsorption of sodium and therefore increases water excretion.

ALDOSTERONE

Increases reabsorption of sodium by distal tubule ∴ retention of water

Increases reabsorption of water by distal and collecting tubules

ANTIDIURETIC HORMONE

OEDEMA

This is an accumulation of excess fluid in the extravascular tissues. Conditions which interfere with the pressure gradients system result in oedema:

1. Rise in capillary hydrostatic pressure, especially at the venous end of the capillary.
2. Fall in blood osmotic pressure.
3. Rise in tissue osmotic pressure.
} Transudate formed (low protein content)

4. Alteration in capillary permeability operates especially in inflammation.
} Exudate formed (high protein content)

LOCAL OEDEMA

Oedema can occur in a very localised form for a variety of reasons. The mechanism is mainly an alteration in the pressure gradient system at capillary level and does not involve general bodily changes. Oedema fluid forming locally usually is associated only with local effects. However oedema of the lungs and brain can be life threatening and are of great importance. They are dealt with separately under 'Cerebral' oedema and 'Pulmonary' oedema.

LOCAL OEDEMA

(a) OEDEMA of VENOUS OBSTRUCTION

This is the commonest form of local oedema and is most frequently seen in venous obstruction of the lower limb.

(b) ASCITES and PLEURAL EFFUSION (accumulation of fluid in the peritoneal and pleural cavities)

These are special forms of local oedema – the common predisposing conditions are cardiac failure, inflammation and tumour growth: ascites is a common complication of hepatic cirrhosis

(c) INFLAMMATORY OEDEMA

In this condition there is intense local congestion and the production of complex chemical agents which alter capillary permeability (see also p.36).

Allergic oedema is a special form of inflammatory oedema. The patient is hypersensitive to particular substances, and the tissues immediately react with the formation of chemicals such as histamine. These induce congestion and alter the capillary permeability.

Both inflammatory oedema and allergic oedema have already been considered when dealing with the inflammatory reaction (p.36 and 111). A similar response is produced by stinging plants and insects.

(d) ANGIONEUROTIC OEDEMA

This is a rare form of local oedema of sudden onset but short duration and unknown cause. Very rarely it may affect the larynx and cause suffocation.

(e) LYMPHATIC OEDEMA

This occurs when there is chronic obstruction to lymphatic flow in an area.

Common causes are:
(a) Destruction of lymphatics by chronic inflammation
(b) Blockage of lymphatics e.g. by cancer cells or parasites such as filaria.

See also page 680.

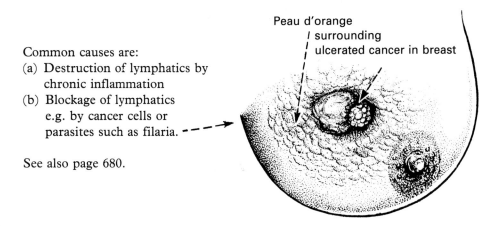

Peau d'orange surrounding ulcerated cancer in breast

LOCAL OEDEMA

PULMONARY OEDEMA

This is the most important form of local oedema since it is associated with serious disease of the heart. It differs from other forms of oedema in that fluid accumulates not only in the tissue spaces but also in the pulmonary alveoli. The results in terms of gaseous interchange are disastrous.

Normal pulmonary fluid interchange
The same factors operate as in other parts of the body. One factor, however, is more important than others — the negative tissue pressure induced by respiration.

Alveolar capillary

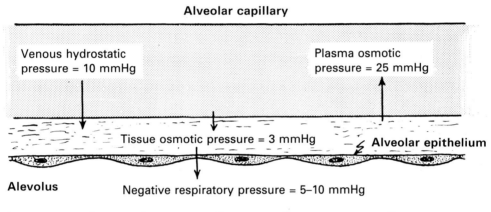

Venous hydrostatic pressure = 10 mmHg

Plasma osmotic pressure = 25 mmHg

Tissue osmotic pressure = 3 mmHg

Alveolar epithelium

Alevolus

Negative respiratory pressure = 5–10 mmHg

Filtration pressure = hydrostatic pressure + tissue osmotic pressure + negative respiratory pressure = 18–23 mmHg
Osmotic reabsorbing pressure = 25 mmHg

The balance between these forces is relatively fine and can be easily upset so that **OEDEMA** can occur rapidly.

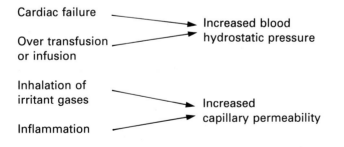

Cardiac failure
Over transfusion or infusion → Increased blood hydrostatic pressure

Inhalation of irritant gases
Inflammation → Increased capillary permeability

GENERAL OEDEMA

In addition to alterations in the capillary filtration process (which have already been described), in generalised oedema there is another important factor — increase in total body water. It is particularly associated with diseases of the heart and kidneys.

CARDIAC OEDEMA

This has already been mentioned under 'Chronic venous congestion'. Three factors are involved:

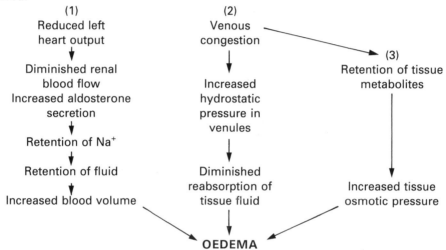

```
        (1)                    (2)
    Reduced left            Venous
    heart output          congestion
         ↓                     ↓              ↘ (3)
  Diminished renal          Increased          Retention of tissue
    blood flow              hydrostatic          metabolites
  Increased aldosterone     pressure in
    secretion                venules
         ↓                     ↓                      ↓
   Retention of Na⁺       Diminished
         ↓                reabsorption of
   Retention of fluid     tissue fluid        Increased tissue
         ↓                                     osmotic pressure
  Increased blood volume          ↓
                              OEDEMA
```

In the early phases of cardiac failure, oedema is slight and is seen where the hydrostatic pressure is greatest — around the feet and ankles. Later, as the condition of the patient deteriorates, fluid gathers in the peritoneal cavity (ascites), in the pleural cavities (hydrothorax) and ultimately becomes generalised (anasarca).

RENAL OEDEMA

Two forms of renal disease are associated with oedema: (a) *acute nephritis* and (b) *nephrotic syndrome*.

The processes involved are different.

	Acute Nephritis	Nephrosis
Degree of oedema	Slight	Marked
Distribution	Loose tissues, e.g. round eyes, ankles	More generalised
Proteinuria	Moderate	Gross
Plasma osmotic pressure	Normal	Reduced
Cause	Retention of fluid	Fall in plasma osmotic pressure

FAMINE OEDEMA

In starvation there is a lack of protein building materials, particularly amino acids. The protein reserves become depleted and, ultimately, the plasma proteins are reduced below the critical level for maintaining the osmotic pressure of the blood.

A special effect of starvation may be the deficiency of vitamin B_1 (thiamine), causing Beri-Beri which is associated with cardiac failure.

SHOCK

Shock is a condition in which the vital functions of the body are depressed due to a severe and acute reduction in cardiac output and effective circulating blood volume. There is progressive cardiovascular collapse characterised by hypotension, hyperventilation and clouding of consciousness. Subsequently there is oliguria.

There are many causes, conveniently grouped under three main headings:

1. **HYPOVOLAEMIC (i.e. diminished blood volume)**

   Associated with:

   (a) **Trauma**
   - (i)   Severe haemorrhage — external or internal
   - (ii) Severe injury — especially fractures of bones and crushing of tissues
   - (iii) Surgical procedures — especially if anaesthesia is not adequate
   - (iv) Burning — especially where extensive surface damage allows loss of a large amount of exudate

   (b) **Dehydration** — in cases of severe vomiting or diarrhoea.

2. **CARDIOGENIC**

   Acute diseases of the heart — especially myocardial infarction — in which there is a sudden fall in cardiac output.

3. **BACTERIAL (Septic, bacteraemic, endotoxic)**

   In serious bacterial infections (especially Gram-negative organisms, e.g. *E. coli* and *bacteroides*).

The loss of effective circulating blood causes tissue and cell damage, and, at the same time, initiates reactive changes in the circulation. These two mechanisms combine to cause the shock syndrome.

SHOCK

REACTIVE CHANGES — EARLY STAGE

These changes are concerned with the maintenance of an adequate cerebral and coronary circulation and are effected by a redistribution of the blood in the body as a whole.

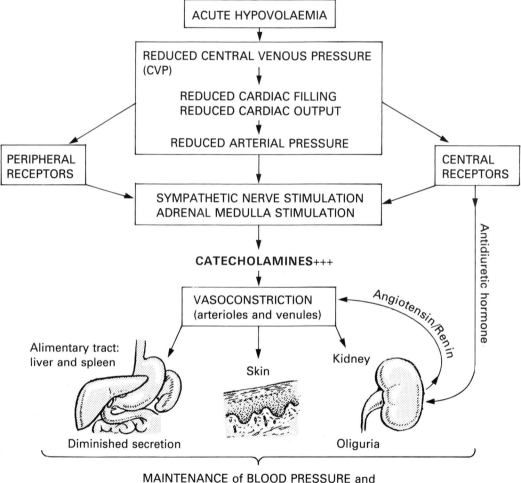

MAINTENANCE of BLOOD PRESSURE and
CONSERVATION of FLUID

At the same time, the circulations in the brain and heart are protected by autoregulatory mechanisms. They are *not* subject to the generalised vasoconstriction.

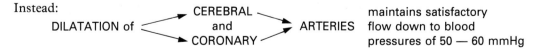

Instead:

DILATATION of → CEREBRAL and CORONARY → ARTERIES   maintains satisfactory flow down to blood pressures of 50 — 60 mmHg

If the loss of circulating fluid volume is great, the limits of the compensatory mechanism are exceeded and the patient goes into a state of severe shock.

SHOCK

ADVANCED STAGE

The patient is now listless, pale and cold, the face is pinched and the lips blue. The pulse is rapid and weak and the blood pressure is low.

Conditions in Vascular bed

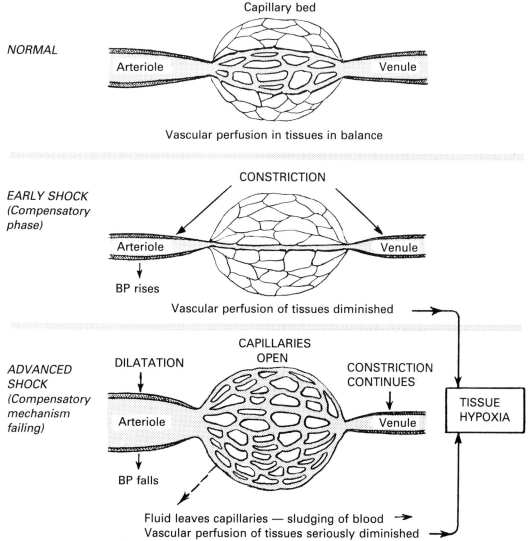

NORMAL

Capillary bed

Arteriole

Venule

Vascular perfusion in tissues in balance

EARLY SHOCK
(Compensatory
phase)

CONSTRICTION

Arteriole

Venule

BP rises

Vascular perfusion of tissues diminished

ADVANCED
SHOCK
(Compensatory
mechanism
failing)

DILATATION

CAPILLARIES
OPEN

CONSTRICTION
CONTINUES

Arteriole

Venule

BP falls

TISSUE
HYPOXIA

Fluid leaves capillaries — sludging of blood

Vascular perfusion of tissues seriously diminished

195

SHOCK — INDIVIDUAL ORGANS

Circulatory changes in the lung (continued)

The mechanisms initiating and progressively augmenting the damage are complex and interacting:

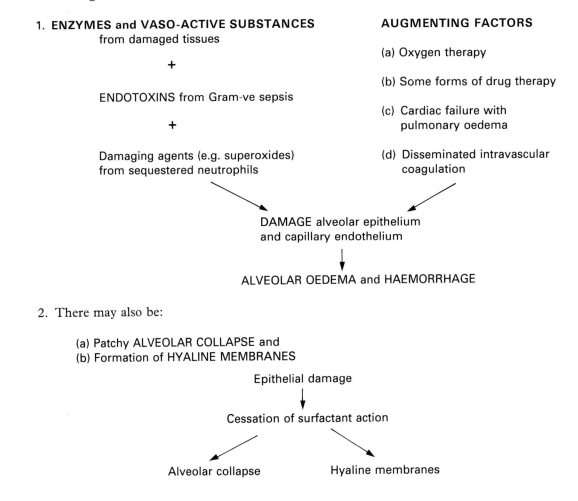

1. **ENZYMES and VASO-ACTIVE SUBSTANCES**
   from damaged tissues

   +

   ENDOTOXINS from Gram-ve sepsis

   +

   Damaging agents (e.g. superoxides)
   from sequestered neutrophils

AUGMENTING FACTORS

(a) Oxygen therapy

(b) Some forms of drug therapy

(c) Cardiac failure with
    pulmonary oedema

(d) Disseminated intravascular
    coagulation

DAMAGE alveolar epithelium
and capillary endothelium

ALVEOLAR OEDEMA and HAEMORRHAGE

2. There may also be:

   (a) Patchy ALVEOLAR COLLAPSE and
   (b) Formation of HYALINE MEMBRANES

   Epithelial damage

   Cessation of surfactant action

   Alveolar collapse   Hyaline membranes

3. If the patient survives, the organisation is followed by fibrosis: the end result in severe cases may be a combination of fibrosis, emphysema and broncheolectasis.

SHOCK — INDIVIDUAL ORGANS

KIDNEYS

The secretory function of the kidneys is always disturbed in shock. This is due to the general circulatory collapse and hypotension, but it may be aggravated by the secretion of renin and angiotensin by the kidney, aldosterone by the adrenal and antidiuretic hormone by the posterior pituitary. These hormones are secreted in an attempt to retain fluid and restore the blood volume, but by inducing vasoconstriction they will tend to increase renal damage.

Mechanism

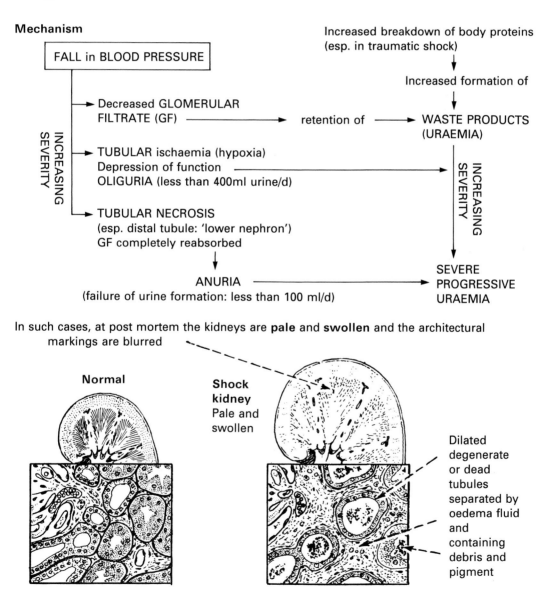

FALL in BLOOD PRESSURE

INCREASING SEVERITY

→ Decreased GLOMERULAR FILTRATE (GF) ──────→ retention of ──────→ WASTE PRODUCTS (URAEMIA)

→ TUBULAR ischaemia (hypoxia)
Depression of function ──────────────→
OLIGURIA (less than 400ml urine/d)

INCREASING SEVERITY

→ TUBULAR NECROSIS
(esp. distal tubule: 'lower nephron')
GF completely reabsorbed

↓

ANURIA ──────────────→ SEVERE PROGRESSIVE URAEMIA
(failure of urine formation: less than 100 ml/d)

Increased breakdown of body proteins
(esp. in traumatic shock)
↓
Increased formation of
↓
WASTE PRODUCTS (URAEMIA)

In such cases, at post mortem the kidneys are **pale** and **swollen** and the architectural markings are blurred

Normal

Shock kidney
Pale and swollen

Dilated degenerate or dead tubules separated by oedema fluid and containing debris and pigment

199

SHOCK — INDIVIDUAL ORGANS

ADRENALS

In addition to the release of **aldosterone** in response to changes in kidney function and fluid electrolyte balance, the adrenal CORTEX secretes increased quantities of **glucocorticoids** and the MEDULLA a great increase of **catecholamines** (adrenaline, etc.).

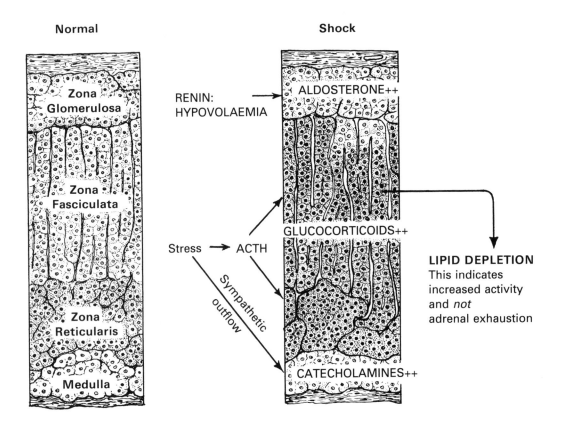

Occasionally in severe shock, adrenal haemorrhage occurs particularly when the blood coagulation mechanism is disturbed or if there is overwhelming bacterial infection.

ALIMENTARY TRACT

Acute ulceration of the stomach and duodenum may complicate shock — the mechanism is not known. (Curling's or stress ulcers.) Haemorrhage of varying severity may also occur, especially from the colon.

SHOCK — INDIVIDUAL ORGANS

BRAIN

During the compensated phase of shock, relatively mild cerebral ischaemia is associated with changes in the state of consciousness. When the blood pressure falls to below 50–60 mmHg, the brain suffers serious ischaemic damage which can amount to actual infarction in the 'boundary zones' of the cerebral cortex (and cerebellum).

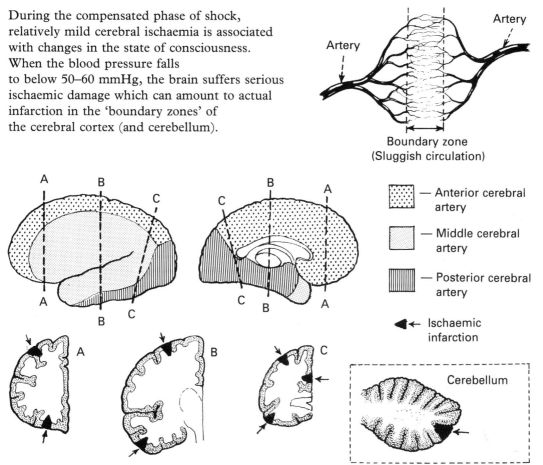

Boundary zone
(Sluggish circulation)

Artery

Artery

— Anterior cerebral artery

— Middle cerebral artery

— Posterior cerebral artery

◄← Ischaemic infarction

Cerebellum

There may also be more diffuse cerebral damage.

POST MORTEM APPEARANCES IN SHOCK

These are very variable.

Often the changes in the organs are not striking, and the continuing presence of the initiating cause of the shock is the most important finding.

Organ damage of the types described above may be present in varying degree and combination.

SHOCK — SPECIAL TYPES

FAINTING (VASOVAGAL) ATTACK — (PRIMARY SHOCK)

What used to be called 'primary shock' is in fact the common fainting attack which is brought on in susceptible individuals by emotional upset or trauma which may be minor, and is mediated by nervous mechanisms. The patient feels 'faint', becomes pale often with a cold sweat and may vomit. The pulse slows and the blood pressure falls: consciousness is lost.

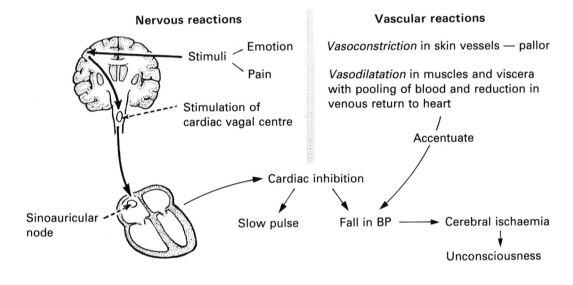

Nervous reactions

Stimuli — Emotion / Pain

Stimulation of cardiac vagal centre

Sinoauricular node

Cardiac inhibition

Slow pulse

Vascular reactions

Vasoconstriction in skin vessels — pallor

Vasodilatation in muscles and viscera with pooling of blood and reduction in venous return to heart

Accentuate

Fall in BP ⟶ Cerebral ischaemia

Unconsciousness

At this stage, nervous reaction quickly begins, and with a simple fainting attack recovery is soon complete. On very rare occasions, sudden death occurs due to complete cardiac inhibition by vagal action.

Because the nervous mechanisms of the fainting attack only play a minor part in the early stages of true shock the term 'primary shock' is now obsolete.

SHOCK — SPECIAL TYPES

SHOCK IN BURNS AND SCALDS

Mechanism
1. The immediate reaction is **NERVOUS — PAIN** and stimulation of afferent nerves, followed by
2. An INFLAMMATORY RESPONSE evoked by the burnt tissues.

Massive exudation and
loss of PROTEIN-RICH fluid   ⟶   HYPOVOLAEMIA   ⟶   SHOCK
(sludging of blood in capillaries)

This mechanism explains why the SEVERITY of the shock is roughly proportional to the exuding SURFACE AREA and not to the depth of the burn, and why PLASMA transfusion is indicated.

Other factors are chemical mediators derived from the burnt tissues.

3. Complications which aggravate the shock.

(a) *Infection*

Burnt tissues ⟶ Susceptible to infection ⟶ BACTERIAL SHOCK
esp. *Staph. aureus*   may be superimposed
Strep. pyogenes
Gram-neg. bacilli
(e.g. *Pseudomonas*)

(b) *Anaemia*

Haemolysis of red cells
at burnt site and later   ⟶   ANAEMIA
if sludging is severe

ANAPHYLACTIC SHOCK
This is an acute reaction caused by hypersensitivity of the host to exogenous protein and is dealt with on page 111.

SHOCK — SPECIAL TYPES

BACTERIAL SHOCK

Causes

1. *Bacteria*

   In modern practice, the GRAM-NEGATIVE BACTERIA, especially the coliform group, are the commonest causes, and the shock is caused by ENDOTOXINS.

   Other organisms which may or may not be associated with endotoxins can also produce shock, e.g. staphylococci, streptococci and menigococci.

2. *Associated conditions*

   (a) Serious *primary* bacterial infection, e.g. septicaemia, peritonitis — potentiated by deficiency in immune status (p.70) and liver disease where detoxification is impaired.

   (b) Bacterial shock may complicate pre-existing shock due to other causes, e.g. burns.

   (c) Bacterial shock may complicate relatively trivial surgical procedures, especially in the gastrointestinal and urinary tracts in the presence of infection.

Mechanism

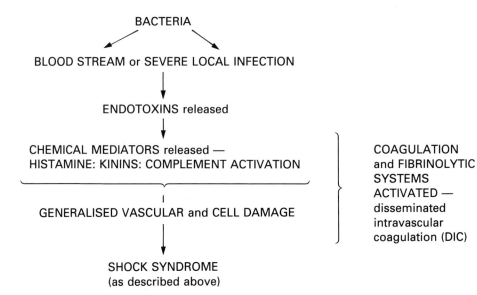

Occasionally, especially in bacterial infection where endotoxin is not produced, there is a generalised arteriolar dilatation with a fall in BP, but the cardiac output is maintained and the patient has a warm, pink skin.

SHOCK — OUTCOME

The OUTCOME of SHOCK

There are 3 possibilities, depending on several factors:

1. RECOVERY
   after convalescence,
   which may be long

2. SURVIVAL
   with permanent damage
   to various organs

3. DEATH

Factors favouring recovery	Factors favouring progression of shock
1. AVAILABILITY of EARLY TREATMENT of (a) the INITIATING CAUSE (b) the HYPOVOLAEMIA	1. DELAY in TREATMENT
	2. FAILURE to REMOVE the INITIATING CAUSE
2. Youth	3. Old age
3. Good general health	4. Poor general health
	5. Pre-existing Cardiovascular and Lung disease
	6. Onset of Complications, esp. Infection and Organ damage

IRREVERSIBLE SHOCK

Theoretically, at some stage in its evolution, shock becomes irreversible due to the severity of vascular impairment and tissue damage. In medical practice, no certain indications are available as to when this point is reached. Measurements of blood pressure and central venous pressure indicate the severity of the vascular disturbance, but many severe cases respond to modern sophisticated treatment. However, the basic essentials remain the early transfusion of fluid and the removal of the original cause of the shock.

CARDIOVASCULAR SYSTEM

ARTERIAL DISEASES

Arterial diseases are very common and are important because of their serious effects on vital organs — particularly the brain, heart and kidneys — accounting for almost half the mortality in Western society.

The two most common are the 'degenerative' diseases.

(1) **ATHEROMA (ATHEROSCLEROSIS)**   ### (2) **ARTERIOSCLEROSIS**

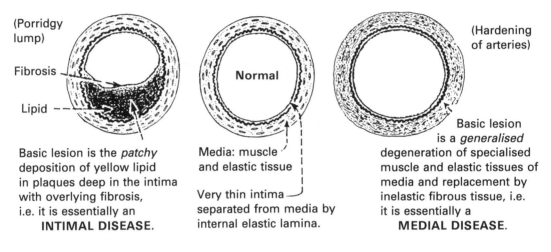

(Porridgy lump)

Fibrosis

Lipid

Normal

(Hardening of arteries)

Basic lesion is the *patchy* deposition of yellow lipid in plaques deep in the intima with overlying fibrosis, i.e. it is essentially an **INTIMAL DISEASE.**

Media: muscle and elastic tissue

Very thin intima separated from media by internal elastic lamina.

Basic lesion is a *generalised* degeneration of specialised muscle and elastic tissues of media and replacement by inelastic fibrous tissue, i.e. it is essentially a **MEDIAL DISEASE.**

These diagrams illustrate the diseases in their pure state. Because both are common diseases and share aetiological factors, they often occur together. However, it is important that they are considered separately since the mechanisms of damage are essentially different. To minimise the chance of confusion we will continue to use the term 'atheroma' rather than 'atherosclerosis'.

In other arterial diseases the important basic changes occur:

in the **intima**   and/or   in the **media**

where fibrous proliferation is common, e.g. in *endarteritis obliterans* — small artery in base of inflammatory ulcer.

where inflammatory or degenerative changes occur e.g. in *polyarteritis nodosa*

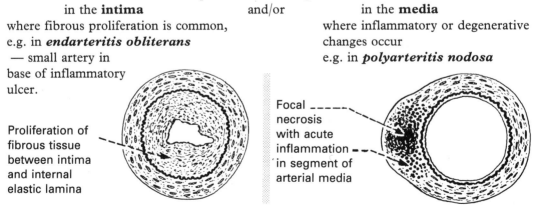

Proliferation of fibrous tissue between intima and internal elastic lamina

Focal necrosis with acute inflammation in segment of arterial media

THROMBOSIS is by far the commonest complication of arterial disease, but haemorrhage and aneurysm formation are also important.

ATHEROMA

Atheroma is a disease of Western countries, of gradual onset but progressive. It may have little effect for many years, but serious chronic disease is often the end result or at any time there may be a dramatic fatal or near fatal episode due to sudden complications such as thrombosis.

Evolution of the disease
(Vessel opened longitudinally)

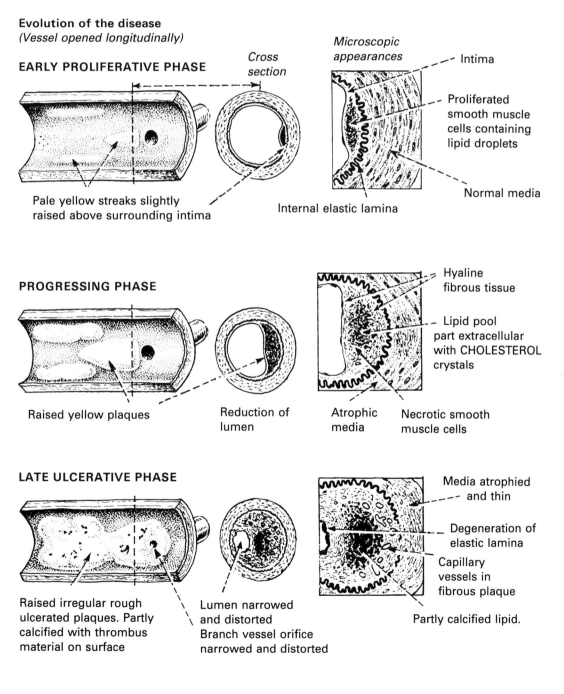

EARLY PROLIFERATIVE PHASE

Cross section

Microscopic appearances

Intima

Proliferated smooth muscle cells containing lipid droplets

Normal media

Pale yellow streaks slightly raised above surrounding intima

Internal elastic lamina

PROGRESSING PHASE

Hyaline fibrous tissue

Lipid pool part extracellular with CHOLESTEROL crystals

Raised yellow plaques

Reduction of lumen

Atrophic media

Necrotic smooth muscle cells

LATE ULCERATIVE PHASE

Media atrophied and thin

Degeneration of elastic lamina

Capillary vessels in fibrous plaque

Raised irregular rough ulcerated plaques. Partly calcified with thrombus material on surface

Lumen narrowed and distorted Branch vessel orifice narrowed and distorted

Partly calcified lipid.

209

ATHEROMA

Fibrosis in the intima and media may lead to aneurysm formation, but the most important complication of atheroma is **THROMBOSIS**.

Local factors at the site of the atheromatous plaque are important:
1. Intimal roughening or distortion with eddying of flow
2. Thin, easily damaged intimal surface
3. Rupture of new capillaries in plaque with haemorrhage into the plaque

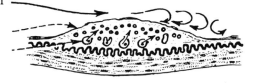

In addition, general factors influencing blood coagulability are important, e.g. smoking affecting vessel contractility and platelet function.

Results

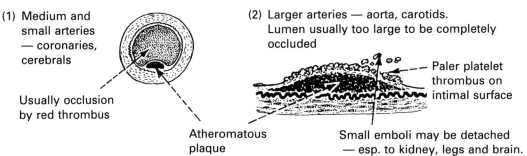

(1) Medium and small arteries — coronaries, cerebrals

Usually occlusion by red thrombus

Atheromatous plaque

(2) Larger arteries — aorta, carotids. Lumen usually too large to be completely occluded

Paler platelet thrombus on intimal surface

Small emboli may be detached — esp. to kidney, legs and brain.

The important sites of atheroma and the effects due to complications are:

CEREBRALS (Circle of Willis or branches)
CAROTIDS
— Generalised chronic ischaemia of brain — senile dementia.

Acute local ischaemia — cerebral softening (infarction).

CORONARIES ——— Chronic ischaemia of heart muscle with fibrosis.
Acute infarction.

ABDOMINAL AORTA ——— ANEURYSM, embolism to legs.

RENAL ARTERIES ——— CHRONIC ISCHAEMIA OF KIDNEYS.

Visceral arteries ——— Chronic ischaemia of bowel.

Lower limb arteries ——— *NB* Collateral circulation is usually good; atheroma
(Upper limb arteries must be very severe before chronic ischaemia with
are rarely affected) intermittent claudication and/or gangrene develop.

In severe cases of atheroma, most of these sites may be affected, but not uncommonly, one particular artery may be much more severely damaged than the others, e.g. coronaries, cerebrals.

ATHEROMA

BACKGROUND AETIOLOGICAL FACTORS

'Background' factors influencing the risk of or susceptibility to atheroma are multiple and interrelated.

Age

Although there is a definite age relationship, age by itself is not a cause of atheroma; it reflects the duration over which other factors have been operative. The most important of these are illustrated in the classical victim of atheroma — the OBESE, HEAVY SMOKING, HYPERTENSIVE, SEDENTARY MALE.

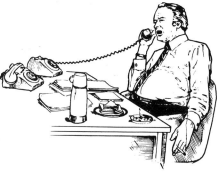

The major background factors may be grouped into two main categories:

1. **Endogenous** ∴ Not modifiable
   (a) SEX (i.e. male > female)
   (b) HEREDITY (i) evidenced in cases with clearly defined abnormalities of lipid metabolism.
   (ii) Single genes controlling aspects of lipid metabolism are now being identified.

2. **Environmental** ∴ Modifiable
   (a) DIET — lipid and carbohydrate metabolism.
   Fibre and anti-oxidants including red wine reduce the risk.
   (b) METABOLIC DISEASES
   (c) HYPERTENSION
   (d) SMOKING
   (e) LACK OF PHYSICAL EXERCISE
   (f) COLD CLIMATE

These background factors may act as follows:

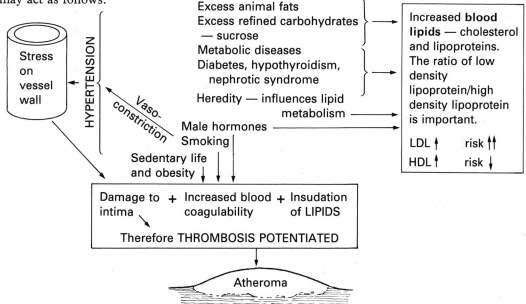

ATHEROMA

BACKGROUND FACTORS (continued)

Population studies indicate that diet is the most important single factor related to *clinical* atheroma (e.g. patients suffering from coronary artery disease). A high intake of saturated fat involving a high cholesterol content is a constant feature in these cases. Other factors such as smoking, sedentary habits, obesity and hypertension are to some extent indicators of life style and probably act in an additive or precipitating manner in the clinical scene.

Atheroma is said to be more prevalent in soft water areas — the reason is not known.

Can modification of the environmental factors influence the progress of atheroma?

Yes, by:
  (a) minimising further deposition of lipid,
  (b) minimising thrombotic complications,
  (c) perhaps allowing removal of some lipid from plaques — but, except in early cases, complete restoration to normal is not possible.

MECHANISMS INVOLVED

1. Endothelial Damage

There is a preferential distribution of lesions, e.g. arch of aorta, coronary arteries, cerebral arteries, carotids, abdominal aorta.
This is determined by local mechanical stresses which potentiate local endothelial damage.

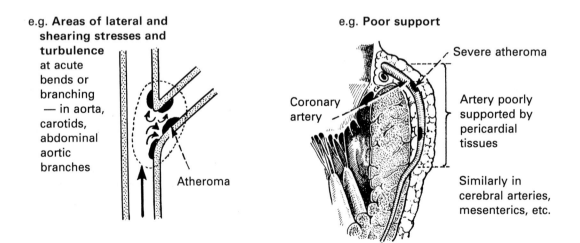

e.g. **Areas of lateral and shearing stresses and turbulence** at acute bends or branching — in aorta, carotids, abdominal aortic branches

Atheroma

e.g. **Poor support**

Coronary artery

Severe atheroma

Artery poorly supported by pericardial tissues

Similarly in cerebral arteries, mesenterics, etc.

ATHEROMA

MECHANISMS INVOLVED

Endothelial Damage (continued)

Other factors may contribute to endothelial damage as follows:

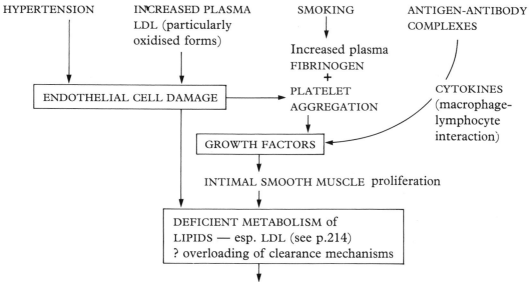

HYPERTENSION   INCREASED PLASMA LDL (particularly oxidised forms)   SMOKING   ANTIGEN-ANTIBODY COMPLEXES

Increased plasma FIBRINOGEN

ENDOTHELIAL CELL DAMAGE

PLATELET AGGREGATION

CYTOKINES (macrophage-lymphocyte interaction)

GROWTH FACTORS

INTIMAL SMOOTH MUSCLE proliferation

DEFICIENT METABOLISM of LIPIDS — esp. LDL (see p.214) ? overloading of clearance mechanisms

ATHEROMA

2. Lipid Deposition

This is related to (a) the ability of the intima to metabolise lipids and
(b) the types of lipid.

The ability of the intima to metabolise lipids:

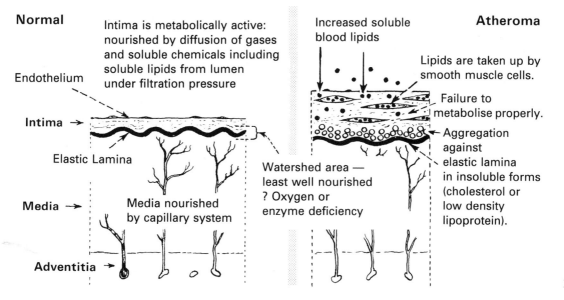

Normal

Intima is metabolically active: nourished by diffusion of gases and soluble chemicals including soluble lipids from lumen under filtration pressure

Endothelium

Intima →

Elastic Lamina

Media →   Media nourished by capillary system

Adventitia →

Increased soluble blood lipids

Atheroma

Lipids are taken up by smooth muscle cells.

Failure to metabolise properly.

Aggregation against elastic lamina in insoluble forms (cholesterol or low density lipoprotein).

Watershed area — least well nourished ? Oxygen or enzyme deficiency

213

ATHEROMA

LIPID METABOLISM in ATHEROGENESIS

As has been indicated previously, CHOLESTEROL and CHOLESTEROL-containing LIPOPROTEINS play an important role in atherogenesis.

The main cholesterol-containing lipoproteins are graded according to their density: the density divisions are arbitrary and represent overlapping averages.

Density ⟶ ↓ related to molecular size	Very low density lipoprotein **VLDL** - - - - - - - - - - Large molecule	Low density lipoprotein **LDL** - - - - - - - - - - Medium	High density lipoprotein HDL - - - - - - - - - - Small molecule
CHOLESTEROL CONTENT	Moderate	**HIGH** **LDL** accounts for 70% of plasma cholesterol	Low

Atheroma is specifically associated with high blood LDL levels (as well as total CHOLESTEROL levels).

LIPID METABOLISM is complex, involving many enzyme systems, receptors and binding molecules (ligands): all with feed-back controls.

The following is a much simplified summary indicating the 3 main sites of activity:

1. **MUSCLES and ADIPOSE TISSUES**

    There are 2 main sources for the supply of TRIGLYCERIDES required for local metabolism:

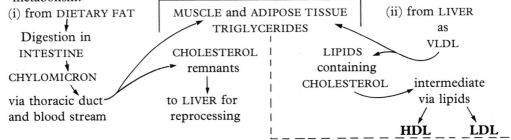

2. The **LIVER** is the main site of synthesis and reprocessing of lipids.

LIVER SYNTHESIS REPROCESSING	⟶ (a) bile acids and cholesterol to intestine. ⟶ (b) VLDL to muscle or adipose tissue. ⟵ LDL and other lipids.

3. The **SOMATIC CELLS** generally require CHOLESTEROL for the synthesis of cell membranes and steroids. LDL is the main source.

    LDL ⟨ majority reprocessed in the liver.
remainder for somatic cell use.

The plasma levels of LDL are conditioned by the delicate balance of these various activities. An understanding of them gives some indication of potential intervention sites.

ATHEROMA

ATHEROGENESIS (continued)

The 2 classical theories of atherogenesis were proposed in the 19th century.

1. The association of high blood cholesterol (and LDL) levels with atheroma gives support to the INSUDATION theory (Verchow). It stated that at sites of intimal damage insudation of lipid occurred and resulted in fat accumulation and fibrosis.

2. The THROMBOTIC theory (Rokitansky) proposed that thrombotic encrustation at the site of intimal injury initiated the atheromatous plaque and that the lipid was derived from the thrombus material (particularly platelets).

Formation of a plaque from platelet thrombus:

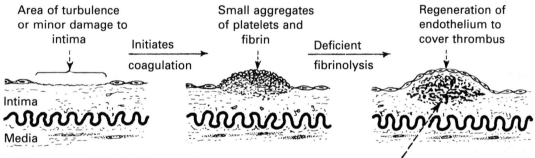

Subsequent similar incidents at the same site augment the atheromatous plaque.

Disintegration of components of thrombus leaving a lipid residue.

ATHEROMA

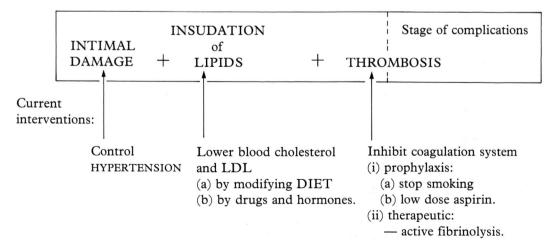

ARTERIOSCLEROSIS

ARTERIOSCLEROSIS usually affects all large and medium vessels.

Elastic and muscular tissues of media — — —

replaced by fibrous tissue impregnated with calcium salts

Sometimes particular individual arteries are affected — e.g. arteries at wrist and temple

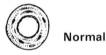

Normal

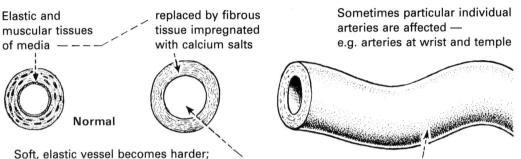

Soft, elastic vessel becomes harder; the collagen stretches so that lumen is **wider** and vessel becomes **tortuous**; as calcium impregnation increases the artery becomes very hard (pipe stem).

HYALINE ARTERIOLOSCLEROSIS affects the small branches of the arterial system (arterioles) — especially in the kidney.

Muscle replaced by hyaline material in media and intima

The arterioles also become tortuous

Normal

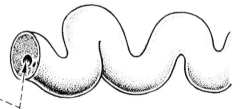

This is due to entry of blood plasma under the endothelium with protein deposition; gradual conversion to collagen occurs. The process is called **plasmatic vasculosis**.

Note that the lumen is usually narrowed so that ischaemia may be an important complication.

CONDITIONS ASSOCIATED

These changes, in mild form, represent the response of the arterial wall to wear and tear. The condition gradually progresses with **AGE**, usually in the arterial system generally, but individual arteries may be particularly affected, e.g. hard, tortuous temporal artery in old age. Certain diseases accelerate and aggravate arteriosclerosis:

1. Hypertension (high blood pressure) — a very important and common condition.
2. Diabetes (the small vessel changes are serious).

HYPERTENSION

HYPERTENSION (High Blood Pressure)

The normal BP in the large arteries of healthy young adult at the level of the heart is normally about 115/70mmHg. These figures are means derived from a range — systolic $\pm$ 20, diastolic $\pm$ 10.

Mechanisms of normal maintenance of BP and the effect of age

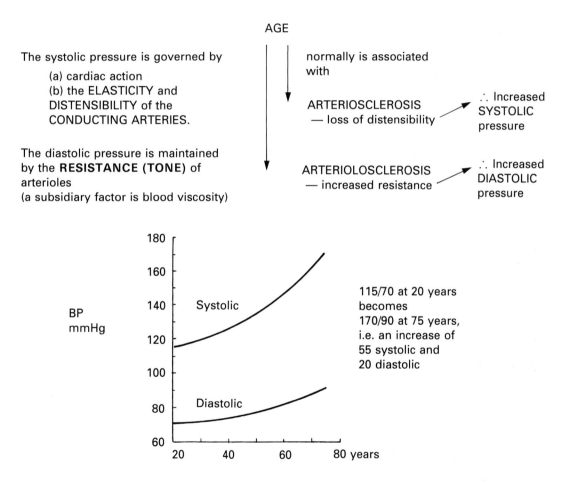

AGE

The systolic pressure is governed by
    (a) cardiac action
    (b) the ELASTICITY and
    DISTENSIBILITY of the
    CONDUCTING ARTERIES.

The diastolic pressure is maintained by the **RESISTANCE (TONE)** of arterioles
(a subsidiary factor is blood viscosity)

normally is associated with

ARTERIOSCLEROSIS
— loss of distensibility

$\therefore$ Increased SYSTOLIC pressure

ARTERIOLOSCLEROSIS
— increased resistance

$\therefore$ Increased DIASTOLIC pressure

BP mmHg

Systolic

Diastolic

20   40   60   80 years

115/70 at 20 years becomes
170/90 at 75 years,
i.e. an increase of
55 systolic and
20 diastolic

Because of this wide range in the normal population, the definition of hypertension is arbitrary.

Sustained DIASTOLIC pressures of 90 mmHg and above are commonly accepted as pathologically high, i.e. HYPERTENSION is present.

HYPERTENSION

AETIOLOGY

Complex interrelated effector mechanisms with feed-back controls regulate arteriolar tone. They are conveniently divided into two main groups:

(1) **Nervous**

(2) **Humoral (Hormonal)**

    (a) Pituitary   (b) SALT and water regulation

Afferent stimuli from:
- External environment,
- Internal environment
  — higher cerebral centres
  — chemoreceptors
  — viscera

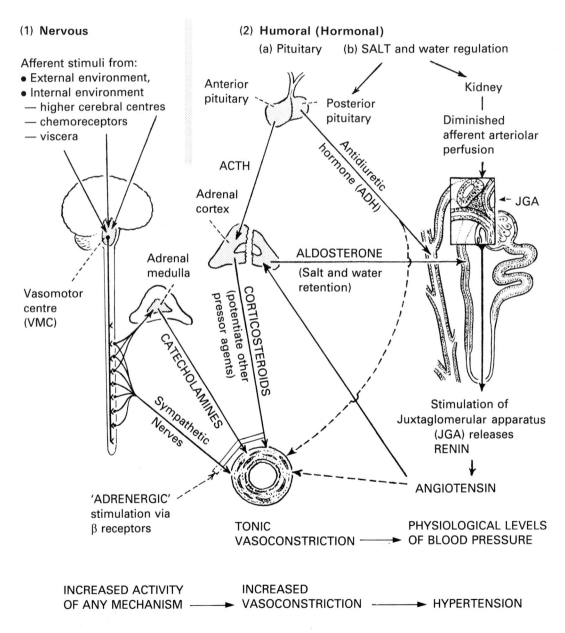

Anterior pituitary

Posterior pituitary

Kidney

Diminished afferent arteriolar perfusion

ACTH

Antidiuretic hormone (ADH)

Adrenal cortex

JGA

Vasomotor centre (VMC)

Adrenal medulla

ALDOSTERONE
(Salt and water retention)

CORTICOSTEROIDS
(potentiate other pressor agents)

CATECHOLAMINES

Sympathetic Nerves

Stimulation of Juxtaglomerular apparatus (JGA) releases RENIN

ANGIOTENSIN

'ADRENERGIC' stimulation via β receptors

TONIC VASOCONSTRICTION ⟶ PHYSIOLOGICAL LEVELS OF BLOOD PRESSURE

INCREASED ACTIVITY OF ANY MECHANISM ⟶ INCREASED VASOCONSTRICTION ⟶ HYPERTENSION

HYPERTENSION

In only 5–10% of all cases of hypertension is any disease which may be associated with disturbance of these mechanisms (see previous page) detectable — such cases are **SECONDARY HYPERTENSION.** Examples:

(a) **Kidney diseases,** especially if renal ischaemia is present, are the commonest cause of secondary hypertension.
(b) **Hyperfunction of** } Cushing's syndrome — corticosteroid excess.
    adrenal cortex } Conn's syndrome — aldosterone excess.
(c) **Tumour of adrenal medulla** (phaeochromocytoma) — catecholamine excess.
(d) **Drugs** may cause hypertension, e.g. the contraceptive pill, corticosteroids, sympathomimetics, monamine oxidase inhibitors if tyramine-containing foods (e.g. cheese) are eaten.
(e) Hypertension occurs in **toxaemia of pregnancy.**
(f) Miscellaneous rare diseases are:
— abnormalities of the vascular system e.g. coarctation (narrowing) of aorta
— increased blood viscosity — e.g. polycythaemia (increased RBC's).

In 90–95% of all cases of hypertension, no cause has been established — such cases are called **essential** or **idiopathic** or **primary.**

A plausible but speculative current theory is that in susceptible individuals the BP is unusually responsive to the afferent STRESSFUL stimuli which would normally be associated only with a mild rise.

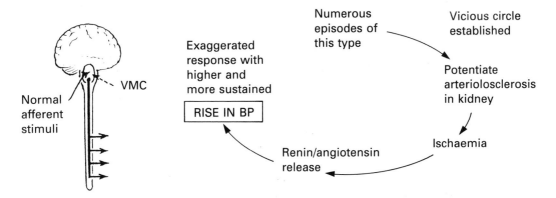

All the above mechanisms are essentially VASO-CONSTRICTOR. The possible roles of VASO-DILATOR mechanisms — for example the effect of NITRIC OXIDE on vascular smooth muscle — are being currently researched.

Genetic and background factors

There is a FAMILIAL incidence and there are very significant racial and geographical variations throughout the world: this is consistent with a polygenetic susceptibility.

HYPERTENSION

CLASSIFICATION

In the classification of hypertension, in addition to the aetiology, two other main factors are considered.

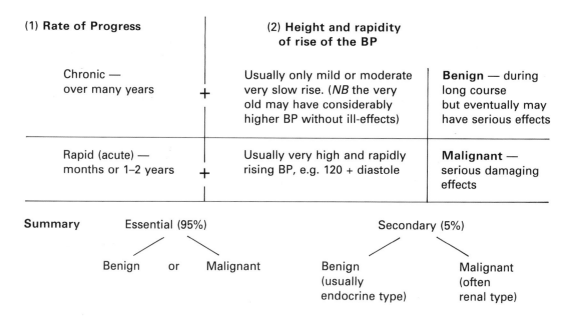

(1) **Rate of Progress**		(2) **Height and rapidity of rise of the BP**	
Chronic — over many years	+	Usually only mild or moderate very slow rise. (*NB* the very old may have considerably higher BP without ill-effects)	**Benign** — during long course but eventually may have serious effects
Rapid (acute) — months or 1–2 years	+	Usually very high and rapidly rising BP, e.g. 120 + diastole	**Malignant** — serious damaging effects

Summary   Essential (95%)   Secondary (5%)

          Benign   or   Malignant   Benign   Malignant
                                           (usually   (often
                                           endocrine type)   renal type)

COMPARISON of BENIGN and MALIGNANT HYPERTENSION

	Benign	Malignant
Aetiology	Usually ESSENTIAL If secondary, commonly of endocrine type	A few cases arise out of benign essential. Majority are SECONDARY TO RENAL DISEASE
Age	Begins younger than 45 years but is prolonged into 6 and 7 decades	Young adults 25–35 years
Sex	Female > Male	Female = Male
Incidence	VERY COMMON — at least 5% of population in Western societies	Rare
Course	VERY SLOW — many years	RAPID — months to 1–2 years
Blood pressure	Diastolic 90–120 mm Hg Very slow rise	120+ Rapid rise

HYPERTENSION

COMPARISON of BENIGN and MALIGNANT HYPERTENSION (continued)

VASCULAR CHANGES

	Benign	Malignant
Arteries	Accelerates ARTERIOSCLEROSIS; POTENTIATES ATHEROMA	Accelerates arteriosclerosis; causes INTIMAL FIBROUS THICKENING
Arterioles	Hyaline thickening	FIBRINOID necrosis of vessel wall and thrombosis, especially affecting kidney and abdominal viscera

Benign diagram: Lumen narrowed but open

Malignant diagram: Necrotic media infiltrated by fibrin; Cellular reaction; Lumen occluded by thrombus

EFFECTS and COMPLICATIONS in VARIOUS ORGANS

	Benign	Malignant
Eyes	Arterial narrowing — retinal exudation.	Papilloedema; arterial narrowing; haemorrhage and exudates
Heart	Hypertrophy of left ventricle	Hypertrophy of left ventricle $\pm$ focal myocardial necrosis
Heart failure	60% of cases	Acute heart failure
Cerebral haemorrhage	Due to rupture of damaged artery — 30% of cases	Encephalopathy (fits and loss of consciousness) due to cerebral oedema
Kidney	Varying degrees of NEPHROSCLEROSIS but usually *not* serious.	Severe renal damage — death in uraemia
Other organs	No significant damage.	Focal necrosis, e.g. gut → perforation.

The effects and complications are proportional to the height of the blood pressure. Therefore drug treatment which lowers the BP lowers the incidence of complications, but the diseased vessels do *not* return to normal and organ perfusion may be inadequate at levels of BP which would usually be considered physiological.

OTHER ARTERIAL DISEASES

Compared with atheroma and arteriosclerosis, which are very common, other arterial diseases are rare. They may be considered within the following broad groups:

(a) **Degenerative,**
(b) **Inflammatory** and
(c) **Miscellaneous.**

DEGENERATIVE ARTERIAL DISEASES

Monckeberg's sclerosis (medial calcification)

This condition which affects elderly people is best regarded as a variant of the arteriosclerosis of old age. The media of the arteries of the legs particularly is the site of deposition of large amounts of insoluble **calcium** salts, at first as circumferential bands but later becoming confluent so that the arteries become rigid tubes of hard chalk (pipe stem).
Note: The striking calcification, best seen on X-ray, is not associated with significant loss of lumen unless atheroma co-exists or is superimposed.

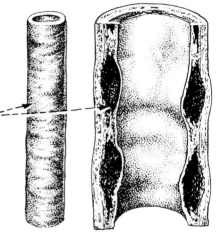

Erdheim's medial degeneration ("cystic medial necrosis")

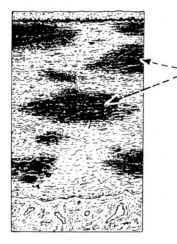

In this rare disease the media of the proximal aorta and occasionally its major branches is abnormal: the musculoelastic tissues are patchily replaced by a weaker mucoid material. The aetiology is unknown, but similar changes in the aorta occur in Marfan's syndrome — an inherited disorder of connective tissue metabolism. Erdheim's degeneration may be an incomplete variant of Marfan's syndrome.

These changes are important because they are the cause of a particularly fatal form of aneurysm (see 'Dissecting Aneurysm', p.228)

ARTERITIS

INFLAMMATORY DISEASES OF ARTERIES — ARTERITIS

(a) Associated with specific infectious diseases, e.g. tuberculosis and syphilis. The endarteritis and periarteritis, sometimes complicated by thrombosis, augment the damage caused by the infecting organisms.

(b) Arterial necrosis and inflammation of less certain or unknown aetiology.

Polyarteritis nodosa

This is a disease affecting the medium and small arteries and arterioles. In the acute phase, there are signs of generalised illness with fever, etc., but the disease often becomes chronic and relapsing so that all stages of the arterial lesion may be present at the same time.

The typical lesion is a focal necrosis of the arterial wall.

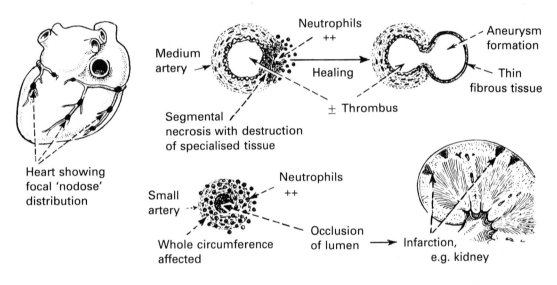

Heart showing focal 'nodose' distribution

Medium artery → Neutrophils ++ → Healing ± Thrombus → Aneurysm formation, Thin fibrous tissue

Segmental necrosis with destruction of specialised tissue

Small artery → Neutrophils ++, Occlusion of lumen → Infarction, e.g. kidney

Whole circumference affected

Any artery may be affected, but damage to the CORONARY or RENAL arteries is particularly important. When the arteries supplying peripheral nerves are affected symptoms of 'neuritis' may be striking.

Other forms of arteritis with some characteristics related to polyarteritis nodosa may occur as *primary disease processes*, e.g. *Wegener's granulomatosis* in which destructive lesions of the nasal mucosa, the lungs and the kidneys result from arteritis.

Arteritis may also complicate other conditions (usually the *connective tissue diseases*, see p.804), e.g. rheumatoid arthritis, systemic lupus erythematosus (SLE).

ARTERIAL DISEASES — MISCELLANEOUS

RAYNAUD'S PHENOMENON and DISEASE

Primary form

The phenomenon is essentially spasmodic attacks of pallor of the fingers (the toes, ears and nose may also be affected) due to intense constriction of the small arteries and arterioles in response to cold.

The condition is not rare and the usual sufferer is the young adult woman.

Mechanism

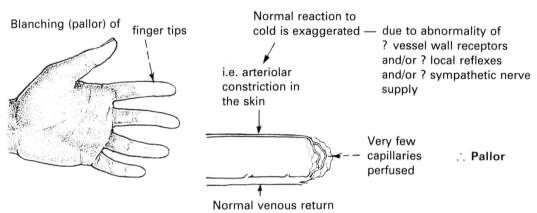

Blanching (pallor) of finger tips

Normal reaction to cold is exaggerated — due to abnormality of ? vessel wall receptors and/or ? local reflexes and/or ? sympathetic nerve supply

i.e. arteriolar constriction in the skin

Very few capillaries perfused ∴ **Pallor**

Normal venous return

In a variant, cyanosis accompanies the attack; neuromuscular control of the small veins is also disturbed.

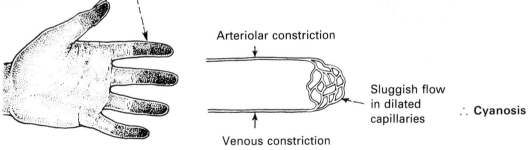

Arteriolar constriction

Sluggish flow in dilated capillaries ∴ **Cyanosis**

Venous constriction

This condition may continue for many years and NO PERMANENT DAMAGE RESULTS.

RAYNAUD'S DISEASE

The simple phenomenon is superseded by organic changes in the vessels — stenosis or occlusion — followed by degenerative changes in the skin and nerves of the fingers. Gangrene occasionally occurs. The term Raynaud's disease may be applied to this condition.

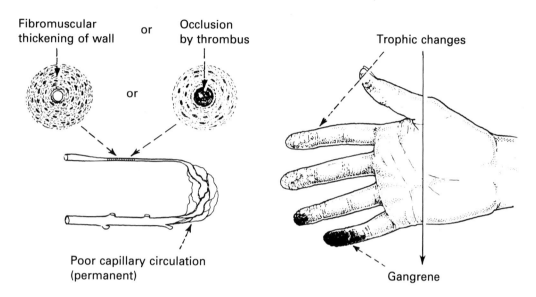

Fibromuscular thickening of wall — or — Occlusion by thrombus

or

Poor capillary circulation (permanent)

Trophic changes

Gangrene

The cause of this condition is unknown.

Secondary form

The phenomenon may occur as a symptom in other conditions, i.e. a secondary form of Raynaud's phenomenon. Examples include the 'connective tissue diseases', systemic lupus erythematosus (SLE) and systemic sclerosis (see p.805); cold agglutinins causing vascular blockage due to agglutination of red cells; the use of heavy pneumatic drills disturbing neurovascular controls in the hands.

In these circumstances the disease is serious and disabling, adding significantly to the damage caused by the primary diseases elsewhere in the body.

DISEASES OF VEINS

Diseases of the veins are important because they can be associated with:

(1) *Acute* severe, sometimes fatal, complications

(2) *Chronic* disability

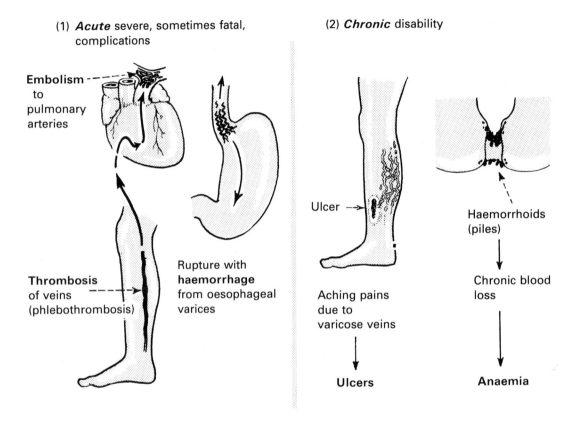

Embolism to pulmonary arteries

Thrombosis of veins (phlebothrombosis)

Rupture with **haemorrhage** from oesophageal varices

Ulcer →

Aching pains due to varicose veins

↓

Ulcers

Haemorrhoids (piles)

↓

Chronic blood loss

↓

Anaemia

ACUTE PHLEBOTHROMBOSIS AND THROMBOPHLEBITIS

The veins of the lower limbs are very common sites of acute thrombosis, especially after surgical operations and during illnesses with enforced recumbancy (see p.170).

In the majority of cases the thrombosis is the primary event and mild inflammation follows as a reaction. Phlebothrombosis is the preferred name.

Thrombophlebitis is reserved for cases in which the thrombosis is secondary to inflammation in or adjacent to the vein.

THROMBOPHLEBITIS

ACUTE PHLEBITIS

Suppurative (pyogenic)

Secondary to bacterial infection
e.g. a rare complication of
appendicitis

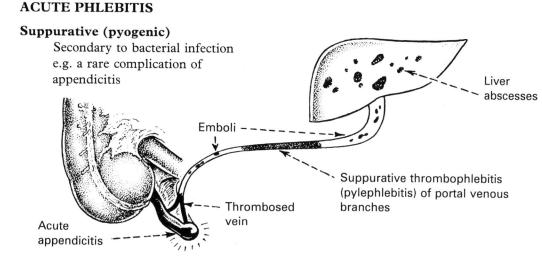

Liver
abscesses

Emboli

Suppurative thrombophlebitis
(pylephlebitis) of portal venous
branches

Thrombosed
vein

Acute
appendicitis

Migratory (thrombophlebitis migrans)

In this rare condition the thrombosis is not confined to the lower limb veins and can affect
veins anywhere in the body. A striking feature is the appearance and disappearance of
thrombosis apparently at random sites.

The mechanism is not fully understood but usually a malignant tumour is in the
background — sometimes the phlebitis is the first clinical sign of an occult tumour but
more often it complicates the terminal stages of tumour growth.

Possible mechanism

Circulating coagulation factors
derived from tumour (tumour
breakdown products or
inappropriate synthesis)

Fibrinolytic
system comes
into action

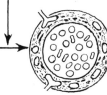

Initiation of
thrombosis in
small venous
radicles or
vasa vasorum
— local precipitating
factors not known

Formation of
loose red thrombus
in main lumen

Lysis of fibrin
coagulum —
restoration to normal

233

THROMBOPHLEBITIS

CHRONIC PHLEBITIS

(a) In small venous radicles it is an integral part of any chronic inflammatory process.

(b) Only occasionally does it affect larger veins.

(c) In **tuberculosis**, direct invasion and destruction of a vein wall can liberate tubercle bacilli throughout the body, causing miliary tuberculosis.

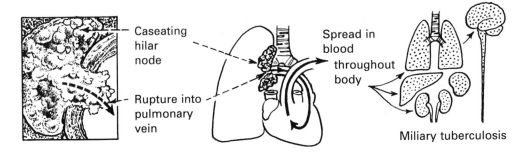

(d) **Hepatic venous occlusive disease** is a special type in which gradual occlusion of the hepatic veins and radicles is the result of gradual fibrous thickening of the venous intima and leads to serious disturbance in the liver. The disease is associated with the ingestion of alkaloids in 'bush' tea, particularly in the West Indies, but the mechanism is not known.

VEINS in MALIGNANT DISEASE

(a) Venules are easily invaded and infiltrated by carcinoma and are an important route in the metastatic spread of the tumour.

(b) Large veins, particularly in the mediastinum and pelvis, may be compressed from outside by the tumour — the resulting obstruction causing serious effects.

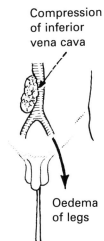

VARICOSE VEINS

This is a very common condition, the incidence increasing with **age**, and particularly high in **females** — often a sequel of pregnancy. The veins become prominent and tortuous and bulge outwards under the skin; the legs are particularly affected.

A **varix** is a localised bulge in a vein analogous to a saccular aneurysm in an artery. It is almost always associated with more generalised varicosity of the vein.

Aetiology

A vein wall, thin and composed of musculoelastic tissues, is designed to conduct blood at low pressures: the physiological movement of the blood is influenced mostly by pressure gradients derived from outside the vein wall.

Varicose veins arise when the vein wall is subjected to an increased expanding pressure (tension) over long periods.

Mechanism

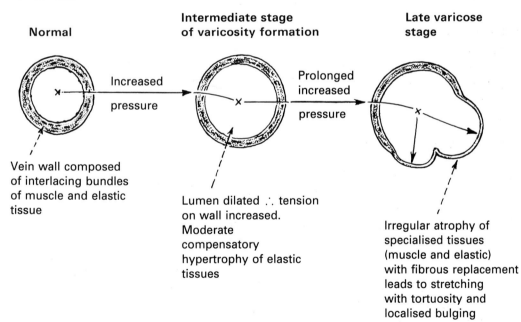

Normal

Intermediate stage of varicosity formation

Late varicose stage

Increased pressure

Prolonged increased pressure

Vein wall composed of interlacing bundles of muscle and elastic tissue

Lumen dilated ∴ tension on wall increased. Moderate compensatory hypertrophy of elastic tissues

Irregular atrophy of specialised tissues (muscle and elastic) with fibrous replacement leads to stretching with tortuosity and localised bulging

VARICOSE VEINS

FACTORS WHICH INFLUENCE THE BASIC MECHANISM

(a) Acting on the vein wall

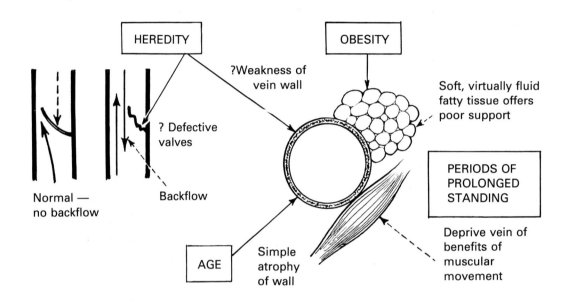

(b) Increasing the intraluminal pressure

1. Obstruction to venous flow
   — usually in the pelvis — by:
   Pregnancy
   Tumour
   Constipation with
   loaded colon
   Thrombosis in veins
   (also may destroy valves)
   Constrictions on limbs.

2. Special anatomical considerations.

Gravitational pressure of a long column of blood

Special communicating veins between deep and superficial systems, if valves not competent, cause backflow into super-ficial veins greatly increasing the pressure within them.

VARICOSE VEINS

Effects

1. Symptoms of leg fatigue and aching pains.
2. Trophic changes — varicose eczema with pigmentation due to haemosiderin deposition — may proceed to ULCERATION: very slow to heal.
3. Haemorrhage is a rare complication.
4. Thrombosis is a frequent complication.
   NB Superficial venous thrombosis is not usually associated with embolism; deep venous thrombosis is the dangerous condition.

VARICOSE VEINS IN SPECIAL SITES

Oesophageal varices

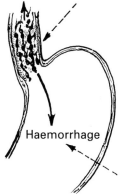

Usually due to portal venous obstruction when portal-systemic venous anastomoses open up.

Haemorrhage

Complicated by serious haemorrhage which may be fatal.

Varicocele

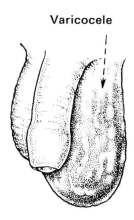

Affects the pampiniform plexus: feels like a 'bag of worms'. It may cause dull aching and, because the increased vascularity raises the scrotal temperature, testicular atrophy is common.

The condition has been incriminated in some cases of infertility.

Haemorrhoids

Varices of the anorectal veins; usually associated with constipation.

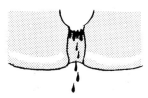

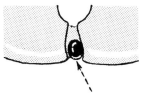

Complications are: 1. *anaemia* due to chronic blood loss

2. acute *thrombosis* with pain (acute thrombotic pile)

DISEASES OF LYMPHATICS

The lymphatic vessels participate in disease processes in two main ways:

1. They afford a natural route by which diseases can spread.
2. They may become obstructed, with serious results.

1. LYMPHATICS as a mechanism by which DISEASE SPREADS

The small lymphatics are delicate vessels formed by a simple endothelial layer with very little supporting tissue.

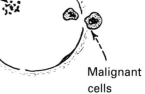

Malignant cells

Large intercellular pores allow entry of bacteria, tumour cells and particulate matter (e.g. dust) which are subsequently transported by the flow of lymph either freely suspended or in phagocytes to the draining node.

The mechanism is important in the spread of

(a) infection and (b) tumour.

Acute lymphangitis

The lymphatics draining an area infected by pyogenic bacteria (especially streptococci) may themselves become acutely inflamed.

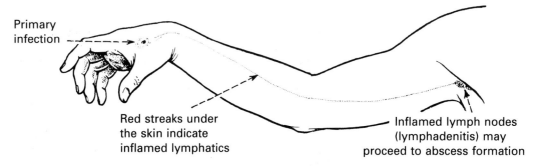

Primary infection

Red streaks under the skin indicate inflamed lymphatics

Inflamed lymph nodes (lymphadenitis) may proceed to abscess formation

Chronic lymphangitis

This is well exemplified by tuberculosis in both the primary and reactivation types.

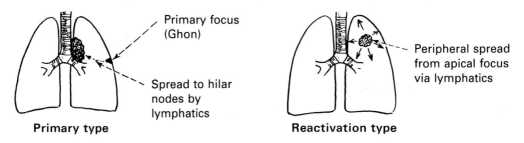

Primary focus (Ghon)

Spread to hilar nodes by lymphatics

Primary type

Peripheral spread from apical focus via lymphatics

Reactivation type

The lymphatics along the route of spread are thickened and show the typical histology of tuberculous granulation tissue.

238

DISEASES OF LYMPHATICS

LYMPHATIC SPREAD (continued)

Spread of tumours

This is an important route of spread of malignant tumours, especially carcinoma.

Disposal of particulate matter

This is well seen in the lungs where inhaled soot, especially in city dwellers, can be seen clearly indicating the lymphatic system under the pleura.

Soot (carbon) is relatively inert, but other dusts may initiate serious disease.

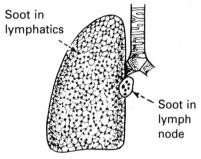

Soot in lymphatics

Soot in lymph node

2. LYMPHATIC OBSTRUCTION

This is usually secondary to acquired diseases. Only very rare cases are due to an inherited defect in the development of the lymphatics. The main causes are:

(a) Tumour growth

1. Obstruction by tumour permeation of lymphatics and/or destruction of lymph nodes, e.g. pelvic and groin nodes.

2. Direct pressure by large tumour mass. e.g.

3. Effects of treatment — scarring following surgery and radiotherapy.

e.g.

Brawny oedema

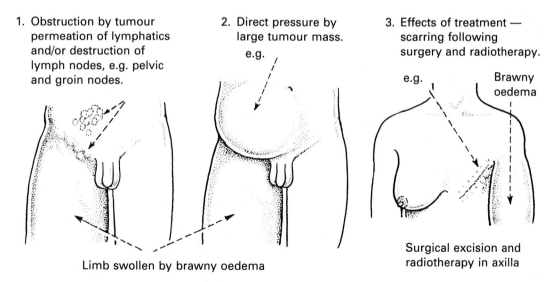

Limb swollen by brawny oedema

Surgical excision and radiotherapy in axilla

(b) Relapsing chronic lymphangitis and chronic inflammation

(c) Blocking by parasites. E.g. the adult worms of FILARIA occurring in the tropics.

DISEASES OF LYMPHATICS

Effects of chronic lymphatic obstruction

1. **Accumulation of fluid** in the tissues causing brawny swelling of the affected part

2. **Low grade inflammation**

Causes fibrosis

Further damage to lymphatics and establishment of a vicious circle

This is called lymphoedema ← Aggravation

Special effects (varieties of lymphoedema)

Peau d'orange — where the lymphatics of the skin are blocked by tumour.

Elephantiasis — where a limb and/ or the scrotum is massively enlarged due to filarial lymphatic blockage.

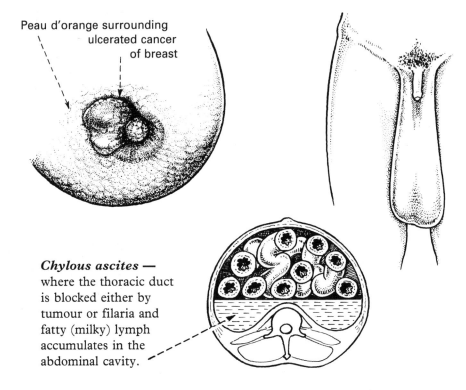

Peau d'orange surrounding ulcerated cancer of breast

Chylous ascites — where the thoracic duct is blocked either by tumour or filaria and fatty (milky) lymph accumulates in the abdominal cavity.

VASCULAR TUMOURS

The benign tumours of vessels are ANGIOMAS — the prefixes 'haem' and 'lymph' indicate the type of vessel involved. They illustrate well the difficulty of adequately defining the border line between true tumours (neoplasms) and hamartomas (developmental anomalies).

Since in many of these conditions vascular dilatation is a feature, the term ANGIECTASIS is sometimes applied and indicates clearly that neoplasia is not involved.

HAEMANGIOMAS are very common, occurring particularly in the skin as one type of birthmark but also in many solid organs. The ordinary tumours of blood vessels have been dealt with on page 152.

SPECIAL VARIETIES of ANGIOMA and TUMOUR-LIKE CONDITIONS

Occasionally specialised structures associated with blood vessels give rise to distinctive tumours:

1. (a) **GLOMANGIOMA** (glomus tumour) — arises from a specialised type of arteriolovenous junction which includes a rich neural component. A common site is the finger tip, perhaps under the nail: a very small but often excruciatingly *painful tumour*. Microscopically it consists of a complex of blood vessels lined by endothelium but cuffed by round clear cells with contractile properties (myoid cells). It is rich in nerve fibres.

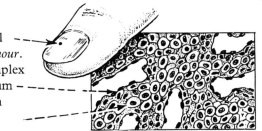

   (b) **ANGIOLEIOMYOMA** (related to glomangioma) is a tumour in which the surrounding cells are clearly of smooth muscle type.

   (c) **CHEMODECTOMA** — this benign tumour arises from specialised chemoreceptors, e.g. (1) glomus jugulare and (2) carotid body tumour.

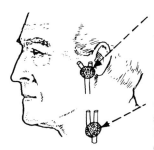

Glomus jugulare arising from jugular bulb and growing into middle ear — may be complicated by severe haemorrhage at operation.

Carotid body tumour — a firm, smooth, ovoid, yellow-brown lump (potato-like) arising at carotid bifurcation.

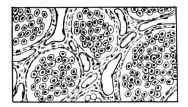

Packets of small chemoreceptor cells separated by sinusoids and capillaries

VASCULAR TUMOURS

2. INFECTED ANGIOMA — PYOGENIC GRANULOMA

There is debate as to whether this is a pre-existing angioma in which infection has supervened, or whether it is granulation tissue in which exuberant capillary growth is the main feature. It is a striking lesion appearing on the skin at a site subject to trauma and infection, e.g. around the finger nails, the nostrils or the tongue.

It grows over several days to form a small red nodular excrescence up to about 1 cm in diameter and is usually ulcerated.

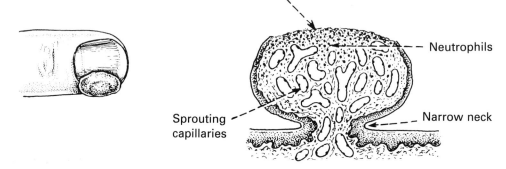

The lesion is entirely benign despite its rapid evolution and responds to simple removal.

3. TELANGIECTASIS

Small localised dilatations of small blood vessels. There are two main types: congenital and acquired.

(a) *Congenital.* In the rare hereditary haemorrhagic telangiectasis, the small lesions occur in the skin and mucous membranes and may be associated with bleeding (especially from the nose).

(b) *Acquired.* The small lesions, affecting the face and neck, are known as **spider naevi**.

The mechanism of their development is probably related to oestrogen excess, since they occur in pregnancy and in serious liver disease (oestrogen catabolism diminished) where they are an important diagnostic sign.

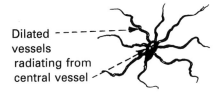

VASCULAR TUMOURS

LYMPHANGIOMA

Lymphangiomas are much rarer than haemangiomas and are usually without serious pathological significance.

Sometimes the abnormal lymphatic vessels become enormously distended and form fluctuant swellings with local pressure effects, e.g. 'cystic hygroma' of neck of babies and children.

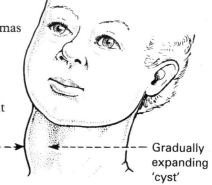

Gradually expanding 'cyst'

SARCOMAS

The extremely rare *malignant tumours* of vessels are classified as **sarcomas** and are true neoplasms.

Haemangiosarcoma (haemangioendothelioma) of the liver is of special interest in that it has occurred in workers in the plastics industry exposed to vinyl chloride.

Kaposi's sarcoma occurs endemically, particularly in tropical African males, as multiple skin lumps followed by extensive visceral involvement. In the West, cases were rare and sporadic until the arrival of AIDS in which Kaposi's sarcoma is now a common associated disease.

Lymphangiosarcoma is a very rare complication of radical mastectomy for breast carcinoma. The destruction of the axillary nodes and lymphatics at the time of operation followed by scarring causes lymphoedema. After many years lymphangiosarcoma may supervene as multicentre subcutaneous nodules. In some cases the differential diagnosis between recurrence of the original breast cancer and a sarcoma of lymphatic vessels is difficult.

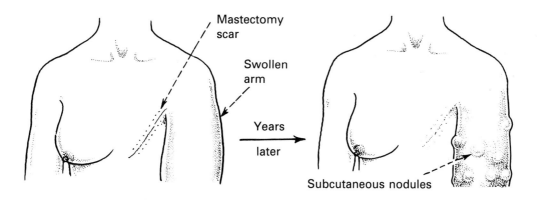

Mastectomy scar

Swollen arm

Years later

Subcutaneous nodules

CARDIAC FUNCTION

The essential function of the heart is to provide the pumping action in a closed circulation.

Comparison with a simple mechanical system is useful and valid provided that it is appreciated that the animal system is infinitely more sophisticated with delicate built-in controls and balances which influence the inotropic (intrinsic contractility) activity of the heart.

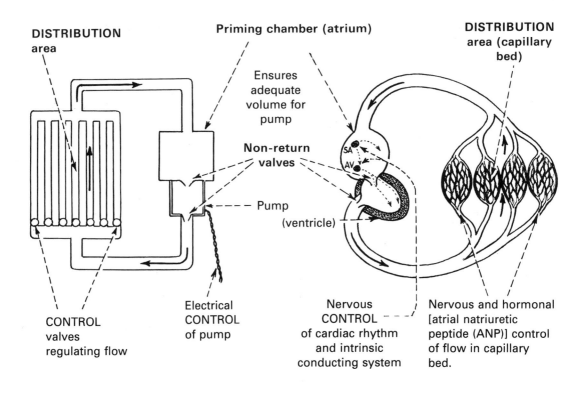

DISTRIBUTION area

Priming chamber (atrium)

DISTRIBUTION area (capillary bed)

Ensures adequate volume for pump

Non-return valves

Pump (ventricle)

CONTROL valves regulating flow

Electrical CONTROL of pump

Nervous CONTROL of cardiac rhythm and intrinsic conducting system

Nervous and hormonal [atrial natriuretic peptide (ANP)] control of flow in capillary bed.

The pump is the essential part of the system: it has to be flexible to accommodate any changes required in the distribution side of the system.

In the animal circulation, very great reserves of ventricular muscle power are available to meet the wide range of metabolic activity required in the distribution area.

HEART FAILURE

Heart failure occurs when the ***ventricular muscle*** is incapable of maintaining a circulation adequate for the needs of the body (usually assessed in terms of O_2 requirement).

Although, in the last analysis, heart failure is the result of myocardial failure, it is useful to separate the situations in which heart failure occurs into two main groups:

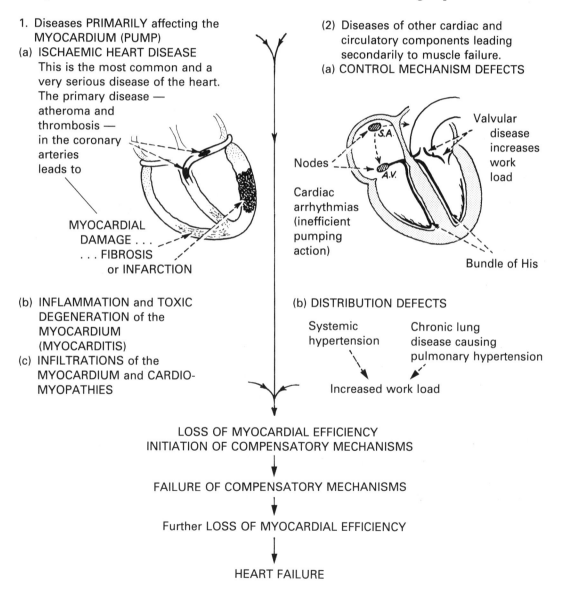

1. Diseases PRIMARILY affecting the MYOCARDIUM (PUMP)

(a) ISCHAEMIC HEART DISEASE
This is the most common and a very serious disease of the heart. The primary disease — atheroma and thrombosis — in the coronary arteries leads to

MYOCARDIAL DAMAGE ...
... FIBROSIS
or INFARCTION

(b) INFLAMMATION and TOXIC DEGENERATION of the MYOCARDIUM (MYOCARDITIS)
(c) INFILTRATIONS of the MYOCARDIUM and CARDIO-MYOPATHIES

(2) Diseases of other cardiac and circulatory components leading secondarily to muscle failure.
(a) CONTROL MECHANISM DEFECTS

Valvular disease increases work load

Nodes

S.A.
A.V.

Cardiac arrhythmias (inefficient pumping action)

Bundle of His

(b) DISTRIBUTION DEFECTS

Systemic hypertension

Chronic lung disease causing pulmonary hypertension

Increased work load

LOSS OF MYOCARDIAL EFFICIENCY
INITIATION OF COMPENSATORY MECHANISMS

FAILURE OF COMPENSATORY MECHANISMS

Further LOSS OF MYOCARDIAL EFFICIENCY

HEART FAILURE

HEART FAILURE

COMPENSATORY MECHANISMS

The myocardial reserve is provided by three main mechanisms:

1. **Increased rate of pumping**
2. **Dilatation** of the ventricular chambers
   (due to increased muscle stretching)
   } are designed to meet the normal physiological reserves
3. **Hypertrophy** is added to these when the pumping load exceeds physiological levels.

   In the heart under pathological strain, all three mechanisms are operative and can compensate for considerable derangement.

DILATATION

In physiological conditions, the volume of the ventricular chamber at the end of diastole directly influences the pumping force of the ventricular muscle thus:

The larger the chamber size
(i.e. the longer the initial fibre length
(i.e. the greater the fibre stretch)
} the greater the contracting force.

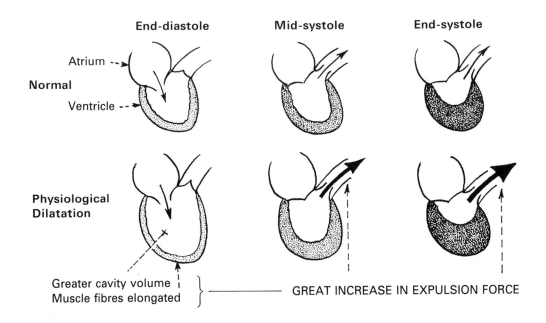

This physiological dilatation also compensates in cardiac disease.

HEART FAILURE

Compensatory mechanisms — Dilatation (continued)

In cardiac disease, particularly in cases of valvular incompetence, dilatation which occurs passively to accommodate the regurgitated blood is an important factor.

Aortic valve incompetence is a good example:

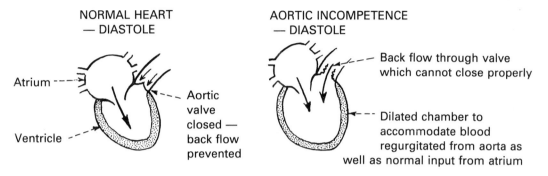

**NORMAL HEART
— DIASTOLE**

Atrium

Ventricle

Aortic valve closed — back flow prevented

**AORTIC INCOMPETENCE
— DIASTOLE**

Back flow through valve which cannot close properly

Dilated chamber to accommodate blood regurgitated from aorta as well as normal input from atrium

HYPERTROPHY involves an increase in muscle fibre bulk; the increased muscle mass is able to deal with a greater work load. In its pure form, hypertrophy is seen best in cases of increased pressure load.

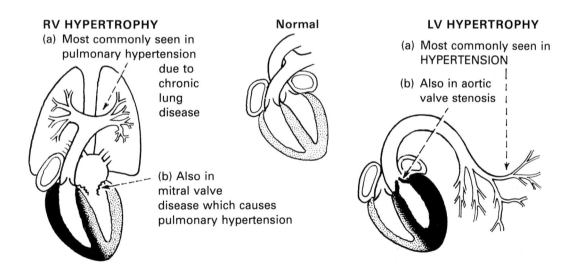

RV HYPERTROPHY
(a) Most commonly seen in pulmonary hypertension due to chronic lung disease

(b) Also in mitral valve disease which causes pulmonary hypertension

Normal

LV HYPERTROPHY
(a) Most commonly seen in HYPERTENSION

(b) Also in aortic valve stenosis

At first the blood supply to the hypertrophied muscle increases to meet the increased metabolic requirements.

HEART FAILURE

FAILURE of COMPENSATORY MECHANISMS

The increased efficiency derived from all three mechanisms is limited, and beyond this limit serious deficiency ensues — HEART FAILURE.

Beyond the critical limit:

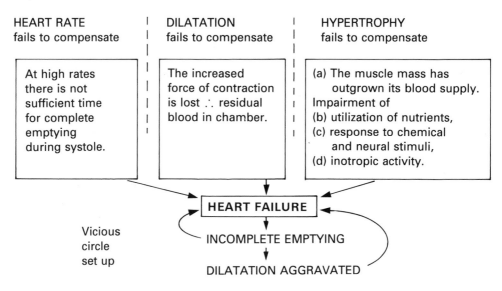

HEART RATE fails to compensate	DILATATION fails to compensate	HYPERTROPHY fails to compensate
At high rates there is not sufficient time for complete emptying during systole.	The increased force of contraction is lost ∴ residual blood in chamber.	(a) The muscle mass has outgrown its blood supply. Impairment of (b) utilization of nutrients, (c) response to chemical and neural stimuli, (d) inotropic activity.

HEART FAILURE

Vicious circle set up → INCOMPLETE EMPTYING → DILATATION AGGRAVATED

Thus in most cases of heart failure there is CARDIAC ENLARGEMENT due usually to a combination of hypertrophy and dilatation.

The **Effects** of heart failure are seen in the peripheral organs and are due to HYPOXIA and VENOUS CONGESTION.

(a) **Hypoxia** is well exemplified in the acute form of left ventricular failure where cerebral function may be seriously disturbed with transient loss of consciousness — Stokes-Adams attacks.

In the chronic forms of heart failure, the **weakness and fatigue** which are so common symptoms are probably effects mainly of **hypoxia**, but damage to organs is more difficult to define since the effects of venous congestion and water retention are added.

(b) **Venous congestion** and the more important complication, **oedema**, have been dealt with on page 184.

Breathlessness (dyspnoea) is almost a constant concomitant of cardiac failure and is essentially due to venous congestion and fluid retention within the lungs.

In severe failure, particularly when bed rest is obligatory, *hypostatic pneumonia* and *pulmonary embolism* (from leg vein thrombosis) may be serious and terminal complications.

HEART FAILURE

ACUTE and CHRONIC

Assignment to a particular category depends on the **suddenness of onset** and **rate of development**.

The causative diseases and the effects are different.

	Acute	Chronic
Time factors	Instantaneous Sudden (Hours — a few days)	January February M 5 12 19 26 2 9 16 23 T 6 13 20 27 3 10 17 24 W 7 14 21 28 4 11 18 25 T 1 8 15 22 29 5 12 19 26 F 2 9 16 23 30 6 13 20 27 S 3 10 17 24 31 7 14 21 28 S 4 11 18 25 1 8 15 22 29 Weeks Months
Causal diseases	(a) ACUTE CORONARY ARTERIAL OCCLUSION with infarction or arrhythmia (b) Pulmonary embolism (c) Severe malignant hypertension (d) Acute toxic myocarditis	(a) Chronic hypertension (b) Myocardial fibrosis (coronary intimal atheroma and hypertension) (c) Chronic valvular diseases (d) Chronic lung diseases (e) Chronic severe anaemia
Effects	May be no time for compensatory mechanisms to be initiated. Acute pulmonary oedema is common. May be acute ischaemic effects in brain and kidneys.	Compensatory mechanisms fully developed — hypertrophy and dilatation. Chronic oedema and chronic venous congestion.

Acute and chronic failure are at opposite ends of a spectrum but may merge into each other in two ways.

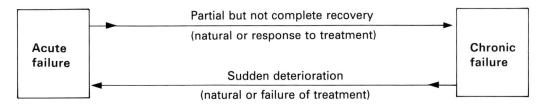

HEART FAILURE

LEFT (LV) and RIGHT (RV) and COMBINED VENTRICULAR FAILURE

The simple diagram on page 244 illustrates a single ventricle and distribution area. In the human, the system consists of two circulations in sequence (series) and the heart acts as both the pump and the connecting link. The right ventricle is the pump for the pulmonary circulation and the left for the systemic circulation. The causes and effects of right and left ventricular failure are different.

The pulmonary circulation

A low pressure system
  Systolic arterial pressure = 24mm Hg
  Pressure gradient, artery/vein = 8mm Hg

The systemic circulation

A high pressure system
  Systolic arterial pressure = 120mm Hg
  Pressure gradient, artery/vein = 90mm Hg

Right ventricular mass   Left ventricular mass
and coronary blood supply < and coronary blood supply

1:4 (approx.)

MAIN CAUSES of:

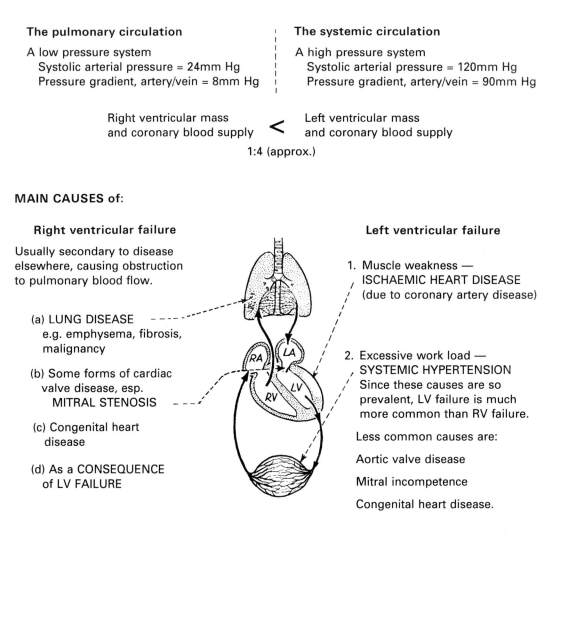

Right ventricular failure

Usually secondary to disease elsewhere, causing obstruction to pulmonary blood flow.

(a) LUNG DISEASE
    e.g. emphysema, fibrosis, malignancy

(b) Some forms of cardiac valve disease, esp.
    MITRAL STENOSIS

(c) Congenital heart disease

(d) As a CONSEQUENCE of LV FAILURE

Left ventricular failure

1. Muscle weakness —
   ISCHAEMIC HEART DISEASE
   (due to coronary artery disease)

2. Excessive work load —
   SYSTEMIC HYPERTENSION
   Since these causes are so prevalent, LV failure is much more common than RV failure.

Less common causes are:

Aortic valve disease

Mitral incompetence

Congenital heart disease.

HEART FAILURE

RV, LV and COMBINED VENTRICULAR FAILURE (continued)

Left ventricular failure is the initiating event in most cases of combined failure.

The main effects are the results of:

(a) low output
(b) 'backward' pressure

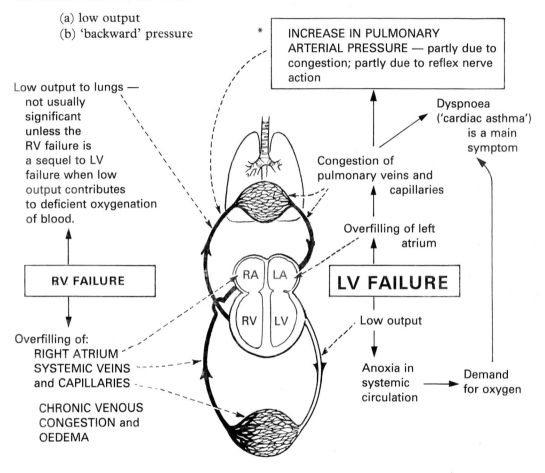

* INCREASE IN PULMONARY
ARTERIAL PRESSURE — partly due to
congestion; partly due to reflex nerve
action

Low output to lungs —
not usually
significant
unless the
RV failure is
a sequel to LV
failure when low
output contributes
to deficient oxygenation
of blood.

Dyspnoea
('cardiac asthma')
is a main
symptom

Congestion of
pulmonary veins and
capillaries

Overfilling of left
atrium

RA LA

RV FAILURE

LV FAILURE

RV LV

Low output

Overfilling of:
RIGHT ATRIUM
SYSTEMIC VEINS
and CAPILLARIES

CHRONIC VENOUS
CONGESTION and
OEDEMA

Anoxia in
systemic
circulation

Demand
for oxygen

Cyanosis is the result
of excess reduced haemoglobin
in capillaries and venules.

* The increase in pulmonary arterial pressure is important because in most cases of chronic LV
failure it eventually leads to RV failure (combined failure).

HEART FAILURE

The distinction between right and left ventricular failure is valid and certainly useful from a clinical point of view.

However, it should be remembered that in health the function of both ventricles is closely integrated in that they have the same capacity, pump virtually synchronously and are constructed in such a way that layers of muscle fibres pass from one ventricle to the other.

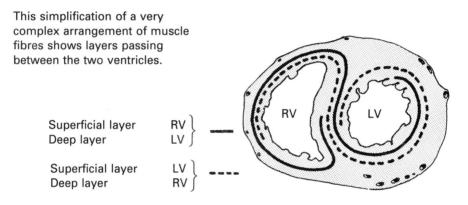

This simplification of a very complex arrangement of muscle fibres shows layers passing between the two ventricles.

Superficial layer   RV ⎱
Deep layer   LV ⎰ ——

Superficial layer   LV ⎱
Deep layer   RV ⎰ - - - -

Thus the action of each ventricle is not isolated; it both influences and is influenced by the action of the other. Therefore, in addition to the combined failure which arises as a later consequence of left ventricular failure, (see p.264), cases which begin and progress as combined failure are not uncommon.

Effects

These are a combination of the separate effects of LV and RV failure which have been described above.

In particular, PLEURAL EFFUSION (Hydrothorax) is a common effect of chronic combined heart failure.

OEDEMA fluid is contributed:

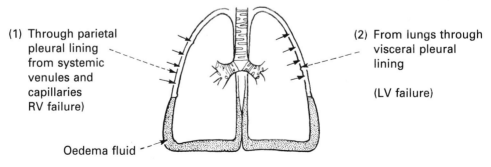

(1) Through parietal pleural lining from systemic venules and capillaries RV failure)

(2) From lungs through visceral pleural lining

(LV failure)

Oedema fluid

HEART FAILURE

LOW and HIGH OUTPUT FAILURE

By definition, in cardiac failure, output is low in respect of body requirements, and in most cases this output is lower than the usual normal output. Such cases are called **Low Output type**.

In a few conditions, the cardiac failure complicates a pre-existing state in which the output before failure was greater than normal. In these cases, the output is not sufficient to meet the body requirements but may still be higher than the normal. Such cases are called **High Output type**.

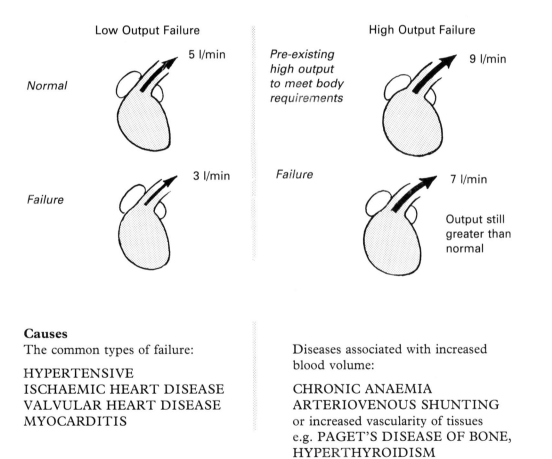

Causes

The common types of failure:

HYPERTENSIVE
ISCHAEMIC HEART DISEASE
VALVULAR HEART DISEASE
MYOCARDITIS

Diseases associated with increased blood volume:

CHRONIC ANAEMIA
ARTERIOVENOUS SHUNTING
or increased vascularity of tissues
e.g. PAGET'S DISEASE OF BONE,
HYPERTHYROIDISM
following TRANSFUSION OVERLOAD.

In both types of failure, venous overfilling is an important sign, but in high output failure, venous overfilling is usually present before failure ensues, reflecting the increased blood volume.

ISCHAEMIC HEART DISEASE

The effects of cardiac ischaemia are of major importance in affluent Western societies, causing severe disability and a large proportion of deaths.

The ischaemia is almost always due to *atheroma* of the coronary arteries and its complications which cause occlusion or narrowing.

The EFFECTS are mainly exhibited in the ventricles, particularly the left.

The ischaemia may be of sudden or gradual onset, depending on the nature of the coronary artery disease.

	Causes	Effects	Clinical Effects
Acute ischaemia	Usually ACUTE CORONARY ARTERY OCCLUSION due to THROMBOSIS	Myocardial necrosis, i.e. INFARCTION, depending on several factors, e.g. site, size etc.	(a) SUDDEN DEATH (b) ACUTE ILLNESS with heart failure, cardiogenic shock, chest pain. (c) ARRHYTHMIAS (d) SILENT
Chronic ischaemia	Usually CORONARY ARTERY NARROWING (STENOSIS) with or without thrombotic occlusion of small vessels	MYOCARDIAL FIBROSIS	(a) ANGINA PECTORIS (b) LV failure RV failure or combined failure from the start

Although acute and chronic ischaemia are properly separated both in respect of their causes and effects, they are often related as follows:

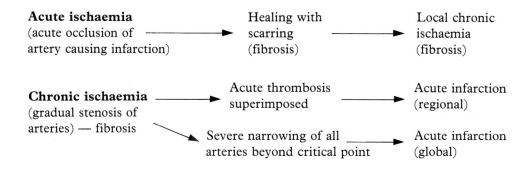

CORONARY ARTERY DISEASE

Atheroma affecting the coronary arteries is essentially the same as atheroma affecting the arteries elsewhere in the body and is subject to the same type of complication and effects. Its major importance is that serious disease of the myocardium is a direct complication.

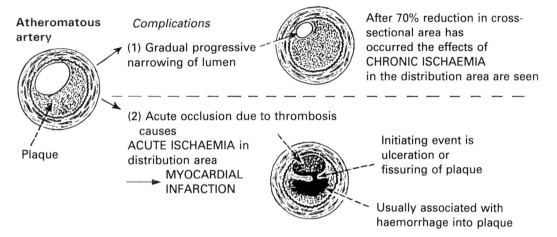

Atheromatous artery

Complications

(1) Gradual progressive narrowing of lumen

After 70% reduction in cross-sectional area has occurred the effects of CHRONIC ISCHAEMIA in the distribution area are seen

Plaque

(2) Acute occlusion due to thrombosis causes
ACUTE ISCHAEMIA in distribution area
→ MYOCARDIAL INFARCTION

Initiating event is ulceration or fissuring of plaque

Usually associated with haemorrhage into plaque

Note: Microemboli from a ruptured plaque may compromise the circulation in the distal arterial distribution, but major coronary embolism and other types of arterial disease are very rare causes of ischaemia.

Distribution of atheromatous plaques

(1) There may be only a few plaques, but because the sites of predilection are in the proximal parts of the arteries (usually within 3 cm of the origin from the aorta), the effects of occlusion are serious.

(2) Very numerous plaques throughout the arborisation on the surface of the heart.
Note: The small terminal arteries penetrating the myocardium are usually not significantly affected.

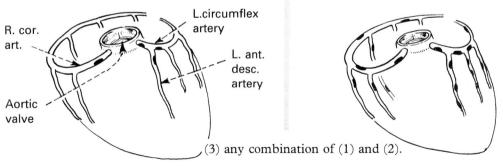

R. cor. art.

L.circumflex artery

L. ant. desc. artery

Aortic valve

(3) any combination of (1) and (2).

The site of ischaemic damage usually represents the distribution area of the diseased arterial branch.

255

ACUTE ISCHAEMIA — MYOCARDIAL INFARCTION

Recently an interesting phenomenon called ISCHAEMIC PRECONDITIONING has been described. It has been shown in animals that brief periods of ischaemia, insufficient to cause necrosis, precondition the heart muscle to withstand episodes of more prolonged ischaemia with very significant reduction in the infarct size. It is possible that such a mechanism is operative in patients with unstable angina due to severe coronary atheroma.

REGIONAL INFARCTION

This is the common type and is the direct result of coronary arterial occlusion usually due to **thrombosis**. (Regional infarction without thrombotic occlusion is very rare.)

GLOBAL OR CIRCUMFERENTIAL SUBENDOCARDIAL INFARCTION

This type is not common. It occurs round the circumference of the left ventricle under the endocardium in cases of severe stenosis of all the coronary arteries and is often without thrombosis.

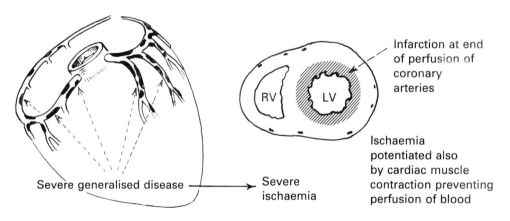

Severe generalised disease ⟶ Severe ischaemia

Infarction at end of perfusion of coronary arteries

Ischaemia potentiated also by cardiac muscle contraction preventing perfusion of blood

Global infarction is a serious, almost invariably fatal condition.

MICROSCOPIC FOCAL INFARCTION

This is necrosis of single or small groups of muscle fibres at the margins of areas of myocardium previously damaged by ischaemia and is a component of progressive chronic ischaemia.

MYOCARDIAL INFARCTION

Time			
0–8 hrs	No change	Normal appearance	No change
8–24 hrs	Minimal change	Slight blotchiness (congestion and pallor) of infarcted area	Slight separation of fibres; slight increase of leucocytes between fibres; slight disturbance of cell cytoplasm *Normal* | *Affected fibres*
24 hrs –3 days	Definite changes in dead muscle	Dead muscle, paler yellow Note: Usually a thin layer of healthy muscle under the endocardium	Dead muscle fibres have lost striations and nuclei; cytoplasm glassy pink (H & E staining); capillary congestion at margin; neutrophils and macrophages increasing in number

MYOCARDIAL INFARCTION

Time			
3–10 days	Healing (organisation) commencing	Margin of congestion (redness) appearing round dead muscle and resorption of muscle becoming visible at the edges	Muscle fibres splitting up and being resorbed; granulation tissue at edges; neutrophils still present
10 days onwards	Healing well advanced	Broad zone of granulation tissue — translucent pink or grey; resorption of dead muscle well advanced	Well established granulation tissue with fibroblastic activity; cellularity now much less
Weeks — months	Scar tissue — healing complete	White fibrous tissue	Scar tissue — may be occasional surviving muscle fibres embedded Scar tissue — may be occasional surviving muscle fibres embedded

These changes represent the uncomplicated continuous process of healing. However, complications are frequent, producing serious, often fatal, effects.

MYOCARDIAL INFARCTION

Time	COMPLICATIONS
Minutes, hours	 **1. ARRHYTHMIAS** (a) *Ventricular fibrillation*, i.e. cardiac arrest (especially liable at onset of infarction and during first few days). (b) *Block of impulse conduction in Bundle of His and/or its branches* — usually causes slowing of ventricular rhythm or upsets the balance of ventricular contraction. **2. CARDIOGENIC SHOCK** Associated with large infarcts.	**Acute heart failure** — *often FATAL*

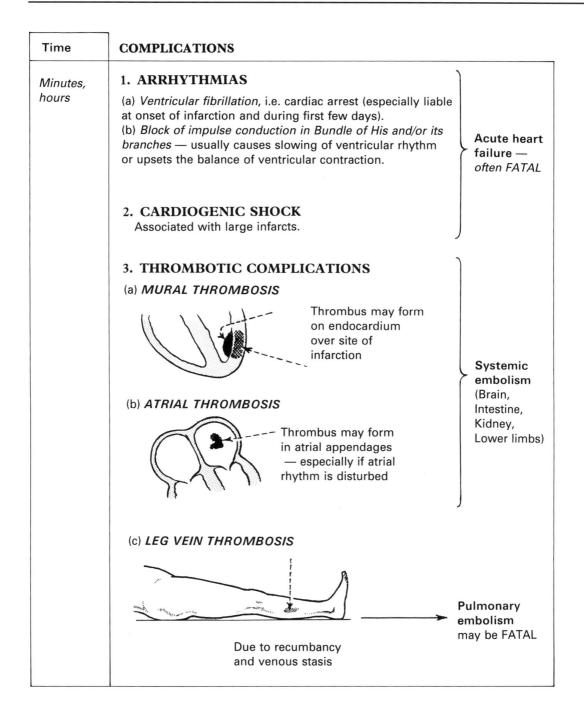

3. THROMBOTIC COMPLICATIONS

(a) *MURAL THROMBOSIS*

Thrombus may form on endocardium over site of infarction

(b) *ATRIAL THROMBOSIS*

Thrombus may form in atrial appendages — especially if atrial rhythm is disturbed

Systemic embolism (Brain, Intestine, Kidney, Lower limbs)

(c) *LEG VEIN THROMBOSIS*

Due to recumbancy and venous stasis

Pulmonary embolism may be FATAL

MYOCARDIAL INFARCTION

Time	COMPLICATIONS (continued)
3–14 days	**4. RUPTURE OF HEART** Potentiated by: (a) infarction of whole wall thickness (b) unusual increased neutrophil activity before organisation is established → softening of dead muscle (myomalacia cordis) **Sites affected and results** (i) *MURAL MYOCARDIUM* 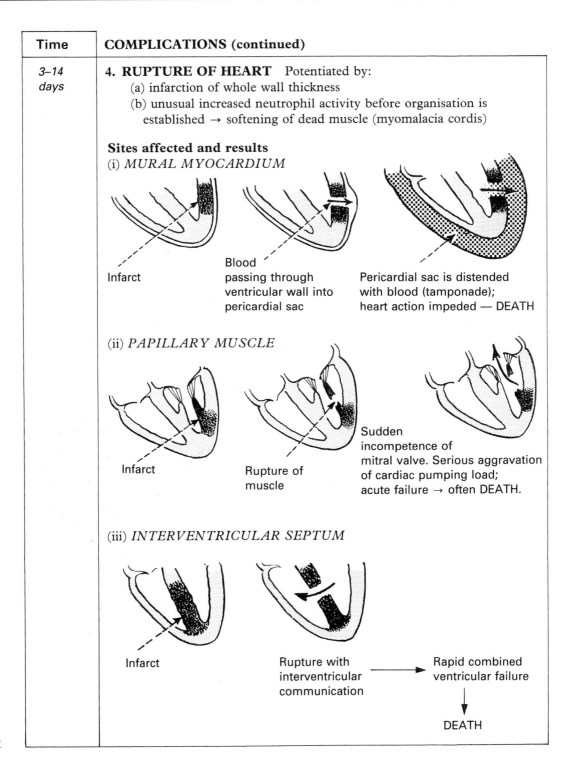 Infarct Blood passing through ventricular wall into pericardial sac Pericardial sac is distended with blood (tamponade); heart action impeded — DEATH (ii) *PAPILLARY MUSCLE* Infarct Rupture of muscle Sudden incompetence of mitral valve. Serious aggravation of cardiac pumping load; acute failure → often DEATH. (iii) *INTERVENTRICULAR SEPTUM* Infarct Rupture with interventricular communication → Rapid combined ventricular failure DEATH

MYOCARDIAL INFARCTION

Time	COMPLICATIONS (continued)
3–14 days	**5. ACUTE PERICARDITIS** This may complicate the infarct.
Weeks	**6. CHRONIC HEART FAILURE** At the stage of fibrosis, chronic heart failure may supervene ($\pm$ ANGINA PECTORIS).
Months	**7. CARDIAC ANEURYSM** 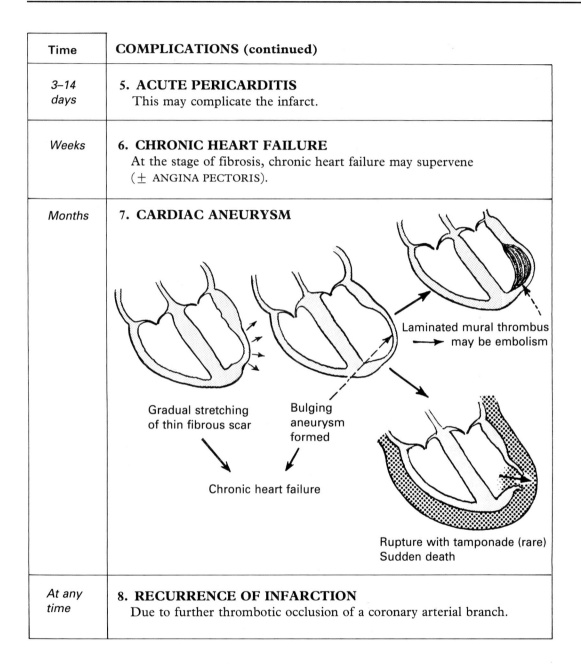 Gradual stretching of thin fibrous scar Bulging aneurysm formed → Chronic heart failure Laminated mural thrombus → may be embolism Rupture with tamponade (rare) Sudden death
At any time	**8. RECURRENCE OF INFARCTION** Due to further thrombotic occlusion of a coronary arterial branch.

CHRONIC ISCHAEMIC HEART DISEASE

The basic pathological process is replacement of the myocardial fibres by fibrous tissue which is laid down in two main ways depending on whether the coronary insufficiency is due to severe generalised stenosis or is the result of local infarction following thrombosis.

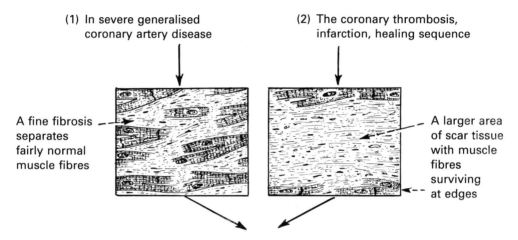

(1) In severe generalised coronary artery disease

(2) The coronary thrombosis, infarction, healing sequence

A fine fibrosis separates fairly normal muscle fibres

A larger area of scar tissue with muscle fibres surviving at edges

However, in many cases both mechanisms are present and lesions merge indistinguishably into each other.

Myocardial fibrosis tends to be progressive, reflecting the progression of the atheromatous narrowing of the arteries.

Myocardial hypertrophy from any cause is an important contributory factor in many cases.

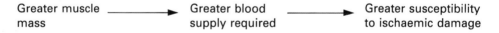

Greater muscle mass ⟶ Greater blood supply required ⟶ Greater susceptibility to ischaemic damage

Thus hypertension, which causes left ventricular hypertrophy, is an important background factor.

ISCHAEMIC HEART DISEASE

CLINICAL, LABORATORY and ELECTROCARDIOGRAPH (ECG) EFFECTS

Cardiac Pain is caused by muscle ischaemia as follows:

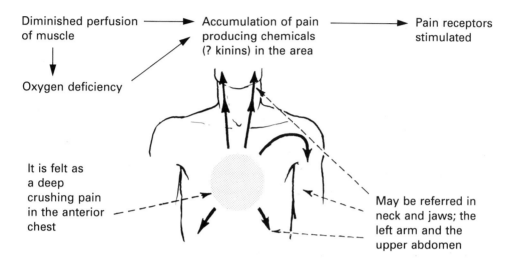

Diminished perfusion of muscle ⟶ Accumulation of pain producing chemicals (? kinins) in the area ⟶ Pain receptors stimulated

Oxygen deficiency

It is felt as a deep crushing pain in the anterior chest

May be referred in neck and jaws; the left arm and the upper abdomen

It occurs in two main circumstances:

1. **In acute infarction** — especially in the early phases before necrosis is complete. It is usually a continuous pain — *not* relieved by rest.

2. **In chronic myocardial ischaemia without infarction,** e.g. ANGINA PECTORIS — episodes of cardiac pain brought on by temporary ischaemia.

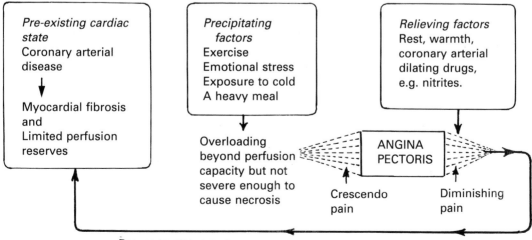

Pre-existing cardiac state
Coronary arterial disease

Myocardial fibrosis and Limited perfusion reserves

Precipitating factors
Exercise
Emotional stress
Exposure to cold
A heavy meal

Overloading beyond perfusion capacity but not severe enough to cause necrosis

Relieving factors
Rest, warmth, coronary arterial dilating drugs, e.g. nitrites.

ANGINA PECTORIS

Crescendo pain

Diminishing pain

Return to status quo

ISCHAEMIC HEART DISEASE

CLINICAL, LABORATORY and ECG EFFECTS (continued)
The blood in myocardial infarction

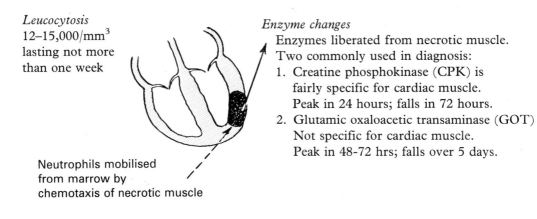

Leucocytosis
12–15,000/mm^3
lasting not more
than one week

Neutrophils mobilised
from marrow by
chemotaxis of necrotic muscle

Enzyme changes
Enzymes liberated from necrotic muscle.
Two commonly used in diagnosis:
1. Creatine phosphokinase (CPK) is
   fairly specific for cardiac muscle.
   Peak in 24 hours; falls in 72 hours.
2. Glutamic oxaloacetic transaminase (GOT)
   Not specific for cardiac muscle.
   Peak in 48-72 hrs; falls over 5 days.

These changes do not occur in angina pectoris since by definition necrosis has not
occurred.

The Electrocardiogram (ECG)

The ventricular changes in ischaemia are reflected in the portion of ECG representing
ventricular activity, i.e. the QRST complex. During excitation, contraction and restitution,
the electrical potentials across the membranes of necrotic muscle fibres are strikingly
different from healthy muscle. The ECG changes may be subtle but three common
patterns are illustrated.

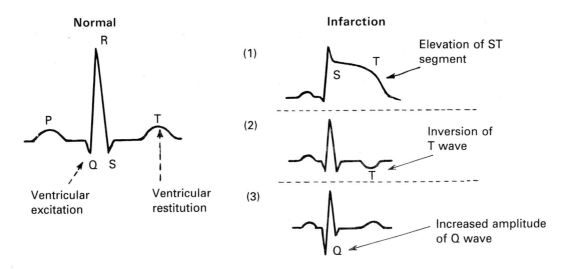

Normal

R

P   T

Q S

Ventricular
excitation

Ventricular
restitution

Infarction

(1) Elevation of ST
     segment
     T
     S

(2) Inversion of
     T wave
     T

(3) Increased amplitude
     of Q wave
     Q

MISCELLANEOUS AFFECTIONS OF THE MYOCARDIUM

MYOCARDITIS

Inflammation of the myocardium is rare but may be caused by a variety of agents. The process is usually acute and may be generalised, regional or focal; the immediate effects are usually serious and cause heart failure, but full recovery is possible.

Agents	Special features	Basic pathology
Bacteria — *pyogenic* Direct invasion either from infected valves or by bloodstream.	Focal suppuration Neutrophils ++	Muscle fibre damage — necrosis and lysis of individual or small groups
Toxins (incl. chemicals) Classical example — diphtheria toxin circulating in blood. Also in other severe infections e.g. typhoid, pneumonia	Usually generalised: muscle damage the main feature	
Viruses E.g. coxsackie B group	Usually generalised: interstitial inflammation the main feature	Interstitial oedema and inflammatory cellular infiltrate

Immunological
   E.g. rheumatic fever — myocarditis is an important component of the disease (see p.272 for details of special pathology).

Note: Nowadays the inflammation which is associated with ischaemia is no longer called myocarditis.

267

MISCELLANEOUS AFFECTIONS OF THE MYOCARDIUM

CARDIOMYOPATHY

This term, which strictly means 'disease of cardiac muscle' and could embrace every type of abnormality affecting the myocardium, has come to be conventionally used for conditions in which ischaemia, valve disease and inflammation have been excluded.

Primary cardiomyopathy

In this group the aetiology is not known.

Two main pathological abnormalities are present:

1. *Muscle hypertrophy* often of a particular anatomical component of the heart: histologically the enlarged muscle fibres show a striking irregularity of orientation.

E.g.
Hypertrophy
of heart with
large septal
cushion
tending to
obstruct outflow
from left ventricle

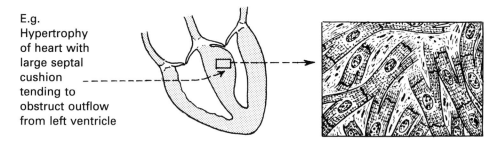

2. *Fibrosis* may be the dominant feature. It is usually diffuse and often subendocardial, forming thick layers of fibroelastic tissue under the endocardium — disease occurs almost exclusively in Africa.

Secondary cardiomyopathy

In a second group, the cardiac muscle abnormality is associated with a miscellany of diseases and conditions. The main groups of associated conditions are:

Nutritional — e.g. Beri-beri (thiamin deficiency)
Chronic alcoholism

Metabolic diseases — Biochemical: (a) potassium and magnesium disturbance.
(b) catecholamines, renin (acute excess).
— Infiltrations of heart muscle: amyloid, iron.
— Storage disease — glycogen.

Endocrine disease — Thyroid abnormality.

The changes in the heart muscle are protean, varying from subtle changes in individual muscle fibres to focal necrosis and fibrosis, and in many situations the mechanism of damage is not known.

MISCELLANEOUS AFFECTIONS OF THE MYOCARDIUM

FATTY INFILTRATION (ADIPOSITY)

The right ventricle is most commonly affected — fatty tissue penetrates between the muscle fibres but only in very severe cases contributes materially to cardiac insufficiency.

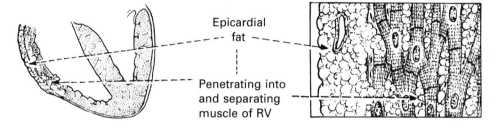

Epicardial fat

Penetrating into and separating muscle of RV

FATTY CHANGE

This reflects serious metabolic disturbance of the muscle cell and is usually caused by the action of toxins or hypoxia, particularly secondary to severe anaemia.

The muscle cells contain microscopic deposits of lipid; the change may be diffuse or in cases of severe anaemia may present as a dappled mottling under the endocardium (thrush breast).

Lipid

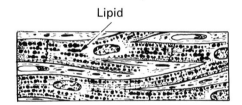

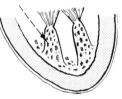

ATROPHY OF HEART

This occurs in cases of starvation and generalised inanition associated with the terminal stages of cancer. The presence of lipofuscin in the muscle cells may give the heart a striking brown appearance.

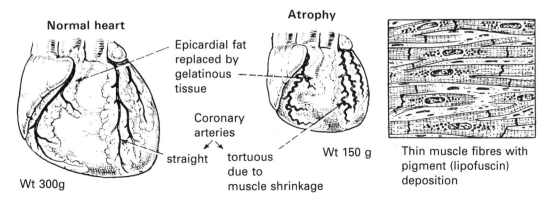

Normal heart

Atrophy

Epicardial fat replaced by gelatinous tissue

Coronary arteries

straight   tortuous due to muscle shrinkage

Wt 150 g

Wt 300g

Thin muscle fibres with pigment (lipofuscin) deposition

269

RHEUMATIC FEVER

In rheumatic fever (acute rheumatism), a disease of children and young adults, inflammation affects the connective tissues at many sites, of which the **heart** is the most important.

Aetiology

There is a strong association with streptococcal sore throat. The streptococcus is important because it may share antigens with human tissues, particularly heart muscle and cardiac valves.

In the current most plausible theory, the inflammation is regarded as being due to immunological cross-reactions since streptococci are not found at the various local sites and the disease follows some 2–4 weeks after the throat infection.

Mechanism

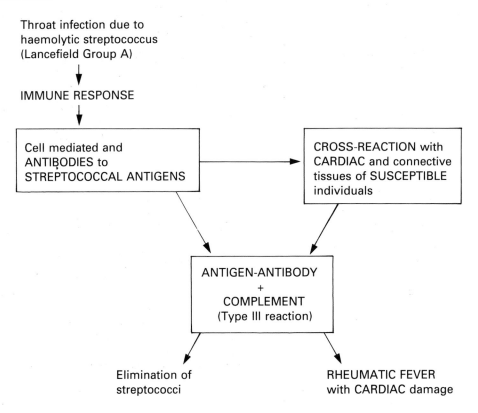

RHEUMATIC FEVER

In addition to the cardiac damage the disease is manifest in the following ways:

1. **General manifestations**
   Fever with sweating and malaise; raised ESR; neutrophil leucocytosis.

2. **Indications of inflammation at local sites**

   (a) *Joints and adjacent musculofascial tissues —* causing arthritis often with effusion, muscle pains and weakness.

   (b) *Serous membranes* Pericardial and sometimes pleural effusion.

   (c) *Skin*
   (i) a surface rash — erythema marginatum
   (ii) small subcutaneous palpable nodules may be present over bony prominences subject to pressure. The histological appearances are striking. It is seen that the palpable nodule is an aggregation of microscopic rheumatic nodules.

The basic process is an acute non-specific inflammation in which exudation of a fibrin-rich fluid is a major component.

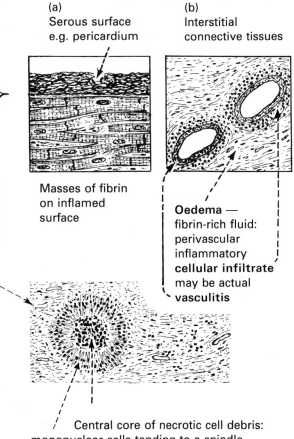

(a)
Serous surface e.g. pericardium

(b)
Interstitial connective tissues

Masses of fibrin on inflamed surface

Oedema — fibrin-rich fluid: perivascular inflammatory **cellular infiltrate** may be actual **vasculitis**

/ Central core of necrotic cell debris: mononuclear cells tending to a spindle shape and arranged in a pallisade. The surrounding tissues show the usual nonspecific inflammation.

   (d) *Central nervous system*
   Chorea — involuntary spasmodic muscular movements.

271

RHEUMATIC FEVER

CARDIAC MANIFESTATIONS

The inflammation is widespread throughout the heart, i.e. there is PANCARDITIS. It is convenient to consider the effects on the three anatomical cardiac layers separately — pericardial, myocardial and endocardial.

1. **Pericarditis** occurs during the acute phase of the illness and is an important cause of pericardial effusion.

2. **Myocarditis** is important during the acute phase and if severe can cause cardiac failure and death. The histological picture is striking and the presence of the Aschoff body is characteristic.

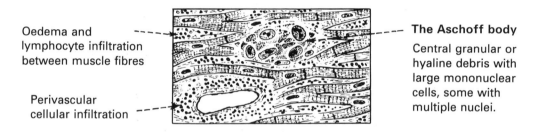

Oedema and lymphocyte infiltration between muscle fibres

Perivascular cellular infiltration

The Aschoff body

Central granular or hyaline debris with large mononuclear cells, some with multiple nuclei.

3. **Endocarditis**. Although there is a widespread histological inflammation, gross changes are seen usually on the endocardial sites subject to the greatest pressures and traumas, i.e. in the left side of the heart at the points of valve closure and at any sites of jet effect in the blood flow. The basic inflammation is complicated by ulceration of the valve surface followed by platelet and fibrin thrombosis in the form of small 'vegetations'.

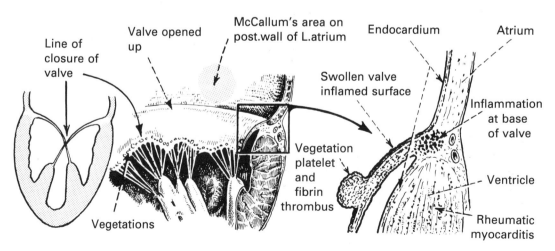

Line of closure of valve

Valve opened up

McCallum's area on post.wall of L.atrium

Endocardium

Atrium

Swollen valve inflamed surface

Vegetation platelet and fibrin thrombus

Inflammation at base of valve

Ventricle

Rheumatic myocarditis

Vegetations

RHEUMATIC FEVER

Progression of the disease

In most cases the acute phase passes off and is followed by healing with various degrees of scarring. In a significant number of cases, no florid acute phase is noticed, and in a small number, a low grade chronic inflammation is present for long periods.

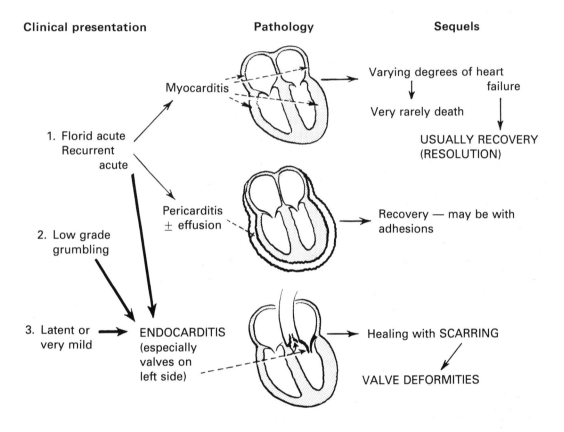

Clinical presentation   **Pathology**   **Sequels**

Myocarditis → Varying degrees of heart failure → Very rarely death → USUALLY RECOVERY (RESOLUTION)

1. Florid acute Recurrent acute

Pericarditis ± effusion → Recovery — may be with adhesions

2. Low grade grumbling

3. Latent or very mild → ENDOCARDITIS (especially valves on left side) → Healing with SCARRING → VALVE DEFORMITIES

Incidence

Since the advent of antibiotics (penicillin particularly), rheumatic heart disease, formerly very common in the temperate zones of the Western world, has declined. This is directly related to the decline in Type A streptococcal sore throat and to the successful prevention of recurrent attacks in susceptible individuals.

Rheumatic fever is still common in countries where antibiotic prophylaxis is not available.

VALVULAR HEART DISEASE

The main causes are RHEUMATIC ENDOCARDITIS and DYSTROPHIC CALCIFICATION. Developmental anatomical abnormality and inherited deficiencies of the ground substance of the valve are rare causes. Nowadays, with the advent of powerful antibiotics, the late effects of healed infective endocarditis are assuming greater importance.

The MITRAL and AORTIC valves, subjected to much greater pressures, are more susceptible to damage than the tricuspid and pulmonic valves. *Rheumatic mitral disease* has been very common in the past and is still seen in middle aged or older patients, but with the decline in rheumatic fever and the increasing age of the population, *calcific aortic disease* is becoming as common.

MITRAL DISEASE

Stenosis is the most common result of rheumatic fever. It is the result of several components of the healing or scarring process occurring either separately or, more usually, together in varying combinations.

Stenosis
Simple adherence of curtains: a diaphragm formed

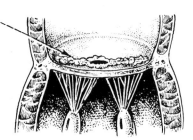

Normal valve
Note thin delicate curtains and chordae tendinae

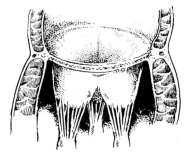

or

Stenosis
Adherence and distortion, thickening, shortening, calcification of valve curtains and chordae resulting in 'funnel' stenosis

[Whole valve replacement required.]

MITRAL VALVE DISEASE

Mitral disease (continued)

Incompetence may follow from the rheumatic process by a similar slow mechanism.

In addition it may develop acutely due to other quite different causes:

1. In cases of left ventricular failure when severe dilatation occurs.

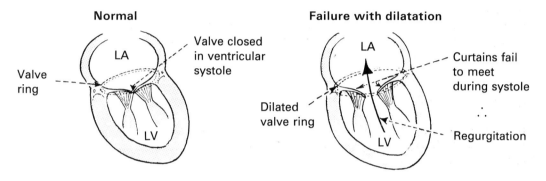

2. Necrosis with rupture of papillary muscle in acute myocardial infarction.

3. Rarely it results from abnormality of the ground substance of the valve — the 'floppy valve syndrome'. More cases of this condition are now being recognised using modern non-invasive techniques to study cardiac valve function in life.

The mechanical effects of mitral disease

Chronic stenosis — pure   *Chronic incompetence — pure (rare)*

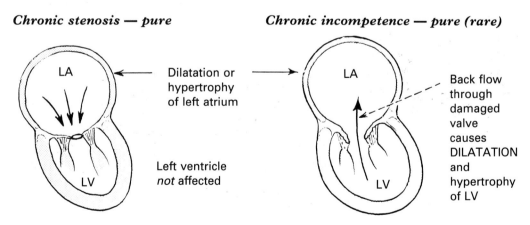

In rheumatic heart disease, pure stenosis is not uncommon; incompetence usually occurs along with stenosis.

MITRAL VALVE DISEASE

Mitral disease (continued)

In mitral disease, the back pressure in the left atrium is transmitted to the pulmonary veins and by raising pulmonary arterial pressure causes effects on the right side of the heart.

(a) Compensated phase

(1) Left atrial dilatation
↓
(2) Pulmonary congestion
↓
(3) Right ventricular hypertrophy

Back pressure

RA

② LA ①

RV

Diseased mitral valve

LV

Pulmonary veins: raised pressure

Pulmonary artery: ③ raised pressure

(b) Congestive cardiac failure

Tricuspid valve

RA

PA raised pressure

RV

Hypertrophied RV

Dilatation →

RA

Back pressure effect

Dilatation of tricuspid ring — functional incompetence of valve
↓
Systemic venous congestion

RV

(3) Right Ventricular Hypertrophy → (4) Dilated RV → (5) Dilated RA

In the acute types of mitral incompetence, the sudden change in the intracardiac haemodynamics very seriously aggravates the heart failure already present due to the primary disease.

Complications of chronic mitral disease

1. Atrial fibrillation is common.
   Fibrillation → Thrombosis in atrial appendage → Systemic embolism
2. Infective endocarditis.

AORTIC VALVE DISEASE

STENOSIS

The main causes are RHEUMATIC SCARRING and CALCIFICATION occurring in a congenitally abnormal valve or one previously damaged by rheumatism or endocarditis (bacterial), but in elderly people there may be no obvious pre-existing disease.

Changes in the valve

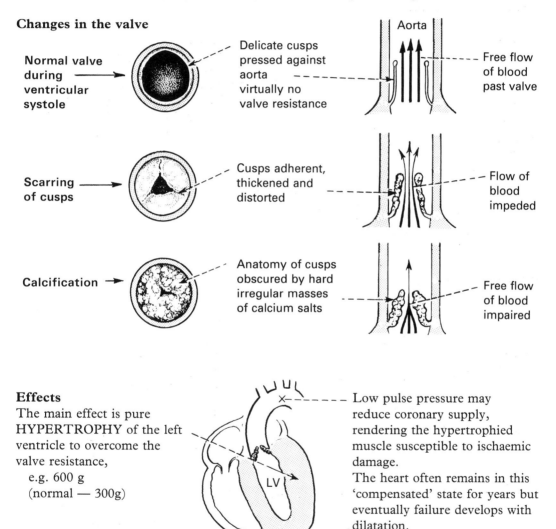

Aorta

Normal valve during ventricular systole → Delicate cusps pressed against aorta virtually no valve resistance — — — Free flow of blood past valve

Scarring of cusps → Cusps adherent, thickened and distorted — — — Flow of blood impeded

Calcification → Anatomy of cusps obscured by hard irregular masses of calcium salts — — Free flow of blood impaired

Effects
The main effect is pure HYPERTROPHY of the left ventricle to overcome the valve resistance,
  e.g. 600 g
  (normal — 300g)

LV

Low pulse pressure may reduce coronary supply, rendering the hypertrophied muscle susceptible to ischaemic damage.
The heart often remains in this 'compensated' state for years but eventually failure develops with dilatation.

However SUDDEN DEATH (without pre-existing signs of failure) is a definite risk at any time, but particularly during exercise in cases of aortic stenosis.

AORTIC VALVE DISEASE

INCOMPETENCE

The main causes are rheumatic and infective endocarditic scarring of the cusps; rarely dilatation of the valve ring due to syphilis or hereditary diesase (e.g. Marfan's syndrome).

Changes in the valve

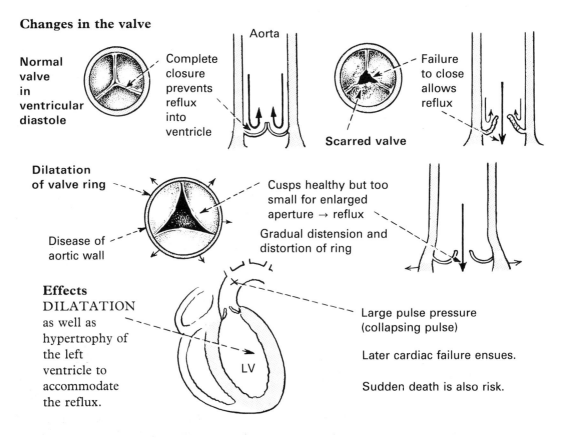

Normal valve in ventricular diastole — Complete closure prevents reflux into ventricle

Aorta

Failure to close allows reflux — **Scarred valve**

Dilatation of valve ring — Disease of aortic wall — Cusps healthy but too small for enlarged aperture → reflux

Gradual distension and distortion of ring

Effects

DILATATION as well as hypertrophy of the left ventricle to accommodate the reflux.

LV

Large pulse pressure (collapsing pulse)

Later cardiac failure ensues.

Sudden death is also risk.

Aortic stenosis and incompetence often exist together and the effects are compounded.

TRICUSPID AND PULMONIC VALVES

Diseases of these valves on the right side of the heart are not common. However functional tricuspid incompetence due to severe cardiac dilatation is an important end stage in progressive cardiac failure.

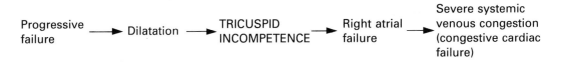

Progressive failure → Dilatation → TRICUSPID INCOMPETENCE → Right atrial failure → Severe systemic venous congestion (congestive cardiac failure)

INFECTIVE ENDOCARDITIS

This is a disease of the heart valves particularly: the mural endocardium is only occasionally affected by late spread from the valves.

In the classical situation, bacteria settle on previously diseased valves. The disease evolves in one of two main patterns depending on the type of bacteria.

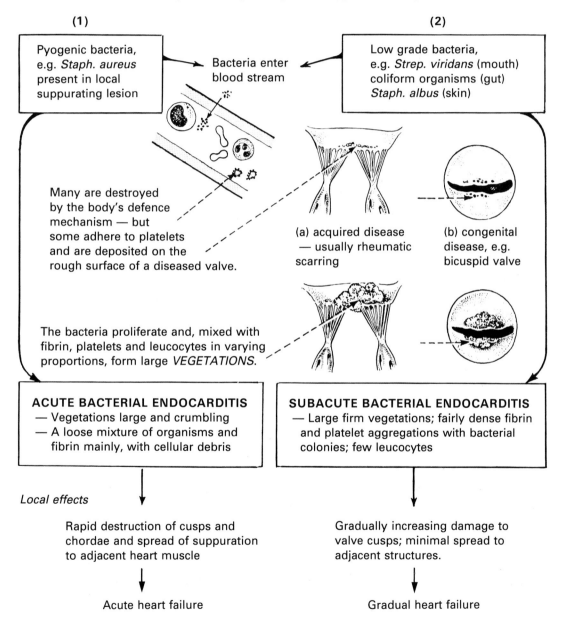

(1)

Pyogenic bacteria, e.g. *Staph. aureus* present in local suppurating lesion

→ Bacteria enter blood stream ←

(2)

Low grade bacteria, e.g. *Strep. viridans* (mouth) coliform organisms (gut) *Staph. albus* (skin)

Many are destroyed by the body's defence mechanism — but some adhere to platelets and are deposited on the rough surface of a diseased valve.

(a) acquired disease — usually rheumatic scarring

(b) congenital disease, e.g. bicuspid valve

The bacteria proliferate and, mixed with fibrin, platelets and leucocytes in varying proportions, form large *VEGETATIONS*.

ACUTE BACTERIAL ENDOCARDITIS
— Vegetations large and crumbling
— A loose mixture of organisms and fibrin mainly, with cellular debris

SUBACUTE BACTERIAL ENDOCARDITIS
— Large firm vegetations; fairly dense fibrin and platelet aggregations with bacterial colonies; few leucocytes

Local effects

Rapid destruction of cusps and chordae and spread of suppuration to adjacent heart muscle

↓

Acute heart failure

Gradually increasing damage to valve cusps; minimal spread to adjacent structures.

↓

Gradual heart failure

INFECTIVE ENDOCARDITIS

In addition to the local effects, the course of the disease is influenced by other important complications.

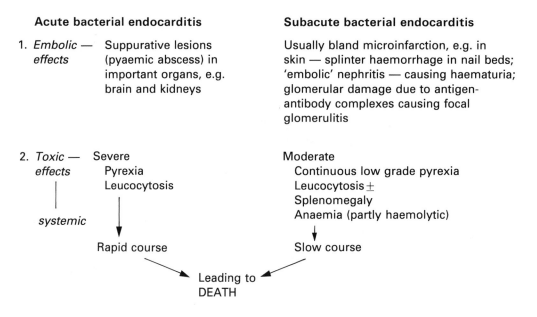

Acute bacterial endocarditis

1. *Embolic — effects*   Suppurative lesions (pyaemic abscess) in important organs, e.g. brain and kidneys

Subacute bacterial endocarditis

Usually bland microinfarction, e.g. in skin — splinter haemorrhage in nail beds; 'embolic' nephritis — causing haematuria; glomerular damage due to antigen-antibody complexes causing focal glomerulitis

2. *Toxic — effects*

systemic

Severe
Pyrexia
Leucocytosis

Rapid course

Moderate
Continuous low grade pyrexia
Leucocytosis $\pm$
Splenomegaly
Anaemia (partly haemolytic)

Slow course

Leading to DEATH

This classical situation is nowadays modified by immunosuppressive drugs, antibiotics and intracardiac prosthesis including catheter lines from peripheral veins.

Immunosuppression
This allows opportunistic infection by a much wider range of organisms, e.g. bacteria not usually pathogenic, and fungi.

Antibiotics
1. Their effects blur the distinction between the two types and allow healing but often with serious scarring of the valve.
2. The structure of the vegetation is important; in some cases the bacterial colonies are protected from the antibiotic.

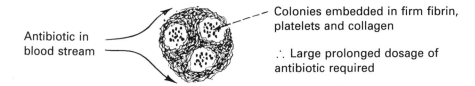

Antibiotic in blood stream

Colonies embedded in firm fibrin, platelets and collagen

∴ Large prolonged dosage of antibiotic required

Cardiac prosthesis and catheter lines act as a focus for bacterial growth and infective endocarditis is a serious complication.

CARDIAC ARRHYTHMIAS

CARDIAC ARRHYTHMIAS and DISEASES of the CONDUCTING SYSTEM

Of the wide variety of cardiac arrhythmias which have now been studied in detail using the electrocardiograph, the majority are due to (A) functional disturbances of the intrinsic excitability of the cardiac muscle at various sites or of the cardiac neurohumoral controls; only a minority are due to (B) organic disease of the conducting system itself. Organic heart disease particularly of ischaemic type is a common concomitant.

(A) Important disorders of cardiac muscle excitability
(1) Atrial fibrillation

In this common disorder, continuous incoordinate movement of the atrial muscle completely negates its role as a priming pump and the atria become functionally inert.

There is no specific pathological change in the atrial wall, but atrial dilatation associated with cardiac disease is usually a precondition.

Predisposing conditions
Rheumatic heart disease
Ischaemic heart disease
Senile heart disease
Thyrotoxicosis
} Atrial dilatation (±atrial muscle hypertrophy) ——→

Increased susceptibility to 'circus' rhythm
↓
——→ Atrial fibrillation

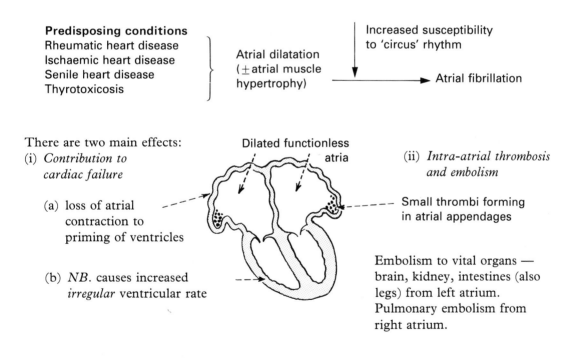

There are two main effects:
(i) *Contribution to cardiac failure*

   (a) loss of atrial contraction to priming of ventricles

   (b) *NB.* causes increased *irregular* ventricular rate

Dilated functionless atria

(ii) *Intra-atrial thrombosis and embolism*

Small thrombi forming in atrial appendages

Embolism to vital organs — brain, kidney, intestines (also legs) from left atrium. Pulmonary embolism from right atrium.

2. Ventricular paroxysmal tachycardia and fibrillation

These very serious conditions are usually superimposed upon and aggravate pre-existing severe myocardial disease — usually ischaemic in type. In fibrillation, a form of 'arrest', cardiac function ceases; it is the terminal event in many fatal diseases.

CARDIAC ARRHYTHMIAS

Cardiac arrhythmia (continued)

(B) Diseases of the conducting system
The usual disorder is slowing of the impulse and it is most often associated with organic disease in the adjacent cardiac tissue.

Associated conditions

Cardiac ischaemia ⟨ Acute infarction ⎫ ———— are the most common
                    ⟨ Fibrosis ⎭   and important

Others are — myocarditis, calcification around the valve rings and drugs, e.g. digitalis, propranolol.

Sites of disorder   **Effects**

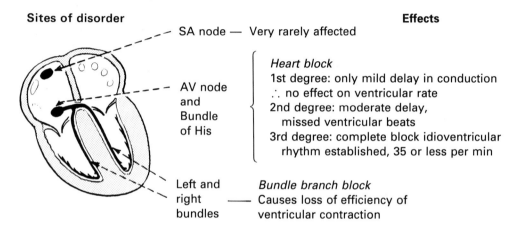

SA node — Very rarely affected

AV node and Bundle of His
Heart block
1st degree: only mild delay in conduction ∴ no effect on ventricular rate
2nd degree: moderate delay, missed ventricular beats
3rd degree: complete block idioventricular rhythm established, 35 or less per min

Left and right bundles
Bundle branch block
Causes loss of efficiency of ventricular contraction

The 3 important components of arrhythmias are:
Tachycardia, bradycardia and irregularity.
The effect of any arrhythmia on cardiac function depends essentially on its effect on ventricular output.

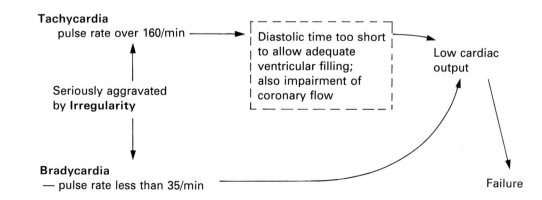

Tachycardia
pulse rate over 160/min

Diastolic time too short to allow adequate ventricular filling; also impairment of coronary flow

Low cardiac output

Seriously aggravated by **Irregularity**

Bradycardia
— pulse rate less than 35/min

Failure

DISEASES OF THE PERICARDIUM

PERICARDITIS

Pericarditis is commonly a complication of diseases of the heart or adjacent structures or of generalised disorders; primary (or idiopathic) inflammation is rare.

In **acute pericarditis,** fibrin exudation is common: sometimes exudation of serous fluid is the main feature. Haemorrhage may be superadded in cases of uraemia and tumour infiltration. Purulent pericarditis complicating bacterial infections is rare.

Fibrinous pericarditis

Cardiac surface covered by shaggy fibrinous exudate

Parietal layer

Tendency for layers to adhere and subsequently organise

Pericardial 'rub' may be heard clinically

Pericarditis with effusion

Varying volume of yellow serous fluid (may be sufficient to embarrass cardiac action)

Very light deposit of fibrin on surfaces

Diseases which may lead to pericarditis

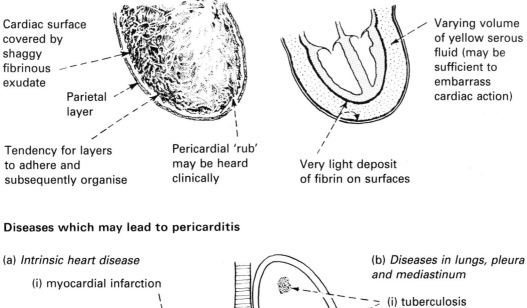

(a) *Intrinsic heart disease*

  (i) myocardial infarction

  (ii) acute rheumatism (pancarditis)

(iii) trauma — esp. surgical

(iv) myocarditis

(b) *Diseases in lungs, pleura and mediastinum*

  (i) tuberculosis

  (ii) carcinoma

  (iii) pneumonia complicated by empyema

(c) *Generalised disorders* (mechanism not known)

  (i) uraemia
  (ii) connective tissue diseases

DISEASES OF THE PERICARDIUM

CHRONIC PERICARDITIS is usually the result of recurrent attacks of rheumatism or allied diseases; occasionally it is insidiously chronic throughout. The basic changes are organisation and calcification. In extreme cases, cardiac function is impaired.

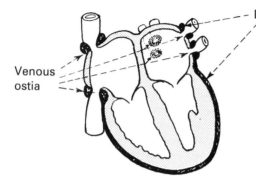

Venous ostia

Dense fibrous calcified tissues —
causing close adherence of the pericardial layers;
preventing proper cardiac filling;
causing stenosis at venous ostia leading
to severe venous congestion
— this extreme condition is called **constrictive pericarditis.**

PERICARDIAL HAEMORRHAGE occurs most commonly as a result of cardiac rupture complicating acute infarction. The other main cause is rupture of aortic aneurysm back into the pericardium.

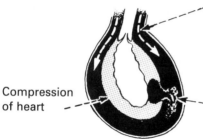

The pericardial sac becomes distended with blood (tamponade) and death follows rapidly due to compression of the heart.

Compression of heart

Cardiac rupture into pericardium

CARDIAC TUMOURS

Primary tumours in the heart are very rare. Secondary tumours, especially from the lungs, affecting the pericardium by direct spread and the heart by blood spread are fairly common and represent terminal stages in malignant disease.

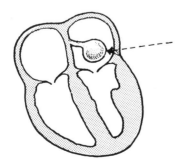

The so-called cardiac 'myxoma' is a rare condition affecting usually the left atrium in which a smooth, pale, soft, rounded mass is attached by a pedicle to the endocardium. It can cause serious effects by occluding the mitral valve opening. It is not certain whether 'myxoma' is a true neoplasm or is the result of organisation of a ball thrombus in a particular way.

CONGENITAL HEART DISEASE

Developmental abnormalities of the heart are relatively common; clinically significant defects occur in 6 per 1000 live births and 2 per 100 of stillbirths. The severity varies from minor aberrations to complex distortions incompatible with life.

Aetiology

This is often obscure. Hereditary factors are of limited importance; possible environmental factors are complex and numerous.

Examples include: virus infection, e.g. rubella; teratogen, e.g. thalidomide; altitude at birth (patent ductus arteriosus is commoner at high altitudes).

The initial damage which is sustained during the early formative stages in the 2nd and 3rd months of pregnancy is modified by later fetal and postnatal growth and development.

Single anatomical abnormalities occur, but often there are multiple defects which are associated in groups of which the more common are given specific names.

Abnormal development occurs:

(1) At the emergence of the great vessels

↓

Stenoses cause impedence to blood flow

(2) During formation of the septa between right and left sides and following failure of closure, e.g. ductus and foramen ovale.

↓

Abnormal apertures allow shunting of blood

Fallot's tetralogy illustrates these main points:

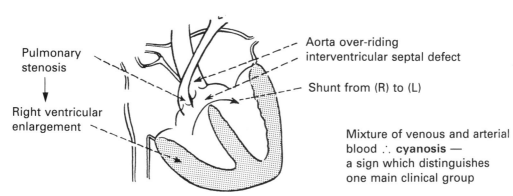

Pulmonary stenosis

↓

Right ventricular enlargement

Aorta over-riding interventricular septal defect

Shunt from (R) to (L)

Mixture of venous and arterial blood ∴ **cyanosis** — a sign which distinguishes one main clinical group

Often complications — pulmonary hypertension, increased blood volume polycythaemia, and occasionally infective endocarditis — increase the disability and failure is progressive.

RESPIRATORY SYSTEM

UPPER RESPIRATORY TRACT

ACUTE INFLAMMATIONS

These are the common inflammations of the nose, nasal sinuses, pharynx, larynx, trachea and bronchi. They are usually mild and self-limiting but may lead to chronic lesions. Generally they exhibit two phases according to the causal agents involved: the *viral infection phase* and the *bacterial phase*.

1. **Viral infection phase**
This phase is characterised by all the features of acute inflammation but without the cellular exudate.

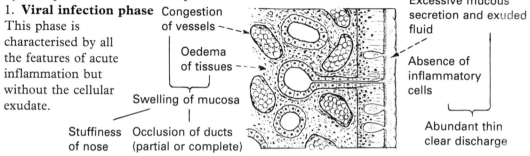

Congestion of vessels
Oedema of tissues
Swelling of mucosa
Stuffiness of nose
Occlusion of ducts (partial or complete)
Excessive mucous secretion and exuded fluid
Absence of inflammatory cells
Abundant thin clear discharge

Viruses involved

A large number of viruses may cause acute inflammation of the upper respiratory tract.

 (i) Rhinoviruses – these are by far the commonest cause of inflammation of the nose (coryza). Coxsackie and Echo viruses may also be a cause. These three are small RNA viruses (picornaviruses).

(ii) Adenoviruses and myxoviruses, e.g. parainfluenza viruses and respiratory syncytial viruses, cause laryngitis, tracheitis and bronchitis. The latter may result in severe bronchiolitis and pneumonia in infants.

Influenza virus is also a myxovirus and may produce severe inflammation of the respiratory tract at any level.

During the viral phase there is some loss of surface epithelium and the viral infection appears to make the mucosa susceptible to secondary infection, thus initiating the second phase.

2. **Bacterial phase**
Bacteria, normally present in the nose and throat, invade the damaged mucosa, and the tissue reaction then shows the classical features of acute inflammation.

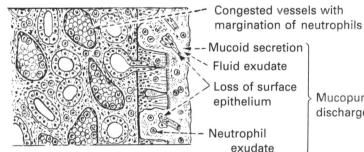

Congested vessels with margination of neutrophils
Mucoid secretion
Fluid exudate
Loss of surface epithelium
Neutrophil exudate
Mucopurulent discharge

The infection is usually mixed; the bacteria commonly involved are *Streptococcus pneumoniae*, *Haemophilus influenzae*, *Streptococcus pyogenes* and *Neisseria catarrhalis*. In institutions where the use of antibiotics has resulted in resistant pathogenic strains colonising the environment, serious respiratory infection may result.

Since these inflammations can be caused by so many different viruses with no cross immunity, and also since immunity is of short duration, repeated attacks are common. Chronic changes may be induced as a result.

RHINITIS

ACUTE CORYZA

This is the commonest form of upper respiratory inflammation (the 'common cold'). In almost all cases the inflammation involves not only the nose but other associated structures.

The two phases, viral and bacterial, are seen typically in this disease.

The drainage from the sinuses, especially the maxillary, is frequently obstructed by swelling of the mucosa. In such a case, a very acute suppurative condition may arise.

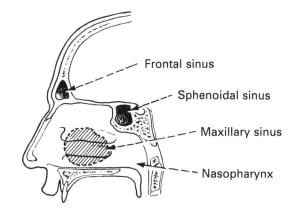

Rhinovirus and parainfluenza virus are the usual initiating agents, but acute rhinitis is also a feature of influenza and measles. The bacteria in the second phase are as previously stated.

Attacks are frequent in childhood and may result in a chronic condition with catarrhal discharge and nasal obstruction.

ALLERGIC RHINITIS

Acute respiratory inflammation is often of allergic type. The reaction has certain characteristics which differentiate it from ordinary, infective inflammation. The nasal form is commonly termed 'hay-fever'.

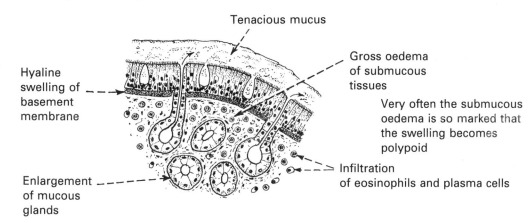

Bacterial infection is commonly superadded and the exudate becomes mucopurulent. The repeated attacks frequently lead to chronic changes in the mucosa with polyp formation.

RHINITIS

NASAL POLYPS

These form particularly
on the middle turbinate
bones and within the
maxillary sinuses.

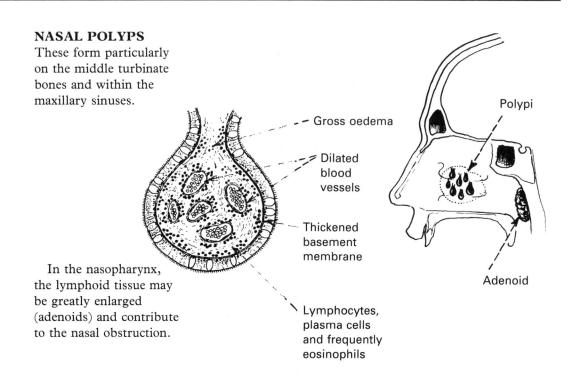

Gross oedema

Dilated
blood
vessels

Polypi

Thickened
basement
membrane

In the nasopharynx,
the lymphoid tissue may
be greatly enlarged
(adenoids) and contribute
to the nasal obstruction.

Adenoid

Lymphocytes,
plasma cells
and frequently
eosinophils

ALLERGIES

Seasonal allergy

This is due to pollens liberated from trees and grass.

Non-seasonal allergy

The main cause is the house dust mite,
Dermatophagoides pteronyssinus, but allergy
may develop to dust-containing animal or
human hair (dandruff), cotton or other fibres.

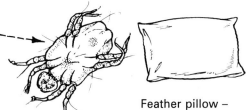

Feather pillow –
invisible infestation

VASOMOTOR RHINITIS

This is a clinical diagnosis. The pathological changes are, to some extent, similar to those
of allergic rhinitis, but the condition is more continuous, less spasmodic. Although the
cause is unknown, viral infections in a polluted atmosphere (usually an urban setting) are
thought to initiate the 'sensitivity' and non-specific stimuli such as bright light and smells
precipitate an attack.

ACUTE LARYNGITIS AND ACUTE TRACHEITIS

These are usually mild conditions due to infection with adenoviruses or parainfluenza virus followed by secondary invaders *Streptococcus pneumoniae*, *Streptococcus pyogenes* and *Neisseria catarrhalis*. The pathological changes are as previously described. A very acute form (croup) due to the parainfluenza virus occurs in children.

Special types

Psedomembranous inflammation
This is an extremely severe form of laryngotracheitis.

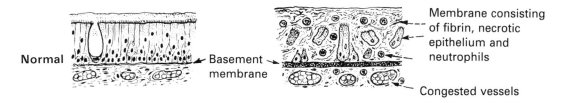

It may be due to secondary invasion by *Staphylococcus aureus*, *Streptococcous pyogenes*, *Streptococcus pneumoniae* or more rarely *Haemophilus influenzae*. Acute fever, enlargement of the local lymph nodes and oedema are common. The larynx or epiglottis may become severely oedematous leading to respiratory obstruction. This is especially apt to happen in childhood. Spread to bronchi is frequent.

Diphtheria, now uncommon in advanced countries, is a special form of pseudomembranous laryngitis. Usually it is due to spread from the pharynx. The corynebacterium diphtheriae is present in large numbers in the fibrinous membrane.

Secondary to endotracheal intubation
This can be a serious complication of treatment in intensive care units.

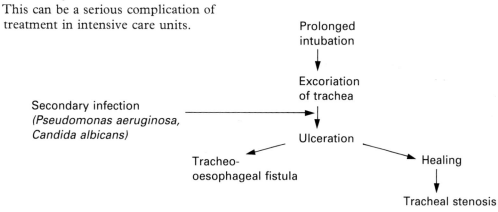

Secondary to specific infections

Serious acute oedema of the glottis (tissues above the vocal cords) may result from infection such as diphtheria, syphilis, typhoid fever, erisypelas, or spread of infection from tonsillitis. It is also a complication of agranulocytosis. Death may occur due to suffocation.

Mild degrees of oedema of the glottis can occur in cardiac and renal disease.

CHRONIC LARYNGITIS AND CHRONIC TRACHEITIS

These lesions are characterised by two changes: (a) change in the lining epithelium and (b) increase in mucous secretion.

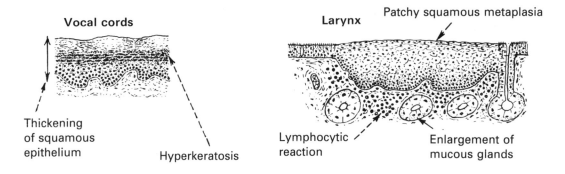

The following sequence of events tends to take place:

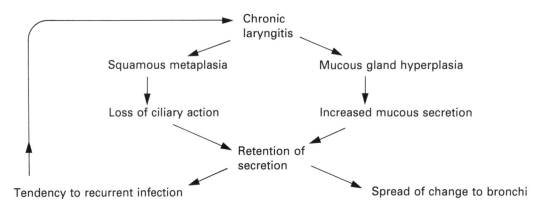

Aetiology

Tobacco smoke is probably the most important factor in initiating and promoting this lesion. Once the metaplastic changes start, other factors such as atmospheric pollution and attacks of acute upper respiratory infection increase the severity of the condition.

Specific chronic inflammations

TUBERCULOSIS. This disease may cause severe ulceration of the larynx, especially in the region of the vocal cords and arytenoid cartilages. It is secondary to pulmonary tuberculosis.

SYPHILIS. Ephemeral lesions, mucous patches and superficial ulcers may be found in the larynx during the secondary phase of syphilis. Gummatous ulceration of the larynx may be caused by tertiary syphilis. Extensive ulceration can take place and the subsequent scarring may lead to stenosis.

292

TUMOURS OF UPPER RESPIRATORY TRACT

SIMPLE TUMOURS

Epithelial   Epithelial tumours take the form of papillomas. They are usually single, but in children, multiple papillomas of viral origin affect various parts of the larynx.

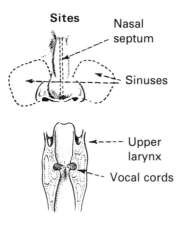

Sites
Nasal septum
Sinuses
Upper larynx
Vocal cords

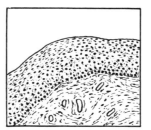

Squamous cell

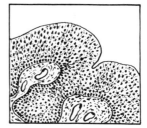

Transitional Cell. The abnormal epithelium grows down the glandular ducts and the name 'inverted papilloma' is applied. Such tumours often recur after incomplete removal. Human papilloma virus is associated with some cases.

Small non-neoplastic nodules of proliferations of both epithelium and connective tissue are common on the vocal cords (Singer's nodes).

Connective tissue

Haemangioma, occurring on the nasal septum, is the commonest and gives rise to persistent nose-bleeds. Other tumours are rare. A special form of angioma, angiofibroma, affects male children. It grows throughout childhood and may cause bone destruction; it usually regresses at adolescence.

MALIGNANT TUMOURS

These are, except in very rare instances, all carcinomata and most are of squamous cell variety.

Sites

The sites are the same as for simple papillomas. Some of them take origin from a transitional-celled papilloma. Changes resembling leukoplakia often precede and accompany malignant growths. In the larynx, those which arise on the true or false cords invade slowly and have a better prognosis. Ulceration destroys the local structures. Infected necrotic tissue may be inhaled and cause pneumonia.

Lymphoepithelioma, a carcinoma accompanied by masses of lymphocytes, is now considered as an anaplastic carcinoma invading local lymph tissue. It is common in Eastern countries and is associated with Epstein-Barr (EB) virus infection.

293

LUNGS – ANATOMY

ACINUS (PRIMARY LOBULE)
This is a sub-unit of pulmonary tissue consisting of respiratory bronchioles with associated alveolar ducts, atria and alveoli. Intercommunications exist between acini, and also between acini and terminal bronchioles. Thus disease can spread from acinus to acinus but, equally, functional deficiency in any part of one acinus can be compensated by by-pass mechanisms via these anastomotic channels.

SECONDARY LOBULE
This is the unit of pulmonary tissue served by a pre-terminal bronchiole. Self-contained and bounded by connective tissue septa, it has no anastomotic connections with other lobules.

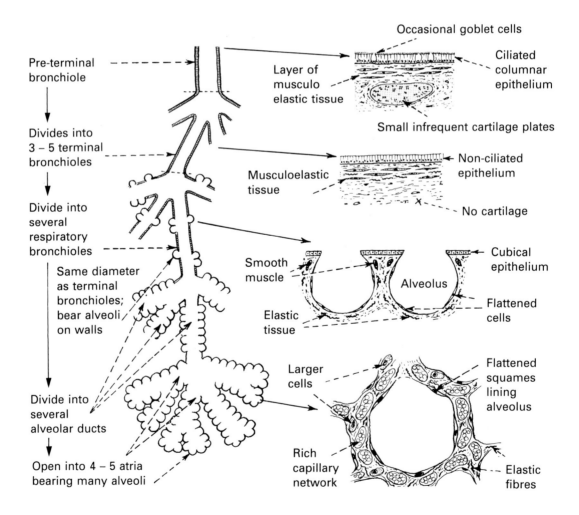

LUNGS – ANATOMY

ANASTOMOTIC CHANNELS in ACINUS

These exist at two levels:

1. Between one or more atria and the related terminal bronchiole.

2. Between alveoli of atria of same respiratory bronchiole and between alveoli related to adjacent respiratory bronchioles.

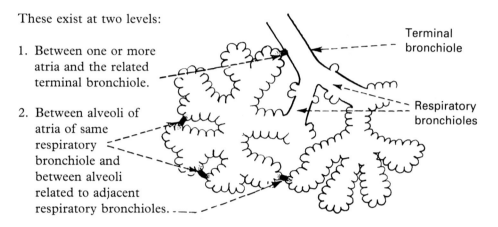

These alveolar connections are known as the pores of Kohn.

HISTOLOGY of the ALVEOLUS

Three types of cell (pneumocytes) line the alveolus.

1. *Membranous pneumocyte (Type I)*
   Nucleus is usually situated at angles of alveolus, and thin cytoplasmic extensions line most of alveolar surface.

2. *Granular pneumocyte (Type II)*
   Project into alveoli and are covered by microvilli. They are essentially reserve cells which undergo hyperplasia when Type I pneumocytes are injured.

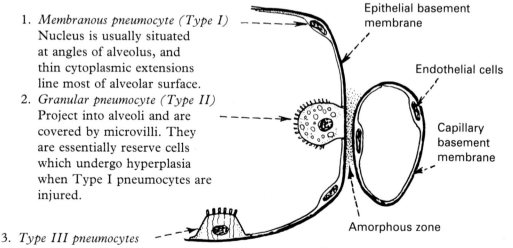

3. *Type III pneumocytes*
   Pyramidal in shape with thick microvilli containing filaments extending through cell body. Resemble chemoreceptor cells.

RESPIRATION

The normal intake of air is around 7 litres per minute; of this, after allowing for non-functioning dead space (trachea, bronchi, etc.), approximately 5 litres per minute are available for alveolar ventilation. A definite flow of air is maintained as far as the terminal bronchiole. Beyond this point the actual flow ceases and gas exchange is effected by diffusion.

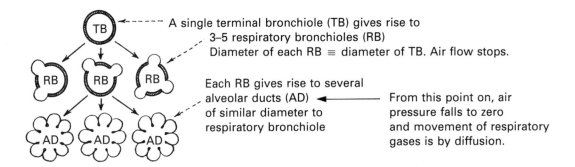

A single terminal bronchiole (TB) gives rise to 3–5 respiratory bronchioles (RB)
Diameter of each RB ≡ diameter of TB. Air flow stops.

Each RB gives rise to several alveolar ducts (AD) of similar diameter to respiratory bronchiole ◄——— From this point on, air pressure falls to zero and movement of respiratory gases is by diffusion.

Three factors are involved in the maintenance of adequate respiration:
1. Adequate intake of air
2. Rapid diffusion along alveolar ducts and through alveolar walls
3. Adequate perfusion of pulmonary circulation
Interference with any of these factors will result in respiratory embarrassment (dyspnoea) and even respiratory failure.

Inadequate air supply to alveoli (hypoventilation)
This may be due to lesions and diseases which interfere with the mechanics of respiration, such as central nervous lesions affecting the respiratory centre, paralysis of muscles of respiration as in poliomyelitis, injuries and deformities of the thoracic skeleton (e.g. fracture of ribs, kyphosis) and pleural disease preventing lung expansion as in pleural effusion or pneumothorax.

Perhaps the most common cause of hypoventilation is bronchial obstruction. This may be due to retained secretions and mucous gland hyperplasia in advanced chronic bronchitis or bronchial spasm in asthma. Local bronchial obstruction can be caused by tumour growth or foreign bodies.

Effects
Fall in alveolar and blood oxygen.
Rise in blood and alveolar CO_2.
The clinical changes mainly due to hypercapnia (increase in systemic arterial carbon dioxide) – rapid pulse, sweating, small pupils and rise in blood pressure.

RESPIRATION

Impaired diffusion of gases

Three mechanisms may interfere with diffusion:

1. Reduction in the total alveolar surface available for diffusion, e.g. consolidated airless lobe in pneumonia, fibrosis of lung, tumour growth, advanced tuberculosis.
2. Increase in distance over which diffusion takes place as in emphysema.

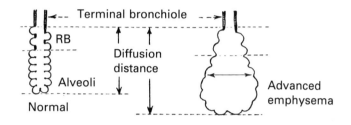

3. Increase in the thickness of the alveolar capillary membrane. Diffusion of gas across the membrane is so rapid this can be of little practical importance. CO_2 is more soluble than O_2 and diffusion through the alveolar wall is 20 times as rapid as O_2, therefore while blood O_2 progressively falls there is no retention of CO_2.

Altered pulmonary perfusion

Interference with the pulmonary circulation may occur in 4 main ways:

1. Occlusion of larger vessels by multiple emboli.
2. Slowing of the pulmonary circulation as in venous congestion due to left heart lesions or congenital left–right shunts.
3. Reduction in the pulmonary capillary bed by diffuse lung disease such as fibrosis, emphysema or extensive tuberculosis.
4. Pulmonary vascular spasm due to hypoxia. Permanent changes can occur in the vessels if the hypoxia is unrelieved.

Note: In addition to hypoxaemia, inadequate perfusion tends to cause retention of carbon dioxide.

In chronic lung disease, ventilation, diffusion and perfusion disorders are present in varying degrees.

Respiratory failure

The essential feature is HYPOXAEMIA (arterial O_2 tension less than 60mm Hg): in its pure form causes Type I Respiratory Failure (clinical) with severe dyspnoea and no cyanosis ('Pink Puffer' syndrome).

In many cases the additional retention of CO_2 (arterial CO_2 tension greater than 45mm Hg) seriously aggravates the condition and gives rise to Type II Respiratory Failure (clinical) with dyspnoea and CYANOSIS ('Blue Bloater' syndrome): progression to pulmonary hypertension and right heart failure (cor pulmonale) is common.

ACUTE BRONCHITIS

This is an inflammation of the large and medium bronchi. The condition may be serious if associated with pre-existing respiratory disease. Mucous and serous glands in the walls of the bronchi provide abundant mucoid secretion during the inflammation. Ciliated epithelia lining the bronchi aid passage of the exudate upward and help prevent spread down to the bronchioles.

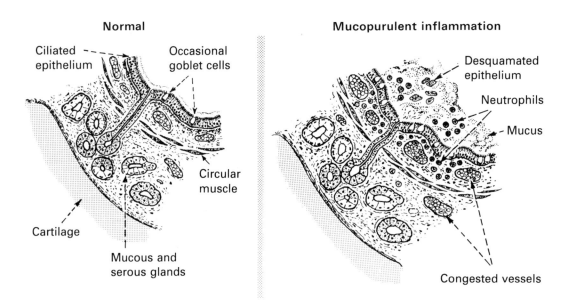

In most cases, the process is initiated by a viral or mycoplasmal infection. It is a common complication of influenza and measles. This initial phase is followed by bacterial invasion. *Streptococcus pneumoniae* and *Haemophilus influenzae* are commonest, but *Staphylococcus aureus* and *Streptococcus pyogenes* may be found, especially in infants.

The condition is usually mild, and spread to the bronchioles is unusual in healthy adults due to the effective ciliary action of the bronchial epithelium. Spread may occur however in children and debilitated people. Bronchiolitis and bronchopneumonia result and can prove fatal. Equally important is the serious effect of repeated attacks of acute infection in patients with chronic bronchitis.

CHRONIC BRONCHITIS

CHRONIC OBSTRUCTIVE AIRWAYS DISEASE (COAD)
This is a clinical syndrome which, as the name implies, is characterised by obstruction to the flow of air in the distal airways. The pathological conditions causing this are: (1) chronic bronchitis, (2) emphysema, (3) asthmatic bronchitis and (4) some cases of bronchiectasis. These conditions usually display considerable overlap.

CHRONIC BRONCHITIS
Clinical definition is based upon the presence of a productive cough over a period of at least 2 years. The pathological counterpart is illustrated.

The essential feature is a change in the epithelial structure of the bronchus.

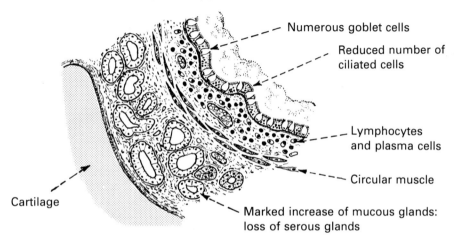

Numerous goblet cells

Reduced number of ciliated cells

Lymphocytes and plasma cells

Circular muscle

Cartilage

Marked increase of mucous glands: loss of serous glands

At first, the bronchial wall is thickened due to the increase in glandular tissue, oedema and congestion. At autopsy, the severity of the disease can be measured using the Reid Index, i.e. the ratio of the submucous layer to the whole thickness. A ratio greater than 1:2 is significant. At a later stage it can become thin as a result of atrophy of all structures.

The effect of these changes is:

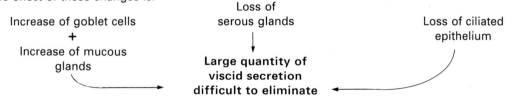

Increase of goblet cells + Increase of mucous glands

Loss of serous glands

Large quantity of viscid secretion difficult to eliminate

Loss of ciliated epithelium

The tendency to retention of secretion encourages bacterial growth and thus a vicious circle may be set up.

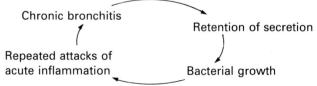

Chronic bronchitis

Retention of secretion

Repeated attacks of acute inflammation

Bacterial growth

Continued chronic irritation may result in squamous metaplasia of the bronchial epithelium.

299

CHRONIC BRONCHITIS

With repeated acute exacerbations of the inflammation and increasing retention of secretion, spread of the chronic changes along the bronchial tree is encouraged.

When the terminal bronchioles are affected, more serious changes take place:

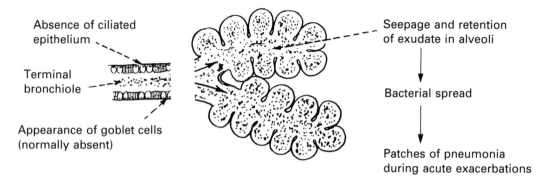

Absence of ciliated epithelium

Terminal bronchiole

Appearance of goblet cells (normally absent)

Seepage and retention of exudate in alveoli

↓

Bacterial spread

↓

Patches of pneumonia during acute exacerbations

The lack of ciliary action makes it difficult to get rid of exudate and hinders resolution. Healing takes place by organisation. The results of this process are as follows:

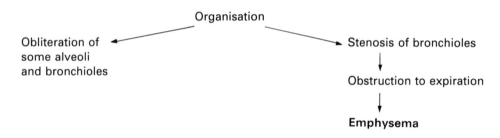

Organisation

Obliteration of some alveoli and bronchioles

Stenosis of bronchioles

↓

Obstruction to expiration

↓

Emphysema

The causes of chronic bronchitis are multiple and form an interacting complex.

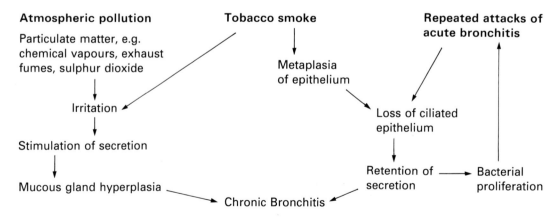

Atmospheric pollution

Particulate matter, e.g. chemical vapours, exhaust fumes, sulphur dioxide

↓

Irritation

↓

Stimulation of secretion

↓

Mucous gland hyperplasia

Tobacco smoke

↓

Metaplasia of epithelium

Repeated attacks of acute bronchitis

Loss of ciliated epithelium

↓

Retention of secretion → Bacterial proliferation

Chronic Bronchitis

Chronic bronchitis is most common in industrial areas with a high rainfall. In its serious form it occurs in males over the age of 40, but the onset can be dated many years earlier.

BRONCHIAL ASTHMA

This condition, of allergic nature, is characterised by spasmodic attacks of severe dyspnoea with some coughing. The difficulty in breathing is mainly related to exhalation due to the plugging of bronchioles with viscid mucus. The lung is rather voluminous but without any real emphysema.

Histological changes are a combination of allergic reaction and muscular hypertrophy, the result of prolonged spasm.

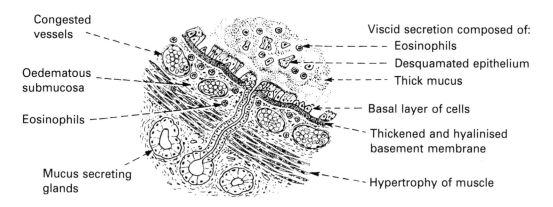

Congested vessels

Oedematous submucosa

Eosinophils

Mucus secreting glands

Viscid secretion composed of:
— Eosinophils
— Desquamated epithelium
— Thick mucus

Basal layer of cells

Thickened and hyalinised basement membrane

Hypertrophy of muscle

The asthmatic attack begins with difficulty in breathing, particularly exhalation, producing loud wheezing noises. Coughing which is non-productive may occur. At the end of the attack, thick viscid sputum is produced.

Sputum

In some cases the following may be seen:

1. *Curschmann's spirals* — appear as small white granules in sputum.

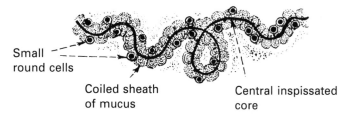

Small round cells

Coiled sheath of mucus

Central inspissated core

2. *Charcot-Leyden crystals* — in association with eosinophils.

Diamond-shaped crystal

Eosinophil

BRONCHIAL ASTHMA

COMPLICATIONS

The repeated attacks of coughing and excessive mucus production may induce a chronic bronchitic condition. This in turn may result in emphysema. An attack may be prolonged and unremitting – **status asthmaticus** and death may occur.

Aetiology: Although two mechanisms are recognised they are not completely separable.

Extrinsic Immune reaction – Type 1 hypersensitivity	Intrinsic Abnormal autonomic regulation of airways
Family history of hypersensitivity common Starts in childhood Preceded by infantile eczema and hypersensitivity to foods Predisposition to form IgE antibodies Allergens recognised – pollen, dandruff, house dust mite Attacks often diminish in later years Chronic bronchitis seldom develops Emphysema unusual No drug sensitivity	No family history Starts in adult life No evidence of atopy IgE antibodies may be formed but no particular predisposition No recognisable allergens Attacks increase in severity Associated with nasal polypi and chronic bronchitis Emphysema commonly develops Drug sensitivity may develop (aspirin, penicillin)

BRONCHIECTASIS

Bronchiectasis means a permanent dilatation of one or more bronchi.

The main bronchi up to the 4th division possess large supporting cartilage rings and the condition only affects bronchi beyond this point. Two main anatomical varieties are described but these may have similar causes and frequently both are found in the same lung.

1. Cylindrical

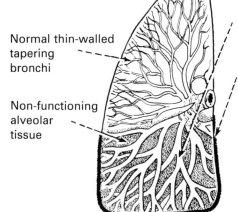

Normal thin-walled tapering bronchi

Non-functioning alveolar tissue

This type is almost always found in the lower lobes. The bronchi are grossly dilated throughout their length. Intervening lung tissue is much reduced and much of it is fibrosed.

The pleura is usually fibrotic and thick with dense adhesions to the chest wall.

There is a foul smell due to the large quantities of secretion containing putrefactive bacteria.

A variation of this type is called 'fusiform' where the bronchi are spindle-shaped, the dilatation affecting part of the length while either end is of normal calibre.

2. Saccular

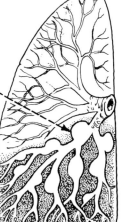

Saccular dilatations usually containing pus

As the name suggests the dilatations tend to be more localised and exaggerated. They are roughly rounded and may be single or multiple. Sometimes they are associated with bronchial obstruction due to tumour, enlarged glands or foreign body. They may also occur in chronic tuberculosis. In these cases, the bronchiectasis may be found in the upper lobe.

BRONCHIECTASIS

Microscopical changes

BRONCHI. The condition usually follows a viral pneumonia in childhood and the initial change is the production of lymphoid aggregations in the bronchial wall.

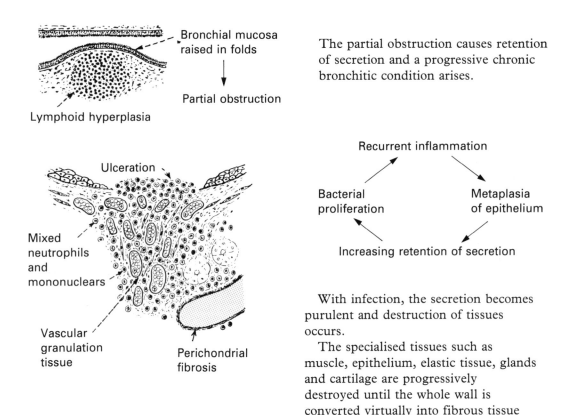

Bronchial mucosa raised in folds

Partial obstruction

Lymphoid hyperplasia

Ulceration

Mixed neutrophils and mononuclears

Vascular granulation tissue

Perichondrial fibrosis

The partial obstruction causes retention of secretion and a progressive chronic bronchitic condition arises.

Recurrent inflammation

Bacterial proliferation

Metaplasia of epithelium

Increasing retention of secretion

With infection, the secretion becomes purulent and destruction of tissues occurs.

The specialised tissues such as muscle, epithelium, elastic tissue, glands and cartilage are progressively destroyed until the whole wall is converted virtually into fibrous tissue with areas of ulceration.

BRONCHIOLES. Frequently these are obliterated by pre-existing disease or may become so due to spread of the inflammatory process along the bronchus. Bands of fibrous tissue are created during healing of these lesions.

ALVEOLAR TISSUE. The alveoli associated with the terminal bronchioles are also obliterated by the inflammatory process or secondary to collapse. In addition, much of the alveolar tissue adjacent to the dilated bronchi is compressed, rendered non-functional and may also be involved by spread of infection.

PLEURA. The inflammatory changes in terminal bronchioles and alveoli extend to the pleura, both layers of which become adherent and fibrotic. More or less continuous bands of fibrous tissue may be formed between the wall of the bronchus and the pleura.

BRONCHIECTASIS

Mechanism of formation

This involves a combination of mechanical factors and concomitant inflammatory changes. The process may be visualised as follows:

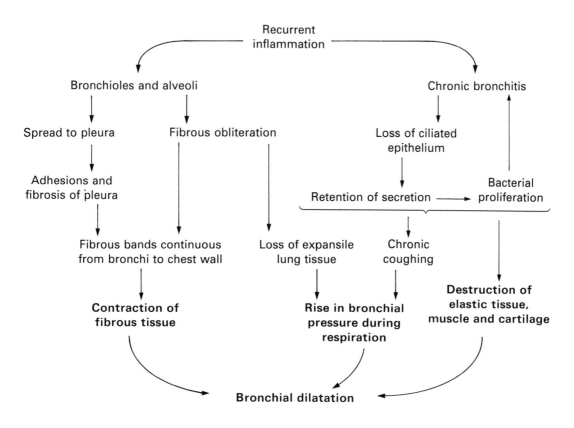

Aetiology

INFECTION. Most cases are initiated by bronchopneumonia which fails to resolve. In children this may be of primary bacterial origin or a complication of specific infections, e.g. measles, whooping cough. Other virus infections, e.g. adenovirus, may be important.

BRONCHIAL OBSTRUCTION. Partial bronchial obstruction by neoplastic growth, enlarged lymph nodes or foreign body, causes retention of secretion and infection leading to localised bronchiectasis.

PNEUMOCONIOSIS. Very occasionally lung fibrosis leads to bronchiectasis.

CONGENITAL DISEASE. Bronchiectasis may complicate maldevelopment of part of the lung or follow acute purulent infections complicating fibrocystic disease (mucoviscoidosis). See page 484.

BRONCHIECTASIS

Effects

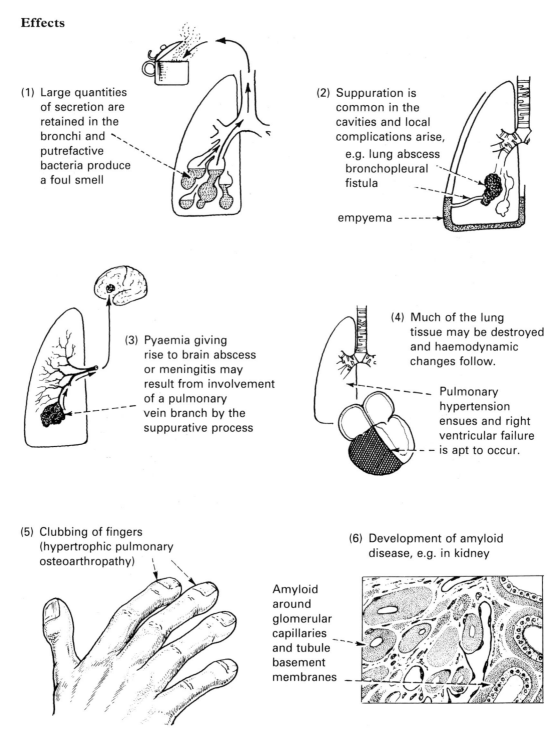

(1) Large quantities of secretion are retained in the bronchi and putrefactive bacteria produce a foul smell

(2) Suppuration is common in the cavities and local complications arise,

e.g. lung abscess
bronchopleural fistula

empyema

(3) Pyaemia giving rise to brain abscess or meningitis may result from involvement of a pulmonary vein branch by the suppurative process

(4) Much of the lung tissue may be destroyed and haemodynamic changes follow.

Pulmonary hypertension ensues and right ventricular failure is apt to occur.

(5) Clubbing of fingers (hypertrophic pulmonary osteoarthropathy)

(6) Development of amyloid disease, e.g. in kidney

Amyloid around glomerular capillaries and tubule basement membranes

EMPHYSEMA

In this condition there is a permanent increase in the size of air spaces distal to the terminal bronchiole with destructive changes in their walls. It causes dyspnoea and is associated with chronic coughing.

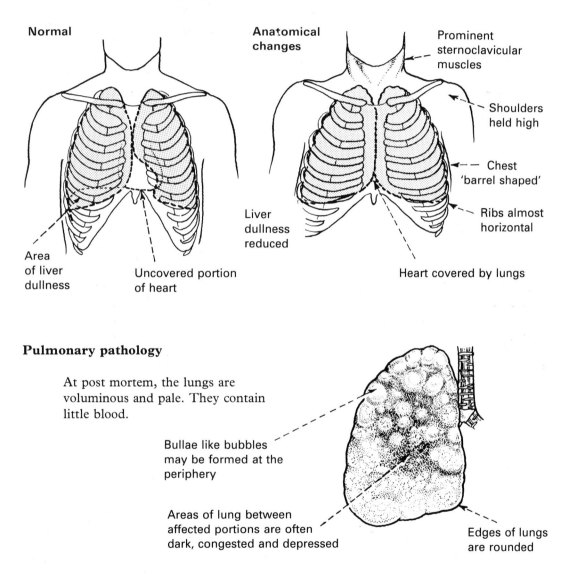

Normal

Area of liver dullness

Uncovered portion of heart

Anatomical changes

Prominent sternoclavicular muscles

Shoulders held high

Chest 'barrel shaped'

Ribs almost horizontal

Liver dullness reduced

Heart covered by lungs

Pulmonary pathology

At post mortem, the lungs are voluminous and pale. They contain little blood.

Bullae like bubbles may be formed at the periphery

Areas of lung between affected portions are often dark, congested and depressed

Edges of lungs are rounded

Section of the lung can reveal two separate patterns:
(1) **alveolar emphysema** and (2) **centrilobular emphysema**.

307

EMPHYSEMA

ALVEOLAR EMPHYSEMA (PANACINAR)

This is the condition which produces the
striking anatomical changes
characteristically associated with
emphysema. Clinically, breathlessness is
striking.

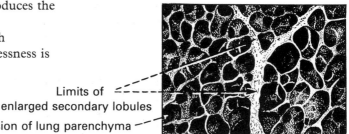

Limits of
enlarged secondary lobules

General distension of lung parenchyma

Histology shows distension of the alveolar tissue.

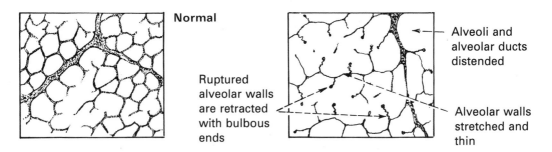

Normal

Ruptured
alveolar walls
are retracted
with bulbous
ends

Alveoli and
alveolar ducts
distended

Alveolar walls
stretched and
thin

Special stains show loss of elastic tissue. The capillaries are stretched and thinned. The
reduction in blood supply is probably a factor in leading to rupture of alveoli.

There is little evidence of bronchiolitis. The voluminous lungs produce characteristic
radiological changes. The distension eventually spreads to involve the respiratory
bronchiole, i.e. the whole acinus is affected — panacinar emphysema.

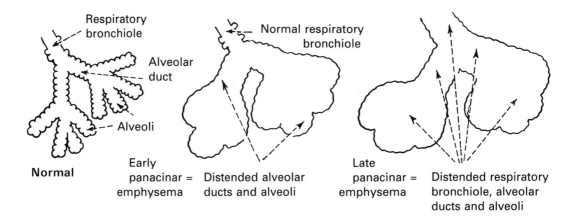

Respiratory
bronchiole

Alveolar
duct

Alveoli

Normal

Early
panacinar =
emphysema

Distended alveolar
ducts and alveoli

Normal respiratory
bronchiole

Late
panacinar =
emphysema

Distended respiratory
bronchiole, alveolar
ducts and alveoli

EMPHYSEMA

CENTRILOBULAR EMPHYSEMA

In centrilobular emphysema, there is no enlargement of the lung and the condition tends to be most marked in the upper lobes. A characteristic pattern is only obvious in cross section of the lungs. In this type hypoxia is severe leading to pulmonary hypertension and right heart failure (cor pulmonale).

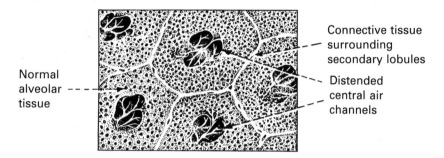

Normal alveolar tissue

Connective tissue surrounding secondary lobules

Distended central air channels

Microscopically, the condition is seen to affect the respiratory bronchioles.

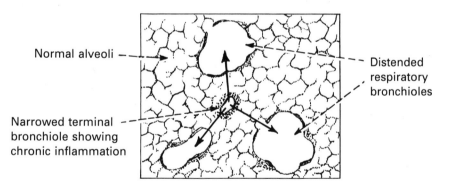

Normal alveoli

Distended respiratory bronchioles

Narrowed terminal bronchiole showing chronic inflammation

The chronic inflammation of the terminal bronchioles is an important feature. In this type of lesion, there is little radiological evidence of emphysema since the alveolar tissue is normal for a considerable time.

Eventually, in many lobules the distension extends to involve the alveolar tissue producing panacinar emphysema.

309

EMPHYSEMA

AETIOLOGY and MECHANISMS

The essential cause is thought to be an imbalance between protease and anti-protease activity at alveolar level. The presence of increased elastase leads to gradual weakening and destruction of alveolar walls.

This is best seen in cases with homozygous α_1-antitrypsin (α_1AT) deficiency where panacinar emphysema develops.

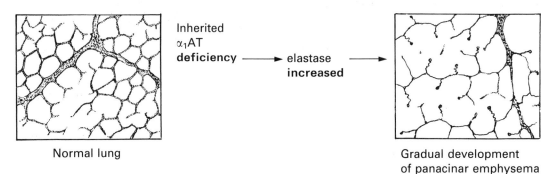

Inherited
α_1AT
deficiency ⟶ elastase
increased ⟶

Normal lung

Gradual development
of panacinar emphysema

Smoking and the coughing associated with chronic bronchitis are connected with centrilobular emphysema.

Centrilobular emphysema (see p.309)

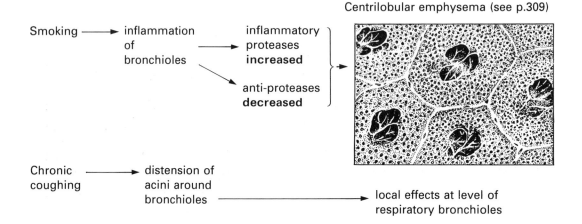

Smoking ⟶ inflammation
of
bronchioles ⟶ inflammatory
proteases
increased

anti-proteases
decreased

⟶ local effects at level of
respiratory bronchioles

Chronic ⟶ distension of
coughing acini around
bronchioles

FUNCTIONAL EFFECTS

Clinically the functional effects are considered under the umbrella title – chronic obstructive airways disease (COAD) (see p.299).

In alveolar emphysema Type 1 respiratory failure is seen initially and the patients are 'Pink Puffers'.

In centrilobular emphysema the bronchiolitis and coughing lead to more serious functional deficiency: the respiratory failure is Type 2 with both hypoxia and cyanosis: the patients tend to be 'Blue Bloaters'.

EMPHYSEMA – OTHER FORMS

FOCAL DUST EMPHYSEMA

This is found in coal miners and is associated with deposition of dust in the walls of bronchioles which become fibrotic and inelastic. Chronic coughing induces stretching of the inelastic bronchiolar walls and a mild form of centrilobular emphysema ensues.

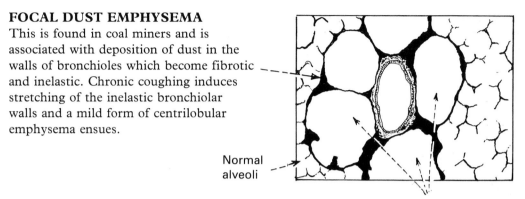

Normal alveoli

Dilated respiratory bronchioles

The deposition of dust around the bronchioles is assumed to trigger the mechanisms for centrilobular emphysema described on previous page.

ATROPHIC or SENILE EMPHYSEMA

This condition occurs in old age and wasting diseases. The lungs are not enlarged and no bullae are formed. The alveolar septa atrophy due to deficient nutrition. It is doubtful if the term emphysema is justified in this condition.

INTERSTITIAL EMPHYSEMA (SURGICAL EMPHYSEMA)

Air may penetrate into the connective tissue framework surrounding the secondary lobules of the lung. It may travel along the septa to the pleura of the lung producing a fine white beaded appearance on the surface. If a large amount of air penetrates the tissues, it can spread via lymphatics and tissue spaces to the mediastinum and to the subcutaneous regions of the neck.

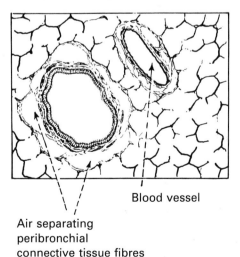

Blood vessel

Air separating peribronchial connective tissue fibres

There are two main causes:

1. Over distension of alveoli due to coughing as in whooping cough, bronchiolitis or Caisson disease or to forced inspiration, e.g. during positive pressure ventilation in the newborn.
2. Trauma. Penetrating and crush injuries of the chest wall.

311

ATELECTASIS

This means failure of the lung to expand at the time of birth.

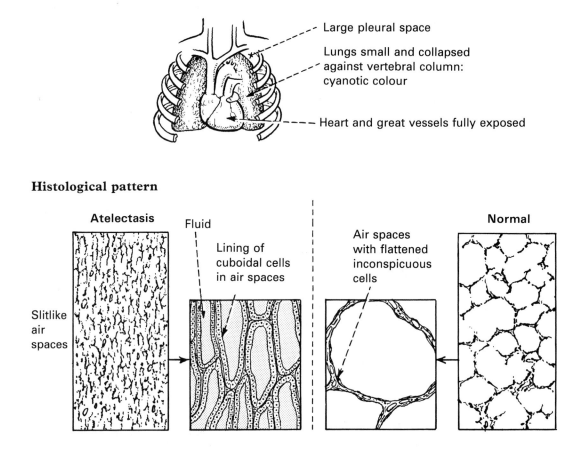

- - - Large pleural space

- - - Lungs small and collapsed against vertebral column: cyanotic colour

- - - Heart and great vessels fully exposed

Histological pattern

Atelectasis

Fluid

Lining of cuboidal cells in air spaces

Slitlike air spaces

Air spaces with flattened inconspicuous cells

Normal

The condition is due to lack of proper inspiration at birth. It occurs in premature infants. Two factors probably operate in varying degree.

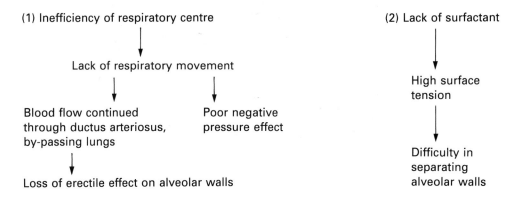

(1) Inefficiency of respiratory centre

Lack of respiratory movement

Blood flow continued through ductus arteriosus, by-passing lungs

Poor negative pressure effect

Loss of erectile effect on alveolar walls

(2) Lack of surfactant

High surface tension

Difficulty in separating alveolar walls

HYALINE MEMBRANE DISEASE

This is a condition of absorption collapse (see p.315) affecting the newborn, with a mortality rate of at least 30%. It differs from atelectasis in its time of onset, the mechanism involved and the bronchiolar changes.

Associated factors

These include prematurity, caesarean section and maternal diabetes.

Respiration is apparently normal at birth, but there is increasing difficulty within a short time, minutes to hours. X-ray examination shows loss of expansion until almost complete collapse occurs.

Clinical effects

These are the result of:

1. Increasing difficulty in obtaining alveolar expansion leading to laboured respiration with use of accessory muscles such as sternomastoid.

2. Lack of oxygenation, hypoxia and cyanosis.

Due to the lack of expansion and the consequent lack of negative alveolar pressure, little blood is drawn into the lungs and there is a continuation of the fetal circulation, i.e. largely a right to left shunt via the foramen ovale and ductus arteriosus.

Pathology

The lungs are very often similar in appearance to those seen in atelectasis. If the changes are less diffuse, the lung shows 'geographical' markings – collapsed congested areas — — — — — — — — surrounded by more normal lung tissue.

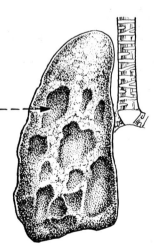

Histologically, the alveoli are collapsed, while the respiratory bronchioles tend to be distended and lined by a prominent pink-staining hyaline membrane of proteinaceous character.

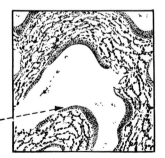

313

HYALINE MEMBRANE DISEASE

Mechanism of production

The main factor is probably immaturity of the lung tissue which, prior to the 34th week of pregnancy, has little ability to secrete lecithin. This is the main component of surfactant, which lowers surface tension. This has two effects:

1. Prevents alveolar walls sticking together and thus allowing easy opening by inspiratory pressure.

2. Allows alveolar fluid to spread as an even film over the walls. This protects surfaces from direct exposure to the air and the cells only have to deal with dissolved gases.

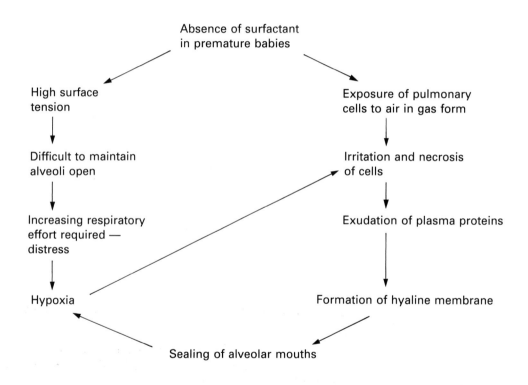

Secondary changes arise as a result of hypoxia – tendency to haemorrhage and disseminated thrombotic episodes.

ADULT RESPIRATORY DISTRESS SYNDROME (ARDS)

The adult lung may show similar changes secondary to a wide variety of disorders: severe shock, inhalation of irritant gases and pure oxygen, paraquat ingestion and uraemia are a few examples.

The condition is illustrated as **shock lung** (see p.197).

COLLAPSE OF LUNG

ABSORPTION COLLAPSE

This is a common condition and
is due to bronchial obstruction

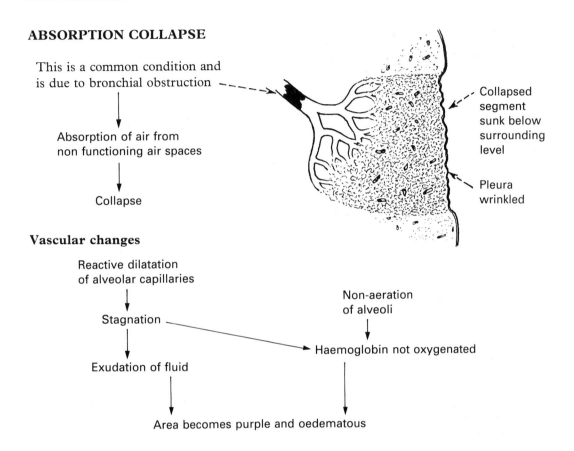

↓

Absorption of air from
non functioning air spaces

↓

Collapse

Collapsed
segment
sunk below
surrounding
level

Pleura
wrinkled

Vascular changes

Reactive dilatation
of alveolar capillaries

↓

Stagnation

↓

Exudation of fluid

↓

Non-aeration
of alveoli

↓

Haemoglobin not oxygenated

↓

Area becomes purple and oedematous

Subsequent development

1. Secretions accumulate behind the obstruction. These frequently become infected and suppuration with abscess formation occurs.

2. In the absence of infection, and if the collapse persists, the granular pneumocytes of the alveoli proliferate and this is followed by progressive fibrosis. Local pulmonary artery branches show narrowing of the lumen due to intimal fibroelastosis.

Causes of obstruction

Acute obstruction

Large bronchi may be blocked by foreign bodies. Small bronchi are frequently blocked by mucus during pulmonary infections.

Chronic obstruction

1. Tumours in the wall of bronchus.
2. Tumours or enlarged lymph nodes pressing on bronchus.

315

COLLAPSE OF LUNG

PRESSURE COLLAPSE
Diffuse collapse may be caused by air or fluid in the pleural cavity.

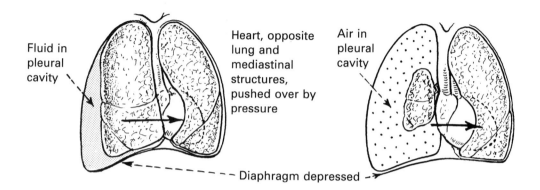

Fluid in pleural cavity

Heart, opposite lung and mediastinal structures, pushed over by pressure

Air in pleural cavity

Diaphragm depressed

Causes

1. Air in pleural cavity – pneumothorax – may result from:
   (a) rupture of emphysematous bulla
   (b) penetrating injury of chest wall, particularly if valve opening produced
   (c) fistulous communication with stomach or oesophagus due to injury or cancer.

2. Pleural effusion due to infection or malignant growth on the pleural surface.

3. Empyema. This condition, now rare in developed countries is usually due to spread of infection from the lung.

4. Haemothorax. Trauma, rupture of a mediastinal aneurysm or haemorrhage from a local cancerous growth may cause effusion of blood into a pleural cavity.

Subsequent development
1. Unlike absorption collapse there is no obstruction to the drainage of pulmonary secretions and therefore no development of new pulmonary inflammation.
2. Inflammation is, however the main problem. Even in pneumothorax, effusion of fluid quickly takes place and secondary infection follows.
3. If the tension within the pleural cavity is unrelieved, healing can occur by organisation of the exudate. Collapse of the lung becomes permanent and pulmonary fibrosis results.

PNEUMONIA – BRONCHOPNEUMONIA

Pneumonia is an inflammatory process involving the alveolar tissue of the lungs. Three main types exist:

1. Bronchopneumonia
2. Lobar pneumonia
3. Interstitial pneumonia

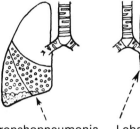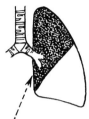

Bronchopneumonia   Lobar pneumonia

BRONCHOPNEUMONIA

Bronchopneumonia caused by a variety of bacteria, is the commonest form. It may affect all ages, but it is particularly frequent in four circumstances:

1. as a terminal event in a chronic debilitating disease
2. in infancy
3. in old age
4. as a manifestation of secondary infection in viral conditions, e.g. influenza, measles.

Bronchopneumonia is primarily a spreading inflammation of terminal bronchioles and their related alveoli.

The lesions are initially focal, involving one or more lobules. First red, then grey, they show a central bronchiole containing pus.

Being a spreading inflammation, the foci are not all at the same stage of the inflammatory process.

The disease starts as a bronchiolitis.

Lesions are usually in the lower lobes

At the lung base the changes are more advanced, coalesce and become confluent

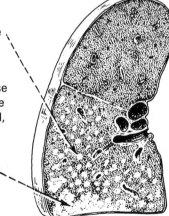

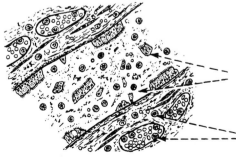

Bronchiole becomes inflamed; ciliated epithelium is destroyed

Congestion of vessels and emigration of neutrophils

317

BRONCHOPNEUMONIA

After the initial bronchiolitis, spread to the alveoli quickly follows.

1. In the early stages, the alveolar walls are congested giving a red colour to the tissues.

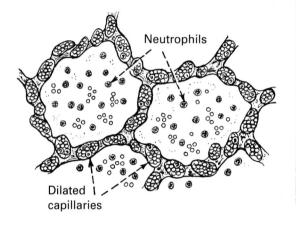

2. At a later stage the exudate becomes fibrinous and neutrophils are extremely numerous. Congestion is less marked and the lesions become pale grey.

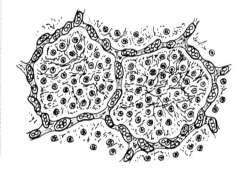

Inflammation spreads through pores of Kohn to adjacent lobules.

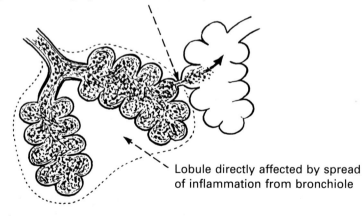

Lobule directly affected by spread of inflammation from bronchiole

The onset is insidious, but marked toxaemia develops. When the inflammation subsides, resolution may take place. The fibrin is dissolved and the exudate is partly absorbed and partly removed by coughing.

BRONCHOPNEUMONIA – COMPLICATIONS

1. **Death** is common since the pneumonia commonly complicates debilitating disease (hypostatic pneumonia).

2. **Resolution** is often incomplete, even if the patient survives. Many consolidated patches end in fibrosis. Granulation tissue is formed as in a healing wound.

Macrophages gradually clear the exudate while fibroblasts and blood vessels grow in from the alveolar septa.

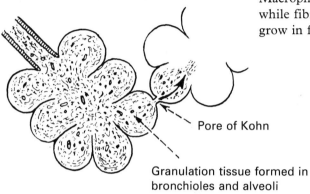

Pore of Kohn

Granulation tissue formed in bronchioles and alveoli

If the resulting fibrosis is gross, the lung structure may be distorted and changes in the larger bronchi cause bronchiectasis. A vicious circle may be set up:

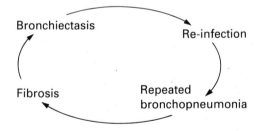

Bronchiectasis

Re-infection

Fibrosis

Repeated bronchopneumonia

3. **Suppurative Changes**
   These are less common with specific antibiotic treatment, but lung abscess and empyema occur in debilitated patients, and especially in cases of aspiration pneumonia.

LOBAR PNEUMONIA

As the name suggests, in this condition a complete lobe or even two lobes of a lung are affected. The most striking changes occur in the alveolar tissue. Although spread of the inflammatory process is via the ducts and not through alveolar walls, changes in the bronchioles are of minor importance. The disease is seen in adult males previously healthy, mainly between 30 and 50 years. It is rare in Western countries but still occurs frequently in underdeveloped countries. One attack gives little immunity. Repeated attacks are common. The sudden onset and pathology suggest an element of hypersensitivity.

Four distinct phases are recognised:

1. Congestion (1–2 days)
2. Red hepatisation (2nd–4th day)
3. Grey hepatisation (4th–8th day)
4. Resolution (8th–9th day).

These are the classic phases seen only in untreated cases. Antibiotic therapy dramatically inhibits the changes described below.

1. Congestion (1—2 days)

The lobe of lung shows the usual early changes of acute inflammation. It is dark red, and frothy, blood-stained fluid can be squeezed from it. Large numbers of the causative bacteria are present in the fluid. Microscopically, the alveolar capillaries are engorged and contain an increased number of neutrophils.

The onset is sudden with fever and rigors.

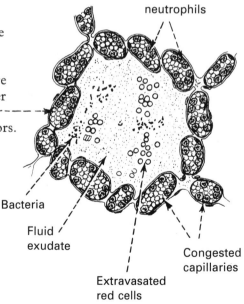

Increase in neutrophils

Bacteria

Fluid exudate

Extravasated red cells

Congested capillaries

LOBAR PNEUMONIA

2. Red hepatisation (2nd–4th day)

The lobe is dry, solid, red and granular. It contains no air. Some fibrin is present on the pleural surface. In addition to the congestion of the previous stage, there is now a well-marked fibrinous exudate, and there are neutrophils in the alveoli.

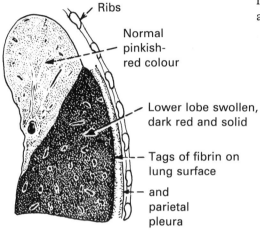

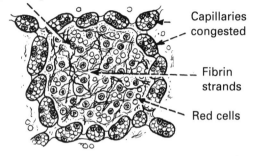

Clinically, there is pain on breathing, due to the pleural exudate, and a productive cough with brown sputum. Leucocytosis occurs early and a positive blood culture is obtained in most cases.

3. Grey hepatisation (4th–8th day)

The affected lobe is even more solid, and the pleural surface is covered by a confluent fibrinous exudate. The cut surface is dry and granular but of a greyish white colour. The alveolar exudate is increased in amount, with dense fibrin strands and very numerous neutrophils. It is this exudate which gives the grey colour to the affected lobe. The congestion of capillaries is now much reduced.

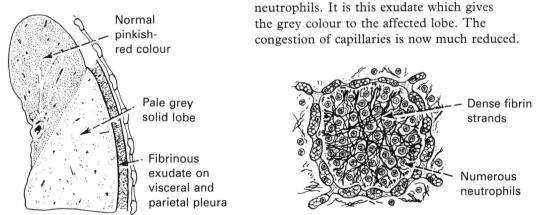

Antibodies to the bacteria appear in the blood at this stage, and the organisms disappear quite rapidly. Coughing is not so marked and less productive. Pain and high fever persist.

LOBAR PNEUMONIA

4. **Resolution (8th—9th day)**

With elimination of the bacteria, the inflammatory process subsides, and since there is no tissue destruction, the lung returns to normal apart from the pleura where the fibrinous adhesions between the visceral and parietal layers tend to undergo organisation with the formation of fibrous adhesions. The fibrin is liquefied by proteolytic enzymes possibly produced in part by the neutrophils. The liquid products together with neutrophils are coughed up – macrophages from the lung tissues invade the alveoli.

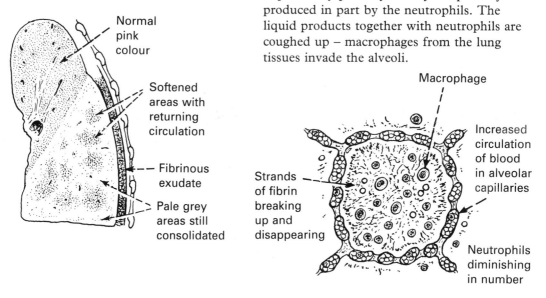

The disease ends in a 'crisis' with sudden drop in temperature.

Bacteriology of lobar pneumonia

The cause of the disease is *Streptococcus pneumoniae*, which has a distinctive morphology.

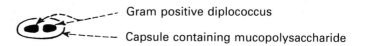

Eight types are recognised, but 90% of cases are caused by seven of these. The following order is an indication of their frequency: I, III, II, V, VII, VIII and IV. Almost 70% of cases are due to Types I, II and III. Type III is found mainly in patients over the age of 50 already suffering from some other disease and the mortality rate is high despite treatment. It has a large amount of capsular substance and this gives a mucoid consistency to the exudate. Complications are more common with this infection, particularly lung abscess.

Types I and II are more commonly found in younger patients.

VIRAL PNEUMONIAS

INFLUENZA

In most cases, influenzal infection is confined to the upper respiratory tract, but in debilitated persons and during epidemics, the whole respiratory tract is affected.

Trachea and bronchi

Intense inflammation with haemorrhage develops.

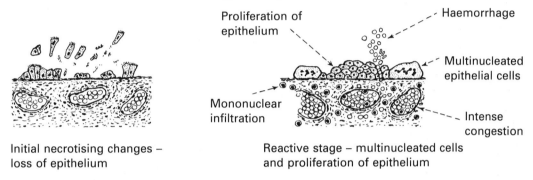

Initial necrotising changes – loss of epithelium

Reactive stage – multinucleated cells and proliferation of epithelium

Pneumonia changes

The lungs are bulky, purple red and exude blood-stained froth when cut. The microscopical changes vary from one part to another.

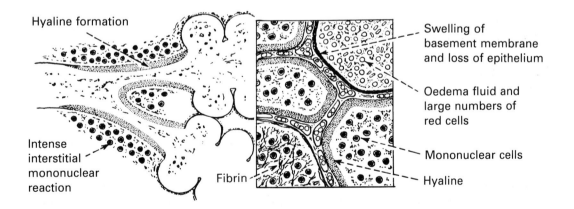

Infective agents

Three main types of influenza virus exist: A, B and C. The A type is the most virulent, and mutants of this type are responsible for most epidemics and the fatalities which occur.

Secondary infection is common, the bacteria most frequently involved being *Haemophilus influenzae, Streptococcus pneumoniae, Streptococcus pyogenes* and *Staphylococcus aureus*.

VIRAL PNEUMONIAS

There are a number of pneumonic conditions due to viruses and virus-like agents in which a common pattern of pathological change is observed.

1. Necrotising bronchiolitis

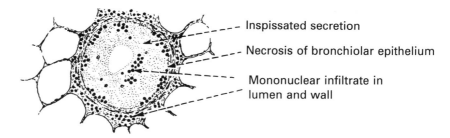

- - Inspissated secretion

- - Necrosis of bronchiolar epithelium

- - Mononuclear infiltrate in lumen and wall

2. Interstitial pneumonia

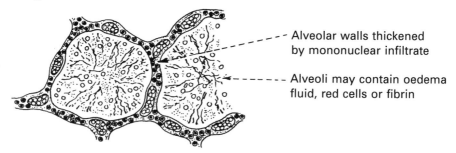

- - Alveolar walls thickened by mononuclear infiltrate

- - Alveoli may contain oedema fluid, red cells or fibrin

3. Reactive changes

The lining epithelial cells of bronchioles and alveoli are stimulated by the presence of the virus.

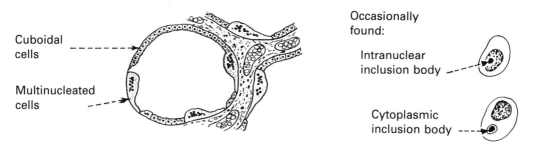

Cuboidal cells

Multinucleated cells

Occasionally found:

Intranuclear inclusion body

Cytoplasmic inclusion body

Variations in the basic pattern occur in different infections. Confluent consolidation is often found in psittacosis and ornithosis (viruses transmitted by birds) and in measles giant cell pneumonia. Interstitial pneumonia is produced by cytomegalovirus and in rickettsial infections such as Q fever (occurring in slaughter house workers infected by animal skins) and 'scrub typhus'. In mycoplasma pneumonia, inflammation spreads from the bronchioles into the lung parenchyma.

LEGIONNAIRE'S DISEASE

Previously confused with pneumococcal pneumonia, Legionnaire's disease occurs in small epidemics, is more common in males and is due to a tiny Gram-negative bacillus – *Legionella pneumophila*. The death rate can be high – up to 20%. Infection is associated with inhalation of aerosol from contaminated water storage systems.

Clinical features

Two phases are recognised:
Prodromal phase – vague flu-like illness lasting about 5 days.

Active phase

A dry cough develops. Vomiting and diarrhoea may be severe.
Patient becomes somnolent, confused and signs of consolidation appear.

Laboratory findings

Hyponatraemia. Lymphopenia. Neutrophils normal.
Signs of disseminated intravascular coagulation may develop.

Pathology

Both lungs are consolidated, dark red, heavy and oedematous. Fibrinous pleurisy or pleural effusion may be found.

Histology

Two stages are evident:

First stage

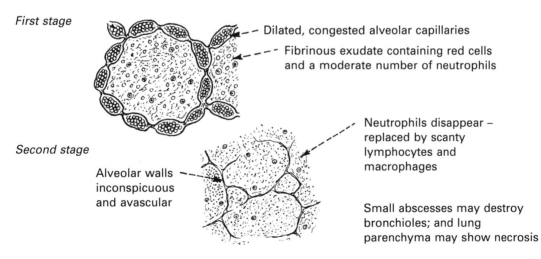

Dilated, congested alveolar capillaries

Fibrinous exudate containing red cells and a moderate number of neutrophils

Second stage

Neutrophils disappear – replaced by scanty lymphocytes and macrophages

Alveolar walls inconspicuous and avascular

Small abscesses may destroy bronchioles; and lung parenchyma may show necrosis

The exudate may organise, causing an increasing interstitial fibrosis with permanent loss of lung function.

325

PNEUMONIA – SPECIAL TYPES

ASPIRATION PNEUMONIA

This is due to inhalation of food or infected material from the mouth or pharynx. It may occur during anaesthesia or coma or may complicate conditions associated with frequent regurgitation e.g. oesophageal obstructions, pyloric stenosis.

In adult cases the inhalation of acid gastric contents may cause an initial shock reaction: in other cases the onset is insidious.

Possible progression is as follows:

Inhalation of foreign material ——————▶ Secondary infection ——————▶ Bronchopneumonia lung abscess

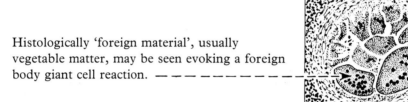

Histologically 'foreign material', usually vegetable matter, may be seen evoking a foreign body giant cell reaction. — — — — — — — — — —

Lipid pneumonia

– The exogenous form is due to long-continued inhalation of small quantities of oily material usually derived from nasal medicaments: it is often clinically silent.

– The endogenous form is derived from tissue lipid debris distal to local bronchial obstruction.

Miscellaneous pneumonias

(1) Opportunistic infections are becoming more common (see p.91).
The causative agents include:
Viruses   – e.g. *Cytomegalovirus.*
Protozoa – e.g. *Pneumocystis carinii.*
Fungi   – e.g. *Aspergillus fumigatus, Candida albicans, Cryptococcus neoformans.*

(2) The use of non-sterile equipment and material for intravenous injection by drug addicts may cause infected emboli with spread of the inflammation into adjacent lung tissue.

LUNG ABSCESS

This is now an uncommon condition. The usual causes are:

1. Inhalation of infected material from the larynx or pharynx.

2. Obstruction of a bronchus by tumour growth or foreign body. Site depends on size of bronchus affected.

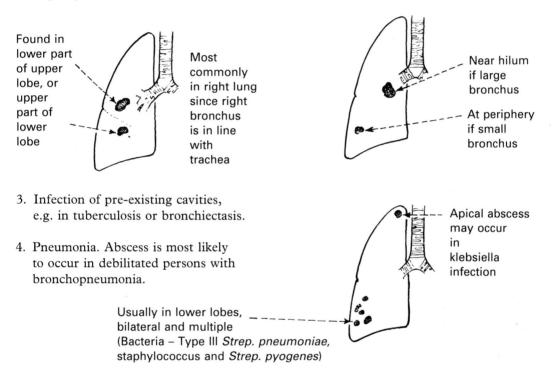

Found in lower part of upper lobe, or upper part of lower lobe

Most commonly in right lung since right bronchus is in line with trachea

Near hilum if large bronchus

At periphery if small bronchus

3. Infection of pre-existing cavities, e.g. in tuberculosis or bronchiectasis.

4. Pneumonia. Abscess is most likely to occur in debilitated persons with bronchopneumonia.

Apical abscess may occur in klebsiella infection

Usually in lower lobes, bilateral and multiple (Bacteria – Type III *Strep. pneumoniae*, staphylococcus and *Strep. pyogenes*)

Rarer causes of abscess are: pyaemia, trauma to lung, extension from suppuration in mediastinum, spinal column or subphrenic region, and infection with *entamoeba histolytica*.

Sequelae of lung abscess

1. Small abscesses may heal.

2. Subpleural abscesses may extend to cause empyema.

3. Bronchopleural fistula resulting in pyopneumothorax is a further complication following on 2.

4. If a large pulmonary vessel is eroded, fatal haemorrhage can occur.

5. On occasion, blood spread leads to meningitis or cerebral abscess.

TUBERCULOSIS

The lungs are more commonly affected by tuberculosis than any other organ. Where tuberculosis is common, infection usually occurs in childhood. In advanced countries where the incidence is lower, the initial lesions of tuberculosis may be delayed until adult life, and certainly the serious forms of this disease are usually found in older individuals.

PRIMARY LESION (GHON FOCUS)

1. Infection is by inhalation

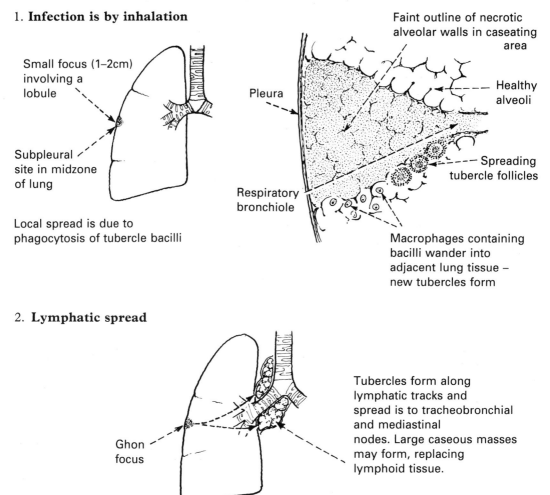

Small focus (1–2cm) involving a lobule

Subpleural site in midzone of lung

Local spread is due to phagocytosis of tubercle bacilli

Faint outline of necrotic alveolar walls in caseating area

Pleura

Healthy alveoli

Respiratory bronchiole

Spreading tubercle follicles

Macrophages containing bacilli wander into adjacent lung tissue – new tubercles form

2. Lymphatic spread

Ghon focus

Tubercles form along lymphatic tracks and spread is to tracheobronchial and mediastinal nodes. Large caseous masses may form, replacing lymphoid tissue.

The combination of the Ghon focus plus hilar nodes is termed the primary complex.

TUBERCULOSIS

SUBSEQUENT DEVELOPMENTS

1. **Healing**
   This is the commonest result.
   Small Ghon focus – complete fibrosis.
   Larger focus – caseous material is encapsulated by fibrous tissue and undergoes calcification. The same changes occur in the hilar nodes.

2. **Spread from the Ghon focus**
   (a) The inflammatory reaction in the adjacent lung tissue may induce an effusion in the pleural cavity.

   (b) Actual tuberculous infection of the pleura may occur resulting in tuberculous empyema.

   Ghon focus

   Lung

3. **Changes due to hilar node involvement**

(a) **Mechanical effect**. Pressure of enlarged nodes on bronchi: bronchial obstruction may lead to collapse, retention of secretion and inflammatory consolidation.

(b) **Spread of tubercles along bronchial lymphatics**

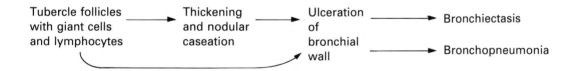

| Tubercle follicles with giant cells and lymphocytes | → | Thickening and nodular caseation | → | Ulceration of bronchial wall | → | Bronchiectasis |
| | | | | | → | Bronchopneumonia |

(c) **Invasion of blood vessels**. This will lead to dissemination via the blood stream giving rise to tuberculous foci simultaneously in many organs (generalised miliary tuberculosis). A modified version of this is seen when tuberculous infection invades one or more branches of the pulmonary artery. Numerous miliary tubercles form in the lung tissue only.

TUBERCULOSIS

SECONDARY TUBERCULOSIS (POST-PRIMARY)

This is a recurrence of tuberculous infection in later life, and may be due to reactivation of the primary lesion or a re-infection by tubercle bacilli.

The lesions tend to appear in characteristic sites:

(a) posterior sub-apical and (b) upper part of lower lobes where the aeration is in relative excess over the blood flow, rendering the tissues susceptible to infection.

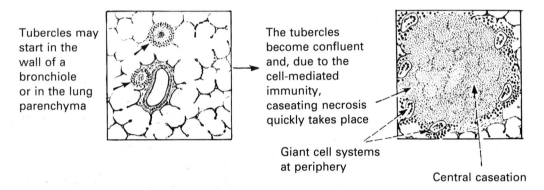

Tubercles may start in the wall of a bronchiole or in the lung parenchyma

The tubercles become confluent and, due to the cell-mediated immunity, caseating necrosis quickly takes place

Giant cell systems at periphery

Central caseation

Spread takes place by lymphatics, but the necrosis induced by the cell-mediated immunity kills many of the bacilli and the macrophages which transport them. Extension of the lesion is therefore very slow, and the hilar lymph nodes are not affected. A kind of granulation tissue heavily infiltrated by lymphocytes and macrophages forms at the periphery. Eventually the fibrous tissue becomes dense.

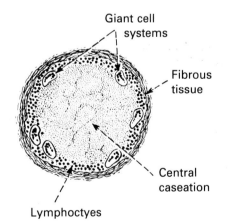

Giant cell systems

Fibrous tissue

Central caseation

Lymphoctyes

At this stage the lesion:

1. May heal leaving a dense grey scar often with central calcification.
2. May become an encysted mass of caseous material and cease to spread. A few tubercle bacilli may persist.
3. May slowly extend by the formation of new tubercles and necrosis of the fibrous barrier. New successive fibrous barriers are formed in advance of the caseating process.

As these lesions extend and coalesce, caseous material may be dislodged via a small bronchus, leaving a CAVITY.

TUBERCULOSIS

SECONDARY TUBERCULOSIS (continued)

Further development

In the untreated case pulmonary tuberculosis tends to be a slowly progressive disease. The following description is of possible further development. Modern antibiotic treatment and chemotherapy usually prevent progression and complications.

Spread may occur via:

1. The bronchial lumens leading to 2. Progressive cavity formation and more widespread fibrosis.

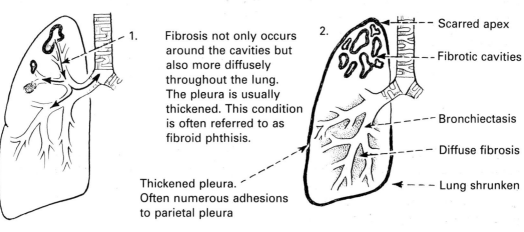

1. Fibrosis not only occurs around the cavities but also more diffusely throughout the lung. The pleura is usually thickened. This condition is often referred to as fibroid phthisis.

Thickened pleura. Often numerous adhesions to parietal pleura

2. Scarred apex
Fibrotic cavities
Bronchiectasis
Diffuse fibrosis
Lung shrunken

Complications

1. Haemorrhage and haemoptysis due to erosion of blood vessels. Occasionally massive haemorrhage from an artery is fatal.

2. Acute tuberculous bronchopneumonia.

3. Acute miliary tuberculosis (rare).

4. Tuberculous ulcers of intestine and larynx due to direct infection from swallowed sputum.

5. Amyloidosis.

Aetiological factors in secondary tuberculosis
1. Occupational hazards (a) exposure to silica dust
                        (b) contact with infected material.

2. Debilitating diseases – e.g. alcoholism, diabetes mellitus.

3. Diminished immune response. *Note*: AIDS and complicating long-continued corticosteroid therapy.

ACUTE TUBERCULOUS BRONCHOPNEUMONIA

This is a complication which may occur in either (a) primary or (b) secondary tuberculous infection.

Primary tuberculous infection

Pneumonic spread may arise from:

1. Extension of the Ghon focus to involve a small bronchus. The caseous material spreads through the bronchial tree.

2. The caseous hilar nodes may ulcerate through the main bronchial wall and sudden spread to main parts of the lung occurs.

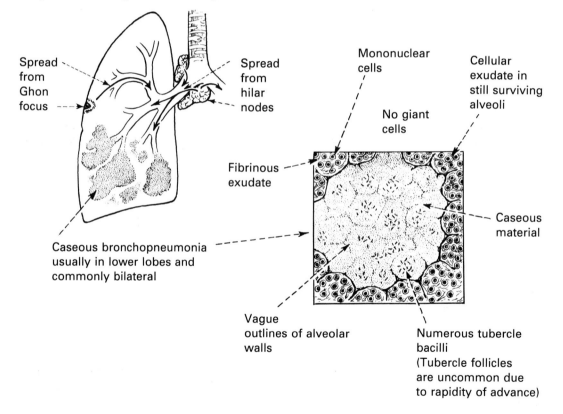

Spread from Ghon focus

Spread from hilar nodes

Mononuclear cells

Cellular exudate in still surviving alveoli

No giant cells

Fibrinous exudate

Caseous material

Caseous bronchopneumonia usually in lower lobes and commonly bilateral

Vague outlines of alveolar walls

Numerous tubercle bacilli (Tubercle follicles are uncommon due to rapidity of advance)

This condition is rapidly fatal. Pneumothorax and pleural effusion are common complications.

ACUTE TUBERCULOUS BRONCHOPNEUMONIA

Secondary tuberculous infection
Tuberculous bronchopneumonia in this instance is always due to evacuation of caseous material from a cavity into the bronchi.

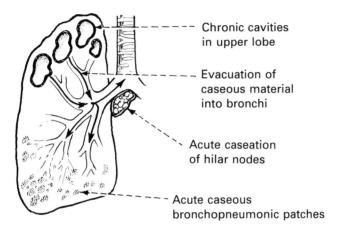

Chronic cavities
in upper lobe

Evacuation of
caseous material
into bronchi

Acute caseation
of hilar nodes

Acute caseous
bronchopneumonic patches

The microscopic
features are similar
to those in
tuberculous
bronchopneumonia
of the primary stage

Usually when caseous material is discharged from a chronic tuberculous cavity into a bronchus, there is no danger of bronchopneumonia. Cell-mediated immunity has destroyed most of the bacilli and their carriers the macrophages. The events leading to bronchopneumonia are as follows:

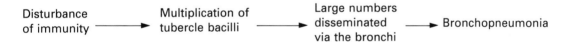

Disturbance
of immunity ⟶ Multiplication of
tubercle bacilli ⟶ Large numbers
disseminated
via the bronchi ⟶ Bronchopneumonia

The causes of disturbed immunological response may be:
  (a) intercurrent disease, e.g. viral infections, diabetes
  (b) malnutrition
  (c) pneumoconiosis
  (d) AIDS

With loss of cell-mediated immunity, spread by lymphatics is once more active, and thus the hilar nodes become caseous. The bronchopneumonic patches break down and discharge via bronchi, leaving ragged, soft-walled cavities and causing further spread.

333

ANTHRACOSIS

This indicates an accumulation of carbon particles in the lung. It is found in a marked form in those who handle soft bituminous coal, particularly coal-miners. Two forms of the condition are recognised: (1) simple coal-worker's anthracosis and (2) progressive massive fibrosis.

Simple coal-worker's anthracosis

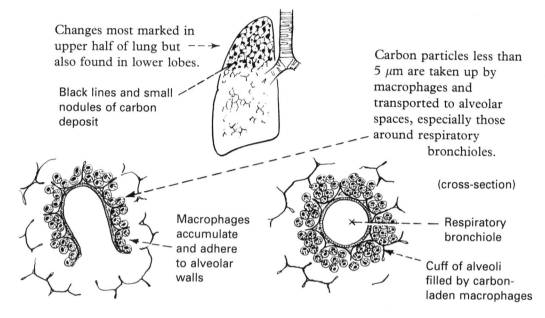

Changes most marked in upper half of lung but also found in lower lobes.

Black lines and small nodules of carbon deposit

Carbon particles less than 5 μm are taken up by macrophages and transported to alveolar spaces, especially those around respiratory bronchioles.

Macrophages accumulate and adhere to alveolar walls

(cross-section)

Respiratory bronchiole

Cuff of alveoli filled by carbon-laden macrophages

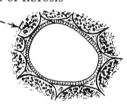

The macrophages die and a limited degree of fibrosis develops around the dust particles.

The respiratory bronchiole becomes inelastic, and with the obliteration of alveoli, the air pressure causes dilatation of the bronchioles. This results in focal dust emphysema (see p.311) which has no significant effect on respiratory function.

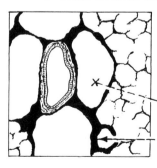

Alveolar epithelium grows over the fibrous masses, the alveoli are obliterated and the specialised structures such as muscle in the bronchiolar wall atrophy.

Distended respiratory bronchiole

Black, obliterated remains of alveoli

ANTHRACOSIS

Progressive massive fibrosis

In a small percentage of workers with simple anthracosis, this further serious change may develop.

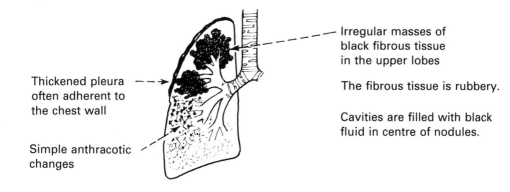

Irregular masses of
black fibrous tissue
in the upper lobes

The fibrous tissue is rubbery.

Cavities are filled with black
fluid in centre of nodules.

Thickened pleura
often adherent to
the chest wall

Simple anthracotic
changes

Tuberculous infection can be demonstrated in some cases. This may be the cause of cavitation in some of the fibrous nodules. In other instances, cavitation may be due to necrosis following obliteration of blood vessels. According to some observers, all of the changes – fibrosis and cavitation – are due to tuberculosis.

The functional effects are severe:

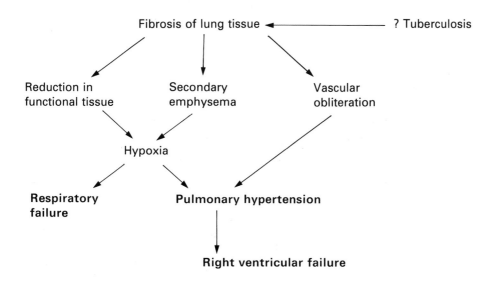

SILICOSIS

Workers exposed to high concentrations of silica dust over a period of years show pulmonary fibrosis of a progressive nature. This can occur in industries such as quarrying of granite, sandstone or slate; mining of anthracite, gold, tin or copper; sandblasting; boiler scaling; glass and pottery manufacture and stonemasonry.

Fine silica particles less than 5 μm are taken up by macrophages which are found in alveoli in the sites previously indicated:
  (a) Peribronchial alveoli
  (b) Perivascular alveoli
  (c) Alveoli around interlobular septa
  (d) Subpleural alveoli.

Macrophages accumulate in these sites and lie undisturbed. Silica-laden macrophages also reach the hilar lymph nodes. A characteristic fibrosis arises in all these sites.

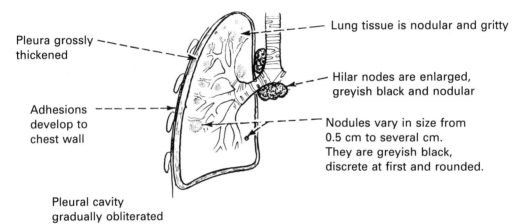

Pleura grossly thickened

Adhesions develop to chest wall

Pleural cavity gradually obliterated

Lung tissue is nodular and gritty

Hilar nodes are enlarged, greyish black and nodular

Nodules vary in size from 0.5 cm to several cm. They are greyish black, discrete at first and rounded.

Histology

The nodules consist of concentric laminae of hyaline, acellular collagen.

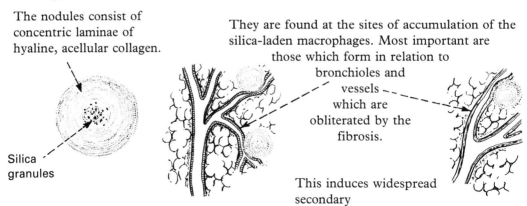

Silica granules

They are found at the sites of accumulation of the silica-laden macrophages. Most important are those which form in relation to bronchioles and vessels which are obliterated by the fibrosis.

This induces widespread secondary changes in the lungs.

SILICOSIS

Silicosis causes progressive respiratory embarrassment due to the destruction of bronchioles and alveoli and the obliteration of pulmonary vessels. Obliteration of the pleural cavity introduces mechanical difficulties in respiration. Death is commonly due to a combination of hypoxia and pulmonary hypertension causing right heart failure.

Tuberculosis and silicosis

Silicosis appears to encourage the establishment of tuberculous infection. The two conditions are commonly associated (reported incidence varies 10–70%). The tuberculous infection spreads rapidly; bronchopneumonia and miliary tuberculosis are common.

Mechanism of action of silica

There are three theories, none of which is entirely satisfactory:

1. *Silica solubility*
   Slow solution of the silica granules is thought to cause fibrosis. The degree of fibrosis does not appear to be related to the solubility of different forms of silica.

2. *Immunologic reaction*
   Silica has been claimed to be antigenic and fibrosis results from the antigen-antibody reaction. There is no evidence for this reaction.

3. *Phospholipid theory*
   Silica-laden macrophages die and release phospholipid which is said to stimulate fibrogenesis. Against this is the fact that macrophages die in other dust diseases, e.g. anthracosis, without causing fibrosis.

Rheumatoid pneumoconiosis

This condition arises in workers exposed to dusts (coal, silica or asbestos) who also suffer from rheumatoid arthritis. Fibrotic nodules up to 5 cm in diameter occur in the lung tissue. These are modified rheumatic lesions and frequently undergo cavitation or calcification.

ASBESTOSIS

Asbestos dust causes severe pulmonary disease. Three distinct types of lesion can be identified, but all of them may occur in the same patient: (1) asbestosis, (2) pleural fibrous plaques, and (3) malignant mesothelioma.

ASBESTOSIS

This term is generally reserved for a process which affects both lungs and leads to progressive destruction of respiratory tissue.

The particles particularly affect the lower lobes and produce a spreading fibrosis.

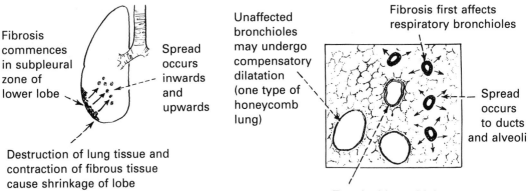

Fibrosis commences in subpleural zone of lower lobe

Spread occurs inwards and upwards

Destruction of lung tissue and contraction of fibrous tissue cause shrinkage of lobe

Unaffected bronchioles may undergo compensatory dilatation (one type of honeycomb lung)

Fibrosis first affects respiratory bronchioles

Spread occurs to ducts and alveoli

Terminal bronchiole

Sequelae

1. The progress is slow and symptoms may be delayed for years.
2. Progressively increasing dyspnoea appears, ending in respiratory failure.
3. Pulmonary hypertension and right heart failure complicate the process.
4. Bronchial carcinoma, usually an adenocarcinoma, arises commonly in the fibrotic lower lobe and is the cause of death in 50% of cases.

PLEURAL FIBROUS PLAQUES

Bilateral pearly white plaques of acellular collagen form on the parietal pleura and upper surface of the diaphragm. They are irregular in shape but well-defined, and circumscribed calcification may follow. They produce no symptoms and are not a precursor of mesothelioma.

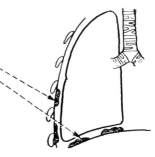

ASBESTOSIS

MALIGNANT MESOTHELIOMA

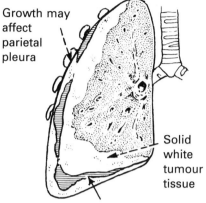

Growth may affect parietal pleura

Solid white tumour tissue

Usually there is localised pleural effusion, often haemorrhagic.

The growth spreads diffusely over the surface of the lung. It forms a thick white membrane which may envelop the whole lung, compressing it. The lung is invaded at a later stage.

This tumour can occur even when the individual is only exposed to a low concentration of asbestos dust for a relatively short space of time. There is, however, a long interval between exposure to the dust and the time of appearance of the tumour. The physical characteristics of the fibres are implicated in the initiation of the carcinogenic process.

ASBESTOS BODIES

Asbestos fibres become coated with mucopolysaccharide and iron. A typical body is brown in colour with bulbous ends. The intervening part is segmented.

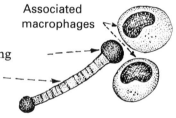

Associated macrophages

These bodies are found in the sputum of individuals exposed to asbestos dust. They occur in the lung tissue whatever type of pathological lesion exists, but are rarely if ever found within the pleural fibrous plaques or in mesothelioma tumour tissue.

Types of asbestos fibres and their industrial uses

1. *Chrysotile* (white asbestos) occurs as soft curly fibres generally retained in the upper respiratory tract. It causes asbestosis but rarely mesothelioma or pleural plaques. Used in making textiles, tiles, brake and clutch linings, gaskets, roofing felt, insulation.

2. *Crocidolite* (blue asbestos)

3. *Amosite* (brown iron-rich asbestos)

Both of these are in the form of rigid fibres which reach the periphery of the lung and are associated with all three types of lesion. Crocidolite is especially associated with mesothelioma. Both are highly resistant to acids and alkalis and are used in insulation work.

Mechanism of fibrogenesis

This is unknown but two suggestions have been made:
1. Macrophages which have ingested asbestos fibres may form a fibrogenic substance.
2. An immunological mechanism may operate. Antinuclear antibody and rheumatoid factor are found in the blood in a quarter of all patients.

341

ORGANIC DUSTS

An increasing number of occupational pulmonary diseases are being recognised in workers handling organic material. The pathological processes are of two varieties:

1. The material being handled may be itself the cause of pathological changes. Byssinosis, due to cotton, flax or hemp, is an example. Exposure to the dust induces chronic coughing. Dyspnoea develops and may end in respiratory failure. The pathological process is one of chronic bronchitis.

Chronic bronchitis ⟶ Hyperplasia of ⟶ Bronchial ⟶ Hypoventilation
mucous glands   obstruction

Intercurrent ⟶   Eventual respiratory
infection   failure

2. In a much larger group, the disease process is related to moulds and fungi contaminating the material handled. Examples are:

Disease	Causative agent
Farmer's lung	Actinomycetes in mouldy hay
Bagassosis	Actinomycetes in mouldy sugar cane bagasse used in paper making
Malt worker's lung	Aspergillus fumigatus in barley in distilleries and breweries
Bird fancier's lung	Moulds and other antigens in bird droppings

Many other industries such as mushroom growing, cork manufacture and maple bark stripping have similar dangers.

Hypersensitivity to the moulds etc. develops and the reaction termed "extrinsic allergic alveolitis" is common to all of these clinical conditions. A high level of precipitating antibody is present in the blood.

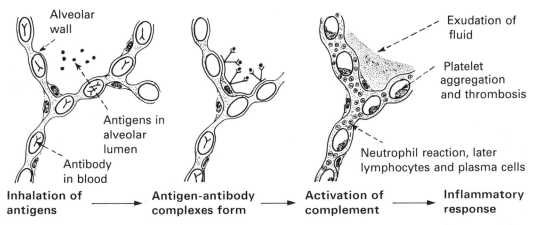

Inhalation of ⟶ Antigen-antibody ⟶ Activation of ⟶ Inflammatory
antigens   complexes form   complement   response

Repeated attacks destroy respiratory tissue and induce a chronic spreading fibrosis. Alveoli and bronchioles are destroyed. Some unaffected bronchioles may undergo compensatory dilatation causing 'honey-comb lung'. Severe respiratory embarrassment occurs which may end in both respiratory and right heart failure.

PULMONARY FIBROSIS

GENERALISED FIBROSIS of LUNGS (CHRONIC INTERSTITIAL PNEUMONIA)

This is the end result of a number of diseases. The pathological changes at this stage are complex, and as a result the aetiology in a large percentage of cases is obscure. Beyond a certain point, the process is not so much a chain of events as a self-perpetuating vicious circle. Three primary mechanisms can be identified.

1. **Alveolar inflammations**. Pneumonias, either bacterial or viral, particularly if attacks are repeated, are important. Toxic fumes such as cadmium and beryllium also act in this way, and prolonged administration of oxygen in high concentration. In these cases, resolution may fail and the exudate is organised.

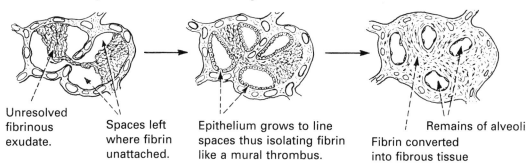

Unresolved fibrinous exudate.

Spaces left where fibrin unattached.

Epithelium grows to line spaces thus isolating fibrin like a mural thrombus.

Remains of alveoli

Fibrin converted into fibrous tissue

2. **Immunological Reactions**. These are exemplified by the reactions to many organic dusts – bagassosis, farmer's lung etc. Pulmonary fibrosis may also occur as a manifestation of rheumatoid disease and scleroderma. An obscure condition known variously as cryptogenic fibrosing alveolitis, idiopathic diffuse interstitial pulmonary fibrosis or Hamman-Rich syndrome appears to be of this nature.

    The hypersensitivity reaction starts in the interstitial tissue but spills over into the alveolar spaces.

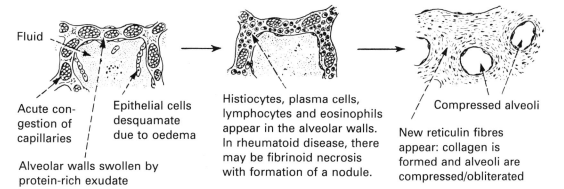

Fluid

Acute congestion of capillaries

Epithelial cells desquamate due to oedema

Alveolar walls swollen by protein-rich exudate

Histiocytes, plasma cells, lymphocytes and eosinophils appear in the alveolar walls. In rheumatoid disease, there may be fibrinoid necrosis with formation of a nodule.

Compressed alveoli

New reticulin fibres appear: collagen is formed and alveoli are compressed/obliterated

3. **Specific fibrogenic irritants**. The inorganic dust diseases (silicosis, asbestosis, haematite miner's lung) illustrate this type of reaction (see p.335 et seq.).

PULMONARY FIBROSIS

GENERALISED FIBROSIS OF LUNGS (continued)

Once the process is initiated, secondary changes take place. In all of them, at least two factors have to be considered:

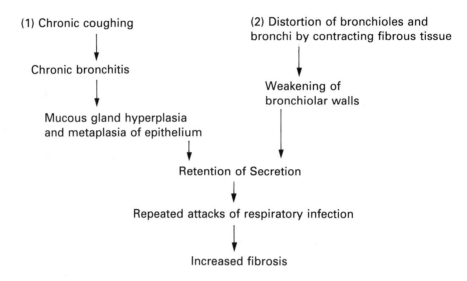

(1) Chronic coughing

↓

Chronic bronchitis

↓

Mucous gland hyperplasia and metaplasia of epithelium

(2) Distortion of bronchioles and bronchi by contracting fibrous tissue

↓

Weakening of bronchiolar walls

↓

Retention of Secretion

↓

Repeated attacks of respiratory infection

↓

Increased fibrosis

It will be realised that in most cases, respiratory infection is a factor inducing a progressive condition whatever the initiating cause. Important changes occur in the pulmonary circulation. Many vessels are destroyed by the fibrosis, while others show endarteritis.

The clinical effects are the same as in all chronic lung diseases which interfere with ventilation and pulmonary circulation. There is increasing respiratory failure, pulmonary hypertension and ultimately right heart failure.

Honeycomb lung

This is the name given to a complication of lung fibrosis, and therefore has the same mixed aetiology.

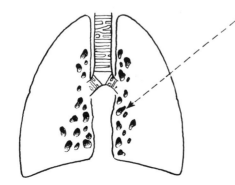

Cysts mainly along anteromedial borders of lungs; 1—2 cm in diameter; smooth linings but often of irregular shape.

The cysts are 'unaffected' bronchioles which have undergone compensatory dilatation following obliteration of others by the fibrosing process. They are lined by columnar or cuboidal epithelium.

CHEMICALS AND DRUGS

Certain chemical poisons induce lung changes resulting in generalised fibrosis indistinguishable from those already described, but the time-scale is very short. The reactions to poisoning with Paraquat (1, 1-dimethyl-4, 4-bipyridilium chloride), a weed killer, are typical of this group of substances.

There is an initial period of general toxicity with mouth ulceration, temporary renal failure due to tubular necrosis, and acute alveolitis.

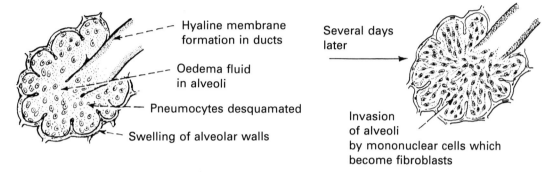

Hyaline membrane formation in ducts

Oedema fluid in alveoli

Pneumocytes desquamated

Swelling of alveolar walls

Several days later

Invasion of alveoli by mononuclear cells which become fibroblasts

As a result of collagen production by the invading fibroblasts, alveoli and bronchioles are obliterated causing progressive respiratory failure. A fatal outcome is common even when the amount consumed is small. It would appear that the chemical stimulates the production of fibrogenic substances.

More important than accidental poisoning is the fact that certain chemotherapeutic agents occasionally cause similar lesions, usually after prolonged treatment. Busulphan, bleomycin, methotrexate – all used in the treatment of cancer – may result in pulmonary fibrosis. Salazopyrin and hexamethonium have also been incriminated. The list of drugs which have this potential in certain patients is bound to grow but, in view of the nature of the diseases which are treated, the dangers must be accepted as a justified hazard.

Oxygen poisoning

This is a hazard in intensive care units where oxygen therapy may be administered over a period of days. The lung lesions, which resemble those of paraquat poisoning, consist of oedema, necrosis of capillary endothelium and alveolar epithelium. Haemorrhagic alveolar exudates are formed which subsequently organise. The fibrous tissue becomes incorporated in the alveolar walls.

Drug sensitivity

A large range of drugs, some complex chemicals like antibiotics, others as simple as aspirin, are sometimes associated with hypersensitivity and may cause asthmatic attacks.

TUMOURS OF LUNG

SIMPLE TUMOURS
Three main varieties are described:

1. PAPILLOMA

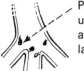

Polypoid tumours, usually multiple, at mouths of large bronchi

Papillomas are similar to the papillary tumours of the larynx. They occur in young people and, on occasion, may cause stridor due to partial obstruction or even aspiration pneumonia.

2. BRONCHIAL ADENOMA

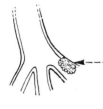

These are relatively common and account for almost 10% of primary lung tumours. They generally appear before the age of 40 and are slightly more common in females. Usually the tumour is situated in a primary bronchus. Commonly it projects into the bronchial lumen and the surface may be ulcerated and haemorrhagic. In some instances it is submucous, growing into the wall of the bronchus and causing obstructive effects.

Histologically, there are two distinctive patterns. The majority are of the 'apudoma' series (carcinoid, see p.397). The remainder are adenomas of the bronchial glands. Very occasionally these may undergo a low-grade malignant change – adenocytic carcinoma.

Clinical features
These may simulate bronchogenic carcinoma when bronchial obstruction occurs. Cough and haemoptysis are the principal symptoms. Obstruction eventually may cause complications:

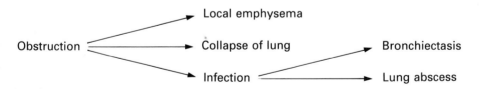

Some patients present with the signs and symptoms of the carcinoid syndrome and excrete 5-hydroxytryptamine in the urine. In these cases, multiple metastases are found in liver and elsewhere.

3. HAMARTOMA

This forms a nodule, usually close to the pleura. It consists of a jumbled mass of tissues usually found in the area – cartilage (often calcified), fibrous tissue, muscle and epithelium lining gland clefts. It usually appears in middle age, more commonly in males, and may be mistaken for carcinoma.

BRONCHOGENIC CARCINOMA

This has now become the most common form of malignancy in Western civilisation.

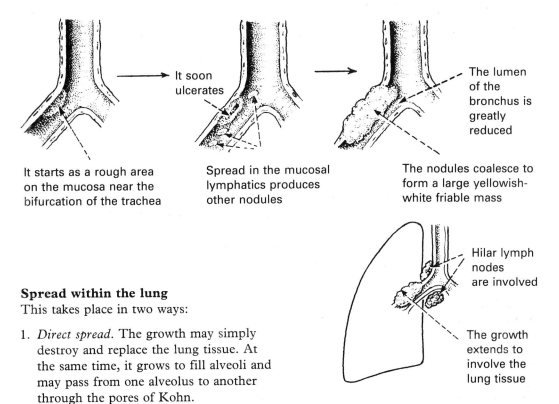

It starts as a rough area on the mucosa near the bifurcation of the trachea

It soon ulcerates

Spread in the mucosal lymphatics produces other nodules

The nodules coalesce to form a large yellowish-white friable mass

The lumen of the bronchus is greatly reduced

Hilar lymph nodes are involved

The growth extends to involve the lung tissue

Spread within the lung

This takes place in two ways:

1. *Direct spread*. The growth may simply destroy and replace the lung tissue. At the same time, it grows to fill alveoli and may pass from one alveolus to another through the pores of Kohn.

2. *Lymphatic spread*. The common mode is spread along peribronchial and perivascular lymph channels.

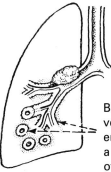

Bronchi and vessels become ensheathed by a white collar of growth

The finer lymphatics of the lobules especially in the subpleural region may be filled by malignant cells producing a network of white lines.

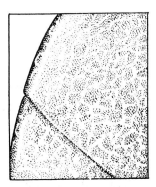

347

BRONCHOGENIC CARCINOMA

Secondary lung changes
These are the result of bronchial obstruction and intercurrent infection.

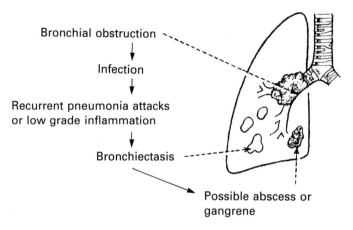

Bronchial obstruction

↓

Infection

↓

Recurrent pneumonia attacks
or low grade inflammation

↓

Bronchiectasis

Possible abscess or
gangrene

Direct spread outside lung and its effects

1. Spread may occur to the
   other bronchus and lung

2. Spread to the pleural and pericardial sacs is common.

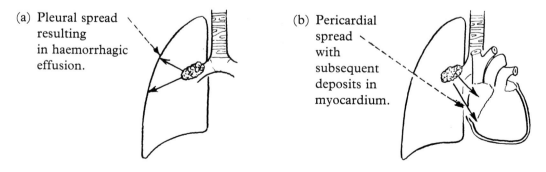

(a) Pleural spread
    resulting
    in haemorrhagic
    effusion.

(b) Pericardial
    spread
    with
    subsequent
    deposits in
    myocardium.

BRONCHOGENIC CARCINOMA

Direct spread outside lung and its effects (continued)

(c) The growth frequently encircles the great vessels.

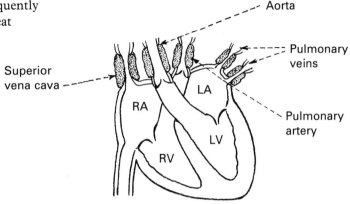

Results

1. Constriction of vena cava: right atrial filling impeded.

2. Pulmonary arteries involved: upset in pulmonary circulation.

3. The pulmonary veins may also be affected, and if the growth permeates the venous wall, malignant thrombi may form giving rise to embolic spread. The aorta is rarely implicated due to the thick musculoelastic wall and the blood pressure.

(d) Nerves may be involved

    1. Recurrent laryngeal ⟶ Paralysis of vocal cords

    2. Phrenic ⟶ Paralysis of diaphragm

    3. Vagus ⟶ Various effects on heart, lungs, etc.

    4. Sympathetic ⟶ Horner's syndrome – ptosis of eyelid, small pupil and absence of sweating on same side of face.

BRONCHOGENIC CARCINOMA

Lymphatic spread outside of lung   This may be widespread.

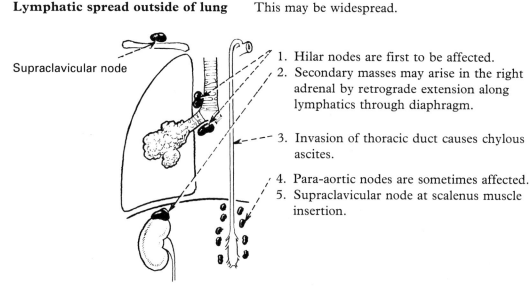

Supraclavicular node

1. Hilar nodes are first to be affected.
2. Secondary masses may arise in the right adrenal by retrograde extension along lymphatics through diaphragm.

3. Invasion of thoracic duct causes chylous ascites.

4. Para-aortic nodes are sometimes affected.
5. Supraclavicular node at scalenus muscle insertion.

Haematogenous spread

This is common. It may be due to direct invasion of a pulmonary vein. Approximately 90% of cases show multiple metastases. The sites and frequency are as follows.

Site	Percentage incidence	
Liver...................	33	
Adrenal................	20–30	– Partly lymphatic spread.
Bones..................	15–20	– Mainly local (ribs, sternum and vertebrae) but may be distant.
Brain	18	– Sometimes first clinical sign of a bronchial tumour.
Kidneys................	10.	

Invasion of a large vessel in the wall of a bronchus occasionally causes severe haemorrhage.

ASSOCIATED METABOLIC and CLINICAL SYNDROMES

Misleading symptoms and signs which suggest well-known clinical syndromes may be exhibited. Some of these are due to elaboration of hormone-like substances by the tumour:

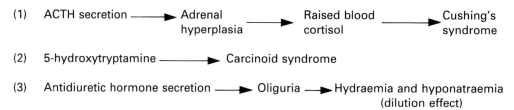

(1)   ACTH secretion ⟶ Adrenal hyperplasia ⟶ Raised blood cortisol ⟶ Cushing's syndrome

(2)   5-hydroxytryptamine ⟶ Carcinoid syndrome

(3)   Antidiuretic hormone secretion ⟶ Oliguria ⟶ Hydraemia and hyponatraemia (dilution effect)

Hypercalcaemia has also been noted, due to formation of parathyroid hormone related peptide. Other curious syndromes are: encephalopathies, cortical cerebellar degeneration, posterior root ganglion degeneration and other neuropathies, myopathy involving wasting of muscles of the limb, girdles and trunk.

BRONCHOGENIC CARCINOMA

HISTOLOGICAL TYPES

Four main varieties are recognised:

1. Squamous cell carcinoma
2. Small cell anaplastic carcinoma (oat cell)
3. Large cell anaplastic carcinoma
4. Adenocarcinoma

These are responsible for 90% of all bronchogenic cancers, and squamous cell carcinoma is the most common of these three.

Squamous cell carcinoma
This shows the usual characteristics of squamous cell carcinoma, but keratinisation is not common.

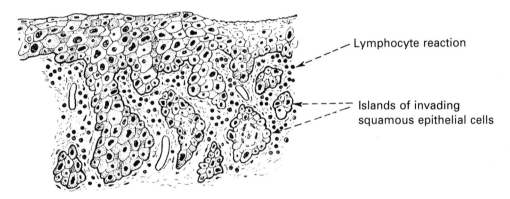

Lymphocyte reaction

Islands of invading squamous epithelial cells

At edge of growth and in unaffected bronchi, squamous metaplasia and Ca in situ are found.

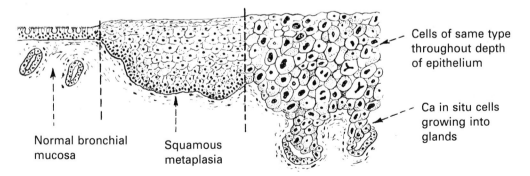

Cells of same type throughout depth of epithelium

Ca in situ cells growing into glands

Normal bronchial mucosa

Squamous metaplasia

Although this type of growth, like all squamous cell carcinomas, is relatively slow growing, it is associated with extensive destruction of local tissues, and the lung lesions due to bronchial obstruction are particularly apt to occur: a high percentage of patients are dead within 1 year.

351

BRONCHOGENIC CARCINOMA

Small cell carcinoma (Oat cell carcinoma)

The cells are relatively uniform: in some cases they are said to resemble oat grains.

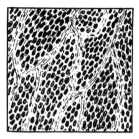

Almost no cytoplasm

Spindle-shaped dark nuclei; may appear to be rounded or oval. May be arranged in sheets, cords or small round aggregates.

On electron-microscopy, cells show argyrophil neurosecretory granules.

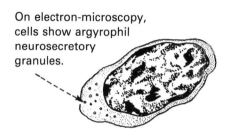

This is the type of lung tumour most commonly associated with endocrine syndromes, and the neurosecretory granules are an indication of this activity. Metastases to lymph nodes may be difficult to recognise initially on histological material because the cells resemble lymphocytes superficially. The growth is of a highly malignant type and widespread metastases occur early. It tends to affect a younger age group more than does the squamous variety. The primary growth may be quite small although numerous blood borne metastases are present.

Large cell anaplastic carcinoma

As the name suggests this tumour shows cells of all shapes and sizes without any distinctive characteristics. Mitoses are frequent and it is highly malignant.

These three foregoing varieties almost always affect bronchi at the hilum and are most common in males. The sex incidence was until recently 8 males to 1 female.

Adenocarcinoma

This form is relatively rare, and at least 50% arise in the peripheral bronchi. Another interesting feature is that there is no sex prevalence, the neoplasm occurring in males and females equally. The gross appearance varies as in all glandular carcinomas.

It may be papillary . . . or solid and scirrhous

Cells are cuboidal or tall columnar and mucus secreting

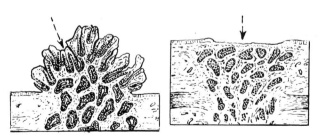

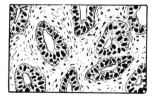

Despite the degree of differentiation, this is usually a highly malignant tumour.

BRONCHOGENIC CARCINOMA

AETIOLOGY

1. Bronchial carcinoma has increased by 500% in the last 25 years.
2. Sex Incidence
   Previously 85% of cases occurred in males over the age of 45, with a sex incidence of 8 males to 1 female. Now the age in males is 30 and the male/female rate is 6 to 1. These facts apply to all histological types of carcinoma except adenocarcinoma which affects males and females equally.
3. Tobacco
   The increase in incidence of bronchial carcinoma is directly related to the number of cigarettes smoked per day. This is most clearly seen in females. The exact carcinogen is unknown but a component of cigarette tar is implicated.
4. Atmospheric Pollution
   Industrial vapours and combusion of oil and petrol are important factors. Bronchial carcinoma is marginally more frequent in towns than in rural areas.
5. Weather
   The incidence is higher in cities with a high rainfall. Noxious agents are concentrated in moisture droplets and in conditions of high humidity remain undispersed.
6. Industrial Causes
   These are related to high atmospheric pollution
       (a) Chromate industry; (b) nickel refining; (c) asbestos manufacture;
       (d) haematite mining and (e) uranium, cobalt mining. Radioactivity is important.

PROGNOSIS

1. Bronchial carcinoma causes 10% of all deaths between the ages of 45 and 64.
2. Only 20% are suitable for surgery, usually squamous cell growths. The 5 year survival rate is 25%, i.e. 5% of all cases survive 5 years. Cytological methods, e.g. brush biopsies may yield earlier diagnosis.
3. Prognosis is poorest with oat cell and anaplastic carcinoma.

SECONDARY LUNG TUMOURS

These are the commonest form of pulmonary malignancy due to the whole blood circulating through the lungs. In addition, lymphatic spread may occur from breast carcinoma and abdominal malignancies.

DISEASES OF THE PLEURA

Diseases of the pleura come under 2 main headings.

1. INFLAMMATION (PLEURISY)

Pleural inflammation is usually secondary to inflammation in the underlying lung.

Fibrinous
Pleurisy

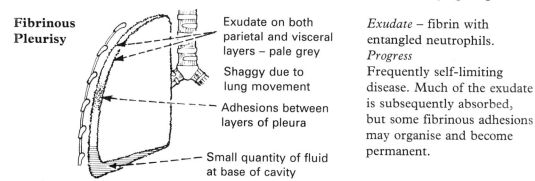

Exudate on both parietal and visceral layers – pale grey

Shaggy due to lung movement

Adhesions between layers of pleura

Small quantity of fluid at base of cavity

Exudate – fibrin with entangled neutrophils.
Progress
Frequently self-limiting disease. Much of the exudate is subsequently absorbed, but some fibrinous adhesions may organise and become permanent.

Progression may take place to pleurisy with effusion (see p.355) or if pyogenic organisms are involved to empyema.

The clinical associations are pain on breathing and audible pleural friction. Note: If progression to effusion occurs, the affected layers are separated and the friction rub eliminated.

Empyema This is now a relatively rare condition since the introduction of antibiotics. It is due to spread of infection from adjacent tissues.

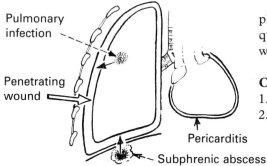

Pulmonary infection

Penetrating wound

Pericarditis

Subphrenic abscess

It is now exceptional for the whole pleural cavity to be filled with pus. Adhesions quickly localise the pus to form a walled-off abscess.

Complications
1. Local spread to lung, pericardium.
2. Embolic brain abscess.

2. TUMOUR GROWTH

METASTATIC tumour affects the pleura in 2 ways:
(1) by direct deposition on the pleural surfaces often in the form of small tumour nodules
    – primary breast carcinoma frequently spreads in this manner.
(2) BRONCHOGENIC CARCINOMA may reach the pleura by direct spread in the lung tissues
    or frequently the inflammatory reaction associated with the tumour reaches the pleura
    evoking an inflammatory reaction (pleurisy with or without effusion) before the
    carcinoma reaches the pleural surface.

354   **MESOTHELIOMA** is the primary neoplasm of the pleura: it is described on page 341.

DISEASES OF THE PLEURA

PLEURAL EFFUSION

The accumulation of fluid within the pleural cavities can be conveniently considered as a form of local oedema. (For the mechanisms see pp.189, 190.)

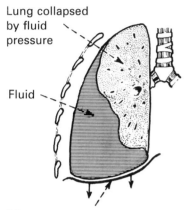

Lung collapsed by fluid pressure

Fluid

Diaphragm depressed

The composition of the fluid is related to the underlying aetiology.

Transudate	*Exudate*
e.g. associated with heart failure.	e.g. associated with underlying lung inflammation.
Specific gravity < 1018	> 1018
Protein content < 4%	> 4% including FIBRIN

Cell content varies considerably and may include lymphocytes, serosal cells, neutrophils and tumour cells.

PNEUMOTHORAX

The effects of the introduction of air into the pleural cavity are variable: the most severe are seen in cases where air can enter during inspiration but does not escape during expiration (TENSION PNEUMOTHORAX).

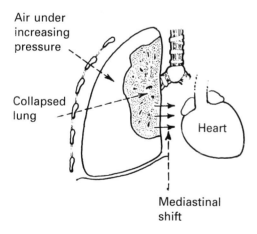

Air under increasing pressure

Collapsed lung

Heart

Mediastinal shift

Causes:
(1) The commonest cause is rupture of an emphysematous bulla.
(2) Traumatic penetrating injury to the chest wall.

Occasionally pneumothorax occurs spontaneously in apparently healthy young males. The cause is thought to be rupture of a congenital bulla in the lung apex.

LIPS AND MOUTH

Acute inflammation

Minor inflammations of the mouth are common due to trauma, hot food or irritants. The lips and mouth are also commonly involved as part of a more general infection such as measles.

An important lesion of modern times is infection by *Candida albicans*. Epidemics may occur in nurseries. It occurs as an opportunistic infection in adults receiving treatment with antibiotics, steroids or cytotoxic drugs.

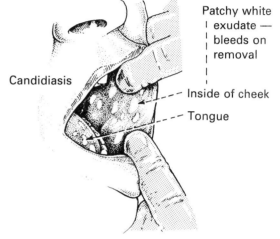

Candidiasis

Patchy white exudate — bleeds on removal

Inside of cheek

Tongue

Aphthous ulceration

Tiny ulcers, whitish in colour and extremely painful are common in the gums, tongue and inside of cheek. The aetiology is unknown.

Chronic inflammation

Specific chronic inflammation such as syphilis and tuberculosis are now rare in most developed countries but occur frequently in underdeveloped regions of the world.

Primary chancre may occur on the lips or tip of tongue. Due to moisture and secondary infection, a softer lesion is produced. In the secondary stage, white areas of cellular infiltration (mucous patches) and irregular silvery lines of ulceration (snail track ulcers) are found. Small gummata which quickly become deep punched out ulcers with a greyish base may form on the dorsum of the posterior third of the tongue.

Tuberculous ulcers are shallow and somewhat ragged with undermined edges. They are due to secondary spread from a pulmonary lesion and are found on the tip of the tongue.

Deficiency diseases associated with anaemia cause cracks and fissures at the angles of the mouth. The tongue is smooth due to loss of papillae — atrophic glossitis. The lack of B group vitamins is the usual cause.

LIPS AND MOUTH

Leukoplakia

This is an ill-understood clinical diagnosis meaning white patches on a stratified squamous epithelium in or near a mucous surface.

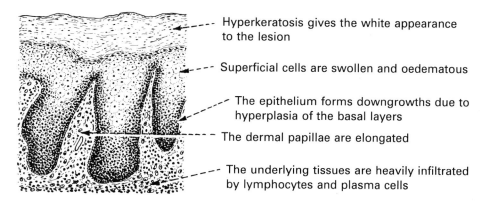

Hyperkeratosis gives the white appearance to the lesion

Superficial cells are swollen and oedematous

The epithelium forms downgrowths due to hyperplasia of the basal layers

The dermal papillae are elongated

The underlying tissues are heavily infiltrated by lymphocytes and plasma cells

The aetiology in many cases is obscure. Some are associated with chronic irritation, e.g. ill-fitting dentures or pipe smoking. The importance of the lesion is that in some individuals the epithelium becomes dysplastic and many cancers in this region have associated leukoplakic lesions.

Pigmentations

Dark pigmentations of the gums are seen in chronic poisoning with heavy metals lead (blue), bismuth (grey), mercury (purplish). Melanotic pigmentation of the mouth is seen in Addison's disease and the Peutz-Jeghers syndrome.

Tumours

Benign tumour masses are not uncommon in the oral cavity. Some of them are of inflammatory origin rather than true neoplasms.

Squamous papilloma is the only epithelial variety. It does not show any tendency to malignant change.

Connective tissue tumours form an interesting group. Haemangioma and lymphangioma are fairly common and give rise to cosmetic problems if on the lips. On the tongue they can interfere with swallowing and severe haemorrhage may be caused.

MOUTH

Granular cell myoblastoma
This is a rare tumour and its importance lies in the fact that it may be mistaken for carcinoma of the tongue.

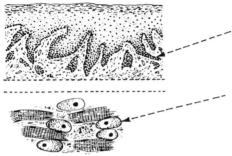

Overlying epithelium shows very irregular downgrowths — but it is not neoplastic (so-called pseudoepitheliomatous hyperplasia)

Large granular cells (thought to arise from Schwann cells or nerves) between and around muscle cells of tongue

Epulis
This is a clinical term applied to swellings at the gum margin. Most of them are granulomas associated with chronic gingivitis. A few are true neoplasms.

Fibrous epulis
This is composed of fibrous tissue but frequently contains bony trabeculae. Usually in the upper jaw, it may be locally invasive and destroy bone.

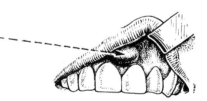

Giant cell epulis

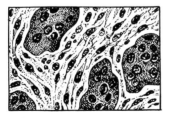

It is problematical if this is a true neoplasm. Histologically, it resembles the giant cell tumour of bone, consisting of giant cells and spindle cells. They are usually found in the mandible of children associated with primary dentition.

Congenital epulis
These tumours are very occasionally seen in the gum of the upper jaw in the newborn. Two types are seen:

1. Soft polypoid tumours containing granular cells like those of the granular myoblastoma.
2. Pigmented tumours which contain cells like neuroblasts and pigmented cubical cells.

MOUTH — MALIGNANT TUMOURS

Squamous cell carcinoma
This is the most important neoplasm, and it may arise on the lip, tongue, floor of mouth, tonsil and fauces, in that order of frequency.

Lip

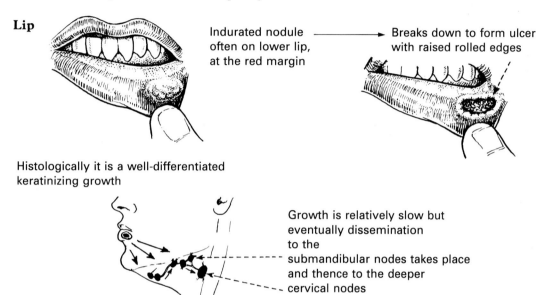

Indurated nodule often on lower lip, at the red margin ⟶ Breaks down to form ulcer with raised rolled edges

Histologically it is a well-differentiated keratinizing growth

Growth is relatively slow but eventually dissemination to the submandibular nodes takes place and thence to the deeper cervical nodes

It is most common in males in the 6th decade, working in outdoor occupations. Exposure to sunlight may be a factor, and in some cases leukoplakia precedes tumour growth. In Eastern countries, cancers of the lip, tongue and inside of cheek are definitely associated with the chewing of a mixture of betel nut and tobacco.

Tongue
Carcinoma of the tongue and other sites within the mouth is a more aggressive growth than tumours of the lips. Starting as a nodule in the buccal sulcus adjacent to the tongue, it quickly breaks down to form an irregular ulcer with ragged edges.

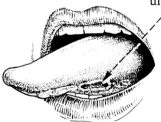

Local infiltration leads to fixation of the tongue. Spread may be extensive to floor of mouth, fauces, pharynx, and into the medullary cavity of the mandible via occlusal ridge gaps particularly in the edentulous patient.

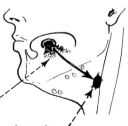

Lymph node involvement occurs early, usually to the deeper cervical nodes.

361

DISEASES OF PHARYNX

Tonsillitis

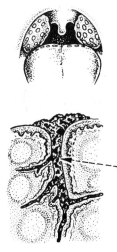

This is a common acute inflammation. It is frequently due to streptococcal infection, but viruses, particularly the adenoviruses, also cause tonsillitis and, due to the use of antibiotics, have become more important. The pharyngeal tissues including the tonsil become acutely swollen and purulent exudate appears at the mouth of the crypts. Occasionally the inflammation is very acute, resulting in suppuration in the tissues — termed quinsy. There is a marked tendency for tonsillitis to recur. Eventually a chronic condition is produced with permanent enlargement of the tonsils.

The crypts are dilated and contain inspissated exudate. During the process, various immunological phenomena arise. The importance of this disease is that it is commonly a precursor of rheumatic fever or one form of glomerulo-nephritis.

Vincent's angina

This is an acute inflammation due to the combined action of fusiform bacilli and a spirochaete — *Borrelia vincenti*. It may cause severe ulceration.

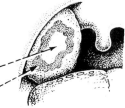

White membrane
Surrounding acute inflammation

Diphtheria

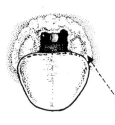

This is now relatively uncommon in most of the world, due to immunisation programmes. It produces an intense superficial inflammation of the fauces, tonsil and soft palate.

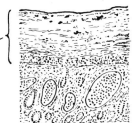

Fibrin strands involving squamous epithelium and underlying dermis producing a membrane difficult to remove.

The infection remains local and the severe clinical effects are due to the powerful exotoxin. In addition to general toxaemia there is specific damage to nerves and myocardium.

Lymphoepithelioma

This is now considered to be a squamous carcinoma heavily infiltrated by lymphocytes. It arises in the pharynx and invasion of the cervical nodes occurs early. These tumours are common in Chinese people and are associated with EB virus infection.

DISEASES OF SALIVARY GLANDS

INFLAMMATION

Simple acute inflammation of these glands is uncommon. It may occur during a prolonged illness, particularly if a calculus has formed in a duct.

More commonly acute inflammation is due to the virus of *mumps*, which produces acute swelling, particularly of the parotid glands, with oedema and mononuclear infiltration of the interstitial tissue. The testes and pancreas may also be inflamed and atrophy may follow.

Chronic inflammation is rare. It may occur as a manifestation of sarcoidosis. The parotid gland becomes swollen and there is an accompanying iridocyclitis. This has given rise to the term 'uveo-parotid fever'. The parotid gland shows a chronic inflammatory reaction with follicular lesions typical of sarcoidosis.

Parotid

Pancreas

Testes

Sjogren's syndrome

In this auto-immune condition there is a destruction of the gland tissue of the salivary, lacrimal and conjunctival glands by an infiltrate of lymphocytes and plasma cells. The duct epithelia often undergo reactive hyperplasia. It results in dryness of the mouth, caries due to lack of saliva and ulceration of the conjunctiva caused by lack of secretion from the lacrimal and conjunctival glands. Polyarthritis is often present and the serum contains autoantibodies and rheumatoid factor.

Very occasionally a B-cell lymphoma arises from the lymphoid proliferation.

Calculus formation

This uncommon condition mainly affects the parotid duct. Blockage of the duct leads to atrophy of the gland. Occasionally acute inflammation may be superimposed.

SALIVARY GLAND TUMOURS

The majority (80%) of tumours arise in the parotid gland and most in this site are benign.

The remaining 20% occur in the submandibular and minor salivary glands — in these sites 30–40% are malignant.

SALIVARY GLANDS — TUMOURS

MIXED TUMOUR [PLEOMORPHIC SALIVARY ADENOMA (P.S.A.)]

This is the commonest tumour of salivary glands, and most occur in the parotid. The mixed elements are of epithelial and 'connective tissue' types and are derived from the epithelial and myoepithelial elements of the glandular acini and ducts.

The tumours vary in size from a few millimetres to several centimetres. They are usually rounded or lobulated; consistency varies with structure.

(a) *Firm* — mainly fibrous

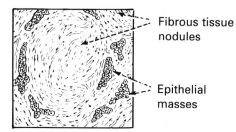

Fibrous tissue nodules

Epithelial masses

(b) *Fleshy* — largely epithelial

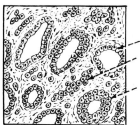

Epithelium arranged in acini or solid strands. Acini often have double layer of cells like normal salivary glands

(c) *Gelatinous* — mucinous matrix

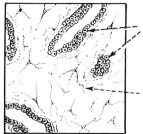

Epithelial structures separated by large areas of myxoid stroma

(d) *Hard* — mainly cartilagenous, sometimes with bony trabeculae

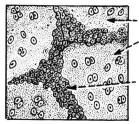

Nodules of chondroid

Strands of epithelium

The epithelium may be arranged as glands, ductules, solid sheets or squamous masses. All epithelial and stromal types may be found in the same tumour.

The tumour is enclosed in a fibrous capsule, but there are frequently microscopic extensions beyond the capsule.

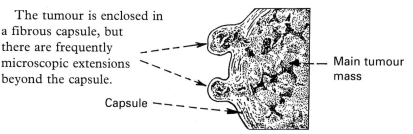

Main tumour mass

Capsule

Tumours which are 'shelled out' tend to recur sometimes years later.

MONOMORPHIC ADENOMA

This is a variant consisting of epithelial elements without any specific stromal change.

ADENOLYMPHOMA is a benign tumour occurring almost exclusively in the parotid glands of usually older men. The tumour is essentially a cystadenoma with a striking lymphoid stroma.

SALIVARY GLANDS — TUMOURS

CARCINOMA of SALIVARY GLANDS
The main types of primary salivary carcinoma are:
1. Acinic cell carcinoma
2. Adenoid cystic carcinoma
3. Muco-epidermoid carcinoma.

Progression of a benign tumour to carcinoma is rare. Squamous cell carcinoma and adenocarcinoma are also rare.

1. **Acinic cell carcinoma**
   Approximately ¼ of all malignant
   parotid tumours are of this type. It grows
   slowly, recurs after removal and sometimes
   there is late extension to the regional
   lymph nodes and distant organs.

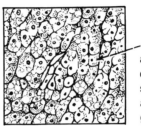

— Closely aggregated cells containing secretory granules and sometimes glycogen.

2. **Adenoid cystic carcinoma**
   This usually occurs in minor salivary glands and accounts for 7% of salivary gland tumours. It extends by direct spread, but metastases occur at a late stage to lymph nodes, lungs and bones.
   There is a special tendency to
   invade nerve sheaths.

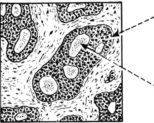

Cribriform pattern. Solid masses of epithelium enclosing small cystic spaces containing mucin. The cells resemble basal cells.

3. **Muco-epidermoid carcinoma**
   The malignancy of this type varies, but all tend to recur and infiltrate locally. More malignant growths metastasise to the lymph nodes and may invade the blood stream.
   They are generally found
   in the major salivary glands
   and form 3 or 4% of all
   tumours of these glands.

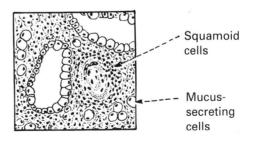

- Squamoid cells

- Mucus-secreting cells

OESOPHAGUS

The oesophagus is a muscular tube lined by stratified squamous epithelium and is highly resistant to damage.

INFLAMMATION

Infection of the oesophagus is rare and is generally due to spread from the pharynx. Herpes may affect infants and opportunistic infection with thrush can occur in states of diminished immunity.

More often, inflammation is due to chemicals and occurs in two circumstances:

1. **Caustic poisoning**

   In strong concentration, widespread necrosis and sloughing of tissues occurs. With weaker poisons, the epithelium is destroyed. Secondary infection and inflammation occur. Healing may lead to fibrous stricture.

2. **Peptic oesophagitis**

   This is the commonest form of inflammation. It is due to reflux of acid from the stomach and is especially apt to happen in any illness involving bed-rest. A more important type is associated with hiatus hernia, particularly where part of the cardia herniates into the thorax.

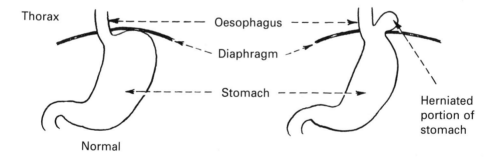

Acid secretion produces inflammation and superficial ulceration of the oesophageal mucosa.

The main complications are *anaemia* due to repeated small haemorrhages and *fibrous stricture* following repeated healing and relapse, and *metaplasia* of the oesophageal squamous epithelium (Barrett's oesophagus).

Barrett's oesophagus is an important PRE-MALIGNANT lesion. 15% of cases progress to carcinomas as follows:

METAPLASIA to GASTRIC or
         INTESTINAL TYPE → DYSPLASIA → ADENOCARCINOMA
         of EPITHELIUM

OESOPHAGUS

OBSTRUCTION is the commonest disorder. Two main types are described.

1. Organic obstruction

Occlusion of lumen. This may be due to tumour growth or foreign body.
Compression of oesophagus by tumours and other conditions in mediastinum.
Stenosis may be caused by scirrhous carcinoma, or strictures following corrosive
poisoning or hiatus hernia.
Neuromuscular incoordination due to destruction of muscles as in systemic sclerosis
or of the autonomic ganglia as in South American trypanosomiasis (Chagas' disease).
Developmental abnormality leading to congenital stenosis.

2. Functional obstruction

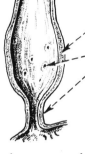

Achalasia of the oesophagus develops in young adults and
may cause severe obstruction.
Above the obstruction the oesophagus is dilated, the
muscle is hypertrophied and the
mucosa may be ulcerated.
Narrowing occurs at the lower end.

It is due to a conduction failure in the peristaltic mechanism, preventing opening of the
cardiac sphincter. Muscle spasm in anaemia of young women (Plummer-Vinson syndrome,
also known as the Kelly-Paterson syndrome) can cause obstruction at the upper end of the
oesophagus.

DIVERTICULA

These are relatively rare and are of two varieties.

1. Pulsion type

Involves pharynx (pharyngeal pouch).
Sac is distended during swallowing of
food. By pushing down behind oesophagus,
it may compress this
structure. Congenital
weakness of
the pharyngeal
muscles is said to
be an aetiological
factor.

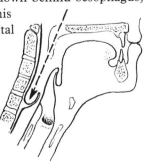

2. Traction type

This is due to traction of fibrous tissue
produced by mediastinal inflammation,
e.g.
tuberculosis
or silicosis of
lymph nodes.

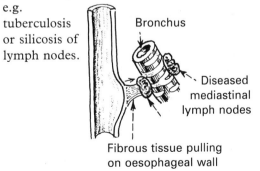

Bronchus

Diseased
mediastinal
lymph nodes

Fibrous tissue pulling
on oesophageal wall

Rarely, there may be a congenital diverticulum at the level of the bifurcation of the
trachea.

367

OESOPHAGUS

OESOPHAGEAL VARICES

These are important lesions which occur secondarily to portal hypertension caused by cirrhosis of the liver (see p. 448).

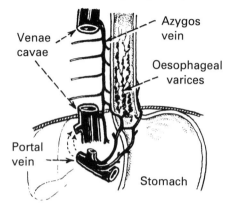

Fibrosis in the liver obstructs the flow of blood from the gastrointestinal tract in the portal system. Anastomotic channels connecting the portal and systemic venous systems open up and become distended. The most important are the oesophageal tributaries of the azygos vein which connect through the diaphragm with the portal system. They become varicose, and are easily traumatised by the passage of food, leading to haemorrhage which can be fatal.

SPONTANEOUS RUPTURE

This is a condition of unknown origin which occurs in healthy men.

A longitudinal slit appears in left posterior aspect of oesophageal wall above the diaphragm. Gastric fluid escapes causing mediastinitis and pleurisy.

It may be due to distension of the oesophagus during the act of vomiting and in some cases is associated with acute alcoholic intoxication. Tears without rupture but causing haemorrhage and haematemesis may also occur (Mallory-Weiss syndrome).

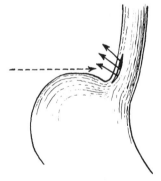

CONGENITAL ABNORMALITIES

Apart from stenosis (already mentioned), atresia is the only other congenital malformation of any note. Two anatomical forms are found:

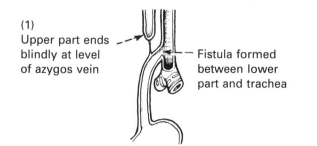

(1) Upper part ends blindly at level of azygos vein — Fistula formed between lower part and trachea

(2) No fistulous communication. This form is very rare.

Regurgitation and inhalation of food or gastric secretions may prove fatal.

OESOPHAGUS

TUMOURS

Benign tumours of the oesophagus are very rare. They are almost always of connective tissue origin and form polyps within the lumen, causing obstruction.

Carcinoma

This is the third most common malignant tumour of the digestive tract, carcinoma of large intestine and stomach taking precedence in that order.

It occurs at three levels:

(1) At level of bifurcation of trachea. This is the commonest site

(2) Upper end of oesophagus at level of cricoid cartilage

(3) Lower end of oesophagus

Seventy-five per cent of those in the upper part of the oesophagus occur in females. In 80% of the remainder, males are affected. The disease is altogether more common in males. Two forms of growth are seen:

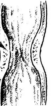

(1) Scirrhous encircling the tube and causing constriction

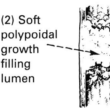

(2) Soft polypoidal growth filling lumen

In both instances the growth tends to extend in a longitudinal manner. Growths at the upper end and at the level of the tracheal bifurcation are usually poorly differentiated squamous cell carcinomas. At the lower end, adenocarcinoma is common, associated with Barrett's oesophagus (see p. 366).

Spread

At the common site, near the tracheal bifurcation, spread may involve the trachea or a bronchus, ulcerating the wall and resulting in aspiration pneumonia. Tumours at other levels will involve the trachea or other mediastinal structures. Death usually results from the oesophageal obstruction, but occasionally the patient may survive long enough for metastases to appear in nodes and other organs, e.g. liver.

Aetiological factors

The incidence shows a geographical variation, being common in China and Africa. The causes are unknown but smoking and dietetic factors including alcohol consumption are thought to be important. Post-cricoid carcinoma in women is a rare late complication of the dysphagia complicating iron deficiency anaemia.

STOMACH

The stomach is divided into five anatomical regions:

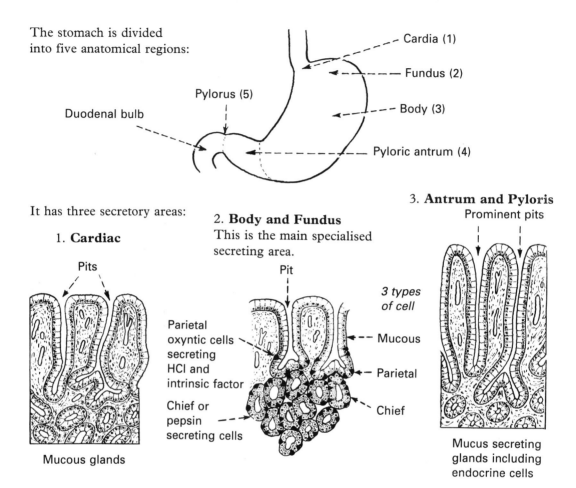

It has three secretory areas:

1. Cardiac

2. Body and Fundus

This is the main specialised secreting area.

3. Antrum and Pyloris

Prominent pits

Pits

Pit

3 types of cell

Parietal oxyntic cells secreting HCl and intrinsic factor

Mucous

Parietal

Chief or pepsin secreting cells

Chief

Mucous glands

Mucus secreting glands including endocrine cells

Note: Mucus is secreted throughout the gastric mucosa: the specialised secretory cells are confined to the body and fundus.

Vascular supply

Along the lesser curvature, run the right and left gastric arteries, which anastomose directly.

The greater curvature shows 3 arterial supplies:

Branches from the splenic artery

Right and left gastroepiploic arteries

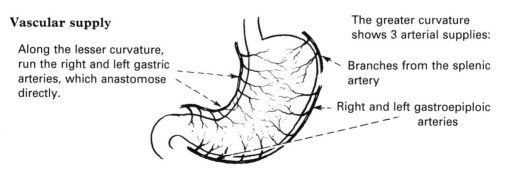

The arteries anastomose freely in the muscular submucous and mucous coats, except along the lesser curvature of the pyloric antrum and including the first part of duodenum. In this area, there is little anastomosis between the terminal branches in the mucosa.

STOMACH

GASTRIC SECRETION

The secretion of gastric juice occurs in two phases under quite different controls.

1. *Reflex nervous phase*   2. *Humoral phase*

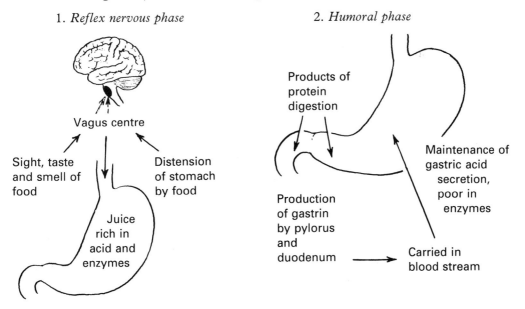

The stomach also produces large quantities of mucus which protects the mucosa from the action of acid and proteolytic enzymes. Both intrinsic factor (IF) which combines with vitamin B_{12} and hydrochloric acid (HCl) are secreted by the specialised parietal cells of the body. Blood group mucopolysaccharide substances are also secreted.

Apart from its secretory activity, one of the important features of the stomach and indeed the whole gastrointestinal tract is the very rapid turnover of epithelial cells.

GASTRITIS

ACUTE INFLAMMATION
Mild acute gastritis is an acute inflammation with neutrophil reaction in the superficial layers of the mucosa. Pain and sickness have a multitude of causes varying from hot fluids, alcohol and aspirin which act as direct irritants, to infections such as childhood fevers, viral infections and bacterial food poisoning.

A more acute form, known as acute haemorrhagic or erosive gastritis, is occasionally seen; it is associated with ingestion of irritant drugs, particularly aspirin and non-steroidal anti-inflammatory drugs (NSAID) and is also a complication of shock states.

Haemorrhagic erosions
These are tiny ulcers, a few millimetres in diameter, which are formed by the digestion of the mucous membrane overlying small haemorrhages. They are usually multiple and affect all parts of the stomach. They occur mostly on the apex of mucosal folds and involve only the mucosa.

Note that the changes are superficial so that restoration to normal can very quickly occur.

Naked eye appearance

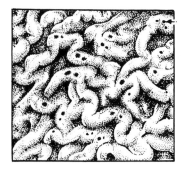

Erosion of mucosa with bleeding and loss of gland duct epithelium

Stress ulcers
Occasionally, particularly in severe shock, there is deeper acute ulceration with considerable haemorrhage and even perforation.

These ulcers are described in more detail on page 375.

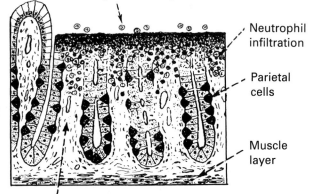

Neutrophil infiltration

Parietal cells

Muscle layer

Oedema resulting in swelling of mucosa and separation of glands

CHRONIC GASTRITIS
Although chronic gastritis is a common disorder it very rarely arises from the types of acute inflammation described above.

Our understanding of the aetiology and mechanisms of GASTRITIS and GASTRODUODENAL ULCERATION has been radically altered by the discovery of a specific infective agent, *Helicobacter pylori*, by Australian workers Marshall et al. (see pp. 374, 380): its role and world wide prevalence have since been confirmed.

GASTRITIS

CHRONIC GASTRITIS (continued)

The SYDNEY SYSTEM is a new classification based on this recent new knowledge. It incorporates two separate divisions: (1) HISTOLOGICAL and (2) ENDOSCOPIC.

The histological classification incorporates three main elements:

(a) AETIOLOGY

(b) TOPOGRAPHY
i.e. site affected:
antrum, body or both.

(c) MORPHOLOGY including information activity, intestinal metaplasia
— graded as mild, moderate or severe.

The two main types of chronic gastritis are examples of this classification in use:

(a) Auto-immune associated chronic pangastritis with severe atrophy (formerly known as Type A gastritis).

(b) H. pylori associated chronic gastritis of the antrum with moderate activity (formerly known as Type B gastritis).

The endoscopic classification uses the same topography and categorises the gastritis in terms of the endoscopic appearances.

AUTO-IMMUNE ASSOCIATED GASTRITIS (Type A)

Prevalence: 5% of chronic gastritis cases are of this type.

Aetiology: Evidence for auto-immune mechanisms:

(1) Presence of antibodies to parietal cells and intrinsic factor.

(2) Associated with other auto-immune disorders, e.g. thyroiditis.

Sites affected: The fundus and body predominantly.

Morphological changes are progressive over several years with gradual thinning of the mucosa.

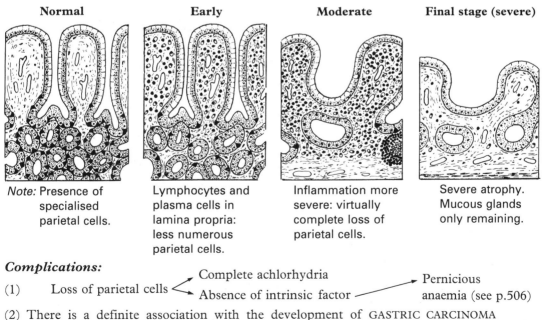

Normal	Early	Moderate	Final stage (severe)
Note: Presence of specialised parietal cells.	Lymphocytes and plasma cells in lamina propria: less numerous parietal cells.	Inflammation more severe: virtually complete loss of parietal cells.	Severe atrophy. Mucous glands only remaining.

Complications:

(1) Loss of parietal cells < Complete achlorhydria
Absence of intrinsic factor → Pernicious anaemia (see p.506)

(2) There is a definite association with the development of GASTRIC CARCINOMA often preceded by INTESTINAL METAPLASIA.

GASTRITIS

Chronic gastritis (continued)

Helicobacter pylori ASSOCIATED CHRONIC GASTRITIS (formerly Type B)

Prevalence: 80% of chronic gastritis cases are of this type. The organism has a world wide distribution.

Aetiology: *Helicobacter pylori* is a Gram-negative vibrio-like ($\smile,\sim$) microbe which is specifically adapted to colonise the gastric mucosa: this continues indefinitely.

Site affected: The antrum and pyloric canal particularly.

Morphological changes are essentially superficial with inflammation involving the upper half of the mucosa.

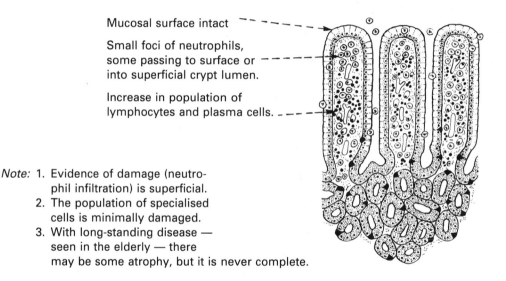

Mucosal surface intact

Small foci of neutrophils, some passing to surface or into superficial crypt lumen.

Increase in population of lymphocytes and plasma cells.

Note: 1. Evidence of damage (neutrophil infiltration) is superficial.
2. The population of specialised cells is minimally damaged.
3. With long-standing disease — seen in the elderly — there may be some atrophy, but it is never complete.

Complications:

(1) Progression to GASTRIC and DUODENAL ulcer (see pp. 375–380).
(2) Progression to CARCINOMA, often preceded by INTESTINAL METAPLASIA.

OTHER FORMS of CHRONIC GASTRITIS

These include eosinophilic gastritis often associated with food allergy, and reflux gastritis due to reflux of duodenal contents.

It is also possible that continuing damage by the agents causing acute gastritis (e.g. drugs) progresses to a chronic form in some cases.

PEPTIC ULCERATION — ACUTE

Peptic ulcers occur only at sites where there is acid-containing gastric juice. The common sites in order of frequency are (1) duodenum, (2) stomach, (3) lower oesophagus, and rarely with heterotopic gastric mucosa, e.g. Meckel's diverticulum.

ACUTE PEPTIC ULCER

This type may be associated with acute gastritis and particularly also with states of severe shock (Stress ulcers, see p. 372).

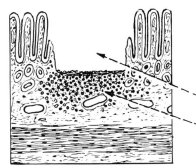

In this type both the mucosa and submucosa are involved. Rarely more than 1 cm in diameter, they may be multiple or single and occur in various parts of the stomach. They have a punched-out appearance.

Mucosa destroyed

Inflammatory cells in submucosa

Healing can be rapid

Occasionally the ulcer extends more deeply.

Erosion of a blood vessel may cause serious haemorrhage

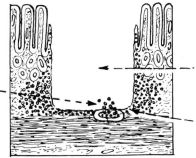

Destruction of mucosa and submucosa

Inflammation extends to edge of muscle

Very rarely is there actual perforation (acute perforating ulcer).

Perforation with little inflammation

Peritonitis

SUBACUTE PEPTIC ULCER

This term is used for ulcers showing greater penetration of the muscularis with more inflammatory reaction and slight fibrosis.

375

PEPTIC ULCERATION — CHRONIC

CHRONIC PEPTIC ULCER

The term 'chronic' is applied when the pathological changes have penetrated and destroyed the muscle coat; they are also, of course, of much longer duration than acute ulcers.

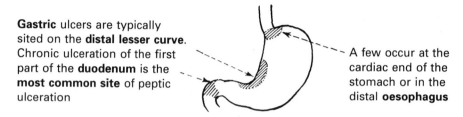

Gastric ulcers are typically sited on the **distal lesser curve**. Chronic ulceration of the first part of the **duodenum** is the **most common site** of peptic ulceration

A few occur at the cardiac end of the stomach or in the distal **oesophagus**

The ulcers are almost always single, but in 5 – 10%, a second ulcer may be found on the opposite aspect of the pyloric canal or duodenum (kissing ulcers).

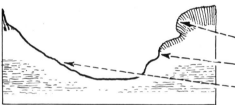

The ulcer is commonly large, 2 – 3 cm, and oval. It has an overhanging lip at the proximal end.
Frequently it has a terraced structure.
The distal end slopes away from the ulcer bed.

The depth of ulceration varies. There are obviously periods of quiescence with attempts at healing and the production of scar tissue.

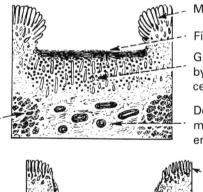

Mucosa

Fibrin and necrotic debris

Granulation tissue infiltrated by lymphocytes and plasma cells

Dense scar tissue replacing muscle. Vessels show endarteritis.

Muscle

Frequently the ulcerative process extends to the serous coat or even beyond.

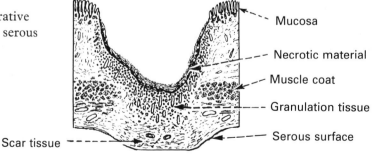

Mucosa

Necrotic material

Muscle coat

Granulation tissue

Serous surface

Scar tissue

Extension of the inflammation to the serous coat may result in adhesion to other organs, e.g. the pancreas, and the ulceration may burrow into the affected organ.
The remainder of the stomach frequently shows chronic gastritis.

PEPTIC ULCERATION — CHRONIC

SEQUELS and COMPLICATIONS

1. **Healing** is common. This is the usual result in acute and probably subacute ulceration. Chronic ulcers frequently, heal.

Healed subacute ulcer

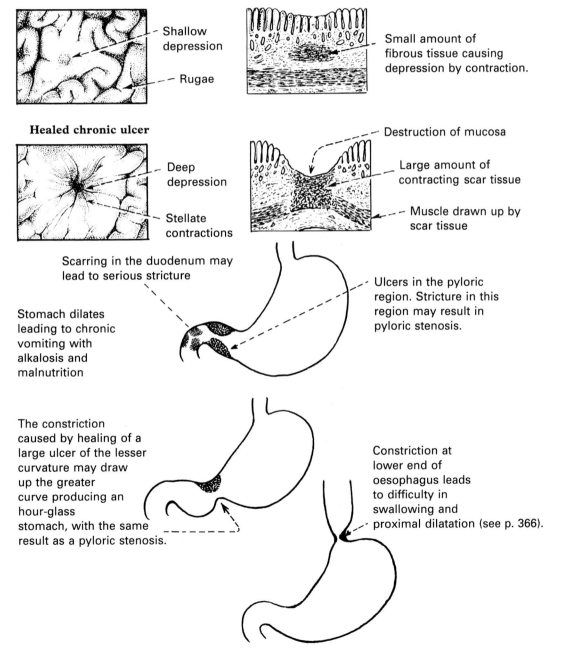

Shallow depression

Rugae

Small amount of fibrous tissue causing depression by contraction.

Healed chronic ulcer

Deep depression

Stellate contractions

Destruction of mucosa

Large amount of contracting scar tissue

Muscle drawn up by scar tissue

Scarring in the duodenum may lead to serious stricture

Ulcers in the pyloric region. Stricture in this region may result in pyloric stenosis.

Stomach dilates leading to chronic vomiting with alkalosis and malnutrition

The constriction caused by healing of a large ulcer of the lesser curvature may draw up the greater curve producing an hour-glass stomach, with the same result as a pyloric stenosis.

Constriction at lower end of oesophagus leads to difficulty in swallowing and proximal dilatation (see p. 366).

377

PEPTIC ULCERATION — CHRONIC

SEQUELS and COMPLICATIONS (continued)

2. Perforation

Acute perforating ulcer
(This is now a rare condition.)

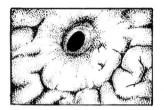

Perforation of a chronic ulcer

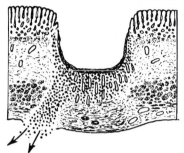

Ulcer has a terraced appearance.
It is probably of subacute type which
has suffered an acute ulcerative
exacerbation.

Acute ulceration occurs diagonally
through the non-scarred soft tissues.

Perforation causes acute peritonitis. Fibrinous adhesions may result in an undiscovered loculus of pus between the liver and diaphragm — subphrenic abscess.

The advancing chronic inflammation of a chronic ulcer frequently causes adhesions to adjacent areas and this prevents perforation.

3. **Haemorrhage**. As in any active ulcerative process, bleeding is frequent. Most commonly it is of minor degree — an oozing from the granulation tissue which can only be detected by testing faeces for occult blood. More marked haemorrhage may actually cause discoloration of the faeces — tarry stools due to the formation of iron sulphides. Vomiting with "coffee-grounds" vomit may also occur. Occasionally a very large haemorrhage may occur, usually from a chronic ulcer.

The pathology is as follows:

Most vessels undergo endarteritis
and serious bleeding is
thus avoided but a large patent
arterial branch in the base of
the ulcer may be attacked by
an acute ulcerative phase. The
scar tissue is an important factor
in causing continued bleeding.

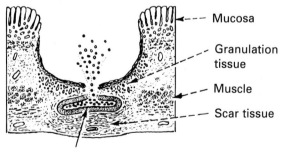

- - - Mucosa

- - Granulation tissue

- - Muscle

- - - Scar tissue

Eroded artery held in fibrous
tissue unable to contract or retract.

4. **Development of carcinoma**. It is now thought that less than 1% of chronic gastric ulcers give rise to carcinoma. It always develops from the surviving mucosa at the edge of the ulcer where there is always active chronic gastritis.

Carcinoma never develops in duodenal ulcer.

PEPTIC ULCERATION

AETIOLOGY

The one essential factor in the causation of peptic ulcer is the presence of ACID, which acts as a continuing 'irritant' resulting in chronic ulceration.

Over 70% of gastric ulcer cases and 90% of duodenal ulcer cases are *H.pylori* positive. The mechanisms by which they act are described on page 380.

For the maintenance of a healthy mucosa there are three essentials:

1. Presence of protective mucus
2. A good blood supply
3. Rapid turnover of epithelial cells to maintain surface integrity.

The diagram illustrates potentially damaging mechanisms:

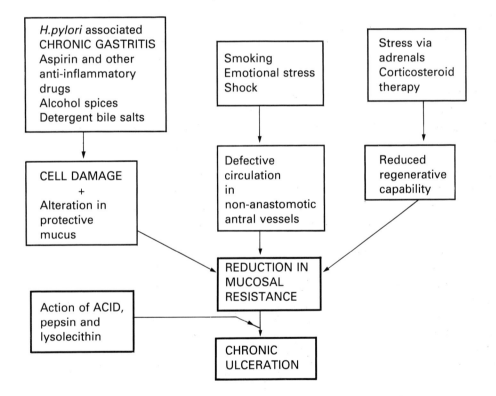

In addition, there is an important genetic component.

PEPTIC ULCERATION

Helicobacter pylori **(continued)**
Infection of the antral mucosa
Chronic gastritis Type II

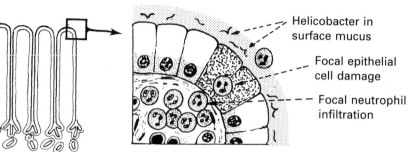

High magnification

Helicobacter in
surface mucus

Focal epithelial
cell damage

Focal neutrophil
infiltration

? Infection is potentiated via glycerolipid mucus.
? Association with non-secretor status of ABO group antigens.

Infection of the duodenal mucosa
This is secondary to the gastric antral infection and depends on the presence of
superficial gastric metaplasia in the first part of the duodenum consequent upon
hyperchlorhydria and rapid emptying of the stomach. With the metaplasia, gastric
mucus appears encouraging helicobacter colonisation.

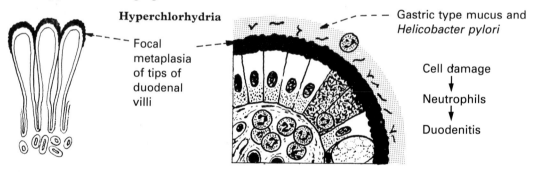

Hyperchlorhydria

Gastric type mucus and
Helicobacter pylori

Focal
metaplasia
of tips of
duodenal
villi

Cell damage
↓
Neutrophils
↓
Duodenitis

This continuing low grade damage establishes conditions suitable for further damage by
acid and digestive enzymes.

Aetiology of duodenal ulceration

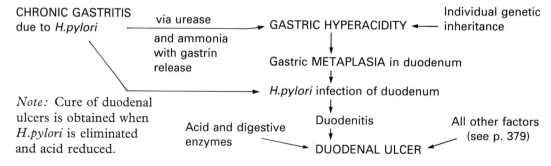

CHRONIC GASTRITIS
due to *H.pylori*

via urease
and ammonia
with gastrin
release

GASTRIC HYPERACIDITY ← Individual genetic
inheritance

↓

Gastric METAPLASIA in duodenum

↓

H.pylori infection of duodenum

↓

Duodenitis

Note: Cure of duodenal
ulcers is obtained when
H.pylori is eliminated
and acid reduced.

Acid and digestive
enzymes

All other factors
(see p. 379)

DUODENAL ULCER

380

GASTRIC CARCINOMA

This is a relatively common form of malignancy, although it occurs less frequently than hitherto.

Approximately 85% of these tumours occur at the pylorus or in the pyloric canal. The remainder may occur in any'part of the stomach. Unlike chronic peptic ulcer, they are not confined to the lesser curvature.

Various types of growth are described:

1. Fungating carcinoma

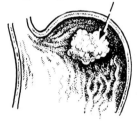

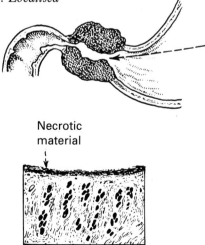

Normal mucus secreting glands

Necrotic material

Adenocarcinoma

Diffuse lymphocyte and plasma cell infiltration

Muscle   Carcinoma

This kind of cauliflower growth is most commonly found in the fundus. It forms a friable mass projecting into the lumen. Necrosis is common and the surface is commonly ulcerated. It remains superficial for a considerable time but eventually grows through the stomach wall and spreads to adjacent structures. Histologically it is usually a typical adenocarcinoma.

2. Scirrhous carcinoma

This occurs in two forms:
1. Localised

Commonest at the pylorus; although it does not protrude into the lumen, constriction is caused by the fibrosis.

Necrotic material

It usually forms a larger ulcer which penetrates to the muscle but not through it. The ulcer is larger and more irregular than chronic peptic ulcer.

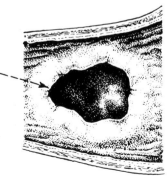

GASTRIC CARCINOMA

Scirrhous carcinoma (continued)

2. *Diffuse*

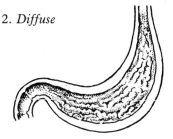

Extension to the oesophagus may occur.
The stomach is reduced in size with a thickened
      firm wall (leather-bottle stomach or linitis plastica).
Ulceration is minimal.
Rugae are prominent.

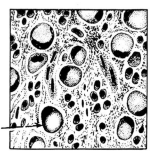

The carcinoma appears to take origin from the deeper glands
and the surface is not involved. The scirrhous reaction is a
pronounced feature. Histologically, it may be an
adenocarcinoma or a signet ring carcinoma. The latter is
distinctive. The cells are rounded and contain a large globule
of mucus pushing the nucleus to one side.

3. Mucoid carcinoma

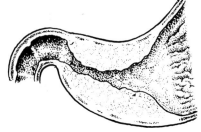

Usually found at the pylorus.
Grows diffusely in wall which
becomes whitish and translucent.
Faint indication of muscle coat.

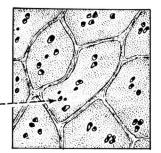

   This growth spreads especially by direct extension and, in the
peritoneal cavity, ensheaths the other organs in a thick gelatinous
mantle. Histologically, it consists of alveoli containing small
numbers of cancer cells suspended in mucus. Sometimes they
may have a signet ring cell structure.

4. Superficial spreading carcinoma

This is an unusual type which forms serpiginous lines of growth spreading in the mucosa
and submucosa.

GASTRIC CARCINOMA

Direct spread
This is usually extensive and various structures may be involved.

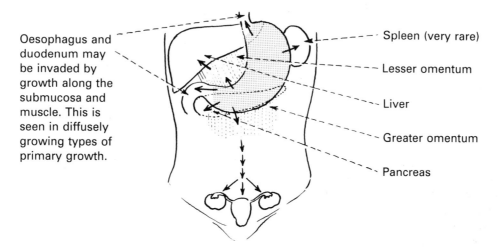

Oesophagus and duodenum may be invaded by growth along the submucosa and muscle. This is seen in diffusely growing types of primary growth.

Spleen (very rare)

Lesser omentum

Liver

Greater omentum

Pancreas

Spread also takes place to the diaphragm and abdominal wall.

Transcoelomic spread is a special type of direct spread. Cells may seed over the peritoneal cavity causing numerous small discrete tumours. The signet ring histological type sometimes causes bilateral hard ovarian tumours by this means — known as Krukenberg tumours.

In mucoid cancer, direct spread gives rise to massive growths in the peritoneal cavity.

Lymphatic spread

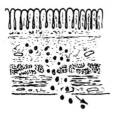

This occurs early and is often extensive, especially in the scirrhous variety. The gastric submucosal lymphatics are first invaded, and this may result in further nodules in the gastric wall. Penetration to the serosal lymphatics soon occurs. The omentum, mesenteries and intestinal walls may be invaded.

Blood spread
In the first instance, this occurs via the hepatic portal system giving rise to metastases in the liver. Later the lung is involved and spread by the systemic circulation results in secondary growths in the brain and bones. Blood spread is commonest with anaplastic growths, less common in mucoid and diffuse scirrhous tumours.

GASTRIC CARCINOMA

Clinical associations

Cachexia and anaemia are usually severe. This may be related in part to the achlorhydria which is almost always present.

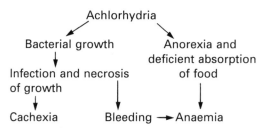

The anaemia is usually of microcytic or normochromic type, rarely macrocytic. Where carcinoma develops in association with peptic ulcer there may be achlorhydria.

Aetiology

The true cause of gastric carcinoma is unknown.

Incidence: Gastric carcinoma was at one time the commonest form of internal cancer in Western civilisation. It appears to be declining in most Western countries except Iceland and Finland. Japan and South American Andean countries also have a high frequency.

Sex: Males outnumber females by 3 to 2.

Social class: The condition is commoner in low income groups but is not related to any particular industry.

Blood groups: A higher incidence has been noted in association with Group A.

Familial factors: Some families show a high incidence but this may be related to socio-economic factors. The cancer is three times commoner in these cases than in the general population.

Chronic gastritis: Both types are associated with an increased risk, especially if intestinal metaplasia is present. Changes described as cellular atypia progressing through dysplasia to localised early carcinoma are seen using endoscopy and biopsy.

Diet: No clear relationship between type of food and gastric carcinoma has been established. More important, perhaps, may be methods of cooking which involve charring of fats etc. as in frying and grilling.

Peptic ulcer: As previously stated, carcinoma only develops in less than 1% of chronic peptic ulcers.

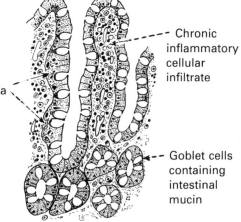

Other forms of malignancy are rare in the stomach. Leiomyosarcoma and malignant lymphoma may occur occasionally.

SMALL INTESTINE

NON-SPECIFIC FORMS of ENTERITIS

Enteritis is a common condition at all ages. The pathological changes may be slight even in the most severe cases. The small intestine is most affected, but the inflammation may extend forward to the large intestine and backward to the duodenum and stomach.

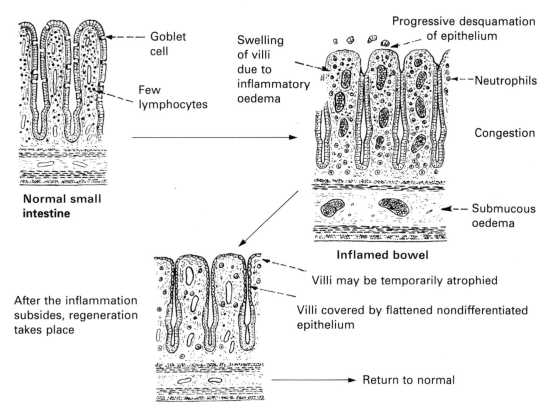

Goblet cell

Few lymphocytes

Normal small intestine

Swelling of villi due to inflammatory oedema

Progressive desquamation of epithelium

Neutrophils

Congestion

Submucous oedema

Inflamed bowel

After the inflammation subsides, regeneration takes place

Villi may be temporarily atrophied

Villi covered by flattened nondifferentiated epithelium

Return to normal

Clinical effects

These are generally mild in adults, unless debilitated. In infants, the condition is often fatal.

1. Loss of fluid into intestinal lumen — diarrhoea and vomiting may be severe enough to cause shock.
2. Electrolyte loss — cardiac irregularities in severe cases, tetany.
3. In the healing stage, the temporary atrophy and loss of function may lead to temporary mild malabsorption.

Aetiology

1. Mild enteritis due to dietary indiscretion occurs in adults and children.
2. Severe enteritis may be caused by poisons such as arsenic and mercury.
3. In infants, a serious variety often assumes epidemic form in nurseries and is frequently fatal. In some instances serological types of *E.coli* have been isolated but usually only from a proportion of cases in the same epidemic. Virus particles have been found in the intestine in many of these patients.

ENTERITIS AND ENTEROCOLITIS

MEMBRANOUS ENTERITIS
This severe acute inflammatory condition is now rare.

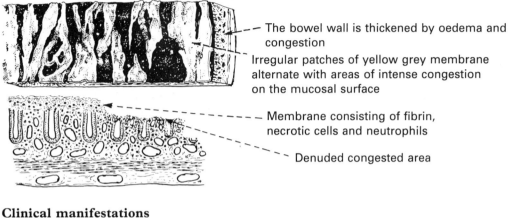

— The bowel wall is thickened by oedema and congestion

Irregular patches of yellow grey membrane alternate with areas of intense congestion on the mucosal surface

— Membrane consisting of fibrin, necrotic cells and neutrophils

— Denuded congested area

Clinical manifestations

Watery diarrhoea ⟶ Dehydration ⟶ Acute circulatory collapse ⟶ Irreversible shock and death

Aetiology Two groups appear to exist:
1. *Ischaemic enterocolitis:* This may occur in states of shock, uraemia or cardiac failure. The lesions are often related to disseminated intravascular coagulation.
2. *Superinfections of intestine:* Prophylactic antibiotic therapy may allow superinfection with *Staphylococcus aureus.*

NEONATAL NECROTISING ENTEROCOLITIS
This lesion occurs in newly born premature infants.

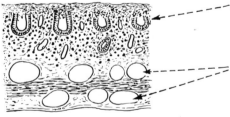

Necrosis and inflammation occur in the bowel wall

The characteristic feature is the occurrence of gas bubbles in the submucosal and muscle layers. These give rise to a characteristic X-ray picture. The gas may enter the portal venous system.

The exact aetiology is not known. Usually the babies, asphyxiated at birth, have required catheterisation of the umbilical vessels. Apnoea causes bowel ischaemia and renders it liable to invasion by gas-forming bacteria. Most babies survive, but stricture may occur during healing leading to intestinal obstruction.

TOXIC ENTERITIS (Toxic food poisoning)
Food contaminated by *Staphylococcus aureus* can contain a large amount of enterotoxin. Cooking kills the bacteria, but the heat resistant enterotoxin causes acute gastroenteritis. *B. welchii* contamination can act in this way also.

CROHN'S DISEASE

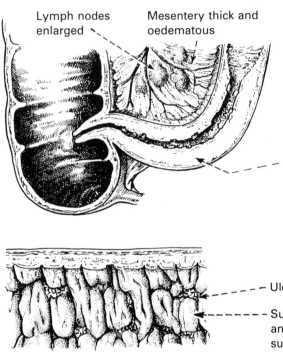

Lymph nodes enlarged

Mesentery thick and oedematous

This is a chronic condition affecting young adults, giving rise to mild diarrhoea and abdominal pain initially.

Typically, it affects the terminal 10 – 20 cm of the ileum and colon but may be found in any part of the intestinal tract, including mouth, oesophagus and anus. The wall is thickened, especially in the submucosa which is oedematous and may have a gelatinous appearance. The lumen is narrowed and there is **ulceration**. The disease has a patchy distribution with areas of normal bowel interspersed.

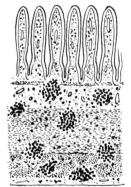

Ulcers are narrow and linear (fissures)

Surviving mucosa is swollen and protrudes as cobbles surrounded by ulcers

Adhesions to other structures occur, and the ulcers frequently penetrate the bowel wall and form fistulous channels.

Microscopic changes

Inflammatory reaction (neutrophils, lymphocytes and plasma cells) extends through whole wall of intestine.

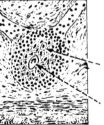

In many cases a granulomatous reaction occurs. Rounded accumulations of epithelioid cells with very occasionally a small giant cell. These resemble the lesions of sarcoidosis.

They occur in association with lymphatic channels causing lymphatic obstruction with dilatation.

Subsequently fibrosis occurs and the mucosa undergoes metaplasia to simple mucus-secreting type resembling that of the pylorus. Secondary infection is common and is responsible for the ulceration and fissure formation.

Note: The important pathological diagnostic features of Crohn's disease of the colon are summarised on page 407.

CROHN'S DISEASE

Aetiology
The aetiology remains unknown: evidence points to an infective agent e.g. an atypical mycobacterium. Immunological abnormalities may determine the susceptibility of the patient, or may develop during the course of the disease. It is a disease of developed countries and it is thought that food processing and chemical additions to food may be potentiating factors.

Possible mechanisms are:

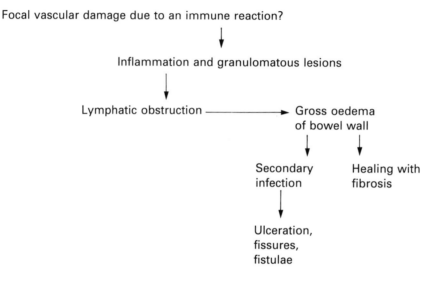

Focal vascular damage due to an immune reaction?

↓

Inflammation and granulomatous lesions

↓

Lymphatic obstruction ⟶ Gross oedema of bowel wall

↓   ↓

Secondary infection   Healing with fibrosis

↓

Ulceration, fissures, fistulae

Complications
1. Intestinal obstruction.

2. Fistula formation either spontaneous or following operation. Perianal fistulae are common.

3. Hypochromic anaemia due to haemorrhage.

4. Macrocytic anaemia caused by interference with absorption.

5. Signs of immunological disorders may be seen — arthritis, uveitis and dermatitis.

TYPHOID

SPECIFIC FORMS of ACUTE ENTERITIS

Salmonella infections
These produce a number of conditions varying in severity from typhoid fever which, untreated, is often fatal, to food poisoning, usually a mild catarrhal inflammation with diarrhoea.

TYPHOID FEVER
Following ingestion of *S. typhi*, the disease process falls into three distinct phases.

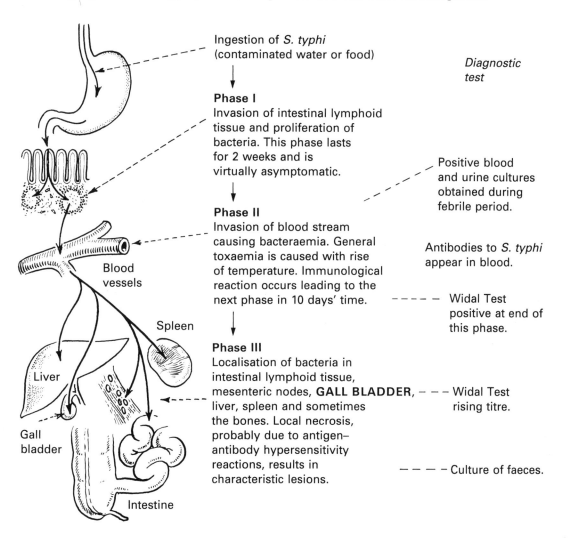

Ingestion of *S. typhi*
(contaminated water or food)

Diagnostic test

Phase I
Invasion of intestinal lymphoid tissue and proliferation of bacteria. This phase lasts for 2 weeks and is virtually asymptomatic.

Positive blood and urine cultures obtained during febrile period.

Phase II
Invasion of blood stream causing bacteraemia. General toxaemia is caused with rise of temperature. Immunological reaction occurs leading to the next phase in 10 days' time.

Antibodies to *S. typhi* appear in blood.

– – – – – Widal Test positive at end of this phase.

Phase III
Localisation of bacteria in intestinal lymphoid tissue, mesenteric nodes, **GALL BLADDER**, liver, spleen and sometimes the bones. Local necrosis, probably due to antigen–antibody hypersensitivity reactions, results in characteristic lesions.

– – – Widal Test rising titre.

– – – – Culture of faeces.

Blood vessels

Spleen

Liver

Gall bladder

Intestine

389

TYPHOID

Intestinal lesions

The ileum is most affected, but lesions may be found in the jejunum and colon.

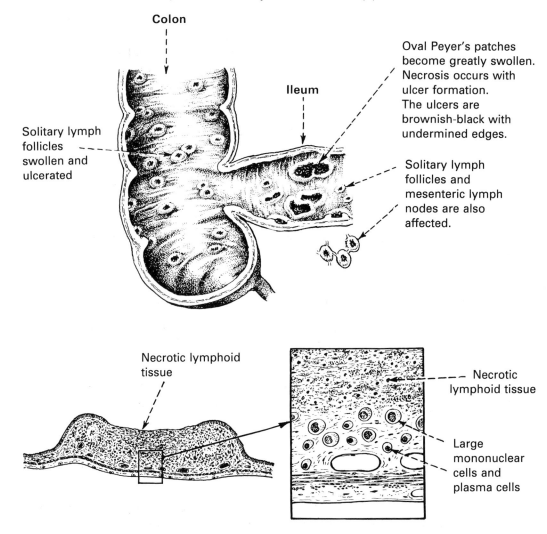

The features of acute inflammation are present, but, instead of neutrophils, large mononuclear cells infiltrate the tissues.

TYPHOID

Other lesions

These are very variable but can be widespread. They are due to:

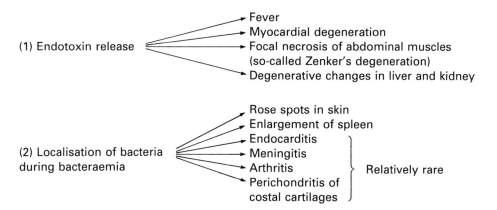

(1) Endotoxin release

- Fever
- Myocardial degeneration
- Focal necrosis of abdominal muscles
  (so-called Zenker's degeneration)
- Degenerative changes in liver and kidney

(2) Localisation of bacteria during bacteraemia

- Rose spots in skin
- Enlargement of spleen
- Endocarditis ⎫
- Meningitis ⎪
- Arthritis ⎬ Relatively rare
- Perichondritis of ⎪
  costal cartilages ⎭

In all lesions there is an absence of neutrophils. The blood shows neutropenia and a relative lymphocytosis.

Sequelae

1. Healing of the lesions is the usual pattern of events. The intestinal ulcers heal with a minimum of scarring.

2. Deep intestinal ulceration sometimes occurs
   - Sometimes severe haemorrhage results.
   - Perforation and general peritonitis (usually fatal).

3. Persistent chronic infection of the gall bladder or urinary tract. In this condition, the patient becomes a 'carrier', constantly excreting the bacilli and serving as a source of further outbreaks of typhoid fever in a community.

PARATYPHOID FEVER

This disease is clinically indistinguishable from typhoid fever but is usually much less severe.

The pathological changes resemble those of typhoid fever but are commonly limited to a small portion of the bowel. Frequently there is an absence of ulceration.

Two serological types of the paratyphoid organism are recognised, A and B. Type B is a common cause of enteric fever in Europe. As in typhoid, patients often become 'carriers'.

CHOLERA

This is due to the exotoxin of the *Vibrio cholerae* which evokes an intense outpouring of watery fluid and electrolytes into the gut lumen, resulting in severe diarrhoea and hypovolaemic shock.

TUBERCULOUS ENTERITIS

Three main pathological forms are recognised:

1. **Primary infection**

   This is due to ingestion of infected milk, usually containing bovine tubercle bacilli, and affects the small bowel. The reaction is similar to that seen in primary tuberculosis of the lung.

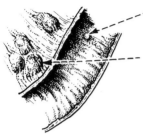

   A tiny lesion, often undiscovered, occurs in the bowel mucosa. This is equivalent to the Ghon focus.

   The infection spreads to the local lymph nodes which are greatly enlarged and caseous (sometimes called tabes mesenterica).

   Usually the condition subsides and the caseous nodes undergo calcification. Infrequently the disease spreads and causes tuberculous peritonitis.

2. **Secondary infection**

   Swallowing of sputum containing large numbers of tubercle bacilli in cases of open pulmonary tuberculosis gives rise to tuberculous lesions in the intestine. Again the small intestine is affected. As in secondary tuberculosis of the lung, the local lesion is prominent and the lymph nodes are less affected. The lesions start in the Peyer's patches and solitary lymphoid follicles.

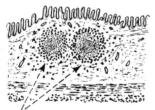

Caseating tubercles form in the mucosa and submucosa

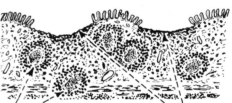

Tubercle follicles in all layers

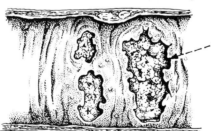

Shallow, ragged ulcers develop which coalesce to form a large ulcer which may encircle the bowel lumen

As in the lung, there is a good deal of fibrous granulation tissue surrounding the caseous lesions and the vessels undergo obliteration. For this reason, perforation and haemorrhage are uncommon. Adhesions to other loops of bowel are common and the caseating process may erode through the walls and cause fistula formation with short circuiting and resulting malabsorption. If the fibrous adhesions are dense, obstruction may arise.

3. **Hyperplastic caecal tuberculosis**

   This rare affection of the caecum involves great fibro-caseous thickening of the bowel wall and numerous pericaecal adhesions.

MALABSORPTION

PRIMARY SYNDROMES

The pathological lesion is very similar in these states. It consists of an atrophy and reduction in the number of villi most marked in the jejunum.

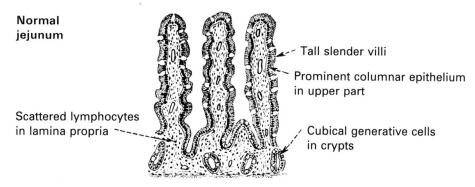

Normal jejunum

Scattered lymphocytes in lamina propria

Tall slender villi

Prominent columnar epithelium in upper part

Cubical generative cells in crypts

The change varies from partial atrophy to almost complete disappearance of villi.

1. Partial villous atrophy

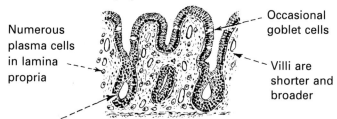

Numerous plasma cells in lamina propria

Occasional goblet cells

Villi are shorter and broader

Many of the villi fuse. To the naked eye, the mucosal surface shows a reduction in the normal folds and there are irregular ridges.

Hyperplasia of the generative cells. This indicates a more rapid turnover in the surface epithelium.

2. Sub-total villous atrophy

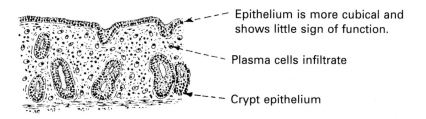

Epithelium is more cubical and shows little sign of function.

Plasma cells infiltrate

Crypt epithelium

In this stage the mucosa appears flat and thin.

The changes occur in several disease states of which the most common are COELIAC DISEASE, TROPICAL SPRUE and AIDS.

MALABSORPTION

COELIAC DISEASE (Idiopathic steatorrhoea)

This affects both children and adults. It is associated with a sensitivity to gluten, a protein from wheat. Diffuse villous atrophy occurs in the jejunum, but the bowel returns to normal both anatomically and functionally if gluten is removed from the diet. There is a familial tendency and patients commonly possess the histocompatibility antigen HLA8. The underlying abnormality appears to be an abnormal immune response to gluten. Splenic atrophy is common and patients frequently show altered immune response to other antigens. Malignant lymphoma of T cell type and adenocarcinoma of the small intestine are rare late complications.

TROPICAL SPRUE

This syndrome occurs in tropical countries with the exception of Africa. It can be very severe with much wasting. Anaemia of macrocytic type due to deficiency of vitamin B_{12} and folic acid is common. Removal from the tropical country effects a cure. Oral broad spectrum antibiotics are also effective, and although the cause is unknown, it is assumed that bacterial colonisation of the small intestine is an important factor.

WHIPPLE'S DISEASE

This is a rare condition. Malabsorption is only one manifestation. There is often lymphadenopathy, arthropathy and skin pigmentation.

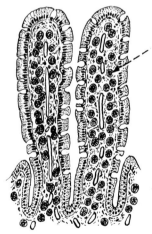

The lesion in the jejunum is characteristic. Large macrophages fill the lamina propria of the villi. These contain mucopolysaccharides staining strongly with periodic acid Schiff (P.A.S.). Similar cells are found in the lymph nodes and sometimes in other organs. Fat accumulates in the lymphatics, possibly due to the obstruction by the macrophages. Bacteria have been found in the macrophages and antibiotics are curative. The disease is almost confined to middle-aged males.

MALABSORPTION

SECONDARY MALABSORPTION
In this instance the malabsorption is secondary to diseases affecting digestion, absorption and transport of nutrients.

Examples are:

1. Interference with absorption
(a) Damage to intestinal mucosa as in Crohn's disease, amyloidosis, systemic sclerosis, radiation damage.
(b) Following bowel resection.
(c) Intestinal stasis due to chronic obstruction and particularly the BLIND LOOP SYNDROME where abnormal bacterial proliferation alters the chemical environment and health of the bowel.
(d) Damage by drugs: e.g. non-steroidal anti-inflammatory drugs (NSAIDs) especially mefenamic acid: cytotoxic drugs.

2. Interference with digestion
(a) Pancreatic or hepatic disease.
(b) Following gastrectomy.

3. Altered transport
(a) Lymphatic obstruction due to neoplasm or tuberculosis.
(b) Disease of mesenteric blood supply.

4. Biochemical abnormality
Disaccharidase deficiency, abetalipoproteinaemia.

The malabsorption in most of these conditions is overshadowed by the primary disease. Fatty diarrhoea, the characteristic feature of coeliac disease, is absent, and the malabsorption is manifested entirely by deficiency states.

The result of the atrophic villous changes is reduction in secretion and absorption which tends to be progressive.

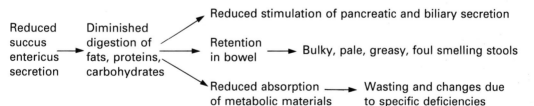

MALABSORPTION

Clinical features of any malabsorption state

The commonest complaint is of diarrhoea due to the bulky, fatty stools, but the presenting signs can vary and specific deficiencies may occur according to the severity and site of the lesions. For example:

Site of lesion	Function affected	Clinical manifestations
Duodenum	Iron absorption	Anaemia
Jejunum	Protein digestion Pancreatic stimulation Emulsification of fats	Wasting Fatty diarrhoea Deficient absorption of fat soluble vitamins — rickets

	Electrolyte and fluid absorption	Dehydration
		Water soluble vitamin
		    deficiencies:
		Vitamin B group
		    Beri-beri, pellagra
		Vitamin C — scurvy
		Folic acid — macrocytic
		    anaemia

Ileum	Absorption of vit B_{12}	Macrocytic anaemia
	Reabsorption of bile salts	Progressive interference with fat absorption

Vitamin deficiencies are particularly liable to occur in children.

TUMOURS OF SMALL INTESTINE

Tumours of all types are uncommon. Simple epithelial tumours are particularly rare.

POLYPI

Multiple tumours of polypoidal structure very occasionally occur as part of a genetic disorder (Peutz-Jeghers syndrome) which includes melanotic pigmentation of lips and mouth. The defect is a Mendelian dominant. The polypi are really hamartomas, consisting of glands, epithelium, muscle, etc. which are normal but arranged in a disorderly fashion.

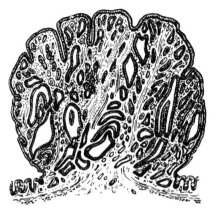

CARCINOMA

This rare lesion is usually found in the jejunum: it is associated with the pathological changes similar to those found in carcinoma of the colon (see p. 413). Carcinoma may arise at the ampulla of Vater and is essentially a bile duct cancer. Clinically, it causes obstruction of the common bile duct and jaundice.

CARCINOID TUMOURS (Argentaffinomas)

These are peculiar tumours which arise in various parts of the body, but the specific clinical features are most commonly exhibited by those found in the ileum.

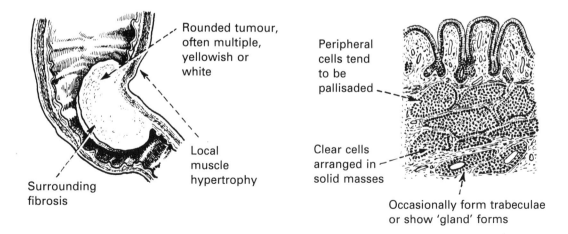

Rounded tumour, often multiple, yellowish or white

Local muscle hypertrophy

Surrounding fibrosis

Peripheral cells tend to be pallisaded

Clear cells arranged in solid masses

Occasionally form trabeculae or show 'gland' forms

The cells have the capacity to reduce silver compounds and are therefore known as argentaffin cells. Cells of a similar type are normally found in the crypts of Lieberkuhn (Kulschitsky cells).

TUMOURS OF SMALL INTESTINE

CARCINOID TUMOURS (continued)

Sites

Appendix
The tip of the appendix is the commonest site for these tumours. They often produce symptoms of acute appendicitis, and it is not clear whether this is due to muscular spasm produced by the secretions of the tumours or to occlusion of the lumen. It is the appendicular form which gave rise to the name carcinoid, since although it infiltrates locally it almost never metastasises.

Ileum
The tumours are frequently multiple and in this case they behave like carcinoma, metastasising to the local lymph nodes and liver. Growth is slow however and the patient may live for many years although secondary spread has occurred. Spread to the liver is frequently associated with the carcinoid syndrome.

Stomach, gall bladder, colon and rectum
Carcinoid tumours are only rarely found in these sites and may be asymptomatic.

Trachea and bronchus
In this site they may be indistinguishable clinically from carcinoma.

CARCINOID SYNDROME

These tumours may secrete a variety of neuroendocrine and paraendocrine substances, in many cases without any apparent clinical functional effects.

However, ileal carcinoids tend to produce two important peptides:
(1) Kallikrein, leading to excessive BRADYKININ production and
(2) 5-hydroxytryptamine (5HT) (serotonin).
These are normally destroyed in the liver and lungs: when metastatic deposits are present in the liver the active agents enter the general circulation and produce the CARCINOID SYNDROME, characterised by episodic flushing, diarrhoea and right heart failure.

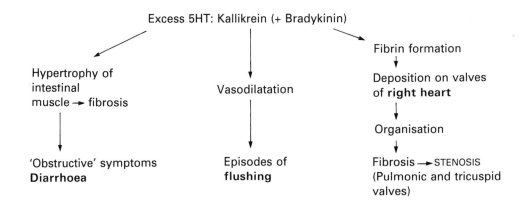

Excess 5HT: Kallikrein (+ Bradykinin)

Hypertrophy of intestinal muscle → fibrosis

Vasodilatation

Fibrin formation
↓
Deposition on valves of **right heart**
↓
Organisation
↓
Fibrosis → STENOSIS
(Pulmonic and tricuspid valves)

'Obstructive' symptoms
Diarrhoea

Episodes of
flushing

TUMOURS OF SMALL INTESTINE

MALIGNANT LYMPHOMA

The extra-nodal lymphoid tissues are collectively known as mucosal associated lymphoid tissues (MALT). The lymphoid tissues of the small intestine are the major component of MALT.

Primary malignant lymphomas are the commonest tumours of the small intestine. B and T cell types are represented.

B cell tumours

(1) Similar types to B cell tumours of nodes: Single or occasionally forming numerous raised nodules (multiple lymphomatous polyposis)

(2) **Mediterranean lymphoma** (α chain disease)

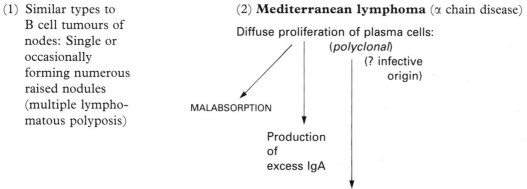

T cell tumours

These tumours occur in late middle age and are associated with enteropathy, particularly coeliac disease.

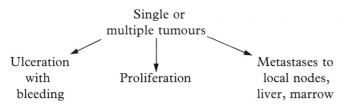

CONNECTIVE TISSUE TUMOURS

These tumours are much more common than epithelial tumours. Smooth muscle tumour (leiomyoma and leiomyosarcoma) sometimes causes an intraluminal swelling which may induce intussusception or, if ulcerated, haemorrhage and anaemia.

APPENDICITIS

Conventionally, three grades of severity of acute appendicitis are described:
(1) Simple acute, (2) suppurative and (3) gangrenous.

SIMPLE ACUTE APPENDICITIS

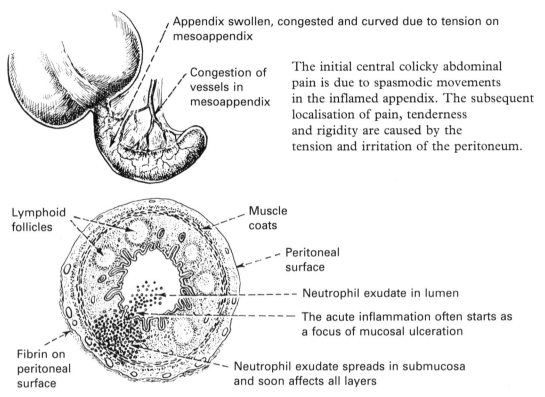

Appendix swollen, congested and curved due to tension on mesoappendix

Congestion of vessels in mesoappendix

The initial central colicky abdominal pain is due to spasmodic movements in the inflamed appendix. The subsequent localisation of pain, tenderness and rigidity are caused by the tension and irritation of the peritoneum.

Lymphoid follicles

Muscle coats

Peritoneal surface

Neutrophil exudate in lumen

The acute inflammation often starts as a focus of mucosal ulceration

Fibrin on peritoneal surface

Neutrophil exudate spreads in submucosa and soon affects all layers

Although the attack can be very acute and lead directly to perforation and peritonitis, the condition may be relatively mild and subside. Repeated attacks are common. The results can be:

(a) Obliteration of the whole appendicular lumen.

(b) Adhesions to surrounding structures. These may lead to complications such as intestinal obstruction.

(c) Local stenosis. By causing retention of waste material more serious inflammation may arise and lead to the second type — suppurative appendicitis.

APPENDICITIS

SUPPURATIVE APPENDICITIS

This may develop from simple acute appendicitis, but often there is a localising factor in the form of a faecal concretion. Less frequently it may be a swallowed foreign body, e.g. vegetable matter or very rarely thread worms which commonly inhabit the appendix.

The pathology may therefore vary.

1. *Complicating simple acute appendicitis*

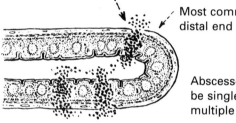

Most commonly the distal end is affected

Abscesses may be single or multiple

2. *Associated with impacted concretion*

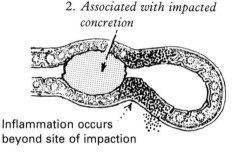

Inflammation occurs beyond site of impaction

In both instances, perforation may occur but is almost inevitable where the abscess is at the site of a concretion. The process can be visualised as follows:

Inflammation
↓
Swelling of tissues + Pressure of concretion
↓   ↙
High tension in tissues ⟶ Vascular supply interrupted ⟶ Necrosis and perforation

GANGRENOUS APPENDICITIS

In the main, gangrene of the appendix tends to develop in two sets of circumstances:

1. *Due to vascular damage*

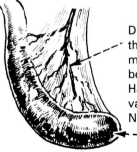

During inflammation the veins in the mesoappendix may become thrombosed. Haemorrhage and vascular stasis follow. Necrosis and gangrene result.

2. *Obstruction of the lumen.* This may be due to a concretion or severe stenosis of the outlet of the appendix. The main factor appears to be distension of the lumen with faecal material. Rapid multiplication of bacteria, especially anaerobes, takes place and this may account for the gangrene. General peritonitis develops early in the process.

SEQUELS OF APPENDICITIS

1. **General peritonitis**

   This is the most important complication since it results in gross toxaemia and may be fatal. It is common with any form of acute appendicitis but almost inevitably happens in the case of gangrenous appendix.

2. **Appendix abscess**

   This arises in the following way:

   Abscess in appendix wall ——→ Perforation + Fibrinous adhesions to adjacent structures (particularly the greater omentum) ——→ Localised abscess in right iliac fossa

   Further complications may arise due to spread of infection:

   (a) Along the right paracolic gutter to produce a subphrenic abscess between the diaphragm and liver
   (b) Into the pelvis to form abscesses around bladder and rectum. In the female the uterus and fallopian tube may be involved.

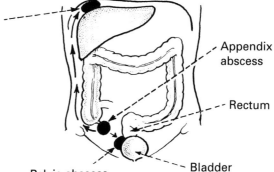

Appendix abscess

Rectum

Bladder

Pelvic abscess

3. **Adhesions**

   Intestinal obstruction may result from constricting bands, or volvulus may be induced.

4. **Liver abscess and portal pylephlebitis**

   These are now rare. They are due to spread of infection to the mesenteric veins resulting in septic embolism. Liver abscesses usually arise from infective emboli, but occasionally there may be a spreading suppurating thrombosis culminating in hepatic sepsis.

APPENDICITIS

Aetiology

1. **Obstruction of the lumen:** In the majority of cases this potentiates distal infection with ulceration. In a few cases no obvious obstruction is evident.

   The usual causes of obstruction are:

(a) Virus infection — this is part of a reaction to alimentary virus infection with reactive hyperplasia of the mesenteric lymph nodes and alimentary lymphoid tissues and is seen particularly in childhood when the lymphoid tissues are prominent. (Infection by *Yersinia enterocolitica* may cause similar changes.)

(b) Inspissated faeces — may form small 'stones' (faecoliths) which obstruct the lumen.

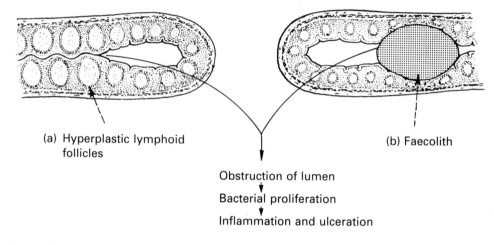

(a) Hyperplastic lymphoid
follicles

(b) Faecolith

Obstruction of lumen
Bacterial proliferation
Inflammation and ulceration

2. **Bacteria:** Those involved are of the normal intestinal flora — coliform bacilli, streptococci and anaerobic organisms.

3. **Inappropriate diet:** Appendicitis is a disease of Western society and the lack of roughage may, by causing stasis, increase the likelihood of attacks.

CHRONIC APPENDICITIS

This is a rather vague condition. In pathological terms, it is synonymous with fibrosis, which may be local or diffuse. The effects may be as follows:

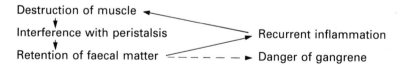

Destruction of muscle
Interference with peristalsis
Retention of faecal matter
Recurrent inflammation
Danger of gangrene

If the fibrosis causes complete obstruction of the lumen, continued mucous secretion may result in cystic dilatation — mucocele. Such a cyst may rupture, giving rise to myxoma peritonei: the mucus-secreting epithelium is spilled into the peritoneal cavity and loculations of mucin and adhesions result.

BACILLARY DYSENTERY

This is an acute inflammation of the large intestine, varying in severity according to the infecting agent.

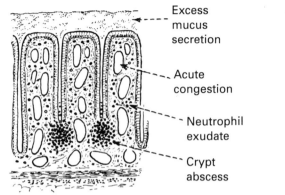

Excess mucus secretion

Acute congestion

Neutrophil exudate

Crypt abscess

Shigella sonnei
Simple acute inflammation of colon.
Common in United Kingdom.

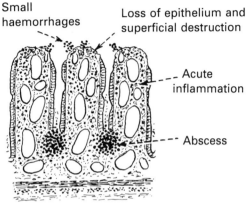

Small haemorrhages

Loss of epithelium and superficial destruction

Acute inflammation

Abscess

Shigella flexneri
Severe acute inflammation.
More common on the continent of Europe.

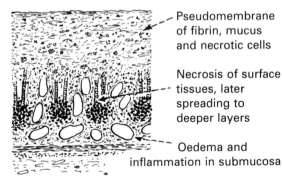

Pseudomembrane of fibrin, mucus and necrotic cells

Necrosis of surface tissues, later spreading to deeper layers

Oedema and inflammation in submucosa

Irregular spreading ulcers with thin shredded margins are formed by shedding of necrotic material.

Shigella dysenteriae
Most severe type, occurs in tropics.

Clinical manifestations

There is acute diarrhoea with abdominal pain, tenesmus and the passage of blood-stained mucus. *S. dysenteriae* infections are often associated with severe toxaemia and sometimes a shock-like condition. Blood mucus and neutrophils are found in the faeces, and in the early stages the bacilli can be isolated.

Healing by resolution with complete restoration of the mucosa is usual. Only in exceptional cases does relapse occur with consequent scarring.

AMOEBIC DYSENTERY

This is due to infection by *Entamoeba histolytica* in food and water.

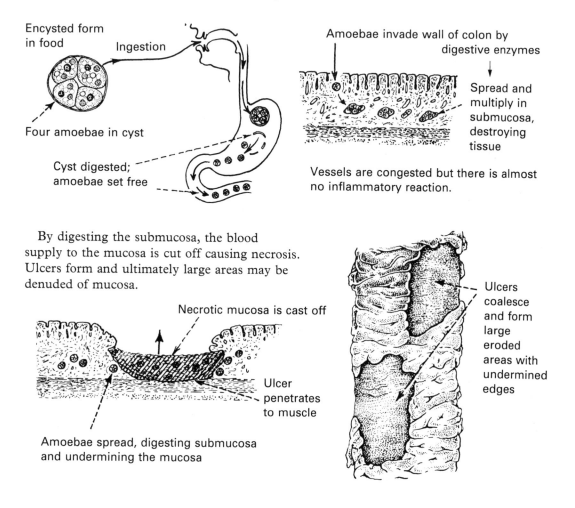

Encysted form in food

Ingestion

Four amoebae in cyst

Cyst digested; amoebae set free

Amoebae invade wall of colon by digestive enzymes

Spread and multiply in submucosa, destroying tissue

Vessels are congested but there is almost no inflammatory reaction.

By digesting the submucosa, the blood supply to the mucosa is cut off causing necrosis. Ulcers form and ultimately large areas may be denuded of mucosa.

Necrotic mucosa is cast off

Ulcer penetrates to muscle

Amoebae spread, digesting submucosa and undermining the mucosa

Ulcers coalesce and form large eroded areas with undermined edges

Healing of the ulcers with fibrosis occurs. The disease persists and overgrowth of fibrous tissue, adhesions to various structures and fistulae may occur. Occasionally the amoebae may invade portal venous tributaries and cause tropical abscess of the liver.

Large numbers of motile amoebae can be found in the faeces during the acute phase of the disease. Later, in the chronic state, they are frequently in an encysted form. Mucus and blood are abundant, but unlike bacillary dysentery, there are no pus cells.

Amoebic abscess
This complication affects the liver (see p. 461).

ULCERATIVE COLITIS

This is an inflammatory condition of the mucosa, primarily of the sigmoid colon and rectum. The inflammation is essentially chronic but acute exacerbations of varying severity are common.

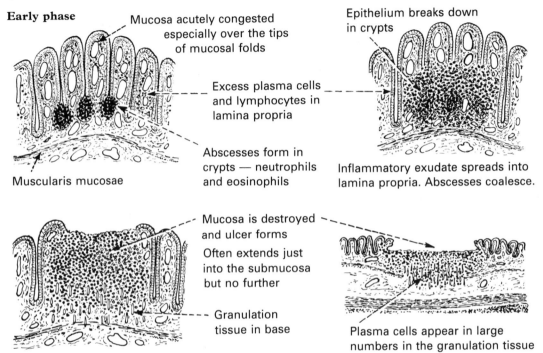

Early phase

Mucosa acutely congested especially over the tips of mucosal folds

Excess plasma cells and lymphocytes in lamina propria

Muscularis mucosae

Abscesses form in crypts — neutrophils and eosinophils

Epithelium breaks down in crypts

Inflammatory exudate spreads into lamina propria. Abscesses coalesce.

Mucosa is destroyed and ulcer forms

Often extends just into the submucosa but no further

Granulation tissue in base

Plasma cells appear in large numbers in the granulation tissue

The ulcers coalesce generally in a longitudinal direction and appear to form over the bands of longitudinal muscle.

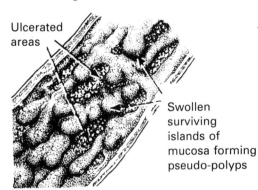

Ulcerated areas

Swollen surviving islands of mucosa forming pseudo-polyps

Periods of remission occur when many of the ulcerated areas heal.

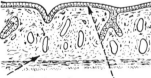

The crypts do not reform completely and show distortion

Granulation tissue

Ultimately the surface may be covered by a simple layer of mucus secreting epithelium with few glands.

Clinical features

Ulcerative colitis is of chronic relapsing nature with periods of remission. It affects young adults and causes episodic diarrhoea with blood and mucus in the stool. Anorexia and weight loss are characteristic of the condition. Protein loss and haemorrhage lead to anaemia.

ULCERATIVE COLITIS

Complications

1. Acute fulminating cases are associated with distension of the colon and perforation is common.
2. Rectal lesions are common, but perianal fistulae are uncommon.
3. Despite granulation tissue formation, fibrosis and stricture are uncommon because the inflammation is restricted to the mucosa.
4. Hepatic cirrhosis is not common.
5. In long-standing cases, carcinoma of the colon frequently develops.
6. Patients frequently show manifestations of hypersensitivity such as erythema nodosum, arthritis, iritis, and haemolytic anaemia and develop sensitivity to drugs easily.

Aetiology

The cause is unknown. It is possible that the intestinal lesions may be due to an autoimmune state.

Macroscopic differences in the pathology of ulcerative colitis and Crohn's disease:

Ulcerative colitis	Crohn's disease (see also p. 387)
1. Lesions continuous — superficial	Lesions patchy — penetrating
2. Rectum always involved	Rectum normal in 50%
3. Terminal ileum involved in 10% (back-wash ileitis)	Terminal ileum involved in 30%
4. Granular, ulcerated mucosa No fissuring	Discretely ulcerated mucosa; cobblestone appearance; fissuring
5. Often intensely vascular	Vascularity seldom pronounced
6. Normal serosa	Serositis common
7. Muscular shortening of colon; fibrous strictures very rare	Fibrous shortening; strictures common
8. Fistulae rare	Enterocutaneous or intestinal fistulae in 10%
9. Inflammatory polyposis common	Inflammatory polyposis not a feature
10. Malignant change — well recognised	Malignant change — doubtful
11. Anal lesions in less than 25%; acute fissures, rectovaginal fistulae	Anal lesions in 75%; anal fistulae; ulceration or chronic fissure

In about 10% of cases it may be impossible to distinguish between ulcerative colitis and Crohn's disease.

COLITIS

PSEUDOMEMBRANOUS COLITIS

Varying lengths of colon show focal inflammation with the formation of surface yellow plaques (pseudomembranes). Most cases are associated with the use in elderly patients of antibiotics, lincomycin, clindamycin and ampicillin.

Microscopic

Foci of mucus, fibrin, epithelial debris and a few neutrophils erupt on the mucous surface

Naked eye appearance

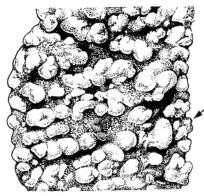

The lesions may coalesce forming typical adherent plaques over large areas, resulting in a fatal outcome. The lesions are caused by toxins from *Clostridium difficile* — an anaerobe normally present in small numbers which proliferate due to elimination of competing bacteria by the antibiotic.

ISCHAEMIC COLITIS

This commonly affects one area of the colon.

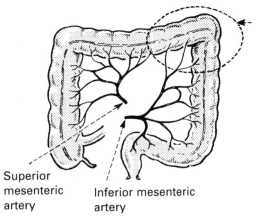

Area of poor anastomosis — watershed zone

Damage is produced by ischaemia. The degree of damage depends upon the duration of ischaemia.

Prolonged ischaemia → necrosis of intestine followed by gangrene

Less prolonged ischaemia → mucosal and submucosal necrosis → bacterial infection. Healing may result in fibrosis and stricture.

Superior mesenteric artery

Inferior mesenteric artery

The ischaemia of the bowel occurs in individuals with arterial disease who suffer a hypotensive episode, e.g. due to shock or cardiac failure.

TUMOURS OF LARGE INTESTINE

Almost all of the tumours of the large intestine are of epithelial origin. Connective tissue neoplasms are rare. Lymphomas are found in the caecum and rectum but less often than in the small intestine.

POLYPI

All of the simple epithelial tumours tend to adopt a polypoidal form. Two of them are of common occurrence:

      1. Tubular adenoma (or adenomatous polyp)
      2. Villous adenoma (or villous papilloma).

The development of these can be visualised as follows.

Tubular adenoma (adenomatous polyp)

Develops from epithelium at base of crypts

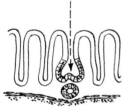

Numerous glands formed

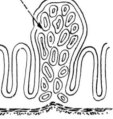

Peristalsis induces formation of pedicle composed of mucosa and muscularis mucosae

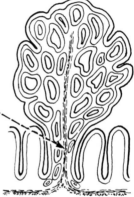

Villous adenoma (villous papilloma)

Develops from superficial epithelium

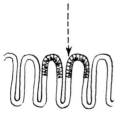

Growth becomes progressively papilliform

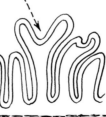

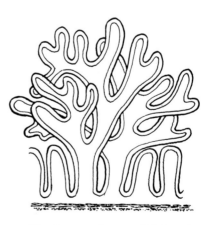

The tumour is superficial and sessile.

TUMOURS OF LARGE INTESTINE

TUBULAR ADENOMA

The majority of tubular adenomas occur in the rectum and sigmoid colon. In the beginning it is a sessile swelling but soon becomes pedunculated.

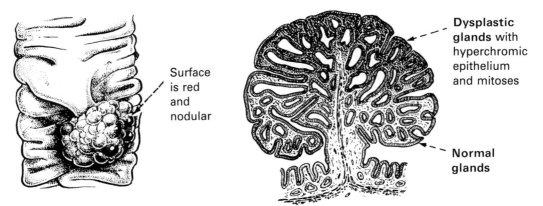

Surface is red and nodular

Dysplastic glands with hyperchromic epithelium and mitoses

Normal glands

They are common in the older age groups and are frequently multiple.

VILLOUS ADENOMA

Villous adenomas are most commonly found in the rectum. They form a sessile mass which may be quite large and have a delicate frond-like structure.

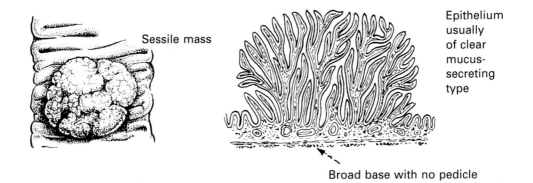

Sessile mass

Epithelium usually of clear mucus-secreting type

Broad base with no pedicle

There is an excessive production of mucus and fluid which may lead to marked loss of potassium, causing muscular weakness.

Many polypi are of mixed variety — part adenomatous, part villous. Both show a tendency to malignant change. If the tumour is of sessile variety invasion of the deeper tissues is immediate. In the pedunculated varieties, invasion of the intestinal wall is delayed.

TUMOURS OF LARGE INTESTINE

METAPLASTIC POLYPI

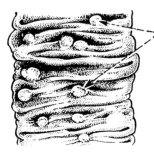

These are usually multiple and present as a small sessile nodule showing unusual feathery metaplastic change in the epithelium. It is found in later life but does not appear to undergo malignant transformation.

JUVENILE POLYPI

These are globular protrusions of the rectal mucous membrane in children. They are usually ulcerated and inflamed but probably represent a developmental abnormality rather than a true neoplasm. They are occasionally multiple.

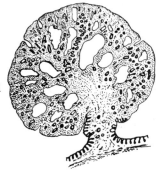

BENIGN LYMPHOID POLYPOSIS of the RECTUM

This is not an epithelial tumour. It consists of masses of lymphoid tissue of normal structure in the submucosa of the rectum in young women. The cause is unknown.

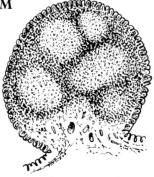

ADENOMATOSIS COLI

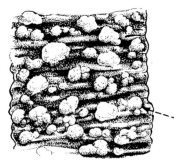

These neoplastic adenomas are a rare hereditary condition which inevitably leads to carcinoma of the colon. Since hundreds of polyps are present, the carcinomas may be multiple and widespread. It is transmitted as an autosomal dominant factor (gene on chromosome 5).
The entire colon is studded with tiny sessile adenomatous polypi. Symptoms appear in late childhood, and carcinoma arises 10 – 15 years later if colectomy is not carried out.

CARCINOMA OF LARGE INTESTINE

This has now taken the place of gastric carcinoma as the commonest form of malignancy of the gastrointestinal tract in Western civilisation.

Site and incidence

Rectum _____ At least 50%
Sigmoid and descending colon ____ Up to 25%
Caecum and ileo-caecal valve _____ Approximately 10%
Ascending colon, hepatic and
          splenic flexures _____ Around 5%
Transverse colon_____ Uncommon.

Types of growth

1. *Fungating polypoid carcinoma*
   This form tends to be more common in the ascending colon. It is frequently a very large, soft, friable growth. Ulceration and haemorrhage are common, leading to anaemia. Infiltration of the base may be slight. Occasionally such a growth is associated with marked loss of potassium leading to muscular weakness.

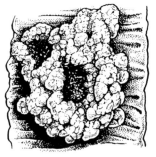

2. *Scirrhous carcinoma*

This is the commonest type of growth and is typical of those neoplasms found in the descending colon. The tumour extends round the circumference of the bowel forming a ring. Fibrous proliferation is marked and results in stenosis with obstruction. The primary growth may be remarkably small and circumscribed even at a late stage.

Hypertrophy and dilatation of proximal bowel

Everted edge

Tumour spread (solid black)

In types 1 and 2 the growth is an adenocarcinoma.

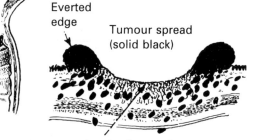

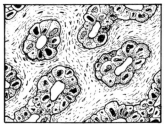

Growth becomes deeply ulcerated

CARCINOMA OF LARGE INTESTINE

3. *Mucoid (colloid) carcinoma*

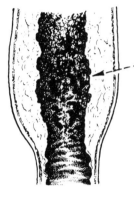

The wall of the colon may be greatly thickened by a gelatinous growth. Almost all of the surface is ulcerated. Bulky secondary masses may form in the omentum and throughout the peritoneal cavity.

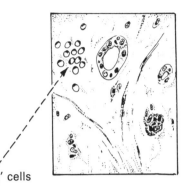

'Signet ring' cells

4. *Diffuse carcinoma*

This type produces a condition similar to that seen in the 'leather-bottle' carcinoma of the stomach.

DEVELOPMENT and SPREAD

1. Lymphatics are the common channel of spread.

Most carcinomas start as an adenoma

Growth extends to submucosa

Submucous lymphatics invaded — bowel encircled

2. Direct penetration of the wall to the peritoneal cavity is also common.

Spread in peritoneum

Invasion of adjacent structures e.g. bladder

Muscularis mucosae

Spread to nearby lymph node

Mesentery

Then to nodes at root of mesentery

3. Blood spread by the portal venous system to the liver occurs later.

413

CARCINOMA OF LARGE INTESTINE

Blood spread

This may lead to secondary deposits in the liver, although these may also be due to spread from affected lymph nodes at the hilum. The lungs, bones and brain are occasionally involved.

Attempts are made to stage the disease since this has an important bearing on prognosis. The following system, which is a modification of the original proposed by Dukes, has been evolved:

Stage		5 year survival figures
A	Tumour confined to mucosa	80%
B_1	Tumour reaching muscularis propria	65%
B_2	Extension through muscularis	50%
C_1	Involvement of paracolic nodes	40%
C_2	Involvement of nodes at root of mesentery	15%

Secondary effects of colonic cancer

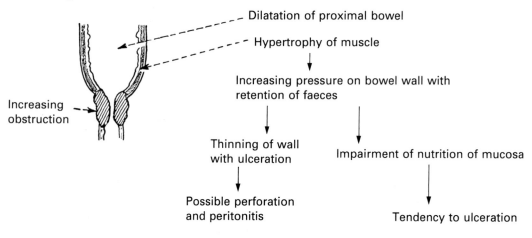

Carcinoembryonic antigen (CEA)

This is a glycoprotein normally produced by fetal endodermal tissues. It is also formed by a number of cancers, among them a proportion of colonic carcinomas, and appears in the blood. It cannot be used as a diagnostic test since it is found in non-neoplastic lesions such as inflammation of the bowel. After treatment, however, changes in the blood concentration of CEA may be used as an indication of recurrence of tumour growth.

Aetiology

The ultimate cause is unknown. A genetic influence is indicated by the fact that the inherited condition, adenomatosis coli, inevitably leads to cancer: the oncogene MSH2 (on chromosome 2) plays an important role in the steps leading to malignancy. (Abnormalities in chromosomes 18, 13 and 1 have also been recorded.)

The nature of the diet and its residue in the colon are also important: a high fibre diet is protective while bile derivatives may be carcinogenic.

DIVERTICULOSIS

Diverticula may form in any part of the intestinal tract but are commonest in the colon.

Small intestine

This is an uncommon site for diverticula. Their importance lies in the fact that bacterial proliferation may occur in them. Vitamin B_{12} is utilised by the bacteria, leading to deficiency and megaloblastic anaemia. Steatorrhoea may also occur. The diverticula occur near the attachment of the mesentery; their thin walls consist of mucosa, submucosa and serosa.

Large intestine

Diverticula are common, especially in the sigmoid colon. At least 10% of adults have this condition.

They form near the mesenteric border of the colon. Closer inspection reveals that they take origin where the blood vessels penetrate the colonic wall.

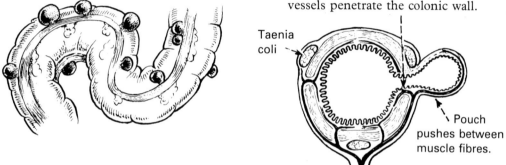

Taenia coli

Pouch pushes between muscle fibres.

The diverticula are often filled with inspissated faeces. The nearby colonic muscle is usually hypertrophied. Inflammation is common in older people. Acute attacks may give rise to symptoms resembling appendicitis but referred to the left side. Abscesses and fistulae may result. Repeated attacks can lead to marked fibrotic thickening of a segment of the colon which may be mistaken for carcinoma. Diverticula in general are only found in adult life. Their prevalence is related to a low residue diet which is thought to cause disturbance of the muscular activity of the colon.

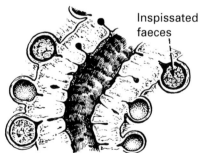

Inspissated faeces

Inflammatory fibromuscular thickening

ACUTE INTESTINAL OBSTRUCTION

This most commonly affects the small intestine due to its mobility and, therefore, its liability to mechanical obstruction in conditions such as hernia, volvulus, intussusception and fibrous adhesions.

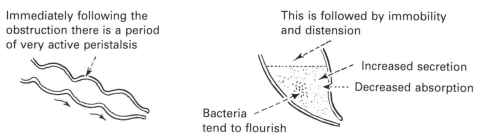

Immediately following the obstruction there is a period of very active peristalsis

This is followed by immobility and distension

Increased secretion

Decreased absorption

Bacteria tend to flourish

Retroperistalsis takes place, the fluid passes back to the stomach and vomiting occurs. The composition of the vomited fluid and the resulting biochemical changes vary with the level of obstruction.

	Pyloric obstruction	Small intestine obstruction
Content of fluid	Acid gastric juice	Saliva, gastric juice, bile, pancreatic secretion, succus entericus
Electrolytes	Chloride lost, sodium retained	Loss of sodium potassium and chloride
CO_2 combining power	Increased due to retained sodium Plasma bicarbonate increased Alkalosis produced	Normal Little change in acid-base balance
Calcium	Alkalosis causes reduction in ionised calcium Tetany may result	Not affected
Potassium	Serum potassium may fall, causing muscle weakness and cardiac irregularity	Not a feature
Fluid balance upset	This may arise late in the process, due to loss of fluid in vomit It may cause oliguria and pre-renal uraemia	Rapid loss of fluid and electrolytes causing fall in blood volume haemo-concentration and shock

CHRONIC INTESTINAL OBSTRUCTION

In this instance the obstruction is incomplete. It is commonly due to changes in the wall of the intestine, e.g. stricture caused by inflammation such as Crohn's disease or scirrhous type of tumour growth, or obstruction of the lumen, e.g. by polypoid growth, or pressure from outside. Since tumour growth and chronic inflammation are more common in large intestine, this is the usual site of chronic obstruction.

1. As the condition develops gradually, the main local change is hypertrophy of the muscle at the proximal part of the bowel.

2. At a later date, obstruction increases and muscle hypertrophy cannot compensate. Marked distension of the proximal bowel occurs with accumulation of gas and fluid.

This gross distension has several effects.

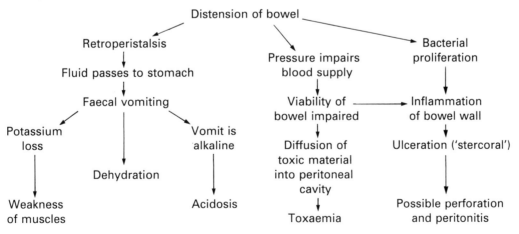

Distension of bowel

Retroperistalsis → Pressure impairs blood supply → Bacterial proliferation

Fluid passes to stomach

Faecal vomiting

Potassium loss

Vomit is alkaline

Dehydration

Weakness of muscles

Acidosis

Viability of bowel impaired → Inflammation of bowel wall

Diffusion of toxic material into peritoneal cavity

Ulceration ('stercoral')

Toxaemia

Possible perforation and peritonitis

417

INTESTINAL OBSTRUCTION

INTUSSUSCEPTION
This is a condition in which the bowel is invaginated into itself.

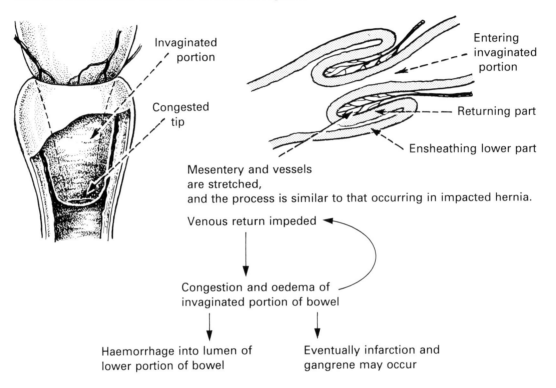

Invaginated portion

Congested tip

Entering invaginated portion

Returning part

Ensheathing lower part

Mesentery and vessels are stretched,
and the process is similar to that occurring in impacted hernia.

Venous return impeded

Congestion and oedema of invaginated portion of bowel

Haemorrhage into lumen of lower portion of bowel

Eventually infarction and gangrene may occur

Sites
The commonest form is the ileocaecal type, the ileum being invaginated into the large intestine with the ileocaecal valve forming the apex. Less commonly, a portion of ileum may pass through the ileocaecal valve. Other sites are occasionally affected, e.g. small intestine or parts of colon.

Clinical manifestations
The patient presents with the signs and symptoms of acute obstruction, a mass in the abdomen and blood is passed per rectum.

Aetiology
It is thought that most cases arise as a result of a swelling in the intestinal wall which is pushed distally by peristalsis, dragging the wall of the bowel with it. Most cases arise in childhood due to swelling of lymphoid tissue produced by virus infection.

Polypoidal tumours of the intestine may cause intussusception in adults.

Very occasionally, adhesions develop between the peritoneal surfaces of the invaginated portion of bowel and the external sheathing portion. The gangrenous invaginated portion may separate and the lesion heal spontaneously.

INTESTINAL OBSTRUCTION

VOLVULUS

As the name suggests, this is a rotation or revolving of the bowel. It affects bowel with a long mesentery. Another factor is the closeness of the ends of the affected loop.

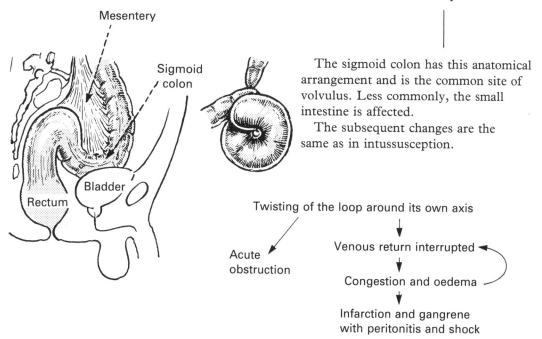

The sigmoid colon has this anatomical arrangement and is the common site of volvulus. Less commonly, the small intestine is affected.

The subsequent changes are the same as in intussusception.

Twisting of the loop around its own axis
↓
Acute obstruction
Venous return interrupted ◄
↓
Congestion and oedema
↓
Infarction and gangrene with peritonitis and shock

Aetiology

In the case of the sigmoid colon, constipation causing loading of the loop in an individual with an abnormally long mesocolon is probably the initiating factor.

Volvulus of the small intestine usually occurs in children. Commonly the mesentery is distorted by disease, e.g. tuberculous nodes.

Very occasionally two loops of bowel may become wrapped round each other.

VASCULAR OCCLUSION

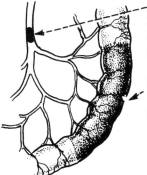

Occlusion of vessels supplying the intestine will result in infarction and subsequently gangrene. A common vascular lesion is thrombosis or embolism of a main branch of the superior mesenteric artery causing infarction of a loop of small intestine.

Due to anastomosis the necrotic segment is usually smaller than might be expected.

Thrombosis or pressure occlusion of the mesenteric veins also leads to infarction.

421

INTESTINAL OBSTRUCTION

PARALYTIC ILEUS

This is an ill-understood condition. The bowel is paralysed and greatly distended. There is usually a thin peritoneal exudate.

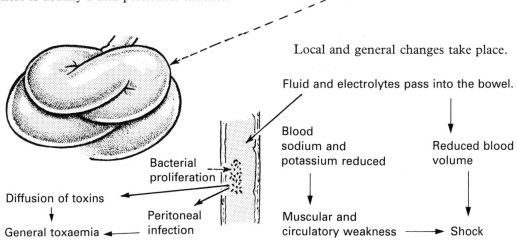

Local and general changes take place.

Fluid and electrolytes pass into the bowel.

Bacterial proliferation

Blood sodium and potassium reduced

Reduced blood volume

Diffusion of toxins

Peritoneal infection

Muscular and circulatory weakness ——→ Shock

General toxaemia ◄——— infection

If the toxic contents of the bowel are not drained and the blood, fluid and electrolytes replaced quickly, death is inevitable. With this treatment the bowel may regain its normal activity.

Aetiology
1. Most commonly it follows abdominal operation, especially if bowel is abused. It may be due to overstimulation of the sympathetic nervous system.
2. Peritonitis from any cause tends to produce paralysis of the intestine.
3. Intestinal infections sometimes have the same effect.

HIRSCHSPRUNG'S DISEASE

Normal ganglion cells

Dilated bowel

Narrow segment

No ganglion cells

Hirschsprung's disease is a rare cause of chronic intestinal obstruction. It is due to a congenital absence of ganglion cells in the parasympathetic Auerbach and Meissner complexes of the rectum.

The aganglionic rectal segment and anus remain contracted due to unopposed action of the sympathetic nervous system, the bowel above becoming grossly distended and hypertrophied.

THE PERITONEAL CAVITY

There are three important features in relation to the peritoneal cavity:

1. Its enormous surface area due mainly to the coils of bowel with their mesenteries
2. A very rich blood supply associated with the abdominal organs, the vessels lying just below the serous surface
3. An equally rich lymphatic drainage.

   These combine to make the area of great importance in relation to fluid exchange and absorption. They influence the pathological changes and clinical effects of any lesions involving the cavity.

Acute inflammation

There are numerous causes of acute peritonitis, almost all of them associated with lesions in the abdominal organs. Examples are:

1. Acute appendicitis
2. Perforating ulcers: peptic ulcers, ulcerative colitis, typhoid ulcers, ulcerated neoplasms
3. Devitalisation of bowel wall: intestinal obstruction, diverticulitis
4. Interference with mesenteric circulation: strangulation of herniae, volvulus, intussusception, mesenteric thrombosis.
5. Cholecystitis, salpingitis, pancreatitis
6. Occasional cases arise during the terminal phases of serious debilitating disease, e.g. uraemia, with no detectable local source.

General peritonitis

This is extremely serious because of the important features mentioned above.

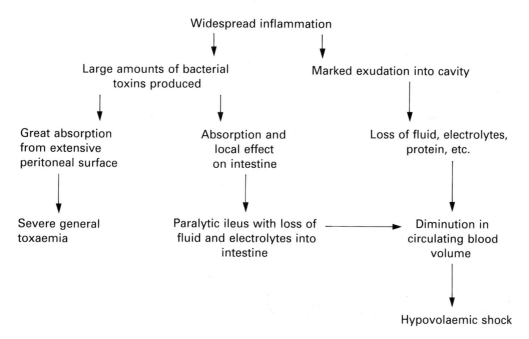

THE PERITONEAL CAVITY

Localised peritonitis

If perforation of the appendix has been preceded by a lesser degree of inflammation on the surface of the appendix, then a localised lesion can result — appendix abscess.

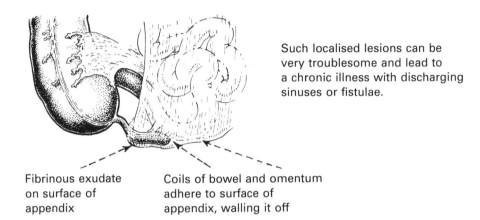

Such localised lesions can be very troublesome and lead to a chronic illness with discharging sinuses or fistulae.

Fibrinous exudate on surface of appendix

Coils of bowel and omentum adhere to surface of appendix, walling it off

Similar pockets of pus may be left behind when a general peritonitis has otherwise resolved with treatment. These are apt to occur in the pelvis or between the liver and diaphragm.

Trouble may arise at a later date if fibrinous adhesions between coils of bowel or between bowel and other structures organise and fibrose. These permanent adhesions interfere with bowel function and may cause obstruction by twisting or kinking of the intestine.

The type of exudate varies with the cause. In most cases which involve the intestines, it is fibrinopurulent. Haemorrhagic exudates tend to be associated with escape of gastric contents or bile into the peritoneal cavity. The exudate is also haemorrhagic in acute pancreatitis but, in addition, opaque yellowish white flecks are seen scattered over the peritoneum. These are small areas of fat necrosis.

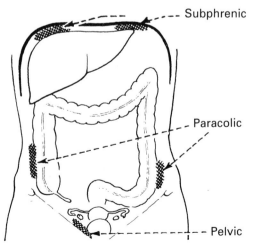

Subphrenic

Paracolic

Pelvic

THE PERITONEAL CAVITY

Chronic peritonitis

The most common type of chronic inflammation involving the peritoneum is that resulting from non-resolution of acute peritonitis.

Tuberculosis of the peritoneum is uncommon in Western civilisation, but frequent in underdeveloped countries. It commonly takes one of the following forms:

1. **Serous effusion.** Small grey tubercles are usually scattered over the peritoneal surface. In addition, the omentum is more extensively involved with the formation of a large fibrous mass in the upper abdomen.
2. **Caseation.** This can vary in extent, from isolated small masses to diffuse caseation involving most of the cavity.
3. **Adhesive peritonitis.** The cavity may be reduced to small pockets containing serous fluid. The source of infection may be caseous lymph nodes, tuberculous salpingitis or tuberculous ulcer of the intestine.

Chronic hyperplastic peritonitis

This is a rare condition of unknown aetiology. It results in marked hyaline thickening of the peritoneum especially over the liver and spleen.

Ascites

Accumulation of serous fluid can occur:

1. As part of a general oedema from any cause such as cardiac or renal failure.
2. Portal venous obstruction as in hepatic cirrhosis, portal thrombosis or compression of the portal vein by tumour growth.
3. Fibroma of the ovary (Meig's syndrome).
4. Tumour of the peritoneum.

Tumours

Primary tumours are rare. Mesothelioma is the most important. It is related to the inhalation of asbestos and the pathology is similar to that of mesothelioma of the pleura, large white plaques of solid growth.

Secondary tumours are common, due to spread of carcinoma from the stomach, ovary and large intestine.

LIVER, GALL BLADDER AND PANCREAS

LIVER – ANATOMY

Conventionally the liver is considered to be composed of regular lobules, each arranged around a central vein with portal tracts at the periphery.

Portal tract

Hepatic artery

Bile duct

Portal vein

Central vein (hepatic venule)

Blood flow

Histologically, it is evident that this is not quite true. The liver in section often has this appearance. The portal tracts and hepatic venules appear to be distributed in a slightly haphazard manner.

Portal tracts

'Central' venules

A new concept of functional structure is now used.

The smallest unit is the simple acinus of varying shape.

The portal venule and hepatic arteriole both send terminal branches into the acinus. They join to form a common trunk which will then contain partially oxygenated blood, and this percolates through the sinusoids to several 'central hepatic venules' (as in diagram).

In terms of oxygen supply and other nutrients, three zones exist:

Zone 1, with the best supply
Zone 2, with a reasonable supply
Zone 3, with the poorest supply which makes it extremely vulnerable to hypoxia.

In Zone 1, glycogen synthesis and glycogenolysis take place. It is also the main area of protein metabolism and formation of plasma proteins. Conjugation of certain drugs takes place.

Portal tract

Pre-terminal hepatic arteriole

Bile duct

Portal venule

Terminal vessels

Zone 3 is associated with glycogen storage, lipid and pigment formation and metabolism of certain drugs and chemicals. Zone 2 shares functions with the other zones.

LIVER – ANATOMY

A complex acinus consists of at least three simple acini organised around the terminal branches of a pre-terminal portal venule, hepatic arteriole and bile duct. The blood circulates through the parenchyma and drains into two or three hepatic venules.

Zones 1, 2 and 3 form roughly concentric layers, zone 1 being the core of the complex acinus. Zone 3 is the outer layer at the periphery of the circulation and, at certain points, can come quite close to the pre-terminal vessels.

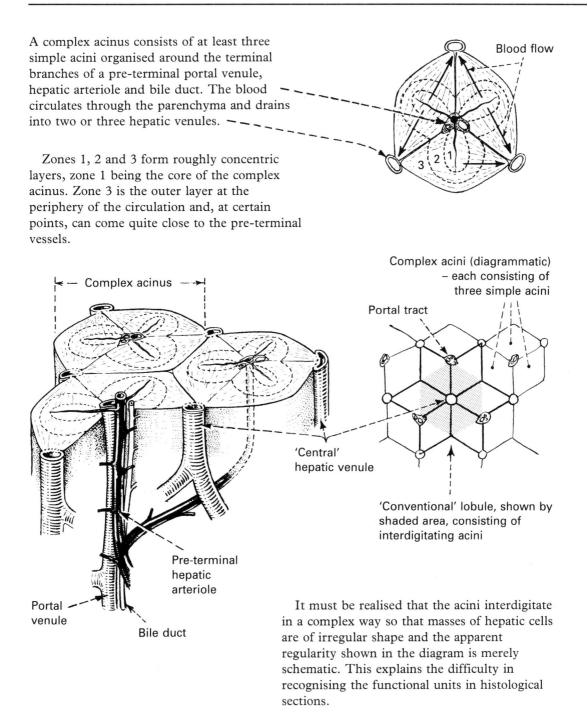

Blood flow

Complex acinus

Complex acini (diagrammatic) – each consisting of three simple acini

Portal tract

'Central' hepatic venule

'Conventional' lobule, shown by shaded area, consisting of interdigitating acini

Portal venule

Pre-terminal hepatic arteriole

Bile duct

It must be realised that the acini interdigitate in a complex way so that masses of hepatic cells are of irregular shape and the apparent regularity shown in the diagram is merely schematic. This explains the difficulty in recognising the functional units in histological sections.

429

LIVER FUNCTION

SECRETORY function

Secretes bile containing: cholesterol; lecithin; bile salts – (detergent action – aid emulsification and absorption of lipids, fat soluble vitamins and cholesterol); bile pigments – products of haemoglobin breakdown – partly excreted, partly recycled.

CONJUGATING function

Steroids, drugs: inactivated and excreted.
Toxins and poisons: inactivation may be attempted but the hepatic cells can be damaged in the process.

METABOLIC function
Protein

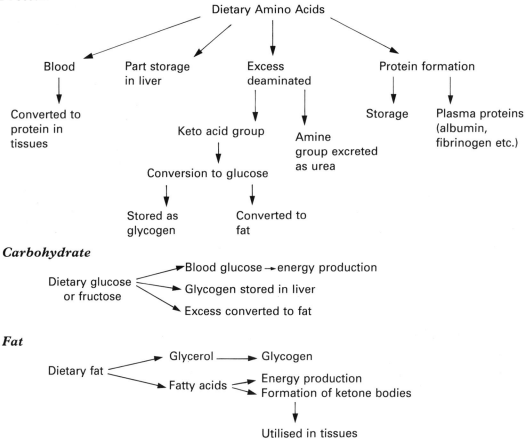

Liver damage will interfere with these functions and this will be reflected in the blood chemistry. Some substances may be increased, e.g plasma amino acids; others may be reduced, e.g. urea. Enzymes may be released from the damaged cells and appear in the plasma.

ANATOMY – HEPATIC LESIONS

The site of hepatic lesions is determined mainly by the microcirculation.
Factors involved are:
1. PO_2 of blood
2. Enzyme functions of the zones
3. Filtration function.

LIVER NECROSIS
In this text the modern description of the liver anatomy is used, providing an explanation of lesions in functional terms. The older conventional lobular nomenclature is shown in brackets.

Perivenular necrosis (Centrilobular necrosis)

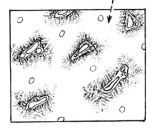

This form is a feature of many apparently unrelated conditions. It is brought about by damage in zone 3 of interdigitating acini (A in diagram). Thus it is a feature of shock due to circulatory collapse reducing the oxygen supply to zone 3. It also occurs in poisoning with chlorinated hydrocarbons (e.g. in chloroform) and drugs, e.g. paracetamol, substances metabolised in zone 3.

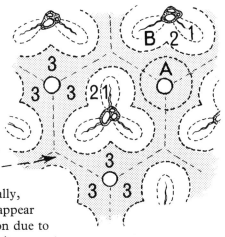

It is important to realise that zone 3, particularly, is continuous from one acinus to another, and in severe cases, the hepatic venules are linked together by necrotic tissues. Microscopically, therefore, the lesions appear irregular in distribution due to differing planes of section.

Mid-zonal necrosis

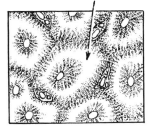

This is uncommon. It is seen in yellow fever and in acute peritonitis; probably the result of toxins affecting zones 2 and 1 (B in diagram).

Periportal necrosis (Peripheral necrosis)
This may represent damage in parts of zone 3 near the portal tracts, or changes in zone 1 due to its metabolism of drugs and chemicals; e.g. phosphorus poisoning causes marked fatty change in the peripheral parenchyma, followed by necrosis.

431

ANATOMY – HEPATIC LESIONS

Massive necrosis

This is an unusual lesion which can follow poisoning due to drugs, industrial chemicals or mushrooms. Rarely it is a complication of viral hepatitis.

Four factors may operate to bring about this necrosis:

1. **Personal sensitivity to the 'poison'.** This has been particularly observed in regard to drugs.

2. **Dosage.** The extent of necrosis is often related to the amount of poison ingested.

3. **Transfer of function.** If one zone becomes necrotic due to the formation of toxic substances when trying to metabolise a chemical, then the task of dealing with the chemical falls upon the adjacent zone. This occurs in paracetamol overdosage and poisoning by chloroform or carbon tetrachloride.

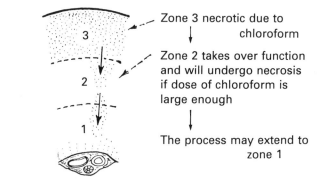

Zone 3 necrotic due to chloroform

Zone 2 takes over function and will undergo necrosis if dose of chloroform is large enough

The process may extend to zone 1

4. **Interference with circulation.** In any necrotic process, the local circulation of blood is bound to be upset, and this will tend to increase the damage which will spread in an increasingly haphazard manner if the cause is still operating.

The following substances are among the most important causing massive liver necrosis:
Drugs: monoamine oxidase inhibitors, paracetamol, halothane.
Industrial chemicals: carbon tetrachloride, tetrachlorethylene, chlorinated naphthalene and nitrobenzene compounds.

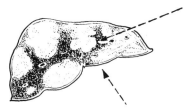

Shrunken liver

In the early stages, the liver is normal in size and is yellow. Soon the dead cells are removed, leaving collapsed dark red areas. Subsequently the surviving cells undergo hyperplasia resulting in a shrunken liver with nodules (multiple nodular hyperplasia) – a form of cirrhosis.

Early acute liver failure may prove fatal. Recovery leaves a liver with gross functional deficiency. The healing fibrotic process and complications inevitably follow.

VIRAL HEPATITIS

Viral hepatitis is the most important form of hepatitis. It is common in Eastern Europe, Africa and Asia. Hospital workers are at special risk and outbreaks are relatively common in mentally handicapped patients in institutions.

Early stage

Liver is enlarged and congested

The histology varies from case to case and from lobule to lobule in the same case.

Ballooning degeneration is the mildest change

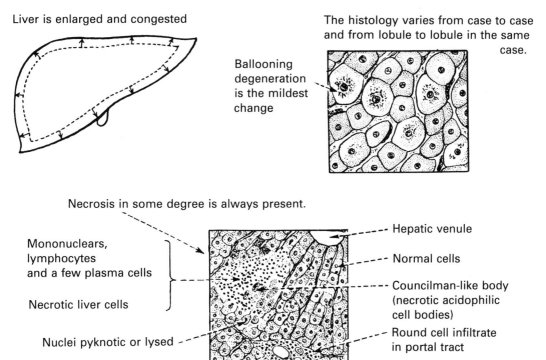

Necrosis in some degree is always present.

Mononuclears, lymphocytes and a few plasma cells

Necrotic liver cells

Nuclei pyknotic or lysed

Hepatic venule

Normal cells

Councilman-like body (necrotic acidophilic cell bodies)

Round cell infiltrate in portal tract

This necrosis may be (a) focal (peripheral or scattered in parenchyma) or more severe (b) forming areas of bridging between vessels (portal to hepatic venule, hepatic venule to hepatic venule) or (c) panacinar: parts or the whole of many acini up to massive necrosis of a large part of the liver occasionally occurs. When it does so, it is usually most marked in the left lobe.

VIRAL HEPATITIS

Later stage

Liver is smaller, yellowish or greenish.

There is evidence of healing with mitotic activity in the hepatocytes.

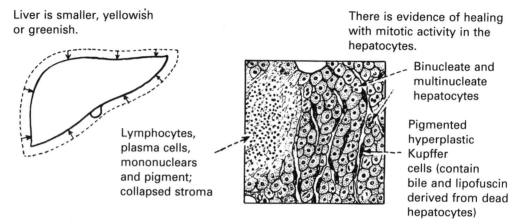

Lymphocytes, plasma cells, mononuclears and pigment; collapsed stroma

Binucleate and multinucleate hepatocytes

Pigmented hyperplastic Kupffer cells (contain bile and lipofuscin derived from dead hepatocytes)

Healing stage

Resolution with complete return to normal is common, e.g in focal and even bridging necrosis. Where necrosis has been severe and extensive with marked inflammatory reaction, the necrotic cells are cleared away, collapse of stroma occurs anbd fibrosis may follow. Surviving adjacent hepatocytes undergo hyperplasia. Lobular structure may become distorted so that vascular relationships, e.g. between hepatic venule and portal tracts, are disturbed and blood flow can be reversed.

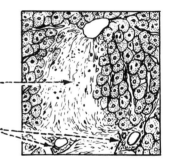

Clinical effects

Pre-icteric phase

The symptoms are those of an acute infection – fever, anorexia, nausea, vomiting, epigastric discomfort, pains in muscles and joints and sometimes a rash. Hepatic enlargement and tenderness are usually present.

Icteric phase

The signs and symptoms are directly due to the changes in the liver. Jaundice increases for 1–2 weeks but frequently disappears in another two weeks. The urine is dark and the stool pale. Leukopenia is followed by lymphocytosis. Splenic enlargement is sometimes present.

VIRAL HEPATITIS

Biochemical changes

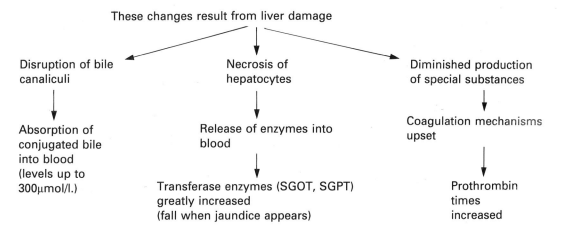

These changes result from liver damage

Disruption of bile canaliculi

↓

Absorption of conjugated bile into blood (levels up to 300µmol/l.)

Necrosis of hepatocytes

↓

Release of enzymes into blood

↓

Transferase enzymes (SGOT, SGPT) greatly increased (fall when jaundice appears)

Diminished production of special substances

↓

Coagulation mechanisms upset

↓

Prothrombin times increased

Clinical progress

1. In most cases, the disease is self-limiting and complete recovery occurs within 4–6 weeks.
2. Death may occur due to massive liver necrosis.
   (a) In the early pre-icteric stage within 10 days – fulminant hepatic failure.
   (b) In 2–3 weeks. The liver is reduced in size.

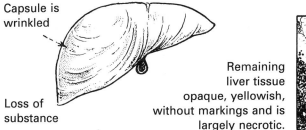

Capsule is wrinkled

Loss of substance

Remaining liver tissue opaque, yellowish, without markings and is largely necrotic.

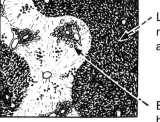

Large necrotic area

Bile duct hyperplasia

This condition is often termed 'acute yellow atrophy'.

(c) Several weeks later. At this stage, regeneration is well advanced in places but function is inadequate and progressive failure occurs.

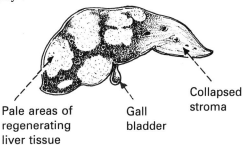

Pale areas of regenerating liver tissue

Gall bladder

Collapsed stroma

435

VIRAL HEPATITIS

Clinical progress (continued)
Secondary pathology due to progressive liver failure occurs in these cases:
Pleural effusion, peripheral oedema, haemorrhagic lesions often in intestinal tract due to upset in prothrombin and vitamin K metabolism, degenerative changes in brain.

3. Chronic hepatitis.

4. Cirrhosis. This may arise in the healing of acute necrosis or result from progressive chronic hepatitis.

Aetiology
Three viruses – A, B and non-A non-B – are the main causes of viral hepatitis, but the pathological changes are similar in all three. (Recently 2 viruses in the non-A non-B category have been isolated and are named Hepatitis C and Hepatitis E viruses.)

	Type A	Type B	Type C	Type E
Virus	RNA Picornavirus family	DNA Hepadnavirus family	RNA	RNA
Mode of spread	Orofaecal, flies, ? parenteral	Parenteral Sexual	Parenteral	Orofaecal
Incubation period	15–40 days	40–180 days	42–90 days	35–40 days
Age of patient	Mostly children	Mainly adults	–	Young adults
Onset	Abrupt	Insidious	Insidious	Abrupt
Viraemia	Transient	Several weeks	Months	Transient
Severity	Mild	Commonly severe	Variable	Mild
Complications	Uncommon	Relatively frequent	Cirrhosis	–
Mortality	Less than 5%	Up to 10%	–	–
Carriers	None	10%	–	–
Immunisation	Passive Pooled human IgG	Active Vaccine on surface viral antigen HBsAg	–	–

VIRAL HEPATITIS

ANTIGENS and IMMUNOLOGY

Hepatitis A

A small cubical RNA virus, 25–28 nm in diameter with a single antigen HAAg. Found in faeces before jaundice occurs. Appears in hepatocytes and Kupffer cells. IgM antibodies appear in the blood during the acute phase and IgG during convalescence. The latter confers immunity and persists for many years.

Hepatitis B

This is a complicated DNA viral structure consisting of a 'core' 37 nm in diameter, the essential infective particle containing several antigens, and a surface protein coat. The core replicates in the liver cell nuclei.

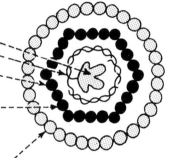

It is composed of central DNA polymerase surrounded by a layer of DNA which in turn is enclosed in a protein coat – the so-called core antigen HBcAg. Associated with this core antigen is another – the e antigen HBeAg.

The surface protein coat is formed in the liver cell cytoplasm and is applied to the core.
This protein is also antigenic – the surface antigen HBsAg. (HBsAg is produced in excess and appears in the blood forming a diagnostic marker.)

The complete virion including the surface protein coat, diameter 42 nm, is known as the Dane particle. The core antigen is never found in blood, but HBsAg, HBeAg and DNA polymerase as well as Dane particles appear during the acute phase.

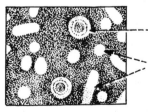

Dane particle

Spheres and tubules of HBsAg in blood

VIRAL HEPATITIS

ANTIGENS and IMMUNOLOGY (continued)

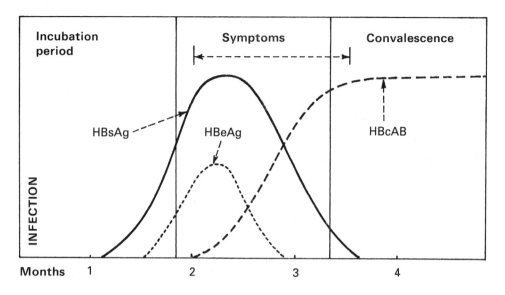

Six weeks after infection the **surface antigen (HBsAg)** appears in the blood, followed two weeks later by the **e antigen (HBeAg)**.

Core antigen (HBcAg) does not enter the blood, but the **antibody HBcAB** is found at the time symptoms appear. This antibody is of IgM variety but later, in convalescence, it changes to an IgG type.

Antibody to the e antigen (HBeAg) rapidly disappears from the blood.

Last to appear is the antibody (HBsAB) to the surface antigen two to three weeks after the symptoms subside and all trace of the antigen is lost. Antibodies to the core and surface antigens persist for many years and confer immunity.

The interpretation of these changes appears to be as follows:
Following infection an immune response is mounted in the liver which damages the hepatic cells and produces the symptoms. Antigens are released during the process and some spill into the blood. The immune response is enhanced leading to neutralisation and disappearance of the antigens with recovery from the illness. The idea that immune response is the cause of the liver damage is suggested by the delay between infection and the onset of symptoms, and by the fact that hepatic B infection in immunosuppressed patients has a very mild course or may be asymptomatic.

VIRAL HEPATITIS

OUTCOME of HEPATITIS B INFECTION

In 90% of cases, there is a vigorous antibody reaction and the patient recovers completely with liver function unimpaired. In the remaining 10%, the illness pursues a variable course, for example:

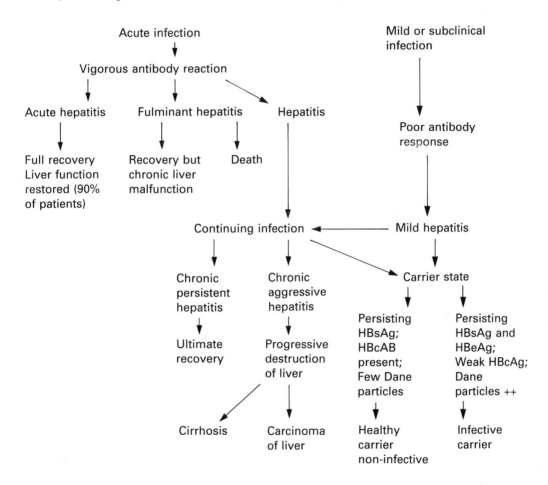

Delta agent

This is a defective RNA virus requiring the presence of HB virus for reproduction. A concomitant infection with HB and Delta agent confers a much more serious prognosis with often fulminant liver damage and subsequent chronic aggressive hepatitis.

Note: Type A rarely leads to severe complications.
   Types non-A non-B are usually mild but in post-transfusion cases may be very severe especially Type C.

439

CHRONIC HEPATITIS

If the condition does not resolve within 6 months it can be assumed that a chronic hepatitis is present. Two types exist:

1. **Chronic persistent hepatitis**
   The patient has poor appetite, vague feelings of ill health, intolerance of fat and alcohol, and transaminase values are slightly elevated. Liver biopsy shows portal tracts expanded by lymphocytic infiltration, but no extension into parenchyma and no destruction of liver cells. Normal lobular formation is retained.

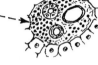

2. **Chronic active or aggressive hepatitis**

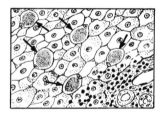

   The symptoms are similar to those of chronic persistent hepatitis but with fluctuating jaundice. It most commonly occurs in men. The histological picture shows progressive destruction of the liver parenchyma: the inflammatory reaction extends from the portal tract into the parenchyma, causing progressive destruction of hepatocytes ('piece-meal necrosis'). 'Ground glass' cells (arrowed) contain an eosinophilic deposit of HBsAg. Bridging necrosis leading to cirrhosis may occur.

In both conditions there is a defective immune response, but the mechanism is unclear. Surface antigen (HBsAg) is commonly found in the blood. In the aggressive type there may be antibodies to the core antigen.

Chronic active hepatitis may also follow infection with the non-A non-B viruses.

A similar pathological process can also arise in conditions of autoimmunity, usually in women. It is important to distinguish between these conditions since the autoimmunity is amenable to immunosuppressive treatment. In this type, autoantibodies are found in the blood, and other systems may be affected – joints, thyroid gland, haemopoietic system, bowel and kidneys.

Chronic hepatitis also occurs in alcoholism, administration of certain drugs such as methyldopa, isoniazid, nitrofurantoin, the laxative oxyphenisatin, and in genetic conditions, e.g. α_1 antitrypsin deficiency and Wilson's disease (an inborn error of copper metabolism).

ALCOHOLIC LIVER DISEASE

Excessive alcohol consumption is associated with several distinct pathological conditions in the liver: (1) **fatty liver;** (2) **alcoholic hepatitis;** (3) **hepatic fibrosis** and (4) **cirrhosis.**

It should be understood however that in many instances the pathology is mixed and all of these changes may be seen.

Fatty liver

This is due to changes in the metabolic activity of hepatocytes and occurs following even a single episode of excessive alcohol intake. The liver is enlarged and in gross cases has a yellow colour.

The accumulation of fat in the liver cells is due to diversion of hepatic enzymes to metabolise the alcohol causing a deficiency resulting in interference with fat and carbohydrate metabolism.

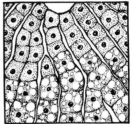

Swollen liver cells
containing globules of fat.

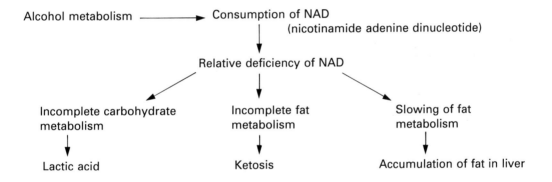

In the early stages of alcohol abuse, the fat accumulating in the liver is mainly derived from the fat deposits of the body.

The main chemical reactions involved are as follows:

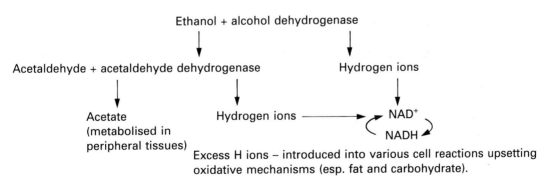

If alcohol abuse continues, further hepatic changes quickly take place, part adaptive, part impairment. The adaptive change is indicated by an increase in the smooth endoplasmic reticulum associated with an increase in microsomal enzymes.

441

ALCOHOLIC LIVER DISEASE

The two processes, adaptation and impairment, act together to increase the effects of alcohol on fat metabolism in the liver.

Increased ability to metabolise alcohol utilises the phosphonucleotide cycle:

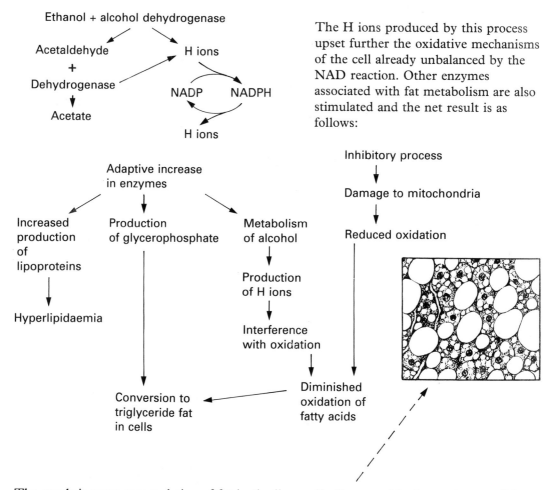

Ethanol + alcohol dehydrogenase

Acetaldehyde + Dehydrogenase → Acetate

H ions

NADP NADPH

H ions

The H ions produced by this process upset further the oxidative mechanisms of the cell already unbalanced by the NAD reaction. Other enzymes associated with fat metabolism are also stimulated and the net result is as follows:

Adaptive increase in enzymes

Increased production of lipoproteins → Hyperlipidaemia

Production of glycerophosphate → Conversion to triglyceride fat in cells

Metabolism of alcohol → Production of H ions → Interference with oxidation → Diminished oxidation of fatty acids

Inhibitory process → Damage to mitochondria → Reduced oxidation

The result is gross accumulation of fat in the liver cells. Even so this change is reversible.

Other enzymes are also increased and side effects may be induced, for example:
- (a) Increased catabolism of drugs which thus become less effective, e.g. warfarin, phenobarbitone, tolbutamide
- (b) Increased catabolism of steroids, e.g. androgens which may lead to a degree of feminisation in males
- (c) Conversion of potential hepatotoxins to active metabolites causing further damage to liver.

Inhibitory activities, mainly damage to mitochondria, can lead to diminished gluconeogenesis and reduced production of albumin and transferrin.

ALCOHOLIC HEPATITIS

Fatty change is reversible even when extensive. In a small proportion of cases, alcoholic hepatitis is superimposed. The essential features are hepatocellular degeneration and necrosis. A peculiar protein, Mallory's hyaline, perhaps produced by the abnormal liver cells accumulates in some of them.

Acute phase

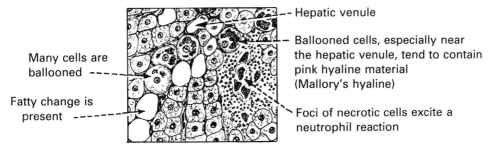

Hepatic venule

Ballooned cells, especially near the hepatic venule, tend to contain pink hyaline material (Mallory's hyaline)

Many cells are ballooned

Fatty change is present

Foci of necrotic cells excite a neutrophil reaction

Clinical features
The patient is acutely ill with fever, nausea, vomiting, and pain in the right upper quadrant. Jaundice may occur, partly due to cholestasis in the bile ductules. Serum transaminases are increased, but the main change is in serum alkaline phosphatase which may reach very high levels. Recently it has been suggested that the increase in glutamic dehydrogenase is directly proportional to the degree of liver damage.

Healing phase
Hyaline fibrous tissue is laid down at an early stage with disappearance of hepatocytes around hepatic venules.

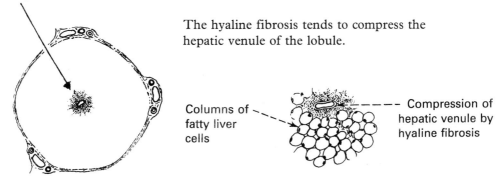

The hyaline fibrosis tends to compress the hepatic venule of the lobule.

Columns of fatty liver cells

Compression of hepatic venule by hyaline fibrosis

ALCOHOLIC HEPATITIS

The hyaline fibrosis, if extensive, may have the following results:

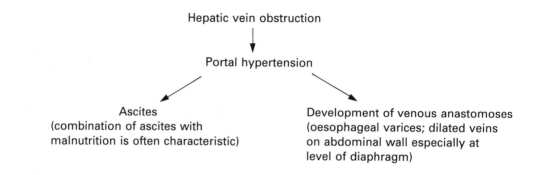

Hepatic vein obstruction

↓

Portal hypertension

Ascites
(combination of ascites with
malnutrition is often characteristic)

Development of venous anastomoses
(oesophageal varices; dilated veins
on abdominal wall especially at
level of diaphragm)

Sometimes the fibrotic changes occur with remarkable rapidity and the hyalinisation process itself produces necrosis ('sclerosing hyaline necrosis') with widespread changes as in the acute phase. There is a neutrophil leucocytosis, progressive ascites and hepatocellular failure.

Aetiology
The aetiology of alcoholic hepatitis is obscure. Several suggestions without adequate proof have been made.
1. Superimposed viral or bacterial infection.
2. Hypersensitivity to alcohol.
3. Delayed hypersensitive reaction to altered proteins produced in hepatocytes, e.g. Mallory's hyaline.
4. Genetic susceptibility. This has been suggested since only a small proportion of alcoholics develop the condition.

ALCOHOLIC FIBROSIS
Focal fibrosis occurs as a result of attacks of alcoholic hepatitis, but in addition there is commonly a piecemeal necrosis at the periphery of the lobules. Spurs of fibrous tissue develop around the portal tracts producing a stellate pattern.

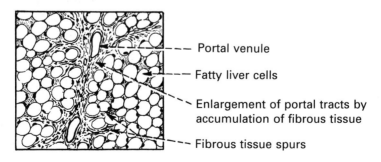

Portal venule

Fatty liver cells

Enlargement of portal tracts by
accumulation of fibrous tissue

Fibrous tissue spurs

Fibrosis sometimes becomes progressive, leading to cirrhosis. This is most apt to happen if there are attacks of alcoholic hepatitis.

CIRRHOSIS

Three macroscopic types are described.

1. **Micronodular**

The liver is usually of normal size or slightly enlarged.

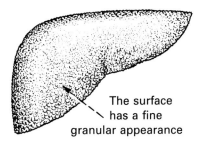

The surface has a fine granular appearance

The nodules of the liver tissue, 1 or 2 mm in diameter, are of fairly uniform size outlined by grey fibrous tissue.

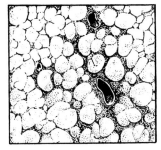

2. **Macronodular**

Liver size tends to vary. Frequently there is irregular shrinkage in parts. The surface shows a coarse nodularity.

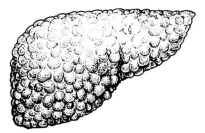

The nodules are larger and may be more than 1 cm in diameter. Often no hepatic venule can be seen in a lobule.

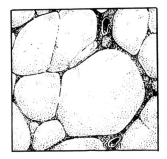

3. **Mixed nodular**

As the name suggests, this pattern is a mixture of the previous two.

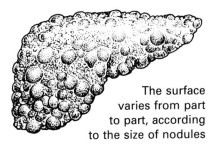

The surface varies from part to part, according to the size of nodules

Similarly the cut surface shows variation in the diameter of the nodules.

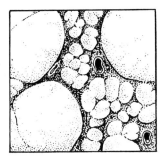

Most cases of cirrhosis end in a mixed nodular condition.

445

CIRRHOSIS

Whatever the cause, four mechanisms are involved in the production of hepatic cirrhosis: (1) hepatocellular necrosis, (2) replacement fibrosis and inflammation, (3) vascular derangement and (4) hyperplasia of surviving liver tissue.

Necrosis, which is often piecemeal, may be:

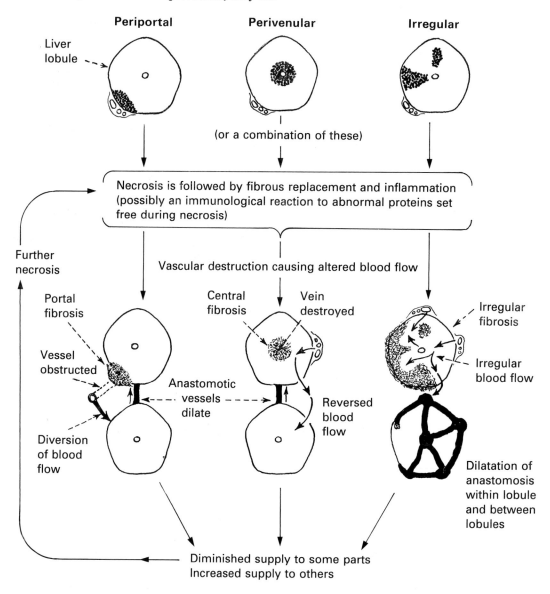

(Illustration of these concepts using the complex acinus as a model would create difficulties. We therefore revert to the 'lobule' for diagrammatic purposes.)

CIRRHOSIS

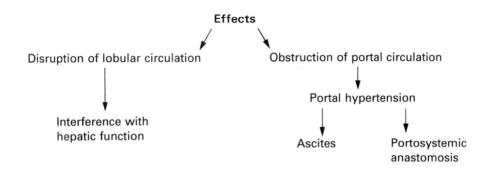

The surviving liver cells undergo reactive hyperplasia forming nodules which further distort vascular distribution. Bile ducts may also undergo hyperplasia.

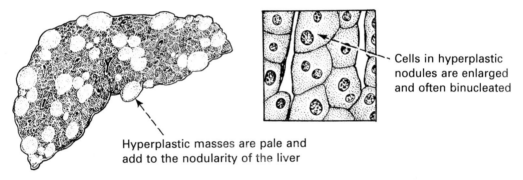

Cells in hyperplastic nodules are enlarged and often binucleated

Hyperplastic masses are pale and add to the nodularity of the liver

Cirrhosis is usually a slow process but inevitably progressive due to:

(a) continued action of the initial damaging factor
(b) development of cytotoxic immune reactions to proteins set free by damaged hepatic cells.

The relative importance of each of these factors varies in individual cases. A vicious circle is set up which maintains the pathological process.

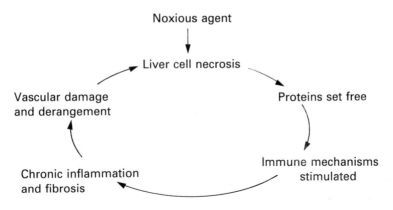

CIRRHOSIS

Complications
Cirrhosis can have three serious effects:

1. ***Portal venous obstruction***
   The process and effects are as follows:

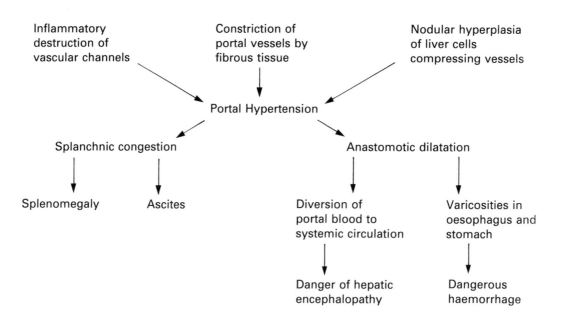

2. ***Hepatocellular failure***
   This is due to a combination of two factors:

   (a) Continuous loss of liver cells
   (b) Increasing distortion of hepatic circulation causing a reduction in effective hepatic blood flow.

   The result is a progressive diminution in hepatic function.

3. ***Liver cell carcinoma***
   This is a late complication in just over 10% of cases of cirrhosis.

CIRRHOSIS

ACQUIRED FORMS

ALCOHOLIC cirrhosis

This is the commonest form of cirrhosis and is most frequent in men over 40. In its early stages, it is a micronodular cirrhosis affecting a large fatty liver.

Periportal cirrhosis with piecemeal destruction of hepatocytes

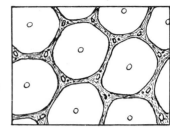

Later, attacks of alcoholic hepatitis lead to peri-venular sclerosis and ultimately a small, non-fatty macronodular or mixed nodular cirrhosis results.

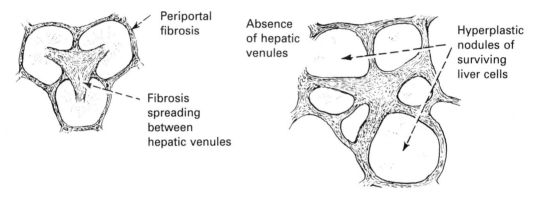

Periportal fibrosis

Fibrosis spreading between hepatic venules

Absence of hepatic venules

Hyperplastic nodules of surviving liver cells

There is little inflammatory change and bile duct hyperplasia is minimal. Mallory's hyaline may be found in hepatic cells.

Clinical effects

Portal hypertension and hepatocellular failure are the main complications. Other changes are anaemia, muscle wasting, polyneuritis and mental changes. Some of these may be due to vitamin lack, especially B and C. Gastritis, peptic ulceration, pancreatitis and Dupuytren's contracture can also occur. Encephalopathy is rare.

INDIAN CHILDHOOD cirrhosis

This affects children aged 1 to 3 years of age. It is of unknown aetiology, but a mycotoxin is suspected. The pathological changes are rather similar to those of alcoholic cirrhosis, and Mallory's hyaline is usually found in the hepatocytes.

CIRRHOSIS

ACQUIRED FORMS (continued)

POST-VIRAL cirrhosis

This is a relatively rare condition. In viral hepatitis, although the hepatocytes undergo necrosis, there is little damage to the supporting tissues which collapse with disappearance of dead cells.

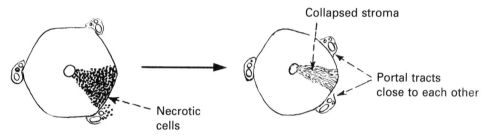

Regeneration is often remarkably complete and normal liver architecture is restored. Cirrhosis is usually the result of continuing inflammation – chronic active hepatitis. It produces a small liver showing macronodular cirrhosis.

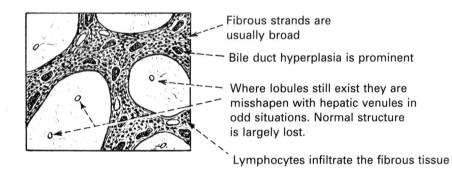

Clinical features

It is commonest in young women. Features of chronic active hepatitis are present and various autoantibodies are found. Prognosis is poor and progress rapid with increasing portal hypertension and hepatocellular failure. Liver cell carcinoma is more common than in alcoholic cirrhosis. It appears to occur particularly in those cases showing a persistence of HB antigen in the blood.

CIRRHOSIS

ACQUIRED FORMS (continued)

BILIARY cirrhosis

Two types of this rare condition occur: primary intrahepatic biliary cirrhosis and secondary obstructive biliary cirrhosis.

PRIMARY INTRAHEPATIC BILIARY cirrhosis

The essential lesion is a chronic inflammation which destroys the small intrahepatic bile ducts.

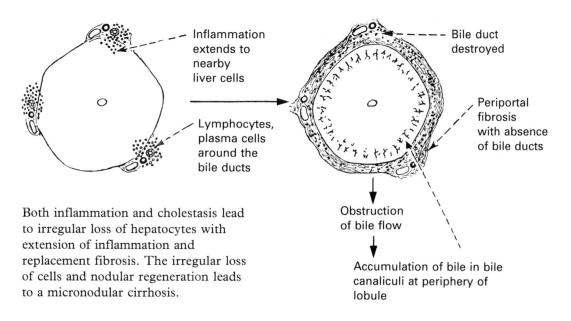

Inflammation extends to nearby liver cells

Lymphocytes, plasma cells around the bile ducts

Bile duct destroyed

Periportal fibrosis with absence of bile ducts

Obstruction of bile flow

Accumulation of bile in bile canaliculi at periphery of lobule

Both inflammation and cholestasis lead to irregular loss of hepatocytes with extension of inflammation and replacement fibrosis. The irregular loss of cells and nodular regeneration leads to a micronodular cirrhosis.

Clinical effects

The disease affects middle-aged women. Symptoms and signs are those of chronic obstructive jaundice. Malabsorption can result in osteomalacia and osteoporosis. The course of the disease is slow, but death is due to the complications of portal hypertension or encephalopathy.

The aetiology is unknown. Antibodies to mitochondria and raised IgM values suggest an immunological process. A few cases appear to be associated with use of drugs such as chlorpromazine. Cholestasis occurs in pregnancy and is known to follow the use of steroids (e.g. contraceptive pill). Some cases may be associated with similar substances.

A similar cirrhosis with obstructive jaundice is the end result of PRIMARY SCLEROSING CHOLANGITIS. There is progressive obliteration of larger bile ducts by fibrosis. The disease occurs predominantly in males and has an association with ulcerative colitis. The aetiology is not known.

451

CIRRHOSIS

SECONDARY OBSTRUCTIVE BILIARY cirrhosis
This is a rare condition which is the end result of chronic impaction of gallstones in the common bile duct or a benign stricture of the duct. The progression is as follows:

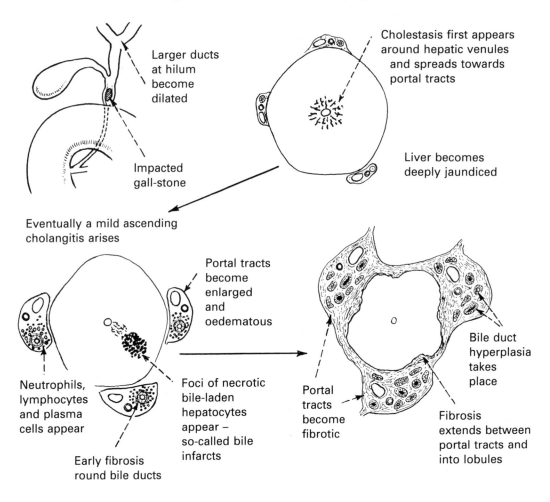

Larger ducts at hilum become dilated

Impacted gall-stone

Cholestasis first appears around hepatic venules and spreads towards portal tracts

Liver becomes deeply jaundiced

Eventually a mild ascending cholangitis arises

Portal tracts become enlarged and oedematous

Neutrophils, lymphocytes and plasma cells appear

Early fibrosis round bile ducts

Foci of necrotic bile-laden hepatocytes appear – so-called bile infarcts

Portal tracts become fibrotic

Bile duct hyperplasia takes place

Fibrosis extends between portal tracts and into lobules

Continuing erosion of the parenchyma and fibrosis lead to a true cirrhosis. The condition may be complicated by liver abscesses due to more acute ascending infection. Death is most often due to liver failure or intercurrent disease. Occasionally there is portal hypertension. Neoplasia, the other cause of bile duct obstruction, usually causes death before cirrhotic changes occur.

CIRRHOSIS

DRUG INDUCED cirrhosis

Isoniazid, methyldopa and oxyphenisatin appear to be associated with a form of cirrhosis showing features similar to those seen in the post-viral type.

Cirrhosis ASSOCIATED with GENERAL DISEASES

Cirrhosis has also been reported in ulcerative colitis, diabetes mellitus, rheumatoid arthritis, scleroderma and hyperthyroidism. A mild fibrosis is associated with chronic congestive cardiac failure. It is not a true cirrhosis and does not cause liver failure.

CRYPTOGENIC cirrhosis

This is a mixed group of conditions of unknown aetiology. The type of cirrhosis varies. As aetiological factors are progressively elucidated this group diminishes.

CONGENITAL FORMS of cirrhosis

Almost all of these are associated with inborn errors of metabolism causing infiltrations and hepatocyte degeneration. The following are examples:

Disease	Metabolic disorder	Type of cirrhosis
Hepatolenticular degeneration (Wilson's disease)	Excessive intestinal absorption of copper – deposition in liver, brain and kidney	Macronodular
Idiopathic haemochromatosis	Excessive absorption of iron – deposition in liver, pancreas and other organs	Micronodular
Galactosaemia	Inability to metabolise galactose Liver cells become distended with fat or glycogen; bile stasis	Micronodular
Glycogen storage disease	Absence of liver glucose-6-phosphatase – inability to break down glycogen to glucose	Micronodular
Alpha 1 – antitrypsin deficiency	Uncontrolled action of proteases in inflammatory states, e.g. hepatitis	Micronodular

Biliary cirrhosis can follow congenital atresia of the bile ducts. Where the atresia affects the large extrahepatic bile ducts, death occurs in a short time before cirrhotic changes occur. Lesser degrees affecting the intrahepatic ducts have a prolonged course and cirrhosis can develop.

CIRRHOSIS

Ascites in hepatic cirrhosis

This is usually a late feature of cirrhosis and is associated with increasing hepatocellular failure. The pathogenesis is thought to be as follows:

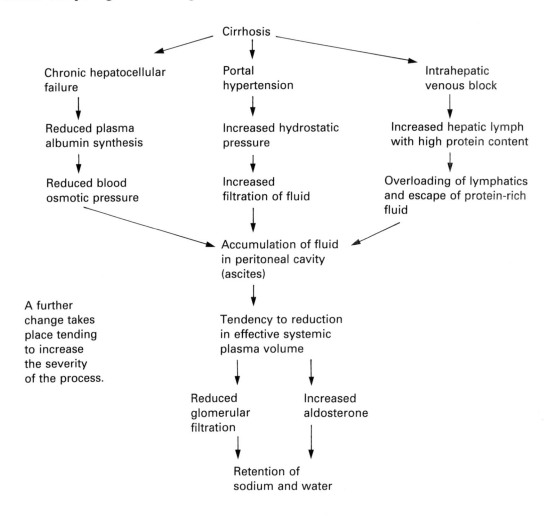

The condition is commonly one of slow accumulation of fluid, but a rapid onset is associated with those factors precipitating liver failure, e.g. haemorrhage from oesophageal varices, operations or bouts of acute alcoholic excess.

HEPATO-CELLULAR FAILURE

Failure of liver function can be:

1. **Acute** with rapid onset, e.g. in cases of massive necrosis due to poisoning (or, less commonly, acute hepatitis).
2. **Chronic** and sometimes recurring, of slow onset, e.g. in cirrhosis or chronic hepatitis.

The mechanism is different in the two types.

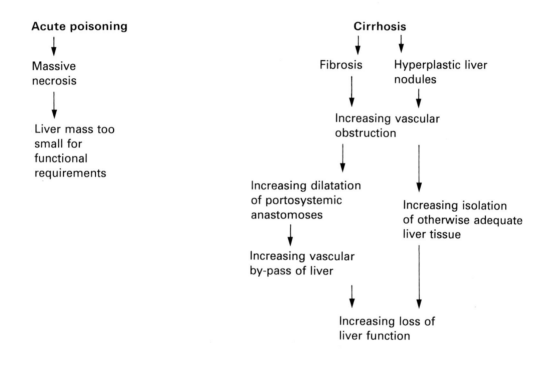

The symptoms and signs tend to be similar in both forms of liver failure but differ in degree. They consist of: jaundice, nervous system disorders, hypoglycaemia, acidosis, bleeding diathesis, renal failure, endocrine disturbances, ascites.

Jaundice

In acute liver failure, jaundice appears early and is related to the extent of liver damage. It arises as a result of lack of conjugation and excretion of bilirubin.

The time of appearance and type of jaundice in cases of chronic liver failure depend on the primary cause. In cases of biliary cirrhosis, the jaundice precedes other signs of liver failure and is of obstructive type, initially at least. Other forms of cirrhosis only give rise to jaundice at a late stage when it is of hepatic type, i.e. due to difficulties in bilirubin conjugation and excretion.

455

HEPATO-CELLULAR FAILURE

Nervous system disorders

These take the form of tremors, behavioural changes, convulsions, delirium, drowsiness and coma, and the syndrome is generally termed hepatic encephalopathy. In the acute form, severe symptoms such as convulsions, delirium and coma develop rapidly, while in chronic conditions milder changes are seen and coma is a late feature, unless a complication arises.

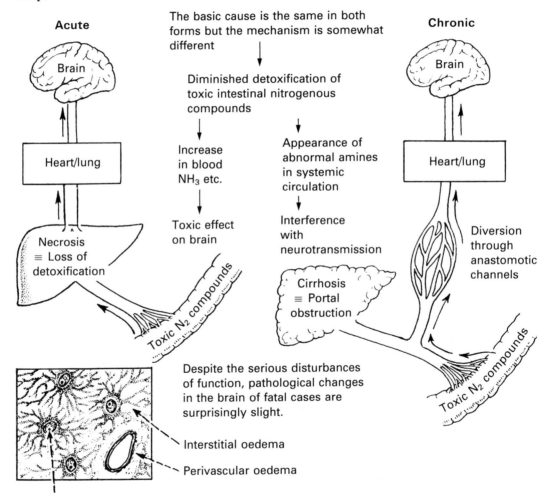

Acute

Brain

Heart/lung

Necrosis ≡ Loss of detoxification

Toxic N₂ compounds

The basic cause is the same in both forms but the mechanism is somewhat different

Diminished detoxification of toxic intestinal nitrogenous compounds

Increase in blood NH₃ etc.

Toxic effect on brain

Appearance of abnormal amines in systemic circulation

Interference with neurotransmission

Chronic

Brain

Heart/lung

Diversion through anastomotic channels

Cirrhosis ≡ Portal obstruction

Toxic N₂ compounds

Despite the serious disturbances of function, pathological changes in the brain of fatal cases are surprisingly slight.

Interstitial oedema

Perivascular oedema

Protoplasmic astrocytes enlarged and increased in number. Nuclei large with prominent nucleoli.

HEPATO-CELLULAR FAILURE

Metabolic and other changes

These may be seen in both acute and chronic liver failure but are variable in their
occurrence. They are again due to deficiencies in the functions of the liver and, in the
chronic state, may be precipitated by some incidental factor such as bleeding, infection etc.
Examples are as follows:

Defective nitrogen metabolism

Defective carbohydrate metabolism

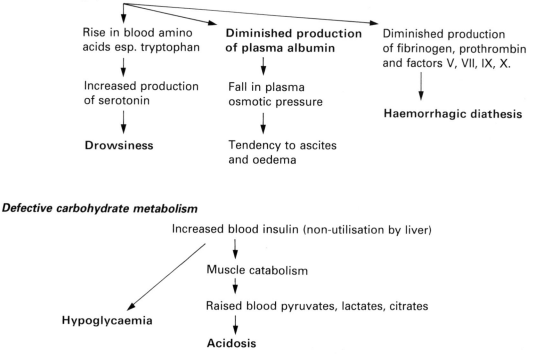

In men, liver failure is associated with gynaecomastia, loss of libido and testicular
atrophy. This is due to defective conjugation of oestrogens.

Renal failure

The reason for renal failure is not certain in all cases. Occasionally it may be due to shock
caused by oesophageal bleeding in cases of cirrhosis, but in acute hepatic failure the
mechanism is obscure.

Anaemia

Three mechanisms may be involved in the causation of anaemia in hepatic failure (usually
the chronic form).
1. Repeated bleeding from oesophageal varices.
2. Hypersplenism. Portal hypertension leads to venous congestion and enlargement of the
   spleen which develops an increased capacity to destroy red cells.
3. Upset in folic acid and B_{12} metabolism in the liver.

HEPATO-CELLULAR FAILURE

Recurrent acute hepatic encephalopathy
This is apt to occur in cases of advanced cirrhosis and is precipitated by:

1. *Gastro-intestinal bleeding*   The mechanism is as follows:

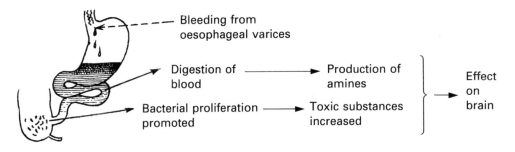

In some patients, even a high protein diet can have the same effect.

2. *Diuretic therapy*

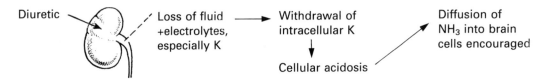

3. *Porta-caval shunt operations*
   These are carried out for relief of portal hypertension, but untoward effects may be encountered.

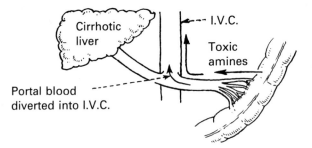

Toxic products from intestines are diverted from the liver and enter the systemic circulation to act on the brain

4. *Narcotic and analgesic drugs*
   These can be very toxic and have a cumulative action due to lack of hepatic drug metabolism.

5. *Intercurrent infections*
   Dehydration, electrolyte imbalance, tissue catabolism and failure of detoxification processes all play a part.

INFECTIONS AND INFESTATIONS

PYOGENIC INFECTIONS

These are now much less common due to the efficient use of antibiotics. Abscess of the liver occurs mainly in two conditions:

1. Ascending cholangitis

Liver abscess

Ascending cholangitis

Common bile duct obstructed (commonly by stone)

2. Suppurative pylephlebitis

This arises from suppurative lesions in the abdominal cavity such as:

Abscesses

Acute appendicitis

Diverticulitis of colon

Inflammation of haemorrhoids

Inflammation

↓

Septic thrombosis of associated veins

↓

Septic emboli in portal veins or spreading pylephlebitis

↓

Liver abscess

ACTINOMYCOSIS

The appendix is the site of the initial lesion. Spread to the liver is via the portal blood but may be direct. The liver lesion is characteristic of *Actinomyces israeli* infection.

Abscesses with shaggy, purulent fibrous walls form a honeycomb structure. The pus contains sulphur granules of actinomyces filaments.

TUBERCULOSIS

This is rare. Miliary tubercles may be seen in generalised infection.

Tuberculoid reactions

Giant cell granulomata are common in sarcoidosis and may also occur in brucellosis, histoplasmosis and early biliary cirrhosis.

INFECTIONS AND INFESTATIONS

SPIROCHAETAL INFECTIONS
Three spirochaetal infections can involve the liver.

1. **Leptospira icterohaemorrhagica (Weil's Disease)**
This organism is associated with the presence of rats and working in wet conditions. It is prevalent among workers in sewers and abbatoirs, miners, agricultural workers and sometimes soldiers on active service. The rat is a reservoir of infection, and rat excreta contain the organism. The disease is characterised by fever, jaundice, haemorrhages into and from various organs, e.g. lungs, kidneys, and renal damage. The liver lesion is characteristic. Death may occur from intrapulmonary haemorrhage or renal failure.

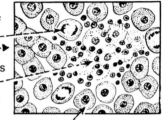
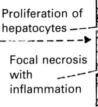

Proliferation of hepatocytes

Focal necrosis with inflammation

Separation of liver cells

2. *Treponema pallidum*
Syphilitic lesions of the liver are now uncommon in this country.
(a) *Congenital infection.* This usually produces a diffuse interstitial fibrosis which isolates individual liver cells and causes ischaemic atrophy. It is accompanied by a striking mononuclear infiltration and tiny areas of coagulative necrosis – miliary gummata. Spirochaetes are often plentiful.
(b) *Acquired infection.* Lesions can occur in the secondary and tertiary stages. In the secondary stage, a diffuse, inflammatory reaction with miliary gummata can occur. Large gummata may occur in tertiary syphilis. Gross scarring with distortion follows healing – hepar lobatum.

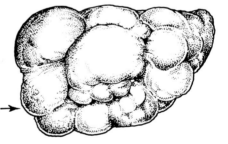

3. **Borrelia**
Borrelia occur in many parts of the world and several species exist – *B. recurrentis* or *B. obermeieri* in Europe, and *B. duttoni* in Africa. They are transmitted by lice and ticks from animals acting as reservoirs, especially rodents. The infections produce peri-venular necrosis of the liver. Jaundice may be severe and liver failure can result in death.

INFECTIONS AND INFESTATIONS

PROTOZOAL DISEASES

Amoebic 'abscess'

This is a complication of amoebic dysentery due to *Entamoeba histolytica*. The 'abscess' is usually single, in the upper right lobe of liver. An irregular fibrous wall encloses what appears to be brownish pus. The 'pus' consists of necrotic liver cells, debris and red cells. Amoebae may be found in the inner wall. There are no pus cells. It may remain localised or track through the diaphragm into the lung, pleural or pericardial cavities.

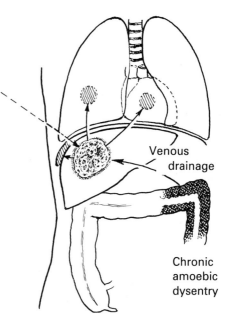

Venous drainage

Chronic amoebic dysentry

Malaria

On initial infection, the parasites develop within the hepatocytes but produce little damage. In chronic malaria, red cells containing parasites are engulfed by Kupffer cells which become hyperplastic and contain brown malarial pigment.

In benign tertian malaria, the parasite can survive for long periods within the liver cells (exoerythrocytic cycle).

Kala-azar

The liver is enlarged due to hyperplasia of the Kupffer cells which phagocytose many Leishman-Donovan bodies.

METAZOAL DISEASES Trematodes (flukes)

Schistosomiasis

S. mansoni is common in Egypt and other parts of Africa. *S. japonicum* is found in China, Japan and the Philippines. Both infections involve the liver.

The schistosomes colonise intestinal tract, the large intestine in the case of *S. mansoni*, while *S. japonicum* infests the small intestine. They invade the intestinal veins; ova are released into the blood stream and embolise the portal venules of the liver. There is a focal granulomatous reaction which may lead to extensive portal fibrosis without cirrhosis. Portal hypertension can result with its attendant dangers.

S. mansoni

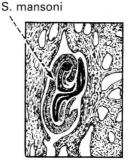

INFECTIONS AND INFESTATIONS

METAZOAL DISEASES (continued)

Two other varieties of fluke disease exist – *clonorchiasis* (Chinese fish fluke) and *fascioliasis* (sheep fluke). Both produce an ascending cholangitis. Clonorchiasis can cause biliary obstruction and marked proliferation of bile ducts. Cholangiocarcinoma may develop. Infestation in both cases is due to eating raw or insufficiently cooked food.

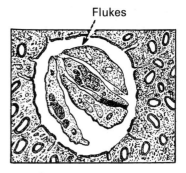

Flukes

Hydatid disease

This is a cystic condition caused by the embryos of *Echinococcus granulosis,* a small tapeworm. The condition is commonest in sheep and may occur in humans in close contact with them. Cattle and pigs may also be affected. Adult worms are found in dogs fed on the infected tissues of sheep, cattle or pigs. Ova are excreted by the dogs and are ingested by other animals including man. The disease is commonest in Australia, New Zealand and South America.

Digestion of the chitinous membrane by gastric juice liberates the embryos which invade the intestinal veins and reach the liver. Sometimes they pass into the systemic circulation and cysts form in the lungs, muscles, kidneys, spleen or brain.

The cyst may be very large, usually multilocular, due to budding of daughter cysts.

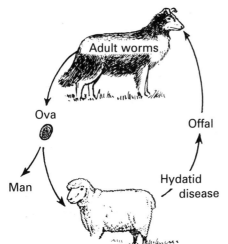

Adult worms

Ova

Offal

Man

Hydatid disease

Ingested by sheep, other domesticated animals and men

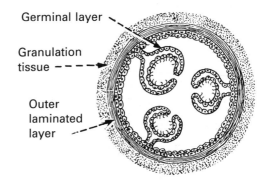

Germinal layer

Granulation tissue

Outer laminated layer

Patients show a hypersensitive reaction to an intradermal injection of hydatid antigen (Casoni test).

PRIMARY CARCINOMA OF LIVER

PRIMARY CARCINOMA is a rare form of malignancy in Western countries but is much more common in South Africa and South East Asia. It occurs in two main forms: hepatocellular carcinoma (75% of cases) and cholangiocarcinoma (25%).

HEPATOCELLULAR CARCINOMA

Three main types of growth are described.

Solitary large tumour	Nodular form	Diffuse growth

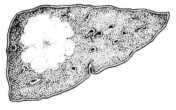 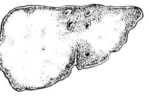

In all three forms the liver is usually cirrhotic.

Histological structure

The cells grow in columns resembling normal liver.

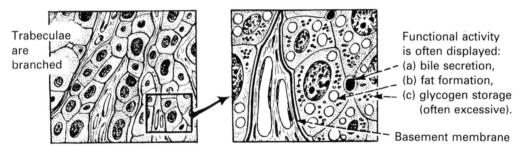

Trabeculae are branched

Functional activity is often displayed:
(a) bile secretion,
(b) fat formation,
(c) glycogen storage (often excessive).

Basement membrane

Some tumours are anaplastic with spindle and multi-nucleated giant cells. Others may show a part acinar structure.

CHOLANGIOCARCINOMA

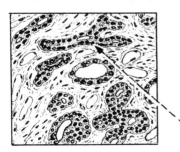

Twenty five per cent of cases arise from the bile ducts. They may develop from small intrahepatic ducts or from the main ducts at the hilum. Two histological types occur. In most instances, the tumour has a tubuloacinar structure. In other cases it is a mucus-secreting adenocarcinoma with a dense stroma. Cirrhosis is rarely present in cholangiocarcinoma.

Cells resemble bile duct epithelium.

PRIMARY CARCINOMA OF LIVER

Spread
Invasion of intrahepatic blood vessels occurs early and results in diffuse growth within the liver. Secondary growths may appear in the lungs, but the massive intrahepatic growth often results in liver failure and death before extrahepatic spread appears.

Clinical features
Many of the clinical findings are related to the underlying cirrhosis. Some unusual features are directly related to the neoplasm.

1. Hypoglycaemia, due partly to the energy requirements of the tumour and partly to its ability to store glycogen.

2. Erythrocytosis. A mild increase in red cells is common in cirrhosis, but it may be exaggerated in hepatoma due to tumour production of erythropoietin.

Other changes are the result of destruction of liver tissue:

1. Upset in blood clotting as a result of disordered production of fibrinogen.

2. Sex hormone effects due to lack of steroid conjugation.

Diagnostic biochemical tests
The usual tests of hepatic function are of little value. Serum alkaline phosphatase may be raised, although the plasma bilirubin remains normal.

Alpha-fetoprotein
This is a protein which is normally only produced in quantity by the fetal hepatocytes. In adult life, very low levels are present in the serum (< 40 ng/ml). It is increased in:

      (a) certain gonadal tumours
      (b) liver cell damage, e.g. in hepatitis
      (c) especially some cases of hepatic carcinoma.

Values above 500 ng/ml indicate carcinoma. This is found in 80% of cases in South Africa and South East Asia, but only 40–50% in Western countries. It is used to monitor progress in those tumours producing the protein.

Alpha-fetoprotein is not produced by the cholangiocarcinoma form of growth.

PRIMARY CARCINOMA OF LIVER

Aetiology

Geography. There is a high incidence in South Africa and South East Asia.

Sex. Hepatic cell carcinoma is much commoner in men. No sex difference has been noted with cholangiocarcinoma.

Cirrhosis. Cirrhosis of macronodular type is present in 60–80% of cases. In Western countries 5–10% of cirrhosis patients develop hepatic cancer, but in South Africa the figure is 60%. Cirrhosis is only rarely associated with cholangiocarcinoma.

Aflatoxins. These are the result of contamination of food, e.g. ground nuts and rice by *Aspergillus flavus*. In Africa the consumption of contaminated food parallels the incidence of hepatic carcinoma.

Hepatitis B surface antigen. There is an association between the presence of this antigen in patients with cirrhosis and the occurrence of hepatoma. The incidence is especially high in South Africa and Far Eastern patients.

The exact relationship between cirrhosis, aflatoxins, hepatitis antigen and hepatic carcinoma is not clear. It would appear that cirrhosis is not necessarily a direct cause of carcinoma but may act as a co-carcinogen.

Liver flukes. In the Far East cholangiocarcinoma is commonly associated with liver flukes in uncooked fish (clonorchis) and mutton (fasciola).

ANGIOSARCOMA

This rare tumour is associated with the use of Thorotrast in radiology, insecticides containing arsenic used in vine cultivation and industrial processes employing vinyl chloride. There is a long latent interval up to 29 years between exposure and tumour development.

HEPATOBLASTOMA

This rare tumour is found in infancy and childhood. It contains a mixture of malignant epithelial and mesenchymal elements. Cartilage, bone and haemopoietic tissue may develop. High plasma levels of alpha-fetoprotein are produced.

TUMOURS OF LIVER

PRIMARY BENIGN TUMOURS
Very few varieties recognised.

1. **Cavernous haemangioma**. This is the commonest type. It forms a dark purple, sharply demarcated geometrical patch on the liver surface. It has the usual structure of a cavernous angioma (see p.152).

2. **Liver cell adenoma**. These small tumours are rare, but an increased incidence has been associated with the use of contraceptive and anabolic steroids. They consist of normal liver trabeculae without normal portal tracts. Intraperitoneal bleeding may occur.

3. **Bile duct adenoma**. These small tumours are extremely rare. They consist of tiny bile duct structures set in loose connective tissue. Occasionally bile duct cystadenomas form large tumours.

SECONDARY
The liver is by far the most frequent site, of all organs, of secondary tumour deposits and they form the commonest type of liver tumour. Approximately 50% of all primary tumours in the portal area spread to the liver and 33% of all disseminated tumours, whatever the source, involve the liver. Apart from the gastrointestinal tract, the lung and breast are the most frequent sites of primary growth. Leukaemic infiltration is also common.

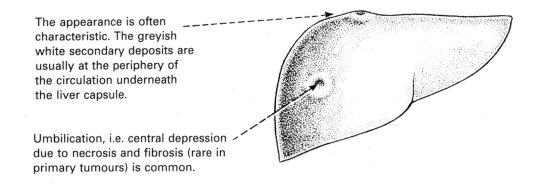

The appearance is often characteristic. The greyish white secondary deposits are usually at the periphery of the circulation underneath the liver capsule.

Umbilication, i.e. central depression due to necrosis and fibrosis (rare in primary tumours) is common.

Variations in appearance are produced by haemorrhage, necrosis and the type of tumour, e.g. mucus-secreting carcinomas.

The secondary tumours grow rapidly and are frequently the main cause of death. An exception are the secondary deposits from a carcinoid tumour which grow slowly over a period of years.

GALL BLADDER AND BILE DUCT – ANATOMY

Anatomy

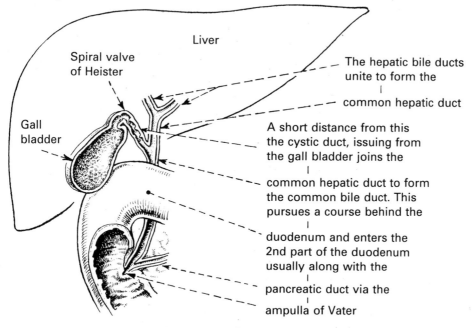

Liver

Spiral valve of Heister

Gall bladder

The hepatic bile ducts unite to form the
|
common hepatic duct

A short distance from this
the cystic duct, issuing from
the gall bladder joins the
|
common hepatic duct to form
the common bile duct. This
pursues a course behind the
|
duodenum and enters the
2nd part of the duodenum
usually along with the
|
pancreatic duct via the
|
ampulla of Vater

The mucosa of the first part of the cystic duct is corrugated to form the spiral valve of Heister.

Histology

Gall bladder

The mucosa is lined by tall columnar epithelium thrown into villous folds

Mucus-secreting glands are found near the neck of the gall bladder

Longitudinal, circular and oblique muscle bundles

Function

Bile is secreted continuously by the liver. The function of the gall bladder is to receive the overflow of bile when it is not secreted into the duodenum. Overdistension is prevented by the ability of the gall bladder to absorb water and electrolytes from the bile, up to 50% of the volume.

467

ACUTE CHOLECYSTITIS

In its mild form, this is a relatively common condition. Severe cholecystitis as a primary condition is uncommon, but it occurs frequently as a complication of chronic cholecystitis and gall-stones. The features are those of acute inflammation.

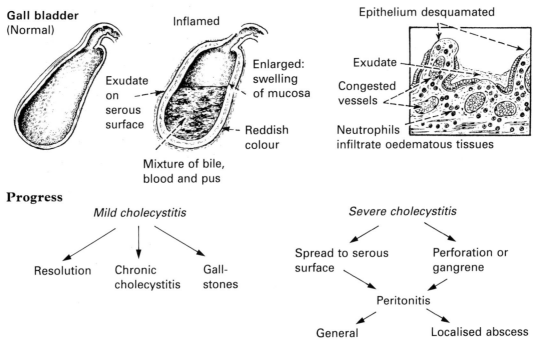

Gall bladder (Normal)

Inflamed

Exudate on serous surface

Enlarged: swelling of mucosa

Reddish colour

Mixture of bile, blood and pus

Epithelium desquamated

Exudate

Congested vessels

Neutrophils infiltrate oedematous tissues

Progress

Mild cholecystitis

Resolution   Chronic cholecystitis   Gall-stones

Severe cholecystitis

Spread to serous surface   Perforation or gangrene

Peritonitis

General   Localised abscess

Aetiology

1. The cause of primary acute cholecystitis is unknown.
2. Bacteria, usually streptococci and staphylococci, or enteric organisms have been isolated, but bacteria have also been isolated from normal gall bladder.
3. Most commonly acute cholecystitis follows occlusion, partial or complete, of the cystic duct by a gall-stone.

Secondary effects of cholecystitis

Inflammation upsets the function of the gall bladder and favours gall-stone formation.

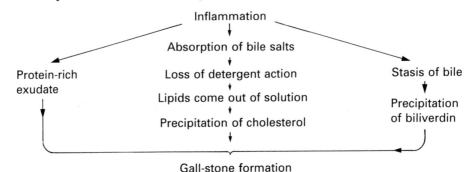

Inflammation

Absorption of bile salts

Loss of detergent action

Lipids come out of solution

Precipitation of cholesterol

Protein-rich exudate

Stasis of bile

Precipitation of biliverdin

Gall-stone formation

CHRONIC CHOLECYSTITIS

Gall-stones are almost always present and this causes a variability in pathology. Two main variations occur:

1. **Hypertrophic**

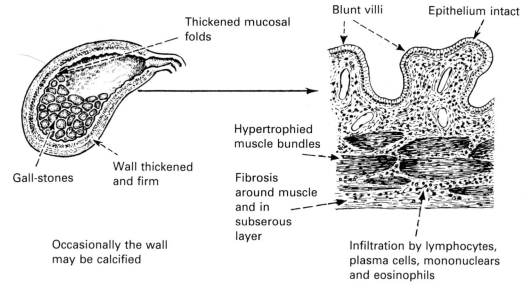

Thickened mucosal folds

Blunt villi   Epithelium intact

Hypertrophied muscle bundles

Gall-stones   Wall thickened and firm

Fibrosis around muscle and in subserous layer

Infiltration by lymphocytes, plasma cells, mononuclears and eosinophils

Occasionally the wall may be calcified

2. **Atrophic**

This occurs when there has been long-standing obstruction of the cystic duct.

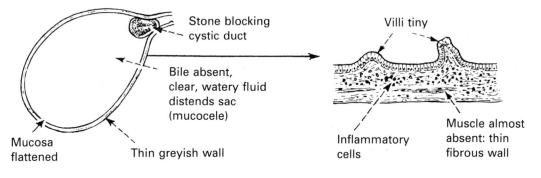

Stone blocking cystic duct

Villi tiny

Bile absent, clear, watery fluid distends sac (mucocele)

Mucosa flattened   Thin greyish wall

Inflammatory cells

Muscle almost absent: thin fibrous wall

Effects

1. Absorptive capacity of gall bladder greatly reduced. Bile is not concentrated and gall bladder is not visualised when radio-opaque substances are given.
2. Tendency to attacks of acute cholecystitis.
3. Further formation of gall-stones following exacerbations of inflammation.

CHRONIC CHOLECYSTITIS

Aetiology

The aetiology of chronic cholecystitis is inextricably associated with that of gall-stones.

1. The condition is said to be most common in females in their late fifties. Usually it is stated that they are fat and fertile but this is questionable.

2. The blood cholesterol is often raised.

3. It may follow an attack of acute cholecystitis, but in most cases no clear history can be obtained other than attacks of 'indigestion'.

4. In some cases there may be evidence of abnormal composition of the bile – excess cholesterol and lack of bile salts and lecithin.

5. By far the commonest single associated factor is the presence of one or more gall-stones.

6. Occasionally cholecystitis may arise in the absence of calculi, in a patient treated with steroids.

CHOLESTEROSIS of the GALL BLADDER (Strawberry Gall Bladder)
This occurs when the cholesterol content of the bile is high.

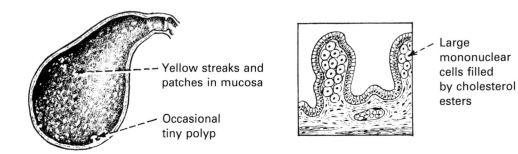

Yellow streaks and patches in mucosa

Occasional tiny polyp

Large mononuclear cells filled by cholesterol esters

The condition is most frequent in females in the 4th and 5th decades. It may be the only abnormality found in the gall bladder but is most commonly associated with the presence of a crystalline cholesterol stone. Cholecystitis frequently complicates the picture and therefore it is also found in chronic cholecystitis when the gall bladder may contain mixed stones.

The cholesterol stone may form around protein during a mild attack of cholecystitis but it is thought that the tip of a tiny cholesterol-containing polyp may break loose and serve as the nidus around which precipitation can occur.

GALL-STONES

The mechanism of formation of gall-stones is not fully understood. Bile consists of bile acids, cholesterol and bile pigment, but it also contains mucin, phospholipids, soaps and fatty acids.

Bile acids, which are detergents and are key substances, have the following metabolic cycle.

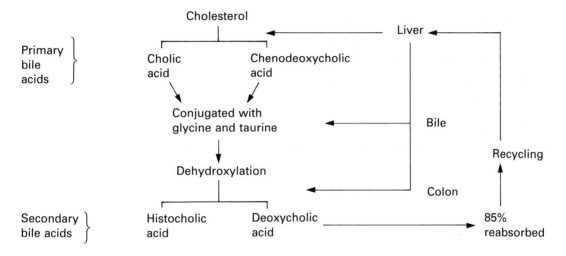

Activities in bile

Solubility of cholesterol. A total pool of 2–4 g of bile acids is required. Micelles soluble in water are formed.

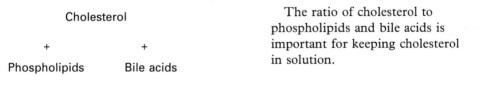

The ratio of cholesterol to phospholipids and bile acids is important for keeping cholesterol in solution.

Activities in intestine

As detergents the bile acids aid in the emulsification and absorption of lipids in the intestines.

GALL-STONES

In the formation of gall-stones, the concentration and solubilities of the various bile constituents are of primary importance.

Three primary types of stone exist:

1. **Cholesterol stone**

   This is the commonest 'pure' stone. It is usually solitary, oval and up to 2 or 3 cm in length.

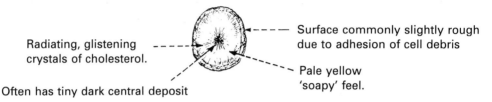

Radiating, glistening crystals of cholesterol.

Surface commonly slightly rough due to adhesion of cell debris

Often has tiny dark central deposit

Pale yellow 'soapy' feel.

Two mechanisms can operate in the formation of this stone:

(a) Excessive cholesterol, e.g. due to diet or metabolic disease such as diabetes. Treatment with 'cholesterol lowering' drugs, e.g. clofibrate, is associated with increased gall-stones due to increased biliary secretion.

(b) Reduction in concentration of bile salts in the bile.

2. **Bile pigment stones**

   These are uncommon. They are always multiple and their presence is associated with excess concentration of pigment in the bile. This may occur in two ways:

   (a) Chronic haemolysis
   ↓
   Excessive biliverdin ⟶ excess bile pigment.
   This is the mechanism when the stones are of primary type.

   (b) Inflammation of gall-bladder.

   Resorption of fluid ⟶ bile concentrated.
   In this condition the stones are secondary to the inflammation.

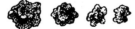 Rarely more than 1 cm in diameter, black and irregular.

3. **Calcium carbonate stone**

   These are rare. They are small, greyish white and crumbling. Sometimes the gall bladder is filled with a paste of calcium carbonate containing the stones. It has been suggested that they are associated with changes in bile pH.

GALL-STONES

Mixed stones

These account for 80% of all cases of gall-stones. Always multiple, they are irregular in shape but faceted due to contact with each other.

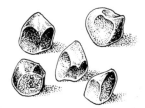

On section they have a laminated structure and the external colour depends on the last layer applied – cholesterol, bile pigment or calcium salts.

Frequently the gall bladder is filled with tightly packed stones. Their varying size indicates formation at different times. Often there is a much larger pure cholesterol stone present – obviously pre-dating the mixed stones.

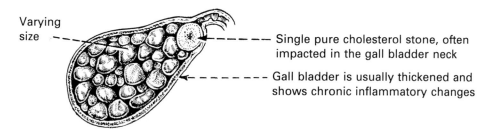

Varying size ---- Single pure cholesterol stone, often impacted in the gall bladder neck

Gall bladder is usually thickened and shows chronic inflammatory changes

Whether chronic cholecystitis is a primary cause of mixed stone formation is not proved but it is an obvious factor in continuing stone formation.

Aetiological factors in stone formation

1. *Diet.* Gall-stones are common in developed countries due to diets rich in cholesterol. The highest incidence is found in North American Indians.

2. *Age.* Stones are almost confined to adult life.

3. *Sex.* It is customary to state that gall-stones occur in women who are fair, fat, forty and parous, but this is certainly wrong. Most gall-stones are discovered accidentally and appear to have little relation to sex or build. It may be that in some female patients parity is coincidentally associated with obesity and increased blood cholesterol which may add a tendency to stone formation.

4. *Cholecystitis.* There is little evidence to suggest that infection is a primary cause of gall-stones but, following formation of a stone, impaction in the gall bladder neck can encourage retrograde infection. This alters the solubility mechanisms and various substances precipitate, forming stones.

5. *Metabolic diseases.* Diabetes is associated with a high blood cholesterol and gall-stones are said to be relatively common.

6. *Haemolytic disease.* This is associated with pigment stone formation.

GALL-STONES

Clinical manifestations and complications

1. Many patients with gall-stones have no associated symptoms, and many more merely have mild dyspepsia.
2. *Impaction* This is common with single cholesterol stones. The stone impacts in the pouch of Hartmann at the neck of the gall bladder. The result depends on whether the blockage is complete or incomplete and intermittent.

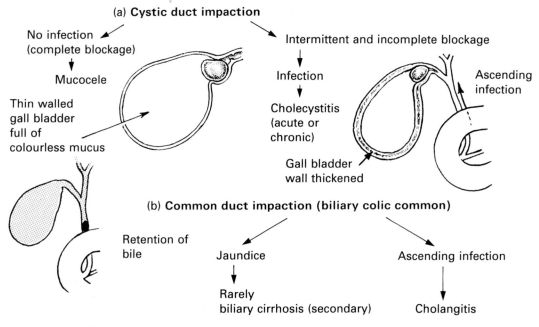

(a) Cystic duct impaction

No infection (complete blockage)
↓
Mucocele

Thin walled gall bladder full of colourless mucus

Intermittent and incomplete blockage
↓
Infection
↓
Cholecystitis (acute or chronic)

Gall bladder wall thickened

Ascending infection

(b) Common duct impaction (biliary colic common)

Retention of bile

Jaundice
↓
Rarely biliary cirrhosis (secondary)

Ascending infection
↓
Cholangitis

3. *Fistulous Communications*. A stone may ulcerate through the gall bladder into intestine and cause obstruction.

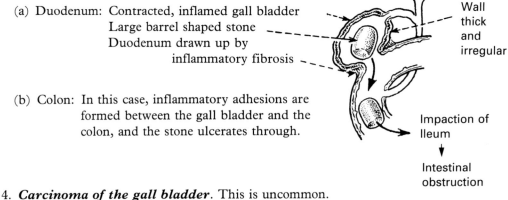

(a) Duodenum: Contracted, inflamed gall bladder
Large barrel shaped stone
Duodenum drawn up by inflammatory fibrosis

Wall thick and irregular

(b) Colon: In this case, inflammatory adhesions are formed between the gall bladder and the colon, and the stone ulcerates through.

Impaction of Ileum
↓
Intestinal obstruction

4. *Carcinoma of the gall bladder*. This is uncommon.
Very rarely the carcinoma arises in the common bile duct.

TUMOURS OF BILIARY TRACT

Simple tumours are exceedingly rare. Fibromas, lipomas and papillomas have been described.

CARCINOMA
This is a relatively rare tumour.

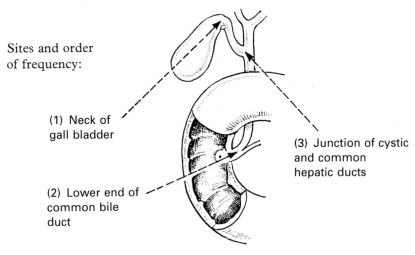

Sites and order
of frequency:

(1) Neck of
gall bladder

(3) Junction of cystic
and common
hepatic ducts

(2) Lower end of
common bile
duct

    The tumour is usually a slowly growing adenocarcinoma. Invasion of the liver and distant metastases occur. In the case of the gall bladder, 80% of cases of carcinoma are associated with gall-stones, but only 2% or less of patients with gall-stones develop carcinoma.

THE EXOCRINE PANCREAS

This is the racemose glandular portion of the pancreas producing its digestive secretion which is delivered to the second part of the duodenum.

Anatomical variations occur in this region.

Commonly the pancreatic and bile ducts fuse as they enter the ampulla of Vater . . .

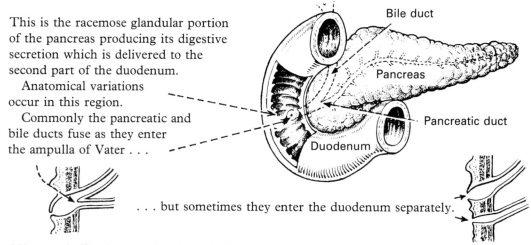

Bile duct

Pancreas

Pancreatic duct

Duodenum

. . . but sometimes they enter the duodenum separately.

Microscopically, the exocrine tissue is similar to salivary glands.

In addition, foci of endocrine islet tissue occur throughout the pancreas

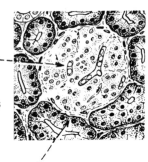

Function: The exocrine pancreas produces an alkaline secretion containing digestive enzymes.
Sodium bicarbonate – gives a pH 7.5–8.0
Amylase – splits starches. Lipase – digests lipids.
Trypsinogen ⎱ converted to active proteolytic
Chymotrypsinogen ⎰ enzymes, trypsin, chymotrypsin.

The islet tissue produces insulin and glucagon.

Exocrine secretory granules

An understanding of the microcirculation is important. The gland has a lobular structure. The larger arteries, veins and ducts course in the fibrous septa between the *lobules*.

This diagram shows the circulation and duct system within the lobule (*intra*lobular).

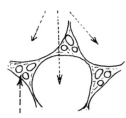

This watershed zone at the *periphery* of the lobule is susceptible when there is a circulatory perfusion deficit

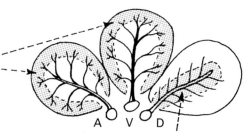

A V D

Interlobular artery, vein and duct

This zone at the centre of the lobule is susceptible if there is damage to the intralobular duct

THE EXOCRINE PANCREAS

CONTROL of EXOCRINE SECRETION

The secretory activity of the pancreas is monitored by the upper intestinal digestive activities and their products.

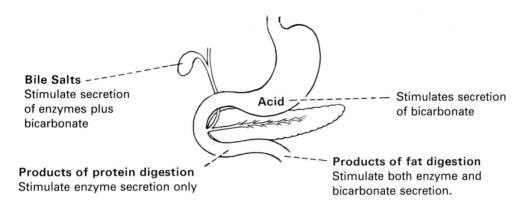

Bile Salts
Stimulate secretion of enzymes plus bicarbonate

Acid ── Stimulates secretion of bicarbonate

Products of protein digestion
Stimulate enzyme secretion only

Products of fat digestion
Stimulate both enzyme and bicarbonate secretion.

These effects are largely mediated through three hormones produced in the intestine – secretin, pancreozymin and cholecystokinin.

Defective secretion

This may be brought about by:

(a) Permanent destruction of pancreatic tissue as in chronic pancreatitis.

(b) Disease of intestine preventing formation of stimulatory hormones.

Insufficiency of exocrine secretion is uncommon. It produces maldigestion and leads to secondary changes in all other processes related to assimilation of food, e.g.

1. *Hyperphagia* which overloads digestive capacity thus exacerbating other effects.

2. *Gastric hypersecretion*. Normally inhibition of gastric secretion is produced by digestive products in the intestine, especially fat. Maldigestion leads to absence of inhibition.

3. *Rapid emptying of stomach*. Lack of digestion leads to loss of the braking effect normally produced by duodenal contents. Acid and pepsin in large quantities reach the duodenum, destroying the enzymes and increasing the maldigestion.

4. *Steatorrhoea and bulky stools* due to maldigestion and lack of absorption of fats.

477

ACUTE PANCREATITIS

There is evidence that mild pancreatitis is not uncommon but, in a significant number of cases, progression to a severe fatal disease occurs. Clinically, there is an acute abdominal emergency with pain and shock.

The essential pathological changes are due to tissue necrosis caused by the action of liberated enzymes on the pancreatic tissues. The severity of the lesion depends on the amount of enzyme set free, the distance it diffuses and the structures affected. The pancreatic damage occurs in two forms:

1. **Periductal necrosis** – in the centre of each affected lobule.

2. **Perilobular necrosis** – affecting the periphery of lobules.

Damage to the epithelial lining of the duct allows diffusion of active enzymes into the adjacent tissues

Small areas of necrosis appear around the ducts of some of the lobules

This type is associated with gall-stones and alcohol.

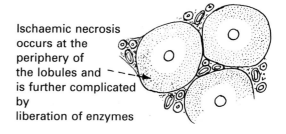

Ischaemic necrosis occurs at the periphery of the lobules and is further complicated by liberation of enzymes

This type is associated with circulatory perfusion failure; severe shock; prolonged operations and hypothermia.

Both types of damage if not inhibited by antitrypsins and α_2 macroglobulins derived from the blood and pancreas itself will progress often very rapidly to the very severe form –

PANLOBULAR PANCREATITIS

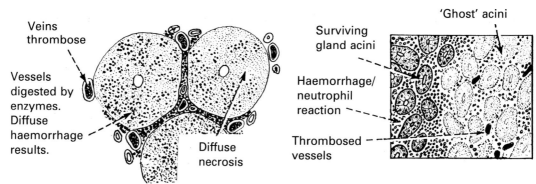

Veins thrombose

Vessels digested by enzymes. Diffuse haemorrhage results.

Diffuse necrosis

'Ghost' acini

Surviving gland acini

Haemorrhage/ neutrophil reaction

Thrombosed vessels

The initial damage is severe, and large quantities of enzymes are liberated, including trypsin, chymotrypsin, lipase, elastase and phospholipase. Locally, these set up a progressive pathological process.

ACUTE PANCREATITIS

SEVERE PANCREATITIS (continued)

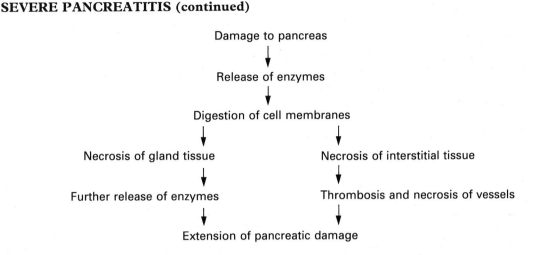

Damage to pancreas

↓

Release of enzymes

↓

Digestion of cell membranes

↓ ↓

Necrosis of gland tissue   Necrosis of interstitial tissue

↓ ↓

Further release of enzymes   Thrombosis and necrosis of vessels

↓ ↓

Extension of pancreatic damage

The released enzymes spread beyond the exocrine tissues of the pancreas:

1. *Via lymphatics to abdominal tissues* especially the omentum and mesenteries

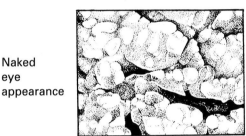

Naked
eye
appearance

Opaque white patches of
necrotic fatty tissue – due to phospholipase
containing   and proteolytic
free   enzymes
fatty acids – lipase splits fat

2. *Locally causing destruction of islet tissue* – hyperglycaemic coma may occur.

3. *Via blood stream.*

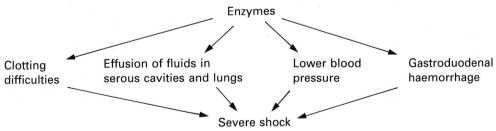

Enzymes

Clotting
difficulties

Effusion of fluids in
serous cavities and lungs

Lower blood
pressure

Gastroduodenal
haemorrhage

Severe shock

These effects are largely due to activation of thromboplastins and formation of vasoactive kinins. Hypoxia due to pulmonary oedema intensifies the shock.

Hypocalcaemia giving rise to tetany may occur due to deposition of calcium soaps in the necrotic fat cells of the omentum and peritoneum.

The appearance of amylase in the blood stream is used as a diagnostic test.

479

ACUTE PANCREATITIS

Aetiology

Two factors are important: (1) gall-stones and (2) alcohol.

Gall-stones

Between 50 and 60% of all cases of severe pancreatitis are associated with gall-stones. Recurrent attacks are common, and in a recent study of known gall-stone patients who developed pancreatitis, gall-stones were found in the biliary tree or stools of 80%.

Two mechanisms are postulated:

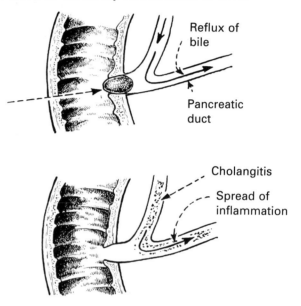

1. ***Bile reflux***
   In most patients, the bile duct and pancreatic duct have a common entrance to the ampulla of Vater. Stones passing down the bile duct could, by blocking the ampulla, cause reflux of bile along the pancreatic duct.

2. ***Bacterial infection***
   In all cases of gall-stone pancreatitis, chronic cholecystitis and cholangitis are present. Infection could spread from the bile ducts to the pancreas.

Bile and bacteria together activate the complement system which can cause cell lysis and initiate the necrotising process.

Alcohol

Acute pancreatitis is common in alcoholics and the incidence of this association is directly related to the consumption of alcohol by the local population, e.g.

Scotland – up to 25%
England – up to 17%
U.S.A. – up to 70%

The causal relationship is obscure, but it is possible that in both gall-stone and alcoholic pancreatitis there is a common pathogenetic mechanism.

ACUTE PANCREATITIS

Inhibitors of pancreatic enzymes are produced by the liver – α_1 antitrypsin and α_2 macroglobulin. Large reserves are found in the normal liver. In the pancreas itself, a trypsin inhibitor is formed.

Fatty change in the liver is present in a high proportion of cases of acute pancreatitis.

Gall-stone cases – 25%

Alcohol cases – 60%

75% of all cases show hyperbilirubinaemia

It is possible that trivial damage may be followed by a necrotising chain reaction in the following way:

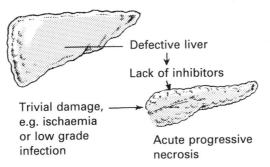

Defective liver

↓

Lack of inhibitors

Trivial damage, e.g. ischaemia or low grade infection

Acute progressive necrosis

Pancreatitis has also been recorded in association with many other conditions, e.g. abdominal surgery, chronic renal failure, renal transplantation, cortisone therapy, cytotoxic therapy, mumps, hyperparathyroidism and familial hyperlipoproteinaemia.

Complications

1. With the frequent presence of cholangitis, the damaged pancreatic tissue is liable to be secondarily infected, and local suppuration is relatively common.

2. During the healing process, fibrosis may cause duct obstruction. Dilatation of the duct and cyst formation follow.

3. Recurrent attacks are common, and this may be one cause of chronic pancreatitis.

Prognosis

Death due to shock occurs in approximately 17% of cases of severe pancreatitis.

CHRONIC PANCREATITIS

The true incidence of this condition is unknown but from post mortem evidence it appears to be quite common. At least two types have been described, but the pathological changes are similar in all cases.

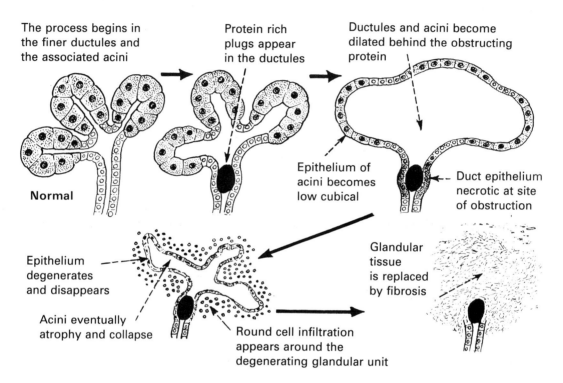

The process begins in the finer ductules and the associated acini

Normal

Protein rich plugs appear in the ductules

Ductules and acini become dilated behind the obstructing protein

Epithelium of acini becomes low cubical

Duct epithelium necrotic at site of obstruction

Epithelium degenerates and disappears

Acini eventually atrophy and collapse

Round cell infiltration appears around the degenerating glandular unit

Glandular tissue is replaced by fibrosis

The change is focal. More and more protein plugs form, some in larger ducts. Obstruction of these may lead to production of cysts.

Ultimately, a large proportion of the exocrine tissue is destroyed.

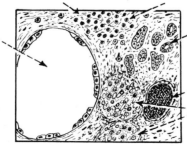

Fibrosis with lymphocytic infiltrate

Cystic dilatation of ducts
Epithelial lining usually atrophic and incomplete

Small ducts, possibly reactive hyperplasia } This may mimic carcinoma in biopsy material

Eosinophilic protein plug in duct

Islet tissue usually survives and may appear to be increased

CHRONIC PANCREATITIS

With progress of the disease, two other developments take place:

1. *Calcification.* This occurs mainly in the protein plugs in the ducts, resulting in the formation of calculi.
2. *Rupture of the duct cysts into the surrounding tissues.* A granulation tissue reaction is set up with formation of a pseudocyst. The result depends on the site of the pseudocyst.

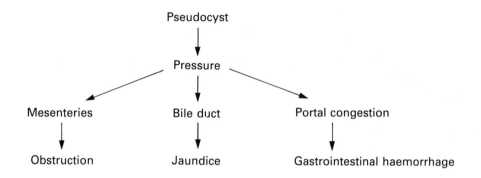

Rupture into the peritoneal cavity causes ascites, frequently haemorrhagic.

Progressive destruction of the parenchyma with fibrosis may ultimately convert the pancreatitis into a thin hard cord.

Effects

Apart from the complications due to cyst rupture, destruction of pancreatic tissue may lead to:

1. Insufficiency of exocrine secretion ⟶ steatorrhoea and wasting.
2. Diabetes mellitus. This is a rare complication due to destruction of islet tissue.

Aetiology

1. The main factor in 75% of cases in Western civilisation is alcohol. Patients have generally consumed more than 150 g daily over a long period of time.
2. In 1% of cases there is biliary disease.
3. Some cases may follow recurrent attacks of acute pancreatitis.
4. A peculiar type of chronic pancreatitis occurs in Africa and South East Asia. It is related to chronic malnutrition with particular deficiency of protein, from infancy. Extensive calcification of the pancreatic tissues occurs. It has been suggested that there is a genetic predisposition to the disease.

CYSTIC FIBROSIS OF THE PANCREAS (Mucoviscidosis)

This is a common autosomal recessive inherited disease due to genetic mutation on chromosome 7; a high percentage (about 4%) of the population are carriers.

The gene involved is called cystic fibrosis transmembrane conductor regulator (CFTR). Its essential function is the control of the transfer of chloride across cell membranes. Many mutations of the gene have been recorded, each being responsible for subtle variations in the evolution of the disorder.

All the exocrine secretory tissues are affected to a greater or lesser degree: the pathological results vary according to which organ is mainly affected – pancreas, bronchi, bowel, biliary tree, testis.

The essential change is as follows:

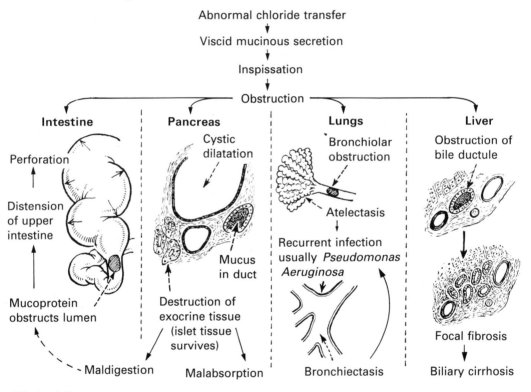

Abnormal chloride transfer
↓
Viscid mucinous secretion
↓
Inspissation
↓
Obstruction

Intestine
Perforation ↑
Distension of upper intestine
Mucoprotein obstructs lumen
Maldigestion

Pancreas
Cystic dilatation
Mucus in duct
Destruction of exocrine tissue (islet tissue survives)
Malabsorption

Lungs
Bronchiolar obstruction
Atelectasis
Recurrent infection usually *Pseudomonas Aeruginosa*
Bronchiectasis

Liver
Obstruction of bile ductule
Focal fibrosis
Biliary cirrhosis

Clinical features

Neonatal
Intestinal obstruction (meconium ileus) may lead to intestinal perforation and fatal peritonitis.

Childhood:
There is failure to thrive due to maldigestion and malabsorption, and steatorrhea is common – all features of pancreatic insufficiency. If the lungs are affected, there is chronic respiratory difficulty with emphysema and bronchiectasis, usually proving fatal at an early age. Liver lesions are of late development.

There is increase of sodium chloride in the sweat of patients and their heterozygote siblings. This provides a diagnostic test which is now being replaced by genetic screening.

TUMOURS OF PANCREAS

Simple tumours of the pancreas are very rare. Occasionally cystadenomas, lipomas and fibromas occur. They may produce symptoms due to pressure on other structures.

CARCINOMA

This is by no means rare, particularly in Western countries and Japan. It is the second commonest gastrointestinal cancer in the U.S.A.

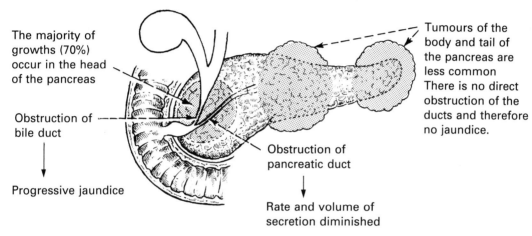

The majority of growths (70%) occur in the head of the pancreas

Obstruction of bile duct

Progressive jaundice

Obstruction of pancreatic duct

Rate and volume of secretion diminished

Tumours of the body and tail of the pancreas are less common There is no direct obstruction of the ducts and therefore no jaundice.

Regional and/or distant metastases are found in 85% of cases at the time of diagnosis and the 5 year survival rate is 1% – the lowest of all cancers.

The growth arises from the duct epithelium and in almost all cases it is an adenocarcinoma. Papillary cystadenocarcinoma, adenosquamous carcinoma and giant cell carcinoma are forms occasionally encountered.

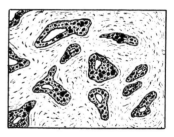

Tumours in the body and tail are commonly larger than tumours of the head, probably due to later diagnosis in the relative absence of symptoms. Thrombosis of unknown cause and at distant sites, e.g. femoral, is apt to occur when the tumour is in the body or tail.

Aetiology

1. Pancreatic carcinoma is most frequent in males in the 5th–7th decades.
2. There is a statistical association with alcohol, cigarette smoking and a diet high in fat and carbohydrate.
3. In the U.S.A., the incidence is higher in the black population and a similar situation is true of the Maoris in New Zealand.

Endocrine Tumours

Islet cell tumours are described on page 824.

485

CHAPTER 12

HAEMOPOIETIC AND LYMPHO-RETICULAR TISSUES

HAEMOPOIESIS

The derivation of blood cells

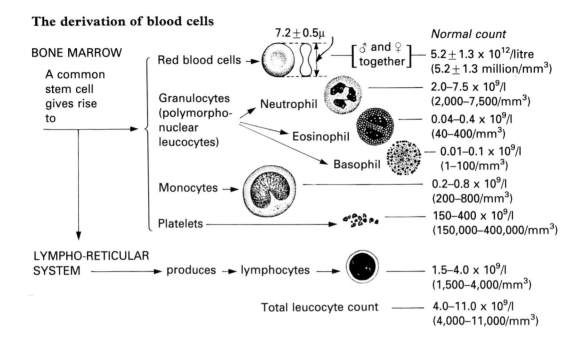

BONE MARROW

A common stem cell gives rise to

Red blood cells →

$7.2 \pm 0.5\mu$

[♂ and ♀ together]

Normal count

$5.2 \pm 1.3 \times 10^{12}$/litre
(5.2 ± 1.3 million/mm³)

Granulocytes (polymorpho-nuclear leucocytes)

Neutrophil

$2.0–7.5 \times 10^9$/l
(2,000–7,500/mm³)

Eosinophil

$0.04–0.4 \times 10^9$/l
(40–400/mm³)

Basophil

$0.01–0.1 \times 10^9$/l
(1–100/mm³)

Monocytes →

$0.2–0.8 \times 10^9$/l
(200–800/mm³)

Platelets

$150–400 \times 10^9$/l
(150,000–400,000/mm³)

LYMPHO-RETICULAR SYSTEM ⟶ produces → lymphocytes →

$1.5–4.0 \times 10^9$/l
(1,500–4,000/mm³)

Total leucocyte count ⟶ $4.0–11.0 \times 10^9$/l
(4,000–11,000/mm³)

Haemopoiesis in bone marrow

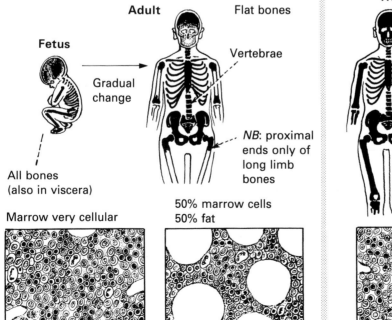

Fetus

Adult   Flat bones

Vertebrae

Gradual change

NB: proximal ends only of long limb bones

All bones (also in viscera)

Marrow very cellular

50% marrow cells
50% fat

When extra blood cells are required MARROW HYPERPLASIA occurs

Extension down long bones

Increased cellularity – obliteration of fat spaces

HAEMOPOIESIS

Mechanisms influencing the production of blood cells

They fall into 2 broad groups: (1) humoral factors and (2) nutrient factors.

Humoral factors with feedback controls

e.g. (a) Erythropoietin stimulates RBC production.

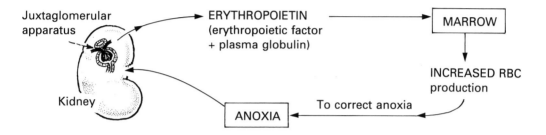

(b) Granulopoiesis is stimulated by crude bacterial and tissue extracts.

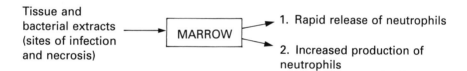

Haemopoiesis is also influenced in a non-specific way by hormones, e.g. thyroid deficiency causes anaemia.

Nutrient factors

These are important and some, e.g. vit. B_{12}, folic acid and iron, have a specific effect.

Most blood diseases are conveniently considered under three headings:

1. Increased numbers of cells, e.g.　erythrocytosis, also known as polycythaemia (RBCs)
　　　　　　　　　　　　　　　　leucocytosis and leukaemia (leucocytes)
　　　　　　　　　　　　　　　　thrombocytosis (platelets)

2. Decreased numbers of cells, e.g. anaemia (RBCs)
　　　　　　　　　　　　　　　　leucopenia (leucocytes)
　　　　　　　　　　　　　　　　thrombocytopenia (platelets)
　　　　　　　　　　　　　　　　pancytopenia (all 3 elements)

3. Dysfunction – may occur alone or as a complication of (1) or (2) above.

DISEASES OF THE RED BLOOD CELLS

Diseases of the red cells are reflected in changes in the composition of the blood. The following measurements are useful and provide values of reasonable accuracy:

1. **HAEMOGLOBIN (Hb) concentration**
Expressed as g/dl whole blood.

(Normal values: male – 15.5 ± 2.5; female – 14.0 ± 2.5.)

2. **PACKED CELL VOLUME (PCV)**
PCV is obtained by centrifugating anticoagulated whole blood in a haematocrit tube.

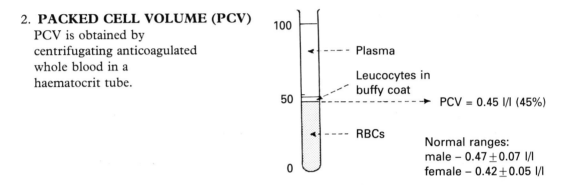

PCV = 0.45 l/l (45%)

Normal ranges:
male – 0.47 ± 0.07 l/l
female – 0.42 ± 0.05 l/l

3. **RED CELL COUNT**
Particle counting machines give reliable measurement.
(Normal values: male – $5.5 \pm 1.0 \times 10^{12}/l$; female – $4.8 \pm 1.0 \times 10^{12}/l$.)
From these basic results the ABSOLUTE VALUES may be calculated.

A. *MEAN CELL HAEMOGLOBIN CONCENTRATION (MCHC)*

Calculation: $\dfrac{Hb}{PCV}$ e.g. $\dfrac{15}{0.45}$ = 33g/dl (Range 30–36)

A low MCHC is due to a low average Hb content in the red cell mass and indicates deficient Hb synthesis.

e.g. Blood film 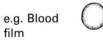 Pale red cells (hypochromic) associated with low MCHC

High MCHCs do not occur in red cell disorders because the haemoglobin concentration is already near saturation point in normal red cells.

Note that because the MCHC is obtained by easy calculation from two simple and accurate measurements – the PACKED CELL VOLUME and the HAEMOGLOBIN – it is extremely useful and widely employed where sophisticated instrumentation is not available.

DISEASES OF THE RED BLOOD CELLS

B. *MEAN CELL HAEMOGLOBIN (MCH)*

This is the average haemoglobin content of each red cell and is measured in pg (picograms).

Calculation: $\dfrac{\text{Blood haemoglobin (g/dl)}}{\text{Red cell count }(10^{12}/l)}$ Normal range = 29.5±2.5 pg

C. *MEAN CELL VOLUME (MCV)*
Measured in fl (femtolitres).

Calculation: $\dfrac{\text{Volume of red cells}}{\text{Number of red cells}}$ Normal range = 85±8 fl

Note: The accuracy of B and C depends on the availability of modern instruments. Where manual methods only are available the MCHC is important.

In addition to changes in the absolute values, valuable information is obtained by examination of blood films stained by a Romanowski method.

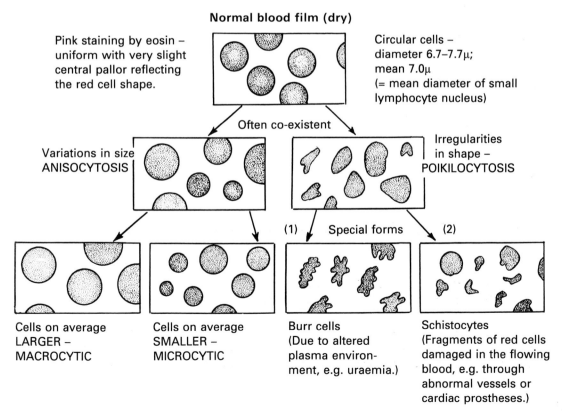

Normal blood film (dry)

Pink staining by eosin – uniform with very slight central pallor reflecting the red cell shape.

Circular cells – diameter 6.7–7.7µ; mean 7.0µ (= mean diameter of small lymphocyte nucleus)

Often co-existent

Variations in size ANISOCYTOSIS

Irregularities in shape – POIKILOCYTOSIS

(1)   Special forms   (2)

Cells on average LARGER – MACROCYTIC

Cells on average SMALLER – MICROCYTIC

Burr cells (Due to altered plasma environment, e.g. uraemia.)

Schistocytes (Fragments of red cells damaged in the flowing blood, e.g. through abnormal vessels or cardiac prostheses.)

DISEASES OF THE RED BLOOD CELLS

Variations in colour (staining)

The haemoglobin content is reflected in the red cell staining.

Normal   *Hypochromic*

Ring staining of cells
indicates poor haemoglobinisation.

Other pathological variations are:

Spherocytes

Small dense red cells
reflect the cell shape.
Loss of biconcavity.

These changes are due to cell membrane
abnormalities which may be
congenital or acquired. The cells
show increased fragility in hypotonic
saline.

Target cells

Centre area of density
with surrounding pallor.
Thin cell with central
bulge.

Sickle cells

Severe distortion of red
cells due to abnormal
aggregation of haemoglobin
molecules in
reduced state.

These changes are associated with
haemoglobinopathies (abnormalities).
Target cells are also seen in liver
disease and after splenectomy.

Red cell inclusions

Any particulate fragments which may form within red cells during the processes of nuclear
maturation and extrusion, and the formation of cytoplasmic haemoglobin are normally
removed by the spleen. Inclusions may be found within the red cells in two main
circumstances:

1. Where red cell maturation and metabolism are disordered

2. When removal by the spleen is defective, e.g. in splenic atrophy and after splenectomy.

DISEASES OF THE RED BLOOD CELLS

Red cell inclusions (continued)

	Appearance	Staining method	Occurrence
Howell-Jolly bodies Fragments of nuclear chromatin 1–2μ		Romanowski (eosin-methylene blue)	In anaemias – esp. macrocytic types
Pappenheimer bodies Small fragments containing iron		Prussian blue stain for iron	Especially after splenectomy
Heinz bodies Refractile crystalline bodies – denatured globin		Supravital staining, e.g. brilliant cresyl blue	Esp. associated with chemical poisons
Punctate basophilia Small particles of RNA		Romanowski (eosin-methylene blue)	In various anaemias, esp. lead poisoning

Nucleated red cells (erythroblasts) in the peripheral blood

Normally nucleated red cells are not seen in the peripheral blood. They appear in many blood and marrow disorders.

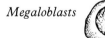

Normoblasts (see p.495) are seen in several types of anaemia but especially when the marrow is actively responding to any demand for new red cells, e.g. after severe acute haemorrhage or haemolysis: also in marrow 'replacement' as part of a leucoerythroblastic anaemia (see p.532).

In seriously ill patients, the appearance of normoblasts in the peripheral blood is a grave prognostic sign preceding death by hours.

Megaloblasts (see p.495) are seen especially in pernicious anaemia and folic acid deficiency.

The nucleated red cells are found with the leucocytes in the haematocrit.

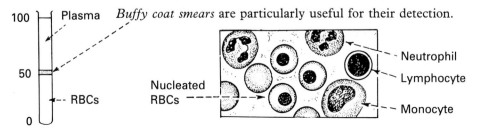

Buffy coat smears are particularly useful for their detection.

DISEASES OF THE RED BLOOD CELLS

The **physical properties** of red cells change in some disorders. The osmotic fragility is altered when the cell shape is abnormal.

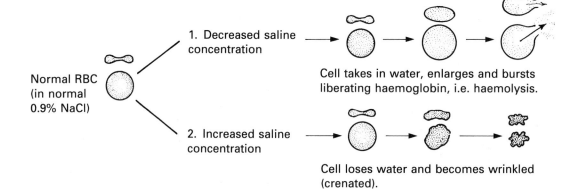

Normal RBC (in normal 0.9% NaCl)

1. Decreased saline concentration

Cell takes in water, enlarges and bursts liberating haemoglobin, i.e. haemolysis.

2. Increased saline concentration

Cell loses water and becomes wrinkled (crenated).

The initial shape of the red cell clearly will influence the amount of water it will take in before it bursts.

In the osmotic fragility test, the lysis of RBCs in varying concentrations of saline is assessed by measuring the haemoglobin liberated. The graph shows typical results.

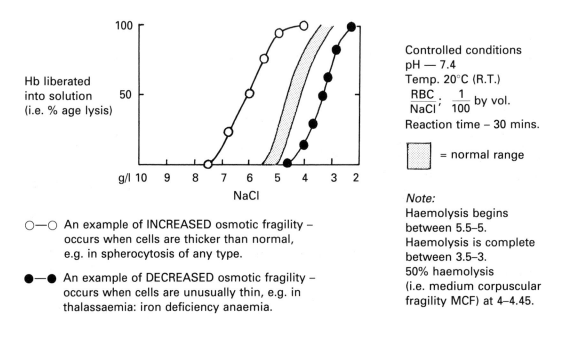

Hb liberated into solution (i.e. % age lysis)

g/l 10 9 8 7 6 5 4 3 2

NaCl

Controlled conditions
pH — 7.4
Temp. 20°C (R.T.)
$\dfrac{RBC}{NaCl}$; $\dfrac{1}{100}$ by vol.
Reaction time – 30 mins.

☐ = normal range

Note:
Haemolysis begins between 5.5–5.
Haemolysis is complete between 3.5–3.
50% haemolysis (i.e. medium corpuscular fragility MCF) at 4–4.45.

○—○ An example of INCREASED osmotic fragility – occurs when cells are thicker than normal, e.g. in spherocytosis of any type.

●—● An example of DECREASED osmotic fragility – occurs when cells are unusually thin, e.g. in thalassaemia: iron deficiency anaemia.

The fragility to mechanical and chemical damage (including changes in pH) also varies in red cell disorders.

DISEASES OF THE RED BLOOD CELLS

BONE MARROW

Erythropoiesis (production of red cells) takes place in the marrow of the flat bones and vertebrae. The process involves mitotic division along with differentiation and maturation from the primitive stem cell.

Normal marrow erythropoiesis is said to be NORMOBLASTIC.

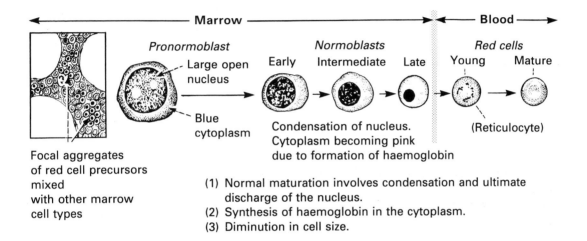

Focal aggregates
of red cell precursors
mixed
with other marrow
cell types

(1) Normal maturation involves condensation and ultimate discharge of the nucleus.
(2) Synthesis of haemoglobin in the cytoplasm.
(3) Diminution in cell size.

When the essential factors vit. B_{12} or folic acid are deficient, the red cell precursors show clear morphological changes – erythropoiesis is said to be MEGALOBLASTIC.

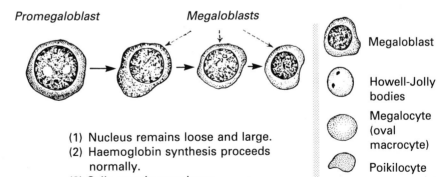

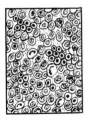

Greatly
increased
marrow
cellularity

(1) Nucleus remains loose and large.
(2) Haemoglobin synthesis proceeds normally.
(3) Cells remain very large, i.e. the nuclear/cytoplasmic maturations are out of phase.

Megaloblast

Howell-Jolly bodies

Megalocyte (oval macrocyte)

Poikilocyte

Abnormal cells in peripheral blood

DISEASES OF THE RED BLOOD CELLS

Reticulocytes

These are the red cells very recently (within 2 days) released from the marrow and may be recognised by the following characteristics:

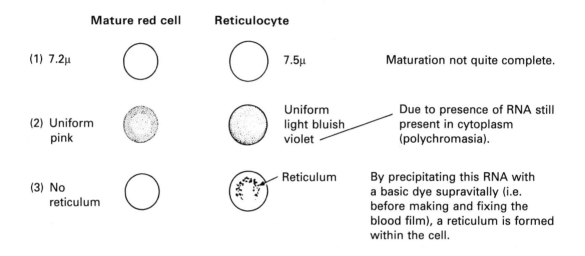

The reticulocyte count (normal range 0.2–2.0%, i.e. 25–$85 \times 10^9/l$) gives an indication of erythropoiesis in the marrow. High counts are seen:

    (a) in haemolytic disorders
    (b) after severe haemorrhage
    (c) when specific therapy is given in megaloblastic anaemias, e.g. vit. B_{12} in pernicious anaemia.

Note: When the reticulocyte count is expressed as a percentage of the RBC count, the results may be misinterpreted when that count is low.

ANAEMIA

The most important function of the red cell is the transport of haemoglobin. The most common and important disorder associated with disease of the red cells is ANAEMIA, which is defined as a reduction below normal of the concentration of haemoglobin in the blood.

Normal Hb concentration: 15.0g/dl (Range: men – 15.5 $\pm$ 2.5; women – 14.0 $\pm$ 2.5).

Effects of anaemia

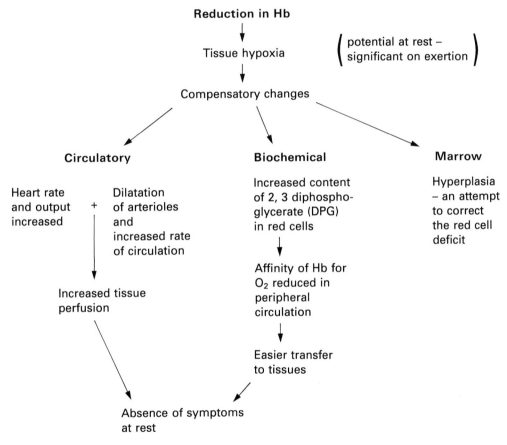

Clinical associations

1. Diminished exercise tolerance, *i.e.* dyspnoea on exertion.
2. Rapid, full, bounding pulse: decreased circulation time.

Note: Pallor is not a reliable sign of anaemia – it may be obscured by the circulatory changes.

ANAEMIA

The effects of anaemia are greatly influenced by its severity, duration and rate of development.

In moderate anaemias of slow evolution, symptoms such as dyspnoea only appear on exertion, and even when the haemoglobin falls as low as 6–7 g/dl, clinical indications may be slight.

Pathological complications of anaemia

1. Effects of degenerative arterial disease are aggravated, e.g. symptoms of ANGINA PECTORIS and lower limb CLAUDICATION are increased.

2. In severe anaemias effects are seen in organs.

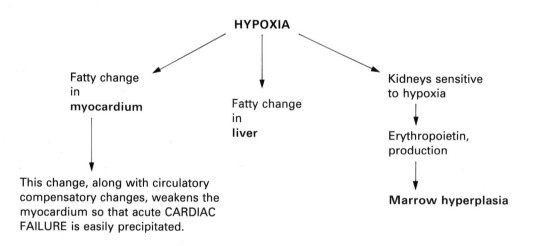

Note: Therefore blood transfusion used in the treatment of anaemia is given ***slowly*** and as ***packed cells***.

In very rapidly developing anaemias, the compensatory mechanisms cannot adjust adequately – the condition merges into SHOCK (see p.193)

ANAEMIA

Aetiology

Although in the last analysis any anaemia is due to the failure of the bone marrow to produce sufficient red cells in any particular circumstance, an understanding of the role of various aetiological agents and of the four main mechanisms by which anaemia develops depends on a knowledge of the basic facts of the life cycle of the red blood cells.

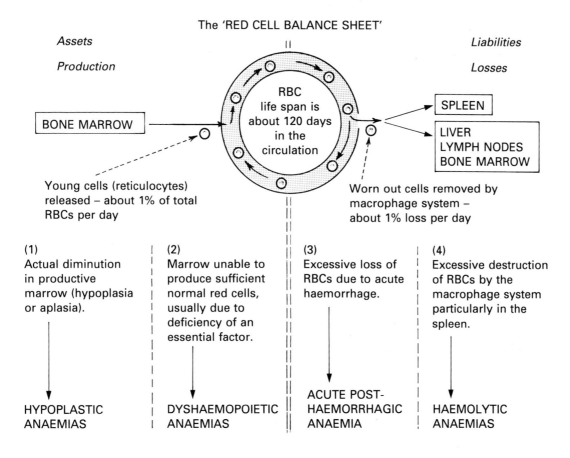

The 'RED CELL BALANCE SHEET'

Assets — *Production* — BONE MARROW → RBC life span is about 120 days in the circulation → SPLEEN / LIVER LYMPH NODES BONE MARROW — *Liabilities* — *Losses*

Young cells (reticulocytes) released – about 1% of total RBCs per day

Worn out cells removed by macrophage system – about 1% loss per day

(1) Actual diminution in productive marrow (hypoplasia or aplasia).

(2) Marrow unable to produce sufficient normal red cells, usually due to deficiency of an essential factor.

(3) Excessive loss of RBCs due to acute haemorrhage.

(4) Excessive destruction of RBCs by the macrophage system particularly in the spleen.

HYPOPLASTIC ANAEMIAS

DYSHAEMOPOIETIC ANAEMIAS

ACUTE POST-HAEMORRHAGIC ANAEMIA

HAEMOLYTIC ANAEMIAS

Note: These are not rigidly exclusive compartments.

e.g. 1. The abnormal cells produced in the hypoplastic and dyshaemopoietic anaemias usually have a shortened life span so that a haemolytic element is superimposed.

2. The anaemia of chronic blood loss is almost wholly dyshaemopoietic in type due to the external loss of iron.

ANAEMIA

HYPOPLASTIC and APLASTIC ANAEMIAS

These are rare conditions and, as the names imply, are due to marrow failure with diminished numbers or absence of haemopoietic cells. Usually all three marrow cell lines are affected, resulting in *pancytopenia* in the peripheral blood.

Marrow failure is dealt with in detail on page 545.

Anaemias associated with miscellaneous chronic diseases ('Secondary' anaemias) are dealt with on pages 543, 544.

DYSHAEMOPOIETIC ANAEMIAS

The usual cause of these anaemias is deficiency of an essential factor required for proper haemoglobin synthesis or erythroblast maturation and development. They are associated with a hypercellular marrow and are divided into two main groups:

(1) normoblastic and (2) megaloblastic, depending on the type of erythroblastic maturation in the marrow.

Deficiency of essential factor

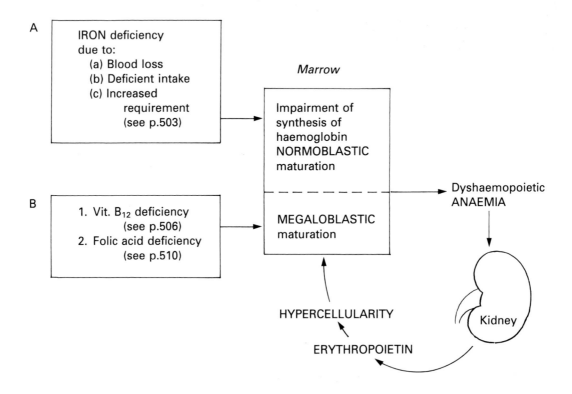

IRON DEFICIENCY ANAEMIA

Without IRON the haem moiety of the haemoglobin molecule cannot be synthesised.

IRON DEFICIENCY
↓
DEFECTIVE SYNTHESIS OF HAEMOGLOBIN
↓
(see p.505)
ANAEMIA

Haem ------>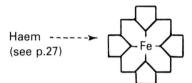
(see p.27)

Changes in the blood are mainly in the red cells which become:
MICROCYTIC (cells smaller – mean diameter $< 6.7\mu$)
HYPOCHROMIC (contain less haemoglobin ∴ less well stained).

Normal

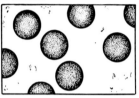

Fairly uniform red cells
– size and shape
(mean diameter 7.2μ)

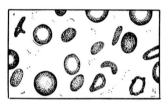

Definite central pallor – ring staining
Variation in size – anisocytosis
Variation in shape – poikilocytosis

MCV (fl) (mean cell volume) is .... LOW (<80)

MCH (pg) (mean cell haemoglobin) is.. LOW (<25)

MCHC (mean corpuscular haemoglobin concentration) is.. LOW: 30%
   derived from Hb and haematocrit PCV: $\frac{Hb}{PCV} \times 100$.   Normal mean = 34%

Serum IRON (normal 13–32 μmol/l) is... LOW(<10)
       (0.7–1.8 mg/l)

Serum FERRITIN (normal 20–100ug/l) is .... LOW (<14)

Serum IRON BINDING CAPACITY (45–70 μmol/l) is .... RAISED (>70)
      (2.5–4.0 mg/l)

Serum IRON SATURATION $\left(\frac{IRON}{Binding\ capacity} \times 100\right)$ (Normal 35%) is................... LOW ($<15\%$)

The reticulocyte count is NORMAL except following episodes of haemorrhage.

Usually there are no changes in the leucocytes and platelets.

The bone marrow is hypercellular and contains many small poorly haemoglobinised
normoblasts; no stainable iron is present.

501

IRON DEFICIENCY ANAEMIA

IRON METABOLISM

Iron is normally conserved and is recycled so that absorption of iron from the diet, which occurs maximally in the duodenum and upper jejunum, is required to replace only the small inevitable losses. Since the diet contains iron in excess of requirements, the intestinal mucosal apoferritin mechanism exists to control absorption.

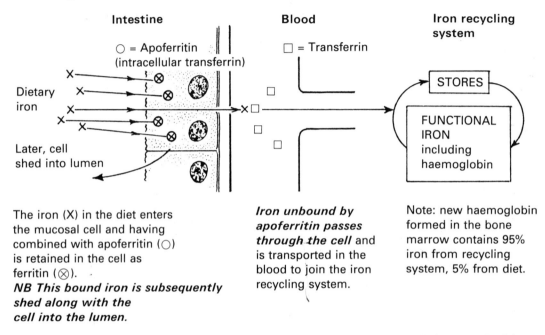

The iron (X) in the diet enters the mucosal cell and having combined with apoferritin (○) is retained in the cell as ferritin (⊗).
NB This bound iron is subsequently shed along with the cell into the lumen.

Iron unbound by apoferritin passes through the cell and is transported in the blood to join the iron recycling system.

Note: new haemoglobin formed in the bone marrow contains 95% iron from recycling system, 5% from diet.

The state of the iron stores controls the apoferritin (a form of intracellular transferrin) content of the intestinal mucosal cell by a feed-back mechanism, thus:

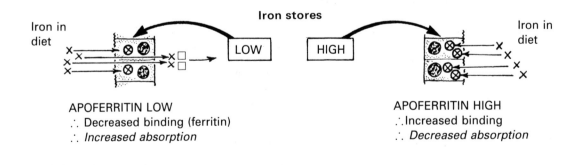

APOFERRITIN LOW
∴ Decreased binding (ferritin)
∴ *Increased absorption*

APOFERRITIN HIGH
∴Increased binding
∴ *Decreased absorption*

ACUTE IRON OVERLOAD

If a large dose of medicinal iron preparations is taken (particularly by children in error) the absorption and transport mechanisms are overwhelmed and free iron radicles exert very toxic effects.

IRON DEFICIENCY ANAEMIA

The *iron balance* may be summarised as follows.

INPUT (Adult male)	BODY IRON Total 3–6g	OUTPUT
Average: 1 mg/day derived from foods (a) animal muscle (b) vegetables. The average diet contains 10–20 mg iron, of which about 10% is absorbed. In the adult female, the average daily input is about 2 mg.	(a) *Functional iron* in haemoglobin, myoglobin, enzyme systems, transferrin } 80% at least (b) *Storage iron* in liver, spleen, bone marrow as ferritin, haemosiderin } 20% or less	Average: 1 mg/day Skin desquamation and miscellaneous secretions *Menstruation* This extra loss of about 0.5 to 1 mg requires extra input in the female

Anaemia results when this delicate balance is upset in one of three main ways.

1. *Increased output* This almost always is caused by blood loss – often small in amount and chronic (1 ml blood = 0.5 mg iron). In the female, uterine bleeding is a common cause, and in both sexes bleeding from the alimentary tract is important.
2. *Decreased input*
   (a) Poor diet (including diets containing substances antagonistic to iron absorption, e.g. phytates, phosphates)
   (b) Malabsorption – due to bowel disease or post-surgical.
3. *Increased body requirement*
   (a) During rapid growth in childhood
   (b) In pregnancy.

Usually anaemia develops slowly (except in cases of serious haemorrhage).

(1) ———————→ (2) ———————————→ (3) ———————————→ (4)

| (1)
Iron deficiency | (2)
Mobilisation of reserves (first haemosiderin then ferritin) | (3)
Exhaustion of reserves

Increased absorption if available in diet may postpone (4) | (4)
Deficient synthesis of haemoglobin
↓
(5) Anaemia |

PREVALENCE of IRON DEFICIENCY ANAEMIA

This is the commonest anaemia on a world basis due to: (a) poor nutrition, (b) intestinal parasites (esp. hookworm) causing bleeding and (c) multiple pregnancies.

In Western countries in the adult male and postmenopausal woman, iron deficiency anaemia is nearly always due to alimentary blood loss and reflects the incidence of the causative diseases, e.g. cancer, peptic ulceration, hiatus hernia, aspirin ingestion, haemorrhoids, etc.

IRON DEFICIENCY ANAEMIA

Associated changes

In addition to the pathological changes due to anaemia per se, the following conditions may be associated with iron deficiency anaemia.

(1) *Angular cheilosis*
    Atrophic glossitis

(2) *Dysphagia* – the Brown-Kelly-Paterson or Plummer-Vinson syndrome

Fissures
at
angles
of
mouth

Smooth
tongue

Incoordinate
movements in pharynx

Sometimes actual
web forms

Occasionally carcinoma
is a late complication

(3)

Thin
mucosa

Hypochlorhydria

↓

Achlorhydria

With gastritis and mucosal atrophy

This aggravates any malabsorption of iron

(4) *Koilonychia*

Brittle
spoon-shaped
nails

(5). *Minimal changes in Peripheral nerves – causing Paraesthesia* (tingling in hands and feet)

These associated changes are in part due to iron deficiency itself, but in many cases are probably the result of deficiencies of other factors in addition, e.g. vitamins and minerals.

THE MEGALOBLASTIC ANAEMIAS

These dyshaemopoietic anaemias are almost always caused by deficiency of either vitamin B_{12} or folic acid which are intracellular co-enzymes, particularly important for the production of nuclear DNA.

The effects of deficiency occur in most organs of the body but are prominent where cell turnover is rapid, e.g. in the marrow.

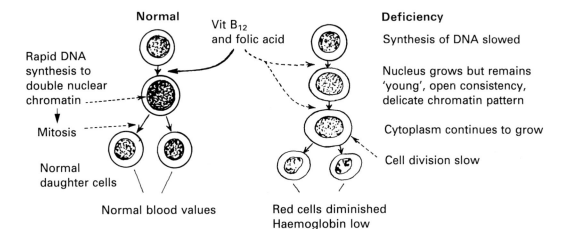

Normal

Vit B_{12} and folic acid

Deficiency

Rapid DNA synthesis to double nuclear chromatin ------

Mitosis ------

Normal daughter cells

Normal blood values

Synthesis of DNA slowed

Nucleus grows but remains 'young', open consistency, delicate chromatin pattern

Cytoplasm continues to grow

Cell division slow

Red cells diminished
Haemoglobin low

Results in organs particularly affected

1. MUCOUS MEMBRANES of alimentary tract and genitalia ⟶ Regenerative activity cannot balance surface cell losses ⟶ THINNING (atrophy) often with functional deficiencies

2. BONE MARROW blood cell precursors of all series affected ⟶ No surface loss: cells not mature enough for release; although many are destroyed locally in the marrow the numbers of abnormal cells increase. ⟶ Hypercellular: megaloblastic

Note:
(a) Vit B_{12} (but not folic acid) has a separate function in the maintenance of the integrity of myelin. Therefore deficiency leads to neuropathies – particularly **subacute combined degeneration** (p. 509).
(b) The marrow and blood appearances are essentially similar in deficiency of vit B_{12} and folic acid from any cause. The classical disease of this type is **pernicious anaemia**.

PERNICIOUS ANAEMIA

This serious and severe anaemia was first described by the English physician Addison in the mid 19th century. At that time it was invariably fatal, but nowadays it can be treated with complete success. It is due to vitamin B_{12} deficiency and is always associated with achlorhydria and gastric mucosal atrophy.

Vitamin B_{12} metabolism and causes of deficiency:

Deficiency of vitamin B_{12}

Normal | **In PA** | **Other causes**

Source:
Food – vit B_{12} in animal products, e.g. meat, eggs.
Daily requirement = 1 μg

— Normal

Dietary deficiency, e.g. strict vegans – takes many years to develop.

Secretion of intrinsic factor (IF) by gastric mucosa – – – –

IF: B_{12} complex formed

IF: B_{12}

Gastric atrophy
No IF
∴ No IF: B_{12} complex

Surgical operations on stomach.

Passage through intestine to terminal ileum

— Normal

Loss during passage in intestine, e.g. utilised by tape worms or bacteria (blind loop syndrome).

Absorption site – can only be absorbed if complexed with IF

No absorption

Disease of ileum, e.g. Crohn's disease.

Storage in liver – up to 10 years' supply

Gradual depletion of liver stores over several years

Released into blood stream to act as important co-enzyme in several intracellular synthetic pathways but particularly of DNA

Especially important to:
(1) Bone marrow
(2) Nervous system

(3) Epithelial coverings

ANAEMIA (MEGALOBLASTIC)
± NERVE CHANGES

± TONGUE } ATROPHY
& VAGINA }

PERNICIOUS ANAEMIA

Blood changes

There is a pancytopenia, i.e. reduction in RBCs, granulocytes and platelets.

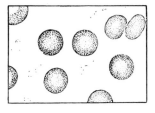

Normal

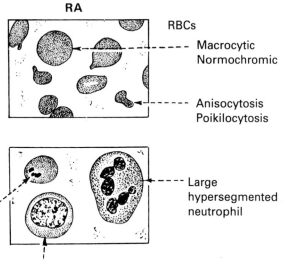

RA

RBCs

- - - Macrocytic
Normochromic

- - - Anisocytosis
Poikilocytosis

Special features

Seen specially in
buffy coat preparations.

Howell-Jolly bodies
(fragments of residual
nuclear material)

- - - Large
hypersegmented
neutrophil

Megaloblast

Absolute values

Red cell count ——————— LOW (may be very low), e.g. 1.0×10^{12}/litre
Hb ——————————— LOW
PCV ————————— LOW
MCV ——————————— HIGH, e.g. (average cell is larger than normal)
MCH ——————————— HIGH   (average cell contains more Hb than normal)
MCHC ——————————— NORMAL (NB average cell contains normal Hb
concentration)

Biochemical

Serum vit B_{12} ———— LOW < 120 (normal > 160 ng/l)
Serum bilirubin ———— Slight increase – due to increased haemolysis of fragile cells.

PERNICIOUS ANAEMIA

Marrow changes

Hyperplasia – often complete cellularity in flat bones and extension down length of femur.

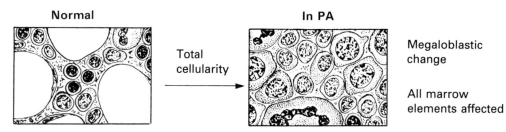

Normal   Total cellularity   In PA

Megaloblastic change

All marrow elements affected

The gastric lesion – The extreme form of diffuse atrophic gastritis (see p.373).

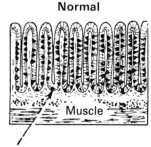

Normal

Muscle

Parietal cells producing both IF and HCl

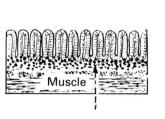

In PA

Muscle

Increased numbers of lymphocytes in lamina propria

Note:
Thin mucosa
No specialised cells
No IF and no HCl
(histamine-fast
achlorhydria)

Mechanism of production of gastritis

PA is an autoimmune disease. The gastric atrophy is caused by an immune reaction against parietal cell cytoplasmic constituents and specifically by antibodies to intrinsic factor (IF).

(1) *Anti-parietal cell immune reaction* gradually causes complete mucosal atrophy including destruction of parietal cells.

(2) *Anti IF antibody* secreted in stomach lumen as well as blood. Specifically blocks any residual IF activity.
(a) Receptor sites for B_{12} complex are blocked.
(b) Receptor sites for ileal absorption are blocked.

IF

There is an increased familial incidence of PA and other autoimmune disease, e.g. Hashimoto's thyroiditis.

PERNICIOUS ANAEMIA

Associated changes

1. *Nervous system*

(a) Subacute degeneration of spinal cord

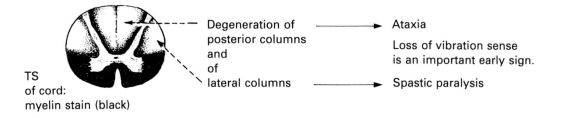

TS
of cord:
myelin stain (black)

Degeneration of posterior columns and of lateral columns ⟶ Ataxia

Loss of vibration sense is an important early sign.

⟶ Spastic paralysis

NB This serious degeneration may occur before clinical anaemia is present, and is aggravated by the administration of folic acid.

(b) Peripheral neuropathy – both sensory and motor loss.

2. *Epithelial surfaces*

Atrophy is common especially in the tongue and vagina – where senile atrophy is aggravated

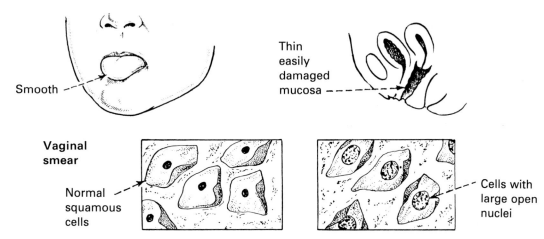

Smooth

Thin easily damaged mucosa

Vaginal smear

Normal squamous cells

Cells with large open nuclei

3. *Effects of long continued haemolysis*

The abnormal cells have a shortened life cycle.

(a) Mild/moderate splenic enlargement.

(b) Iron deposition in liver, kidney, spleen and marrow.

(c) Increased bilirubin in blood (mild jaundice).

509

FOLIC ACID DEFICIENCY

FOLIC ACID (Pteroyl-glutamic acid) DEFICIENCY

Normal metabolism	Deficiency

Normal metabolism

Source
Polyglutamines in
green vegetables, cereals,
meat, fish and eggs
(not milk)

Minimum daily requirement
50 μg

Body reserves   50–100 days

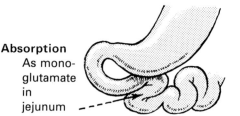

Absorption
As mono-
glutamate
in
jejunum

Utilisation
for DNA synthesis with
vitamin B_{12}
as 5-tetrahydrofolate (5THF)

Deficiency

Dietary
Anorexia, alcoholism, poverty (elderly),
infants (late weaning)

Increased requirements
Pregnancy (fetal growth)
Infancy and childhood (rapid growth)
Haemolysis
Malignancy

Malabsorption
Coeliac disease: sprue
Surgical by-pass
Associated with dermatitis herpetiformis
Drugs (e.g. anti-convulsants)

Utilisation block
Drugs e.g. specific antagonists
e.g. in cancer chemotherapy,
also anti-convulsants.

Note:
(1) Since the marrow and blood changes in folic acid and vitamin B_{12} deficiency are
   similar, the differential diagnosis has to be obtained by other laboratory tests –
   particularly the measurement of vit B_{12} in the serum and of folic acid in the serum and
   RBCs. Special tests of absorption of vit B_{12} (e.g. Schilling test) are available.
(2) Since the causes of vit B_{12} and folic acid deficiency are often non-specific and
   associated with malabsorption, other deficiencies (e.g. iron) may also occur at the same
   time (see p.533)
(3) All megaloblastic anaemias are macrocytic, but *not all* macrocytic anaemias are
   megaloblastic.
(4) There is an association with folic acid deficiency in PREGNANCY with congenital neural
   tube defects.

ACUTE POST-HAEMORRHAGIC ANAEMIA

ACUTE POSTHAEMORRHAGIC ANAEMIA

The effects of severe acute haemorrhage are considered under two main headings:

1. The adaptive haemodynamic changes which are usually at least partly successful in maintaining perfusion of vital organs – see section on SHOCK (p.195).
2. The changes reflecting the body's reactions to restore the blood constituents.

The rate and volume of the blood loss are important influences on both types of effect. For example – in a young healthy adult male (assume blood volume = 5000 ml):

Blood loss ml	%vol.	Duration of loss	Effects	
500 e.g. Blood donation	10%	15 min	Nil or negligible	
1700	33%	3 hrs	Shock ↓ usually survival	**Aggravating factors** (a) pre-existing cardiac or debilitating disease
2500	50%	3 hrs	Severe shock ↓ usually death	(b) old age (c) anxiety associated with vasovagal stimulation – especially if haemorrhage is external and visible
2500	50%	36 hrs	Shock ↓ usually survival	

While the bleeding is continuing, the shock syndrome is predominant, and although the marrow begins to react to the anoxia, the full haematological effects – particularly the ANAEMIA – are not seen until the haemorrhage is controlled or stops and the plasma volume begins to be restored.

ACUTE POST-HAEMORRHAGIC ANAEMIA

In the following example the effects of a severe haemorrhage – 2500 ml (50%) in 36 hours – in a healthy young adult male are seen. It is assumed that blood transfusion has not been given – a rare circumstance nowadays.

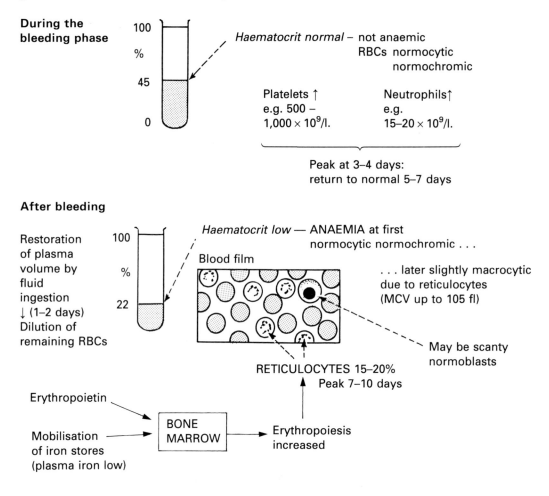

During the bleeding phase

100
%
45
0

Haematocrit normal – not anaemic
RBCs normocytic
normochromic

Platelets ↑
e.g. 500 –
1,000 × 10⁹/l.

Neutrophils↑
e.g.
15–20 × 10⁹/l.

Peak at 3–4 days:
return to normal 5–7 days

After bleeding

Restoration of plasma volume by fluid ingestion ↓ (1–2 days) Dilution of remaining RBCs

100
%
22

Haematocrit low — ANAEMIA at first
normocytic normochromic . . .

Blood film

. . . later slightly macrocytic
due to reticulocytes
(MCV up to 105 fl)

May be scanty
normoblasts

RETICULOCYTES 15–20%
Peak 7–10 days

Erythropoietin

Mobilisation of iron stores (plasma iron low)

BONE MARROW

Erythropoiesis increased

The plasma proteins and other biochemical constituents are restored rapidly – 2–3 days. The full red cell restoration may take up to 6 weeks.

Note: With recurrent less severe haemorrhages the picture merges into that of **iron deficiency anaemia**.

THE HAEMOLYTIC ANAEMIAS

HAEMOLYTIC ANAEMIAS

In all haemolytic anaemias, the basic pathological change is a reduction in the life span of the red cells; another way of expressing this is that there is an increased rate of red cell destruction – haemolysis.

The balance between the increased haemolysis and the consequent increased production of red cells by the bone marrow may be illustrated in three main situations:

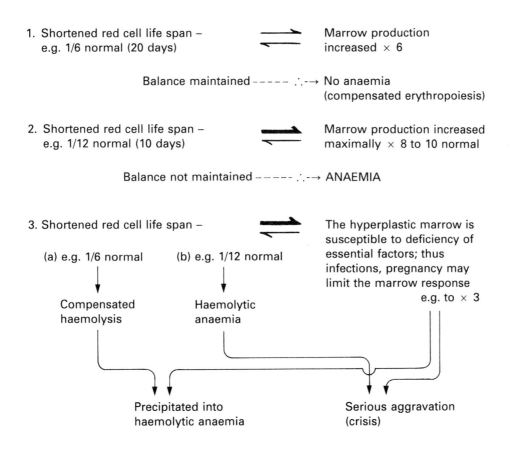

1. Shortened red cell life span – e.g. 1/6 normal (20 days)   ⟶⟵   Marrow production increased × 6

Balance maintained – – – – ∴–→ No anaemia (compensated erythropoiesis)

2. Shortened red cell life span – e.g. 1/12 normal (10 days)   ⟶⟵   Marrow production increased maximally × 8 to 10 normal

Balance not maintained – – – – ∴–→ ANAEMIA

3. Shortened red cell life span –   ⟶⟵   The hyperplastic marrow is susceptible to deficiency of essential factors; thus infections, pregnancy may limit the marrow response e.g. to × 3

(a) e.g. 1/6 normal → Compensated haemolysis

(b) e.g. 1/12 normal → Haemolytic anaemia

Precipitated into haemolytic anaemia

Serious aggravation (crisis)

THE HAEMOLYTIC ANAEMIAS

The pathological changes associated with haemolytic anaemia are conveniently considered under two main headings:

1. Associated with the shortened   2. The bone marrow reaction.
    RBC life span (increased haemolysis).

1. **RBC LIFE SPAN**

   (1a) **Measurement of red cell life span by radioactive sodium chromate**

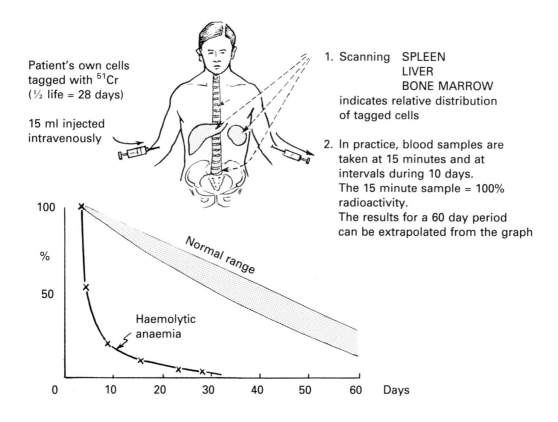

Patient's own cells tagged with ^{51}Cr (½ life = 28 days)

15 ml injected intravenously

1. Scanning   SPLEEN
                  LIVER
                  BONE MARROW
indicates relative distribution of tagged cells

2. In practice, blood samples are taken at 15 minutes and at intervals during 10 days. The 15 minute sample = 100% radioactivity. The results for a 60 day period can be extrapolated from the graph

Normal range

Haemolytic anaemia

Note:
   In *normal* curve, gradual loss of radioactivity 50% level at 30 days.
   In *haemolytic* anaemia, rapid loss of radioactivity 50% at 3 days.

THE HAEMOLYTIC ANAEMIAS

(1b) Effects of the increased degradation of haemoglobin

In most haemolytic conditions, the red cells are removed and the haemoglobin degraded in the usual way, i.e. by phagocytosis by the macrophage system.

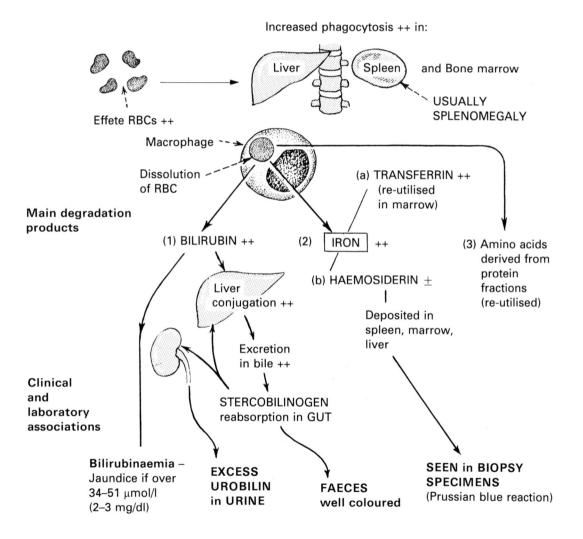

Note: 1. The bilirubin is unconjugated and is attached to protein so that renal excretion does not occur – **acholuric jaundice**.

2. Unconjugated bilirubin is toxic to the central nervous system of neonates; **kernicterus** (see p.523) is a serious complication of haemolytic disease of the newborn.

515

THE HAEMOLYTIC ANAEMIAS

(1c) Effects of liberation of haemoglobin

In all haemolytic processes, small amounts of haemoglobin are liberated into the blood stream. The free haemoglobin rapidly forms a complex with **haptoglobin** – an α globulin.

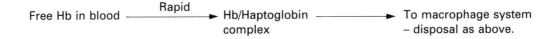

Free Hb in blood $\xrightarrow{\text{Rapid}}$ Hb/Haptoglobin complex $\longrightarrow$ To macrophage system – disposal as above.

The complex is protective against damaging effects of the free haemoglobin, particularly on the kidneys.

In severe intravascular haemolysis, e.g. severe malaria, incompatible blood transfusion and with the toxic action of chemicals and bacteria, the mechanism may be overloaded.

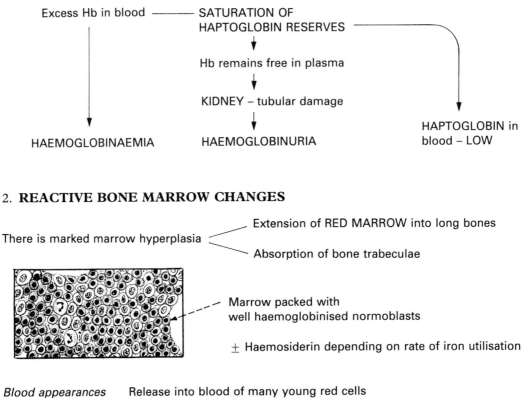

Excess Hb in blood ——— SATURATION OF HAPTOGLOBIN RESERVES

Hb remains free in plasma

KIDNEY – tubular damage

HAEMOGLOBINAEMIA   HAEMOGLOBINURIA   HAPTOGLOBIN in blood – LOW

2. REACTIVE BONE MARROW CHANGES

There is marked marrow hyperplasia

— Extension of RED MARROW into long bones

— Absorption of bone trabeculae

— Marrow packed with well haemoglobinised normoblasts

± Haemosiderin depending on rate of iron utilisation

Blood appearances   Release into blood of many young red cells
20–30% RETICULOCYTES – occasional normoblasts.
Film – normocytic: may be mild macrocytosis due to young cells.
– normochromic: may be polychromasia due to young cells.

The blood film may of course reflect the specific red cell abnormality responsible for the anaemia, e.g. spherocytosis.

INTRINSIC HAEMOLYTIC ANAEMIAS

The causes of shortened red cell survival are divided into two main groups:
(1) INTRINSIC (defects of the red cells) and (2) EXTRINSIC (factors outside the red cells).

INTRINSIC DEFECTS ——— Usually hereditary.

In (i) cell membrane (ii) enzymes (iii) molecular structure of haemoglobin (haemoglobinopathies).

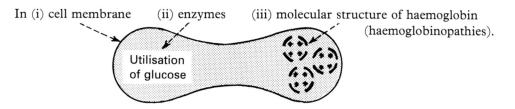

Utilisation of glucose

(a) Cell membrane defects

1. ***Hereditary spherocytosis:*** the majority of cases are familial (autosomal dominant).

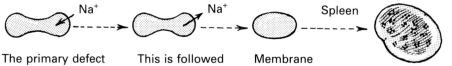

The primary defect allows excessive permeability of Na⁺.

This is followed by increased glycolysis to maintain the sodium pump.

Membrane *weakened* by secondary loss of intrinsic lipid. Cell becomes spheroidal.

Premature sequestration in splenic pulp (see p.569). Splenomegaly is a constant association.

Note: Splenectomy is usually 'curative' but the red cell defect remains.

The severity of the haemolysis is variable; many cases are compensated and not anaemic, but crises are common. Intercurrent infections may precipitate increased red cell destruction with jaundice or temporary bone marrow hypoplasia with severe anaemia.

The laboratory diagnosis depends on:
          (1) typical blood film with spherocytes,
          (2) high reticulocyte count and
          (3) increased osmotic fragility of RBCs.

2. ***Hereditary elliptocytosis*** is similar to spherocytosis in many respects, but it is usually not severe enough to cause anaemia or jaundice.

3. ***Hereditary abetalipoproteinaemia:*** a rare disease in which the red cell membranes are abnormal and the cells become spiky (acanthocytes).

4. ***Paroxysmal nocturnal haemoglobinuria*** – a rare, acquired condition in which the red cell membrane is particularly susceptible to the action of complement (usually activated by the alternative pathway) at low pH.

517

INTRINSIC HAEMOLYTIC ANAEMIAS

INTRINSIC DEFECTS of the RED CELLS (continued)

(b) Enzyme defects

Usually hereditary. Glucose is the source of energy with which the red cell metabolism is maintained. Glycolysis is effected by two classical enzyme pathways.

The following simplified diagram outlines the pathways and indicates only the main enzymes and substrates.

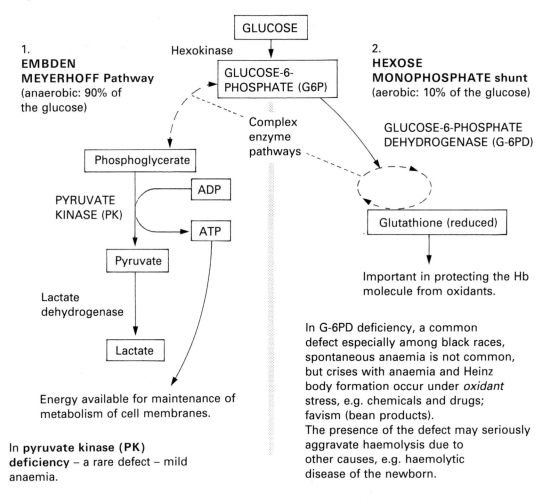

1. EMBDEN MEYERHOFF Pathway (anaerobic: 90% of the glucose)

Hexokinase

GLUCOSE

GLUCOSE-6-PHOSPHATE (G6P)

2. HEXOSE MONOPHOSPHATE shunt (aerobic: 10% of the glucose)

Complex enzyme pathways

GLUCOSE-6-PHOSPHATE DEHYDROGENASE (G-6PD)

Phosphoglycerate

PYRUVATE KINASE (PK)

ADP

ATP

Pyruvate

Lactate dehydrogenase

Lactate

Glutathione (reduced)

Important in protecting the Hb molecule from oxidants.

Energy available for maintenance of metabolism of cell membranes.

In **pyruvate kinase (PK) deficiency** – a rare defect – mild anaemia.

In G-6PD deficiency, a common defect especially among black races, spontaneous anaemia is not common, but crises with anaemia and Heinz body formation occur under *oxidant* stress, e.g. chemicals and drugs; favism (bean products).
The presence of the defect may seriously aggravate haemolysis due to other causes, e.g. haemolytic disease of the newborn.

G-6PD deficiency shows X-linked inheritance so that in the male the defect is fully expressed, while in the female heterozygote there are two populations of red cells in the blood (1) normal cells and (2) defective cells.

In both these defects and in the rare defects of other enzymes in the pathways which have been described the expression of the abnormal gene is very variable from case to case.

INTRINSIC HAEMOLYTIC ANAEMIAS

INTRINSIC DEFECTS of the RED CELLS (continued)

(c) Haemoglobinopathies

In some hereditary disorders, the molecular structure of haemoglobin is abnormal.

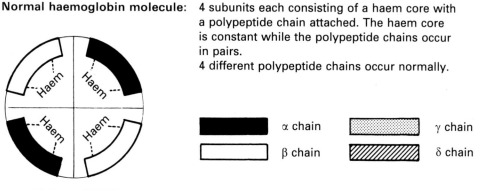

Normal haemoglobin molecule: 4 subunits each consisting of a haem core with a polypeptide chain attached. The haem core is constant while the polypeptide chains occur in pairs.
4 different polypeptide chains occur normally.

■ α chain   ▦ γ chain

□ β chain   ▨ δ chain

Mol. wt.=68,000

There are 3 types of normal haemoglobin.

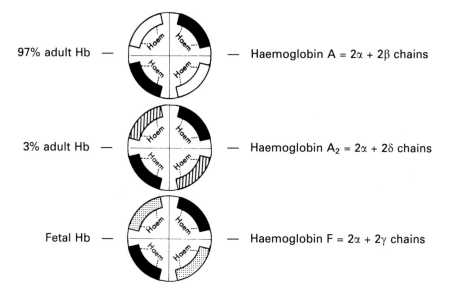

97% adult Hb — — Haemoglobin A = 2α + 2β chains

3% adult Hb — — Haemoglobin A$_2$ = 2α + 2δ chains

Fetal Hb — — Haemoglobin F = 2α + 2γ chains

Fetal haemoglobin is replaced by adult haemoglobin during the first year. Note that the α chain occurs in all normal haemoglobins.

INTRINSIC HAEMOLYTIC ANAEMIAS

Very many abnormal haemoglobins have now been described. Only a few have serious consequences.

Abnormal haemoglobins may be formed in two ways:

(1) Due to variation in the amino acid content and sequence of one of the chain pairs.

e.g.

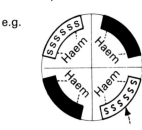

Haemglobin-S
β chains are abnormal –
SICKLE CELL DISEASE results

|
Sickle cell disease

Hb-S molecules stack abnormally and cause sickling in reduced O_2 state – serious haemolysis.

Sickle cell trait – heterozygote – symptoms mild but trait can be detected by in vitro sickling using a reducing agent or electrophoresis of Hb.

NB: falciparum malaria resistant.

(2) By a slowing or failure to synthesise

α *chains*   or   β *chains*

This leads to an excess of β chains which form a tetramer called Hb-H.

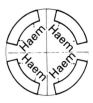

This disease is termed
α-*THALASSAEMIA*

This leads to an excess of α chains.

These do *not* form tetramers.
∴ No abnormal Hb formed.

The deficiency of Hb A is compensated for by an increase in Hb A_2 and F.

The disease is designated

↓

β-*THALASSAEMIA*

Thalassaemia

Major – homozygous.

Serious haemolytic anaemia; 'target cells'; increased osmotic resistance.

Minor – heterozygous –
presents as hypochromic microcytic anaemia.

Note: The anaemias resulting from the haemoglobinopathies are usually at the same time *both* dyshaemopoietic and haemolytic in type.

EXTRINSIC HAEMOLYTIC ANAEMIAS

In extrinsic haemolytic anaemias, the premature destruction of red cells is caused by agencies arising outside the cells. They are usually acquired and may be idiopathic (i.e. with no known cause) or secondary to some other disorder (i.e. symptomatic).

They will be considered in five main groups:

        1. ANTIBODIES to RBCs
        2. INFECTIONS
        3. DRUGS and poisonous chemicals
        4. TRAUMATIC DAMAGE to RBCs
        5. MISCELLANEOUS

(1a) DESTRUCTION of RBCs due to ISO-ANTIBODIES

In these, the antibodies act against antigens which are derived from another individual of the same species.

Incompatible ABO blood transfusion is a classical example.

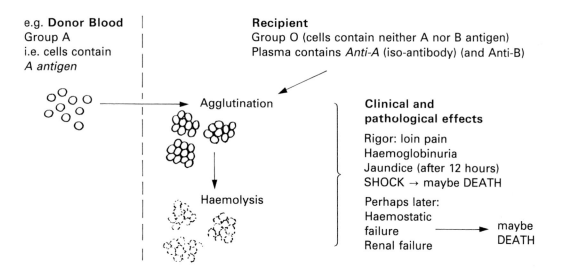

e.g. Donor Blood
Group A
i.e. cells contain
A antigen

Recipient
Group O (cells contain neither A nor B antigen)
Plasma contains *Anti-A* (iso-antibody) (and Anti-B)

Agglutination

Haemolysis

Clinical and pathological effects

Rigor: loin pain
Haemoglobinuria
Jaundice (after 12 hours)
SHOCK → maybe DEATH

Perhaps later:
Haemostatic
failure   → maybe
Renal failure   DEATH

Notes:

(a) The severity of the effects is influenced by (1) the transfusion rate and (2) the strength (titre) of the antibody.

(b) Only rarely does incompatible donor plasma destroy the recipient red cells because the plasma antibodies are rapidly diluted in the recipient circulation.

EXTRINSIC HAEMOLYTIC ANAEMIAS

DESTRUCTION of RBCs due to ISO-ANTIBODIES (continued)

Incompatibilities within the Rh blood group systems cause haemolytic disorders in two main circumstances: (a) Incompatible blood transfusion and (b) haemolytic disease of the newborn.

(i) Blood transfusion

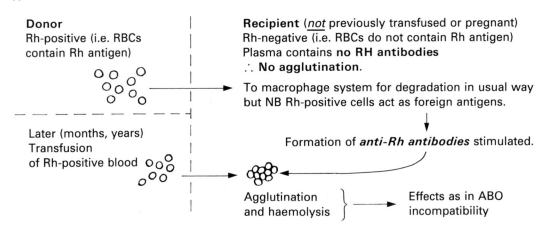

Donor
Rh-positive (i.e. RBCs contain Rh antigen)

Recipient (*not* previously transfused or pregnant)
Rh-negative (i.e. RBCs do not contain Rh antigen)
Plasma contains **no RH antibodies**
∴ **No agglutination.**

To macrophage system for degradation in usual way but NB Rh-positive cells act as foreign antigens.

Later (months, years)
Transfusion
of Rh-positive blood

Formation of *anti-Rh antibodies* stimulated.

Agglutination and haemolysis ⎫ Effects as in ABO incompatibility

Note: In Rh-negative males anti-RH antibodies can only be stimulated by the parenteral injection of Rh-positive blood. In Rh-negative females pregnancy with an Rh-positive fetus is an additional and more common mechanism.

(ii) **Haemolytic disease of the newborn (HDN).** This occurs in Rh-positive fetuses conceived by Rh-negative mothers. The usual mechanism is as follows:

First pregnancy: Rh-positive fetus in Rh-negative mother – no antibodies present;
∴ *Healthy Baby*

But during this pregnancy, iso-immunisation of the mother may occur.

Towards term and particularly during labour the placental barrier is breached and fetal RBCs enter the maternal circulation.

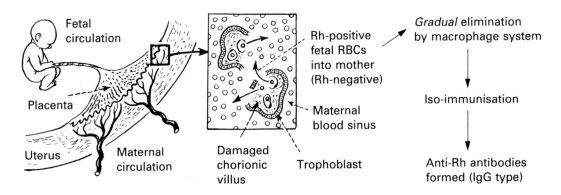

Fetal circulation

Placenta

Uterus   Maternal circulation

Damaged chorionic villus

Trophoblast

Rh-positive fetal RBCs into mother (Rh-negative)

Maternal blood sinus

Gradual elimination by macrophage system

Iso-immunisation

Anti-Rh antibodies formed (IgG type)

522

EXTRINSIC HAEMOLYTIC ANAEMIAS

Haemolytic disease of the newborn (continued)

The basic mechanism is influenced by three important factors:

(a) The maternal immune response tends to be proportional to the number of fetal cells entering the circulation.

(b) The maternal immune response is boosted in successive Rh incompatible pregnancies – the highest maternal antibody titres are found in the latest of multiple pregnancies.

(c) Fetal/maternal ABO compatibility influences the Rh immune response.

e.g. *ABO compatible*		*ABO incompatible*	
Fetus	*Mother*	*Fetus*	*Mother*
Group O Rh+	Group O Rh-	Group A Rh+	Group O Rh-
Gradual elimination of fetal cells		*Rapid* destruction of fetal cells	
∴ *Maximum* immune response		∴ *Minimum* immune response	

Subsequent pregnancies: All Rh-positive fetuses conceived by a mother who has acquired anti-Rh antibodies either during previous pregnancies or by blood transfusion (in this case the first fetus also) are at risk.

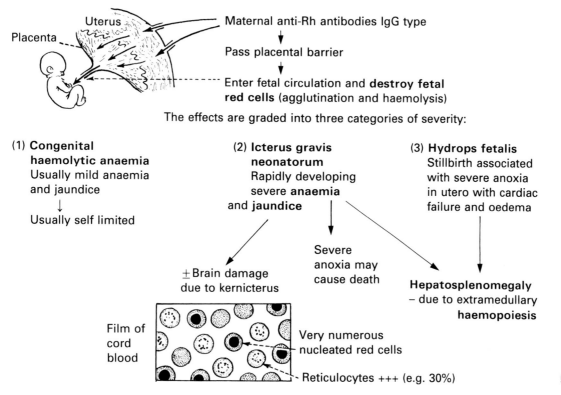

Placenta / Uterus — Maternal anti-Rh antibodies IgG type

↓

Pass placental barrier

↓

Enter fetal circulation and **destroy fetal red cells** (agglutination and haemolysis)

The effects are graded into three categories of severity:

(1) **Congenital haemolytic anaemia**
Usually mild anaemia and jaundice
↓
Usually self limited

(2) **Icterus gravis neonatorum**
Rapidly developing severe **anaemia** and **jaundice**

±Brain damage due to kernicterus

Severe anoxia may cause death

(3) **Hydrops fetalis**
Stillbirth associated with severe anoxia in utero with cardiac failure and oedema

Hepatosplenomegaly – due to extramedullary **haemopoiesis**

Film of cord blood

Very numerous nucleated red cells

Reticulocytes +++ (e.g. 30%)

523

EXTRINSIC HAEMOLYTIC ANAEMIAS

The autoimmune haemolytic anaemias are divided into two main groups depending on the temperature at which the reactions occur.

1. *Warm antibody type*
   Reaction at normal temperature (37°C)
   ⅄ = Antibody usually IgG type

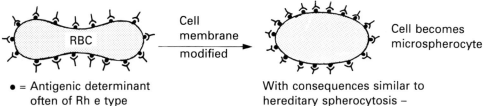

• = Antigenic determinant
often of Rh e type

Cell membrane modified →

Cell becomes microspherocyte

With consequences similar to hereditary spherocytosis – early sequestration in spleen etc.

Clinically presents as chronic haemolytic anaemia ± crises.

2. *Cold antibody type*
   Reactions at temperatures usually below 30°C ∴ they occur in peripheral circulation and in cold weather.

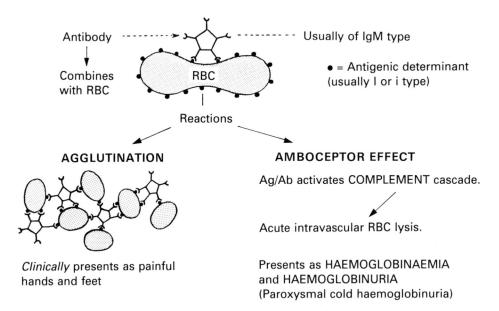

Antibody ·······➤ ⅄ ·········· Usually of IgM type

↓

Combines with RBC

RBC

• = Antigenic determinant (usually I or i type)

Reactions

AGGLUTINATION

Clinically presents as painful hands and feet

AMBOCEPTOR EFFECT

Ag/Ab activates COMPLEMENT cascade.

Acute intravascular RBC lysis.

Presents as HAEMOGLOBINAEMIA and HAEMOGLOBINURIA (Paroxysmal cold haemoglobinuria)

Note: The classical paroxysmal haemoglobinuria associated with syphilitic infection is rare nowadays. It is due to an IgG antibody, and the antigenic determinant on the red cell is usually P type.

EXTRINSIC HAEMOLYTIC ANAEMIAS

2. INFECTIONS

There are three mechanisms by which infections cause haemolysis:

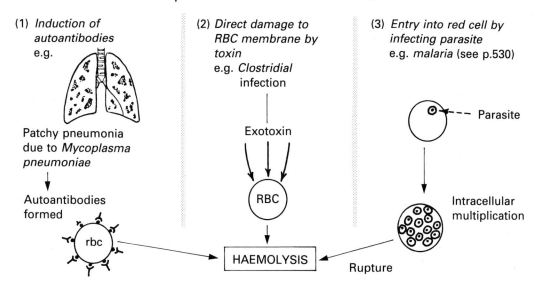

(1) *Induction of autoantibodies* e.g.

Patchy pneumonia due to *Mycoplasma pneumoniae*

Autoantibodies formed

(2) *Direct damage to RBC membrane by toxin* e.g. *Clostridial* infection

Exotoxin

RBC

(3) *Entry into red cell by infecting parasite* e.g. *malaria* (see p.530)

Parasite

Intracellular multiplication

rbc

HAEMOLYSIS

Rupture

3. DRUGS AND CHEMICALS

The three main mechanisms by which drugs and chemicals cause haemolysis are:

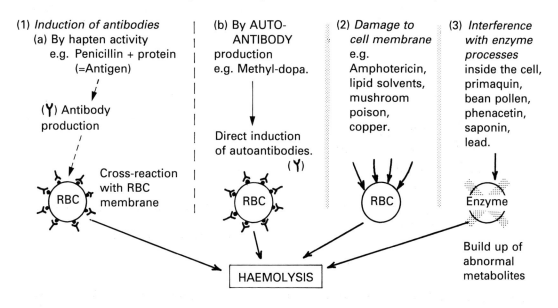

(1) *Induction of antibodies*
(a) By hapten activity e.g. Penicillin + protein (=Antigen)

(Y) Antibody production

RBC

Cross-reaction with RBC membrane

(b) By AUTO-ANTIBODY production e.g. Methyl-dopa.

Direct induction of autoantibodies. (Y)

RBC

(2) *Damage to cell membrane* e.g. Amphotericin, lipid solvents, mushroom poison, copper.

RBC

(3) *Interference with enzyme processes* inside the cell, primaquin, bean pollen, phenacetin, saponin, lead.

Enzyme

Build up of abnormal metabolites

HAEMOLYSIS

527

EXTRINSIC HAEMOLYTIC ANAEMIAS

4. MECHANICAL TRAUMA

The results of damage to red cells within the circulation are:

(1) Intravascular haemolysis

Haemoglobinuria

(2) Formation of red cell fragments (schistocytes)

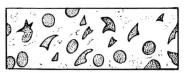

seen in blood film as 'burr', 'triangle', 'helmet' cells

The main circumstances in which red cells are damaged are:

(a) In the **heart and great vessels**

When the blood flow is subjected to undue turbulence or jet effect. An important example nowadays is with prosthetic valves in left side of heart.

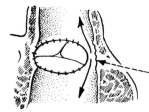

RBCs damaged by shearing stresses where valve seating is defective

Other examples are:
Aortic stenosis and regurgitation
Arterio-venous shunts.

Note that in this chronic situation, iron is lost in the urine so that *iron deficiency anaemia* is often superimposed.

(b) In the **microcirculation**

(i) When the blood flow in arterioles is impeded by strands of fibrin.

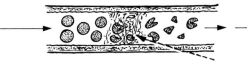

(1) Liberation of haemoglobin
(2) Emergence of fragments

RBCs being distorted and cut by fibrin sieve

This condition is called MICROANGIOPATHIC HAEMOLYTIC ANAEMIA and occurs in many disease states involving small blood vessels and/or intravascular coagulation.

(ii) When blood vessels are subjected to direct trauma. This is seen classically in military recruits marching long distances in hard soled boots, when the blood vessels of the soles of the feet are squeezed with every step – **march haemoglobinuria**. The condition is also seen in karate exponents when the hand is repeatedly struck against hard objects.

The haemolysis is usually not severe enough to be of clinical significance, but haemoglobinuria may cause alarm.

EXTRINSIC HAEMOLYTIC ANAEMIAS

5. EXTRINSIC – MISCELLANEOUS

1. Hypersplenism (see p.569)

In enlargement of the spleen from any cause, the sequestration of red cells is increased so that haemolytic anaemia may result.

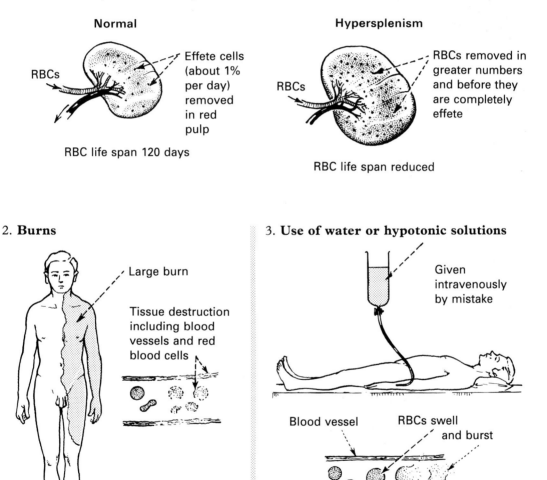

Normal

RBCs

Effete cells (about 1% per day) removed in red pulp

RBC life span 120 days

Hypersplenism

RBCs

RBCs removed in greater numbers and before they are completely effete

RBC life span reduced

2. Burns

Large burn

Tissue destruction including blood vessels and red blood cells

In severe burns haemolysis is an important component of the acute anaemia which develops.

3. Use of water or hypotonic solutions

Given intravenously by mistake

Blood vessel

RBCs swell and burst

Intravascular haemolysis

EXTRINSIC HAEMOLYTIC ANAEMIAS

MALARIA

Malaria is an endemic disease in many parts of Africa, Asia, Central and South America. Many millions of cases occur each year and the mortality is at least 1%. The disease is particularly severe in non-immune subjects from temperate climates; in endemic areas where the 'herd' immunity is high, a low grade chronic illness is common.

Female anopheline mosquitos act as intermediate hosts in the life cycle of the parasite, a protozoon (genus *Plasmodium*).

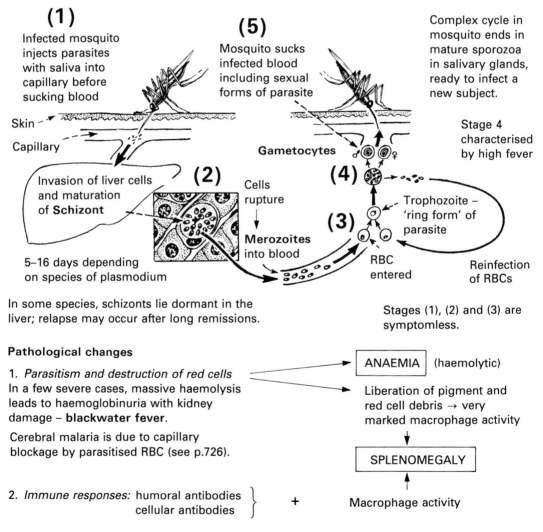

(1)
Infected mosquito injects parasites with saliva into capillary before sucking blood

(5)
Mosquito sucks infected blood including sexual forms of parasite

Complex cycle in mosquito ends in mature sporozoa in salivary glands, ready to infect a new subject.

Skin

Capillary

Stage 4 characterised by high fever

Gametocytes

(2) Invasion of liver cells and maturation of **Schizont**

Cells rupture

(4)

(3) Trophozoite – 'ring form' of parasite

Merozoites into blood

RBC entered

Reinfection of RBCs

5–16 days depending on species of plasmodium

In some species, schizonts lie dormant in the liver; relapse may occur after long remissions.

Stages (1), (2) and (3) are symptomless.

Pathological changes

1. *Parasitism and destruction of red cells*
In a few severe cases, massive haemolysis leads to haemoglobinuria with kidney damage – **blackwater fever**.

Cerebral malaria is due to capillary blockage by parasitised RBC (see p.726).

→ ANAEMIA (haemolytic)

→ Liberation of pigment and red cell debris → very marked macrophage activity
↓
SPLENOMEGALY
↑
Macrophage activity

2. *Immune responses:* humoral antibodies } + cellular antibodies }

3. *Associations:*
   (a) Recurrent attacks of malaria potentiate EB virus infection progressing to B-cell lymphoma (see p.160).
   (b) The sickle cell gene protects against falciparum malaria (see p.520).

ANAEMIAS – MISCELLANEOUS

There remain anaemias of which the causative mechanisms are obscure or complex and the morphological details indeterminate.

This miscellaneous group can be subdivided as follows:

1. **Anaemias associated with chronic disease states**

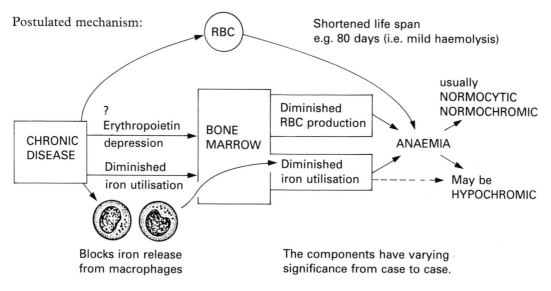

Postulated mechanism:

The chronic disease states commonly associated with anaemia of this type are:

(a) Chronic infections and inflammations e.g. tuberculosis: rheumatoid arthritis.

(b) Renal disease – in addition the following factors are often important:

Renal — RBC survival is inversely proportional to severity of uraemia
— Burr cells (e.g. in renal disease with vascular fibrin deposition)
— Erythropoietin specifically lost.
In dialysis, folate and iron loss.

(c) Liver failure – additional factors are:

Liver — Bleeding Varices
— Deficiency of coagulation factors
— Hypersplenism
— Alcoholic – other nutritional deficiencies.

In addition, malignant tumour growth may cause anaemia by two more specific mechanisms.

(a) Chronic bleeding from the surface of an ulcerated tumour – especially from the alimentary tract.

(b) Actual invasion of the bone marrow by malignant tumour.

ANAEMIAS – MISCELLANEOUS

2. The sideroblastic anaemias

In these rare anaemias, failure of synthesis of the haem component of the haemoglobin molecule is indicated by the presence of a ring of iron granules around the normoblast nucleus.

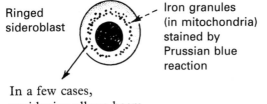

Ringed sideroblast

Iron granules (in mitochondria) stained by Prussian blue reaction

In a few cases, pyridoxine allows haem synthesis to proceed normally

The condition arises secondarily in many of the chronic disease states mentioned on previous page, or as a result of drug treatment or chemical poisoning (e.g. lead). A few cases are 'primary' – possibly representing a form of myelodysplasia.

The anaemia is usually *dimorphic*; i.e. showing hypochromic and macrocytic features combined.

3. Anaemias associated with endocrine deficiencies

These anaemias have no specifically identifying features and their mechanism of production is obscure.

The anaemia of hypothyroidism is often macrocytic.

4. Refractory anaemias

These rare anaemias of unknown aetiology fail to respond to many various treatments. They are usually macrocytic. As the aetiology of anaemias is elucidated, the number of 'refractory' cases diminishes.

5. Leucoerythroblastic anaemia

In this condition, primitive myeloid cells as well as nucleated red cells appear in small numbers in blood film; the cause is usually a serious bone disorder often due to infiltration by malignant tumour or fibrosis.

The foregoing classification is based on the basic aetiological mechanisms, and although in some cases the mechanisms overlap, the classification is fundamental to rational treatment.

ANAEMIA – MORPHOLOGICAL CLASSIFICATION

The initial investigation of any anaemia consists of an examination of blood (and/or marrow) films and determination of absolute values. A morphological classification is therefore very useful.

The three broad divisions which depend on the red cell size may be further subdivided in respect of haemoglobin content of the cell:

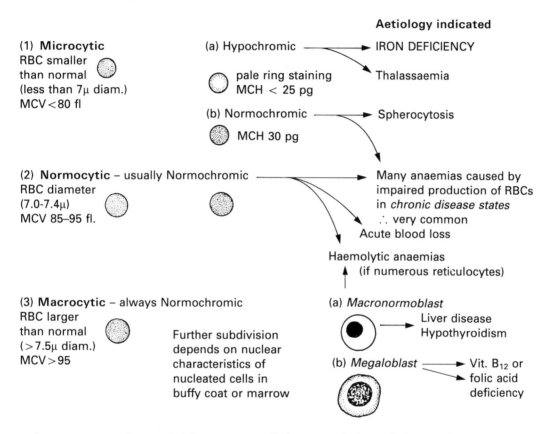

Aetiology indicated

(1) Microcytic
RBC smaller than normal (less than 7μ diam.) MCV < 80 fl

(a) Hypochromic ⟶ IRON DEFICIENCY
pale ring staining MCH < 25 pg ⟶ Thalassaemia
(b) Normochromic ⟶ Spherocytosis MCH 30 pg

(2) Normocytic – usually Normochromic ⟶ Many anaemias caused by impaired production of RBCs in *chronic disease states* ∴ very common
RBC diameter (7.0-7.4μ) MCV 85–95 fl.
Acute blood loss
Haemolytic anaemias (if numerous reticulocytes)

(3) Macrocytic – always Normochromic
RBC larger than normal (>7.5μ diam.) MCV >95
Further subdivision depends on nuclear characteristics of nucleated cells in buffy coat or marrow

(a) *Macronormoblast* ⟶ Liver disease / Hypothyroidism
(b) *Megaloblast* ⟶ Vit. B$_{12}$ or folic acid deficiency

In some cases of anaemia, there are two distinct populations of abnormal red cells (e.g. microcytic/hypochromic and macrocytic/normochromic). These DIMORPHIC anaemias are usually caused by double deficiencies.

The logical use of these classifications in the investigation of anaemia:

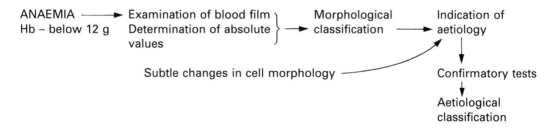

ANAEMIA ⟶ Examination of blood film / Determination of absolute values ⟶ Morphological classification ⟶ Indication of aetiology
Hb – below 12 g

Subtle changes in cell morphology ⟶ Confirmatory tests ⟶ Aetiological classification

POLYCYTHAEMIA

POLYCYTHAEMIA

Polycythaemia (erythrocytosis) is defined as a sustained increase in red cell mass: the haematocrit is always elevated.

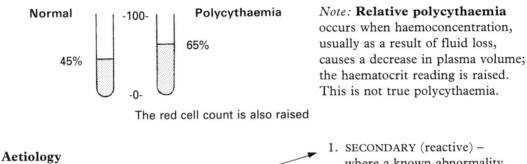

Normal

45%

-100-

-0-

Polycythaemia

65%

The red cell count is also raised

Note: **Relative polycythaemia** occurs when haemoconcentration, usually as a result of fluid loss, causes a decrease in plasma volume; the haematocrit reading is raised. This is not true polycythaemia.

Aetiology

There are two main types

1. SECONDARY (reactive) – where a known abnormality causes the red cell increase.
2. PRIMARY (rare) – where the increase is autonomous and without explanation.

SECONDARY POLYCYTHAEMIA

The red cell increase is the result of increased stimulation of marrow by erythropoietin. Two main groups of conditions are associated with this:

1. (Commonly) Conditions causing tissue HYPOXIA:

    (a) Living at high altitudes
    (b) Chronic cardiac disease especially R → L shunts
    (c) Chronic respiratory disease
    (d) Presence of abnormal haemoglobin causing defective release of O_2 to tissue – usually hereditary, sometimes due to drugs.

2. (Rarely) Renal tumours and ischaemia; occasionally tumours of other organs.

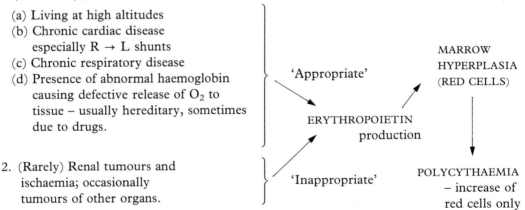

'Appropriate'

ERYTHROPOIETIN production

'Inappropriate'

MARROW HYPERPLASIA (RED CELLS)

POLYCYTHAEMIA – increase of red cells only

PRIMARY POLYCYTHAEMIA (*Polycythaemia Rubra Vera*)

The red cell increase in this rare condition is autonomous. It may be associated with an increase in other marrow elements and is grouped within the myeloproliferative disorders (see p. 545). Splenomegaly is always present.

POLYCYTHAEMIA

Effects of polycythaemia
(a) There is usually a distinctly florid complexion.
(b) Increased blood viscosity causes: (i) **hypertension** and (ii) a tendency to **thrombosis**.
(c) Increased marrow activity → increased uric acid metabolism → tendency to gout.

Comparison of SECONDARY and PRIMARY polycythaemias

	Secondary	Primary
Prevalence	Lesser degrees COMMON	RARE
Cause	Underlying disease – especially HYPOXIA	Not known (associated with non specific chromosome aberrations)
Erythropoietin	++	Not increased; may be decreased
Marrow	Increased cellularity but some fat spaces remain: pure red cell hyperplasia	Total cellularity – including increase in myeloid elements and megakaryocytes → May terminate as acute **myeloid leukaemia** → Marrow fibrosis may follow
Blood	RBCs normal	Leucocyte count often increased Platelet count often raised RBCs may be hypochromic
Splenomegaly	None	+ +
Hypertension	+	+ +
Tendency to thrombosis	+	+ +
Tendency to gout	+	+ +
	Increased cellular breakdown in marrow causes uricaemia	
Progress	Where the erythropoietin excess is 'appropriate' the outcome depends on the progress of the basic disease	Without treatment – **poor** Progressive deterioration over a few years

THE WHITE BLOOD CELLS

NEUTROPHIL Polymorphonuclear Leucocyte (Neutrophil granulocyte)

The essential function of these cells is protection against microbial infection by phagocytosis and killing. They are produced alongside red blood cells, platelets and monocytes from a common stem cell in the marrow.

Marrow Production – stained by a Romanowski method

	Stem cell (Primitive-multipotential)	Myeloblast (committed)	Promyelocyte	Myelocyte	Metamyelocyte	Neutrophil in marrow and blood
% age	<1	<5	<15			
Size (Diameter) 15–25μ		10–18μ	12–18μ	12–18μ	12–15μ	10–15μ
Nucleus Spherical; even dispersal of chromatin		Spherical; even dispersal of chromatin	Spherical; chromatin slightly condensed	Ovoid; condensation of chromatin	'Band' of 'stab' shape; chromatin condensed	2–5 lobes; Chromatin condensed
Nucleoli Several		2–4	2–4	None	None	None
Cytoplasm Blue (High RNA content)		Blue (High RNA content)	Blue	Less blue	Less blue Glycogen++	Less blue Glycogen++
Granules None		None	Scanty large granules; contain *myeloper-oxidase* and *hydrolases*	Many small granules; alkaline *phosphatase,* various lytic enzymes	→ → → →	

WHITE BLOOD CELLS IN DISEASE

NEUTROPHIL POLYMORPHONUCLEAR LEUCOCYTOSIS

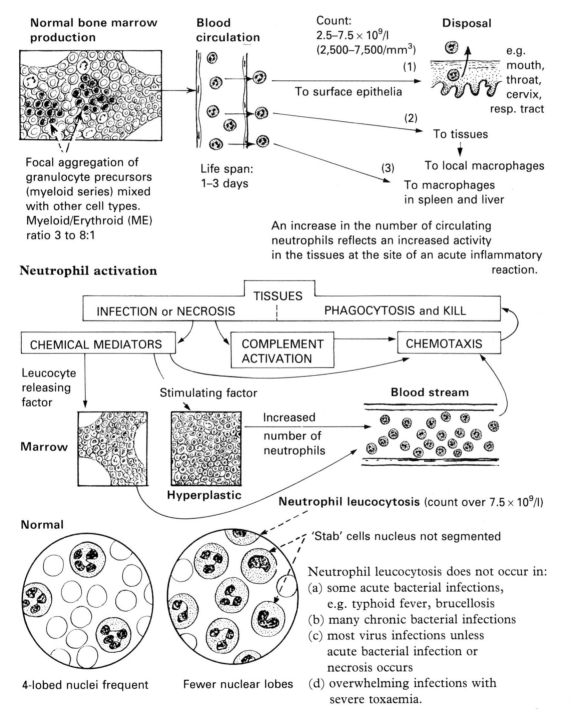

Normal bone marrow production

Focal aggregation of granulocyte precursors (myeloid series) mixed with other cell types. Myeloid/Erythroid (ME) ratio 3 to 8:1

Blood circulation

Life span: 1–3 days

Count:
2.5–7.5 × 10⁹/l
(2,500–7,500/mm³)

(1)

To surface epithelia

(2)

To tissues

(3)

Disposal

e.g. mouth, throat, cervix, resp. tract

To tissues
↓
To local macrophages

To macrophages in spleen and liver

An increase in the number of circulating neutrophils reflects an increased activity in the tissues at the site of an acute inflammatory reaction.

Neutrophil activation

TISSUES

INFECTION or NECROSIS | PHAGOCYTOSIS and KILL

CHEMICAL MEDIATORS → COMPLEMENT ACTIVATION → CHEMOTAXIS

Leucocyte releasing factor

Stimulating factor

Blood stream

Marrow

Hyperplastic

Increased number of neutrophils

Neutrophil leucocytosis (count over 7.5 × 10⁹/l)

'Stab' cells nucleus not segmented

Normal

4-lobed nuclei frequent

Fewer nuclear lobes

Neutrophil leucocytosis does not occur in:
(a) some acute bacterial infections, e.g. typhoid fever, brucellosis
(b) many chronic bacterial infections
(c) most virus infections unless acute bacterial infection or necrosis occurs
(d) overwhelming infections with severe toxaemia.

537

DISORDERS OF NEUTROPHILS

In most disorders, increased susceptibility to infection is the important sequel and clinical presentation.

Absence (agranulocytosis) or diminished numbers – $<2.5 \times 10^9/l$ $(2,500/mm^3)$ (neutropenia). There are two main mechanisms which often co-exist.

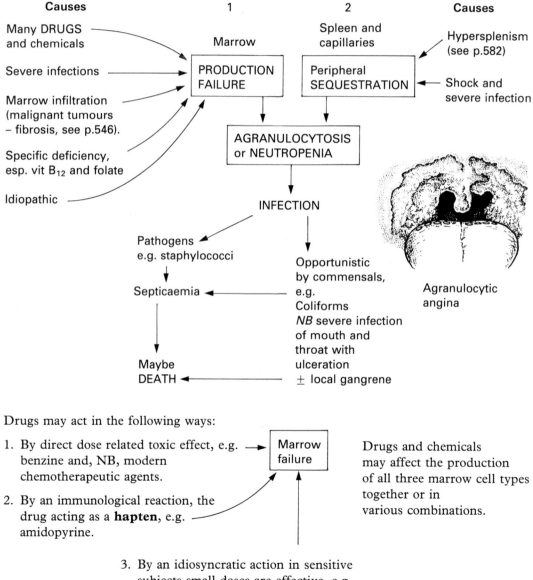

Causes   1   2   **Causes**

Many DRUGS and chemicals

Severe infections

Marrow infiltration (malignant tumours – fibrosis, see p.546).

Specific deficiency, esp. vit B_{12} and folate

Idiopathic

Marrow

PRODUCTION FAILURE

Spleen and capillaries

Peripheral SEQUESTRATION

Hypersplenism (see p.582)

Shock and severe infection

AGRANULOCYTOSIS or NEUTROPENIA

INFECTION

Pathogens e.g. staphylococci

Septicaemia

Maybe DEATH

Opportunistic by commensals, e.g. Coliforms
NB severe infection of mouth and throat with ulceration ± local gangrene

Agranulocytic angina

Drugs may act in the following ways:

1. By direct dose related toxic effect, e.g. benzine and, NB, modern chemotherapeutic agents. → Marrow failure

2. By an immunological reaction, the drug acting as a **hapten**, e.g. amidopyrine.

3. By an idiosyncratic action in sensitive subjects small doses are effective, e.g. chloramphenicol.

Drugs and chemicals may affect the production of all three marrow cell types together or in various combinations.

DISORDERS OF NEUTROPHILS

Disorders of neutrophil function

Divided into three groups: (1) chemotaxis, (2) microbial phagocytosis and (3) microbial kill.

Chemotaxis and phagocytosis may be defective due to:

(a) an intrinsic defect of the neutrophils e.g. lazy leucocyte syndrome
(b) plasma deficiency of chemotactic factors and opsonins – seen especially when there are deficiencies in the complement cascade.

Microbial kill fails when there is an intracellular enzyme defect e.g. in *chronic granulomatous disease* (CGD) and the Chediak-Higashi syndrome where the neutrophils contain abnormal giant granules.

The normal sequence following phagocytosis is:

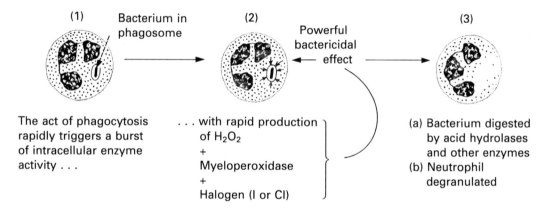

(1) Bacterium in phagosome

(2) Powerful bactericidal effect

(3)

The act of phagocytosis rapidly triggers a burst of intracellular enzyme activity . . .

. . . with rapid production of H_2O_2
+
Myeloperoxidase
+
Halogen (I or Cl)

(a) Bacterium digested by acid hydrolases and other enzymes
(b) Neutrophil degranulated

In CGD, the rapid production of H_2O_2 is defective (in the neutrophils and also in macrophages – ? due to cytochrome deficiency).

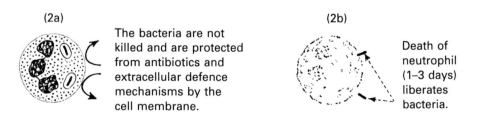

(2a) The bacteria are not killed and are protected from antibiotics and extracellular defence mechanisms by the cell membrane.

(2b) Death of neutrophil (1–3 days) liberates bacteria.

DISORDERS OF NEUTROPHILS

CHRONIC GRANULOMATOUS DISEASE (CGD)
CGD is a rare hereditary disorder in which the neutrophils have normal phagocytic function but are unable to kill certain bacteria.

Presentation
The disease is fully expressed only in males. It presents as multiple chronic abscesses and granulomas affecting skin, lungs, bones, spleen and liver. The abscesses contain abundant debris derived from tissue breakdown. This is seen as fatty material and pigment within macrophages and illustrates the unimpaired phagocytic capacity.

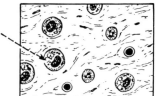

Bacteriology:
Infection is by a limited range of organisms –
e.g. staphylococci, coliforms (no H_2O_2 production).
Organisms, e.g. streptococci, which naturally produce H_2O_2 contribute this missing factor and are themselves killed and the infection is eliminated.

Inheritance
The disease is X-linked.

(Ⓧ = affected chromosome)

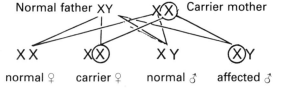

Normal father XY   Carrier mother XⓍ

X X   XⓍ   X Y   ⓍY

normal ♀   carrier ♀   normal ♂   affected ♂

Note 1. Affected males die of chronic infection before the age of sexual maturity.
    2. The carrier female may present with minor skin inflammation.
    3. The carrier female has two approximately equal populations of neutrophils:
        (a) with normal ability to kill bacteria.
        (b) with defective ability to kill bacteria.

The Lyon hypothesis states that in the female, the **XX** chromosomes are randomly inactivated during cellular growth and differentiation. The neutrophils of the carrier female support this hypothesis.

(a) If Ⓧ is inactivated, the normal X remains active and the neutrophil has normal ability to kill.

A small drumstick-like projection from the nucleus carries the inactivated sex chromosome.

(b) If X is inactivated, the defective Ⓧ remains active and the ability to kill is defective.

These are rare defects and usually have a hereditary basis.

    Other acquired abnormalities of neutrophil function are more difficult to pinpoint but are probably relevant in the increased rate of infection seen in diseases such as diabetes mellitus, rheumatoid arthritis and glomerulonephritis.

EOSINOPHILS

EOSINOPHIL Polymorphonuclear Leucocyte
These cells circulate in the blood (normal count 0.04–$0.4 \times 10^9/l$ or 40–$400/mm^3$) and are found in the tissues, particularly near points of external environmental contact.

Production is in the bone marrow as a component of myeloid haemopoiesis.

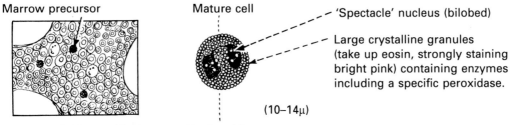

Marrow precursor   Mature cell   ‒ ‒ ‒ 'Spectacle' nucleus (bilobed)

‒ ‒ ‒ Large crystalline granules
(take up eosin, strongly staining
bright pink) containing enzymes
including a specific peroxidase.

(10–14μ)

Myeloblasts→Myelocytes→Eosinophil
(Analogous to neutrophil series)

Although their basic function is similar to that of neutrophils and they are found in small numbers in inflammatory cellular infiltrates, they exhibit specialised functions in certain disorders:

1. They protect against 'foreign' substances – especially the foreign proteins of infesting helminths.
2. They exert a controlling influence on mast cells and the effects of histamine release at the site of Type I antigen-antibody reactions.

There are several specific eosinophil chemotactic agents, particularly those derived from mast cells, which activate the release of chemotactic lymphokines from T cells.

Eosinophilia (an increased number of eosinophils in the blood) is seen in:

1. Parasitic infestations – e.g. ankylostomiasis, schistosomiasis

2. Hypersensitivity (atopic) reactions – both generalised and local, e.g. asthma and hay fever; food and drug sensitivity

3. Chronic eczema of the skin (probably due to antigen-antibody reaction)

4. Occasionally in association with malignant tumours – but particularly in Hodgkin's disease.

'Allergic' nasal polypi

The typical cellular infiltrate consisting of numerous eosinophils and plasma cells under mucosa in a loose myxomatous stroma.

541

LYMPHOCYTES

The main function of lymphocytes is concerned with the immune responses occurring in the lymphoid organs, and the immune reactions occurring at surfaces and adjacent tissues (see p.99). Their presence in the blood is only one component of their complex circulation.

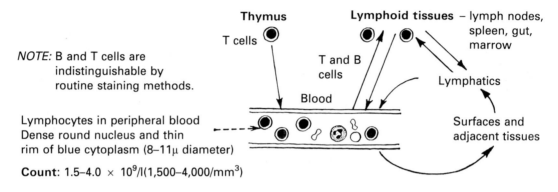

NOTE: B and T cells are indistinguishable by routine staining methods.

Lymphocytes in peripheral blood Dense round nucleus and thin rim of blue cytoplasm (8–11μ diameter)

Count: 1.5–$4.0 \times 10^9/l (1,500$–$4,000/mm^3)$

In many diseases there may be significant changes in the functional activity of lymphocytes, but these are seldom reflected in lymphocyte counts and lymphocyte morphology. Age has an important effect on blood lymphocyte counts, probably reflecting the amount and activity of the lymphoid tissues which gradually atrophy with age – as exemplified in thymus, tonsils and appendix. In childhood, there are active immune responses to a host of first contact antigens.

Infants: $3.5 \pm 1.5 \times 10^9/l$. *Children:* $7.0 \pm 1.5 \times 10^9/l$. *Adults:* 1.5–$4.0 \times 10^9/l$.

Lymphocytosis – (a) *Relative.* If the neutrophil numbers decrease it is unusual for the lymphocyte numbers to fall also: a differential WBC in these circumstances shows an increased ratio (% age) of lymphocytes. This relative lymphocytosis must not be confused with   (b) an *Absolute* lymphocytosis, i.e. count $> 4.0 \times 10^9/l$.
This occurs in many virus infections in children, and in adults in GLANDULAR FEVER and smallpox as well as in typhoid fever and brucellosis. *NB* In the late middle aged and elderly, an absolute lymphocytosis should always raise the suspicion of a *neoplastic proliferation of lymphocytes* (leukaemia, lymphoma, see p.579).
Lymphopenia (count $< 1.5 \times 10^9/l$). Apart from rare hereditary diseases seen in childhood, lymphopenia is commonly seen in medical practice during therapy using ionising radiation, cytotoxic drugs and corticosteroids.
Morphological changes are seen in blood film particularly in virus infections.

Normal lymphocyte: dense spherical nucleus with thin rim of cytoplasm

Larger cell with loose-textured nucleus with clear foamy cytoplasm; can easily be mistaken for monocyte.

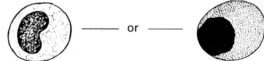

— or —

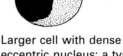

Larger cell with dense eccentric nucleus: a type of plasma cell (Turck cell).

The changes in Glandular Fever (infectious mononucleosis) are described on page 88.

MONOCYTES

These cells, derived from stem cells in the bone marrow, are the circulating members of the mononuclear phagocyte system. Their main function is to replace local macrophages (see p.109).

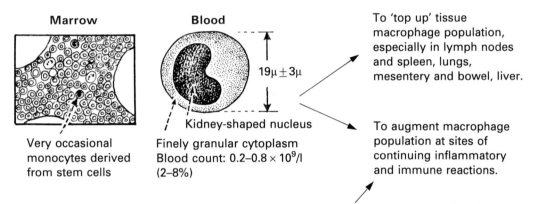

Marrow

Blood

$19\mu \pm 3\mu$

Kidney-shaped nucleus

Very occasional monocytes derived from stem cells

Finely granular cytoplasm
Blood count: 0.2–0.8×10^9/l
(2–8%)

To 'top up' tissue macrophage population, especially in lymph nodes and spleen, lungs, mesentery and bowel, liver.

To augment macrophage population at sites of continuing inflammatory and immune reactions.

Although many macrophages may be present at these sites, only occasionally is the monocyte blood count significantly increased. The following are examples of conditions in which there may be a monocytosis.

Infections:			Immunological disease	Chemical poisoning
Bacterial	Rickettsial	Protozoal		
Subacute bacterial endocarditis	Typhus fever	Malaria Kala-azar Trypanosomiasis	Systemic lupus erythematosus (SLE)	Tetrachlorethylene

Little is known about disease associated with abnormal monocytic function.

Note: The abnormal cells seen in the blood in 'glandular fever' (infectious mononucleosis) are transformed 'T' lymphocytes and not monocytes.

THE LEUKAEMIAS

Increased numbers of any one type of leucocyte or its precursors are seen in most cases of leukaemia – a neoplastic proliferation of white blood cells.

The various types of leukaemia are dealt with on pages 573–580.

BLOOD PLATELETS

These small, non-nucleated discs, derived from the cytoplasm of the bone marrow megakaryocytes, are released into the blood stream by a budding process.

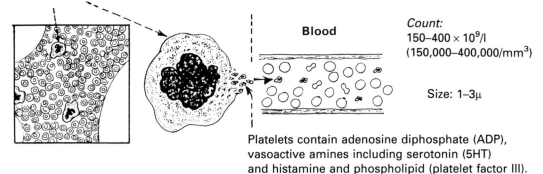

Blood

Count:
$150–400 \times 10^9/l$
$(150,000–400,000/mm^3)$

Size: 1–3μ

Platelets contain adenosine diphosphate (ADP), vasoactive amines including serotonin (5HT) and histamine and phospholipid (platelet factor III).

Their main role is concerned with haemostasis:

1. By aggregating to form the **haemostatic plug**.

and 2. by activating and augmenting the coagulation cascade.

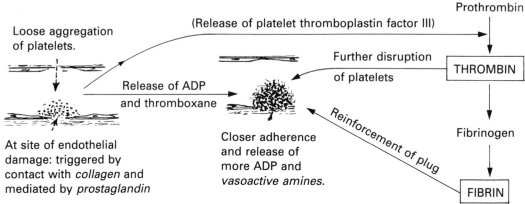

A prostaglandin (prostacyclin) synthesised by endothelium is antagonistic to platelet 'release' and normally prevents intravascular coagulation.

Disorders of the platelets include:

1. (a) deficiencies of number – thrombocytopenia
   (b) defective function
   } lead to **purpura** (see p.554)

2. Increased *adhesiveness* with or without increased numbers (thrombocytosis) occurs as a reactive state in many conditions – after haemorrhage, trauma and operations, childbirth, myocardial infarction, pulmonary embolism, splenectomy and during the use of the contraceptive pill. This change in platelet function is an important factor in the aetiology of **thrombosis** (see p.170).

DISEASES OF THE BONE MARROW

The role of the bone marrow and the reactive changes occurring in it in disorders of the blood cells have been described.

Primary disorders of the bone marrow are also important. There are 3 main groups: (1) marrow hypoplasia, (2) myelodysplastic disorders and (3) myeloproliferative disorders.

1. MARROW HYPOPLASIA or APLASIA (diminished or absent haemopoietic cellularity)

The marrow throughout the body has a pale, fatty gelatinous appearance.

Microscopically the haemopoietic cells are reduced or absent.

Sparse foci of lymphocytes or plasma cells remain.

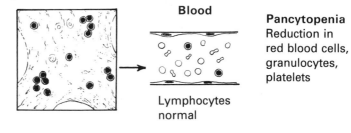

Blood

Pancytopenia
Reduction in red blood cells, granulocytes, platelets

Lymphocytes normal

Congenital and idiopathic forms are rare. Most cases are ACQUIRED as the result of therapy:

   (a) marrow toxic drugs and radiations used in the treatment of cancer
   (b) idiosyncratic reactions to a wide range of drugs – chloramphenicol is a good example.

The effects of the pancytopenia are serious (severe anaemia, susceptibility to infection and haemorrhage) and usually fatal unless the marrow activity is resumed or marrow transplant is successful.

2. MYELODYSPLASTIC SYNDROMES (MDS)

These are primary disorders of stem cells associated with several different chromosomal abnormalities. They lead to ineffective haemopoiesis of varying types, with the appearance in the peripheral blood of abnormal cells. A significant number progress to LEUKAEMIA.

3. MYELOPROLIFERATIVE DISORDERS (increased cellularity)

The various acquired reactive states of the bone marrow already described are specifically excluded from this category which embraces proliferations of the various marrow cellular components in a purposeless way and without known cause. It is important to note that a significant number of cases of myeloproliferative disorders terminate in acute leukaemia. The leukaemias and other primary marrow neoplasms will therefore be described separately in order to avoid confusion in classification.

The disorders included in the group comprise proliferations of:

   1. All haemopoietic cells including fibrous tissue
   2. Erythroid cells predominantly
   3. Megakaryocytic cells.

545

DISEASES OF THE BONE MARROW

Myeloproliferative Disorders (continued)

MYELOFIBROSIS

In this rare affection of the elderly, the haemopoietic cellular proliferation is overshadowed by progressive FIBROSIS of the marrow; SPLENOMEGALY (often of massive proportions) due to EXTRAMEDULLARY HAEMOPOIESIS (myeloid metaplasia) is an invariable concomitant.

Marrow: ordinary marrow puncture usually results in a 'dry tap', therefore trephine or cutting needle biopsy is required.

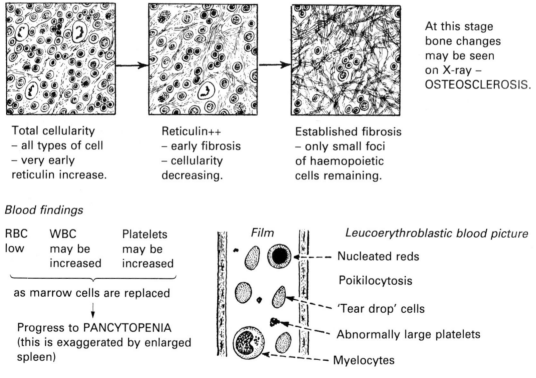

Total cellularity
– all types of cell
– very early
reticulin increase.

Reticulin++
– early fibrosis
– cellularity
decreasing.

Established fibrosis
– only small foci
of haemopoietic
cells remaining.

At this stage
bone changes
may be seen
on X-ray –
OSTEOSCLEROSIS.

Blood findings

RBC	WBC	Platelets
low	may be increased	may be increased

as marrow cells are replaced

↓

Progress to PANCYTOPENIA
(this is exaggerated by enlarged spleen)

Film   *Leucoerythroblastic blood picture*

– – Nucleated reds

Poikilocytosis

– 'Tear drop' cells

– Abnormally large platelets

– Myelocytes

Note: The Philadelphia chromosome is absent (cf. chronic myeloid leukaemia).

POLYCYTHAEMIA VERA

In this condition, erythroid proliferation predominates (see p.534).

THROMBOCYTHAEMIA (ESSENTIAL)

In this condition, megakaryocytic proliferation is associated with increased circulating platelets. The signs of the disease which range from spontaneous bleedings to thromboses are associated with abnormality of platelet function.

In these chronic myeloproliferative disorders, progress to marrow fibrosis is a common end result.

546

DISEASES OF THE BONE MARROW

Myeloproliferative Disorders (continued)

EXTRA-MEDULLARY HAEMOPOIESIS (Myeloid metaplasia)

When the blood forming capacity of the bone marrow is impaired, the primitive stem cells, still resident in the extra-medullary sites of haemopoiesis of fetal life, may be stimulated.

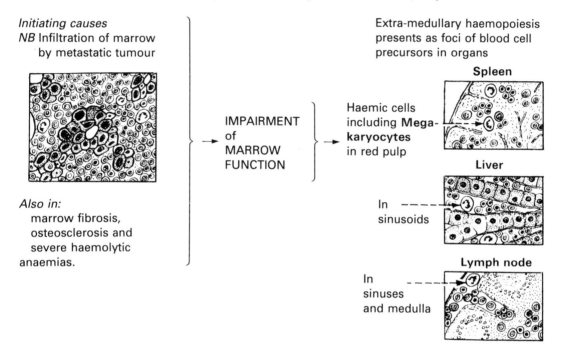

Initiating causes
NB Infiltration of marrow by metastatic tumour

Also in:
marrow fibrosis, osteosclerosis and severe haemolytic anaemias.

IMPAIRMENT of MARROW FUNCTION

Extra-medullary haemopoiesis presents as foci of blood cell precursors in organs

Haemic cells including **Megakaryocytes** in red pulp

Spleen

In sinusoids

Liver

In sinuses and medulla

Lymph node

In these conditions extra-medullary haemopoiesis is compensatory.

The most extreme forms of splenic enlargement due to extra-medullary haemopoiesis are seen in **MYELOPROLIFERATIVE DISORDERS** at the **MARROW FIBROSIS** stage.

Two factors combine:

1. Compensation for fibrosis of marrow
2. Stimulation of extra-medullary haemopoiesis by the unknown mechanism which is responsible for the myeloproliferation.

NB Hypersplenism due to the enlarged spleen aggravates the pancytopenia.

COAGULATION DEFICIENCY DISEASES

FIBRINOLYSIS

Clotting of blood naturally occurs in vessels, even after trivial injury. To control this process another mechanism – the fibrinolytic system – exists which limits clot deposition by lysing fibrin.

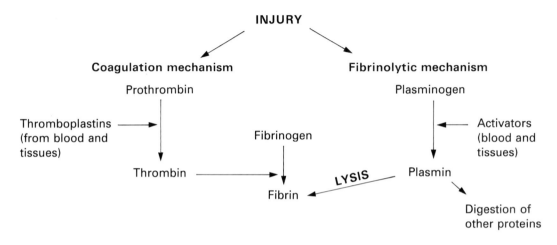

Normally these two mechanisms are activated at the same time and are in dynamic equilibrium. The lytic activity modifies the coagulation process preventing excessive or continued clotting. The fibrinolytic process is also activated during repair of wounds and helps to remove the fibrin scaffold when no longer required.

Sometimes the balance between coagulation and lysis is upset. This is particularly apt to happen in those conditions leading to acquired afibrinogenaemia. Not only is coagulation progressively reduced but the clots formed are of poor quality.

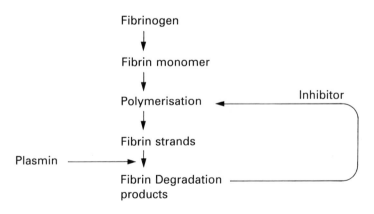

550   The poorly formed fibrin is more susceptible to fibrinolysis and a vicious circle ensues.

COAGULATION DEFICIENCY DISEASES

FIBRINOLYSIS (continued)

As the lytic activity intensifies, the patient often shows symptoms of stress in a degree quite unrelated to the severity of the causal condition. The mechanism may be as follows:

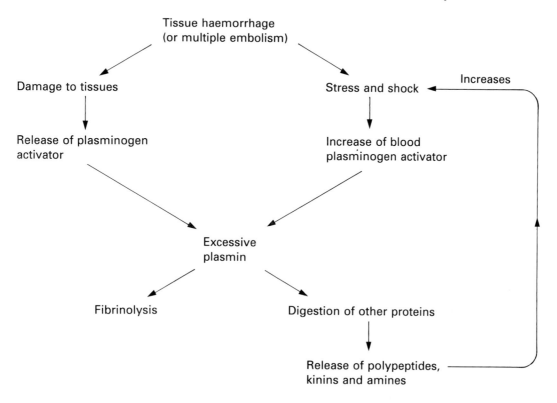

Kinins are produced by digestion of α_2 globulins. They cause pain, increased permeability of capillaries, contraction of some smooth muscles and relaxation of others.

As a result of these complex interlocking mechanisms, the patient becomes increasingly shocked and the incoagulable condition of the blood is difficult to correct.

ANTI-COAGULANT THERAPY

Dicoumarol has already been mentioned (p.549). Heparin, commonly used therapeutically as an anticoagulant, inhibits the conversion of prothrombin to thrombin and also the action of thrombin on fibrinogen. Overdosage with heparin will result in incoagulability of the blood and possible haemorrhages from mucous membranes.

THROMBOCYTOPENIA

Although the normal platelet count ranges from $150\text{--}400 \times 10^9/l$, a risk of dangerous spontaneous haemorrhage is unusual unless the count falls below $30 \times 10^9/l$.

The causes of thrombocytopenia fall into two main groups:

1. Deficient marrow production

Hypoplasia or aplasia
Replacement } of marrow
(e.g. leukaemia, fibrosis)

Dyshaemopoiesis
(e.g. Vit B_{12} deficiency)

2. Increased destruction

Platelets damaged by *drugs*, *immune mechanisms*

Platelets sequestered in *hypersplenism*

Platelets utilised in coagulative disorders (e.g. DIC)

NB Marrow examination throws light on the possible mechanism.

In (1) megakaryocytes are reduced in number (except in vit. B_{12} deficiency)

In (2) megakaryocytes are increased and immature in an attempt to make good the platelet loss

Idiopathic thrombocytopenia (ITP) occurs particularly in children and is usually self limiting; evidence has accumulated that platelet antibodies are responsible. The marrow picture is characteristic with numerous megakaryocytes.

PURPURA

This is the term used for disorders involving bleeding from capillaries, with the production of small petechial spots. In severe cases, more massive bleeding occurs; the subarachnoid space, the alimentary and renal tracts are particularly vulnerable. Thrombocytopenia is the most common cause, but abnormalities of the capillary walls are also due to a variety of agents, e.g. vit C deficiency, allergic immune reactions (Henoch-Schönlein purpura), drugs acting both directly and also as haptens, infections and intoxications and the hereditary condition, haemorrhagic telangiectasis. In the purpuras, the clinical tests for increased capillary fragility are usually positive, while the laboratory tests of coagulation function are normal.

BLOOD TRANSFUSION

Two antigenic group systems, ABO and Rhesus, are of paramount importance, but blood is a complex mixture of many antigenic substances and the increasing use of blood and blood products can give rise to new antibodies with the danger of reactions.

ABO system

One of three alleles, A, B or O, is borne on each of two chromosomes. There are thus six possible genotypes – AA, BB, AB, AO, BO and OO. The O allele is nonantigenic and therefore individuals can be divided into four groups – A, B, AB and O. Plasma contains natural antibodies to the A and B antigens according to the rule: – the particular antibody, anti-A or anti-B, is present in the plasma, provided the red cells do not contain the corresponding antigen. Thus:

Blood group	Antigens on cells	Isoantibodies in plasma
A	AA or AO	Anti-B
B	BB or BO	Anti-A
AB	A + B	none
O	None	Anti-A + Anti-B

AB individuals having no antibodies in their plasma could receive blood of any group and have been termed 'Universal Recipients'. Similarly, group O blood possessing no antigens could be given to any person and is termed 'Universal Donor'. Except in dire emergencies, however, neither of these actions should be taken.

The distribution of these blood groups varies with geography. In Western Scotland, the incidence of the various groups is as follows:

Group O – 53% Group A – 33%
Group B – 11% Group AB – 3%

The distribution is changing due to population movement and immigration.

Rhesus system

This is another sequence of red cell antigens – first discovered in Rhesus monkeys. There are three pairs of alleles, C or c, D or d, E or e, one of each pair occupying a position on one chromosome, i.e. if C is absent c is present, D absent d present, E absent e present, and vice versa. With any three of the six alleles transmitted by each parent, the genetic make-up is very varied.

BLOOD TRANSFUSION

Rhesus system (continued)

The most frequent groupings of three alleles on one chromosome in the United Kingdom are: CDe, cde, cDE. The most common genotypes are:

(Abbreviated notation) ‒ ‒ ‒ ➤	CDe/CDe – 17.5% (R R)	cde/cde – 15.0% (r r)	cDE/cde – 5.0% (R r)
	CDe/cde – 16.0% (R r)	CDe/cDE – 6.0% (R R)	Other combinations are rare

The D antigen has the strongest antigenic power and individuals possessing it are termed Rhesus positive. Those who have no D antigen (homozygous for d) are termed Rhesus negative and are at greatest risk of developing antibodies if given Rhesus positive blood. The C antigen also has strong antigenic activity and it is important to test for this antigen and its corresponding antibody.

There are no natural antibodies to Rhesus antigens. They only arise when red cells bearing Rhesus antigens foreign to the patient are introduced into the circulation. They develop in two particular situations:

1. After a Rhesus incompatible transfusion, especially if the transfused cells contain the D antigen and the patient is Rhesus negative.
2. In a proportion of pregnant Rhesus negative women, Rhesus positive (D derived from the father) fetal red cells escape into the maternal circulation inducing antibody formation. The antibody crosses the placenta and causes haemolysis of fetal red cells (see p. 522). Rhesus positive blood must never be given to a Rhesus negative patient.

In emergency, where Rhesus grouping is impossible, Rhesus negative ABO compatible blood is given.

Grouping and cross-matching
ABO grouping

1. Standardised anti-A and anti-B sera are used.
2. The test red cells are mixed with the appropriate antiserum.
3. Controls are set up with the individual's RBC versus:
      Group O serum (contains both anti-A and anti-B) and versus:
      Group AB serum (contains no antibodies and should cause no reaction).
The whole set of tests is carried out at room temperature.

Agglutination reaction

	Anti-A	Anti-B	Group O	Group
Patient's RBC	+	–	+	A
or	–	+	+	B
Donor's RBC	+	+	+	AB
	–	–	–	0

BLOOD TRANSFUSION

Grouping and cross-matching (continued)

Rhesus grouping

Anti-C and anti-D are both used. These antisera are collected from sensitised donors and standardised. A mixture of the two antisera previously absorbed to remove anti-A and anti-B is used, and the reactions must be carried out at 37°C.

Despite tests for ABO and Rhesus groupings, mistakes can still occur due to:

1. Faulty testing – very infrequent
2. Irregular antibodies
3. Clerical errors – wrong identification of patients, donors, specimens, containers, storage.

A final cross-matching test is carried out before transfusion. The red cells of each donor unit of blood are tested against the patient's plasma for the possibility of an antibody reaction against them.

DANGERS of blood transfusion

In addition to incompatibility, other dangers arise in transfusion practice:

1. *Reactions occurring during or very shortly after transfusion*

   (a) Fever – may be due to pyrogens in the blood or allergies to degradation products of leucocytes.

   (b) Biochemical disturbances – particularly in massive transfusions or if out-dated blood is used.
   (i) Hypocalcaemia (citrate in blood binds Ca^{++}).
   (ii) Hyperkalaemia (lysed RBCs contribute excess K^+).

   (c) Circulatory overload – in cases of anaemia or incipient cardiac failure where transfusion is too rapid or excessive.

2. *Delayed infections*

   Hepatitis B, AIDS and other infections, e.g. syphilis and malaria are potential risks.

THE LYMPHO-RETICULAR TISSUES

The basic function of these tissues is FILTRATION of a variety of materials varying from 'foreign' microorganisms and particles to the degradation products of cells and metabolism.
Filtration occurs at the following sites:

Lymph nodes – tissue fluids
Nasopharynx – tonsils and adenoids
Alimentary tract – submucous lymphoid aggregations } – surfaces
Spleen – blood.

In the two remaining important lymphoid organs, filtration is not an important function:

Thymus – T lymphocyte processing.
Bone marrow – site of (a) mature lymphoid aggregates
(b) lymphoid stem cells.

In addition, microscopic aggregates of lymphoid cells are scattered throughout the body.

The LYMPH NODES in DISEASE
The basic anatomy reflects the primary function.

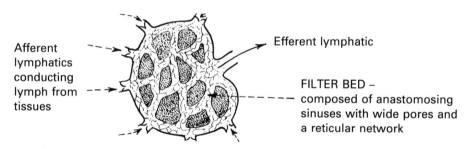

Afferent lymphatics conducting lymph from tissues

Efferent lymphatic

FILTER BED –
composed of anastomosing sinuses with wide pores and a reticular network

In addition, the presence of special cells reflects functions superimposed on filtration.

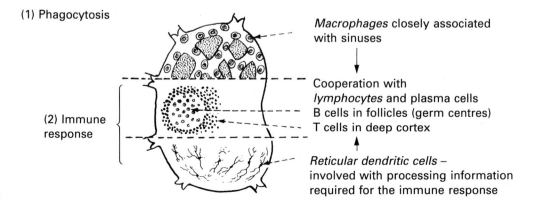

(1) Phagocytosis

Macrophages closely associated with sinuses

Cooperation with *lymphocytes* and plasma cells
B cells in follicles (germ centres)
T cells in deep cortex

(2) Immune response

Reticular dendritic cells – involved with processing information required for the immune response

DISEASES OF THE LYMPH NODES

The LYMPH NODES in DISEASE (continued)

In physiological conditions, the lymph nodes are small and show minimal evidence of functional activity: the major contribution towards disposal of particles derived from metabolic processes is performed by the spleen.

Very shortly after infection occurs or when the nodes begin to filter noxious particles, **reactive changes** occur – usually causing enlargement of the nodes.

The changes may be **general** - - - - or - - - - **local** – reflecting disease in the
in systemic INFECTIONS drainage area, e.g. simple chronic gastric
– bacterial or viral, ulcer (enlarged reactive nodes in omentum)
e.g. syphilis, measles – local low grade inflammation;
$\pm$ absorption of foreign particles.

The changes include three basic and several subsidiary:

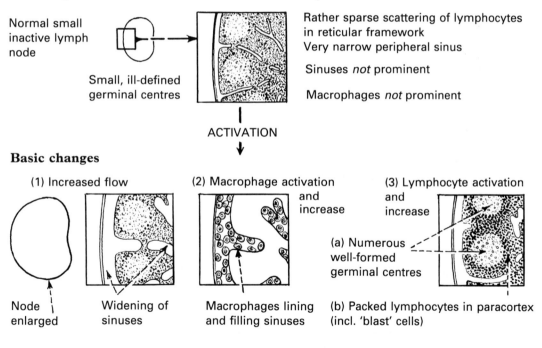

Normal small inactive lymph node

Small, ill-defined germinal centres

Rather sparse scattering of lymphocytes in reticular framework
Very narrow peripheral sinus

Sinuses *not* prominent

Macrophages *not* prominent

ACTIVATION

Basic changes

(1) Increased flow

Node enlarged | Widening of sinuses

(2) Macrophage activation and increase

Macrophages lining and filling sinuses

(3) Lymphocyte activation and increase

(a) Numerous well-formed germinal centres

(b) Packed lymphocytes in paracortex (incl. 'blast' cells)

Subsidiary changes

1. Infiltration by neutrophils (in acute inflammation)
2. Increased blood flow (prominent venules)
3. Increased plasma cells
4. Increased eosinophils
} → Chronic inflammation

The qualitative and quantitative variations and combinations of these changes are very numerous; in most reactive states the appearances are non-specific. In only a few instances do particular patterns of response reflect a specific stimulus.

559

ACUTE LYMPH NODE ENLARGEMENT

This is usually due to acute infections causing **ACUTE LYMPHADENITIS**.

(a) In many bacterial infections neutrophil infiltration is a feature.

Typhoid fever is an exception – mesenteric node.

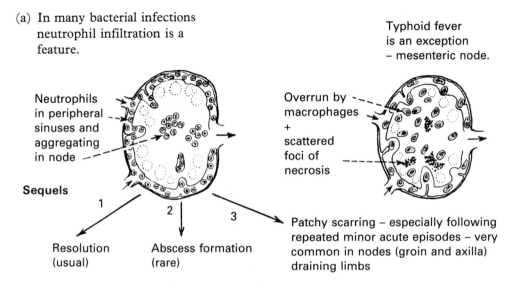

Neutrophils in peripheral sinuses and aggregating in node

Overrun by macrophages + scattered foci of necrosis

Sequels

1
2
3

Resolution (usual)

Abscess formation (rare)

Patchy scarring – especially following repeated minor acute episodes – very common in nodes (groin and axilla) draining limbs

(b) In the majority of acute virus infections, neutrophils are absent and the nonspecific reactive changes previously described are seen.

In **GLANDULAR FEVER** (Infectious mononucleosis), a virus infection (Epstein–Barr virus) of young adults, the cervical lymph nodes are particularly involved.

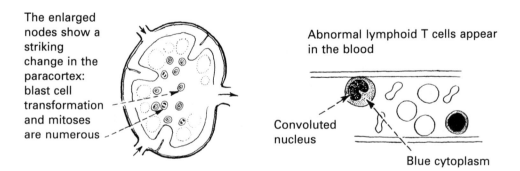

The enlarged nodes show a striking change in the paracortex: blast cell transformation and mitoses are numerous

Abnormal lymphoid T cells appear in the blood

Convoluted nucleus

Blue cytoplasm

Similar changes are seen in the pharyngeal lymphoid tissues, the spleen and bone marrow.

ACUTE LYMPH NODE ENLARGEMENT

Diagnostic tests
In addition to virus-specific antibodies, the infection evokes the production of non-specific antibodies. These are detected using the agglutination of animal red cells as indicators.

The Paul Bunnell test – sheep erythrocytes in tubes.
The Monospot test – formalinised horse and sheep erythrocytes on a slide.

In **MEASLES**, the reactive nodes and lymphoid tissues generally contain unusual, multinucleate **giant cells** (Warthin-Finkeldey).

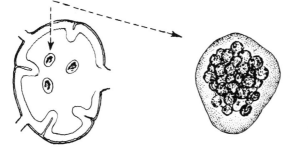

This is a good example of virus fused cells

In **LYMPHOGRANULOMA VENEREUM (LGV)**, the enlarged lymph nodes show a striking histological appearance.
LGV is an infection by a **chlamydial** organism. The portal of entry is by venereal contact and the disease runs a subacute course.

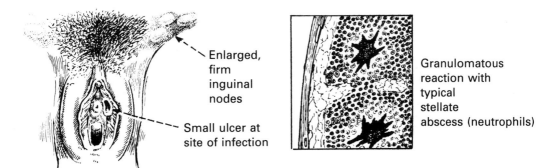

Enlarged, firm inguinal nodes

Small ulcer at site of infection

Granulomatous reaction with typical stellate abscess (neutrophils)

The diagnosis has to be confirmed by a skin test (Frei test) or a complement fixation test.

In **CAT SCRATCH FEVER**, the nodes draining the scratched area show similar histological changes but the organism has not yet been identified.

561

CHRONIC LYMPH NODE ENLARGEMENT

This common and important clinical sign may give rise to difficulty in diagnosis in practice.

Aetiology

The many and varied causes are considered under three main headings:

1. **Enlargement due to low grade chronic INFLAMMATION, local or general**
   In most cases, the enlargement is due to reactive hyperplasia and the morphological changes are essentially similar so that the aetiology cannot be deduced from the histological appearance of the node.

   Specific diagnosis depends on identification of the infecting organism (a) by direct staining and/or (b) by culture and/or (c) by serological tests for specific antibodies.

   In only a few conditions do the histological appearances give a clue to the aetiology, e.g. (a) tuberculosis and sarcoidosis and (b) toxoplasmosis.

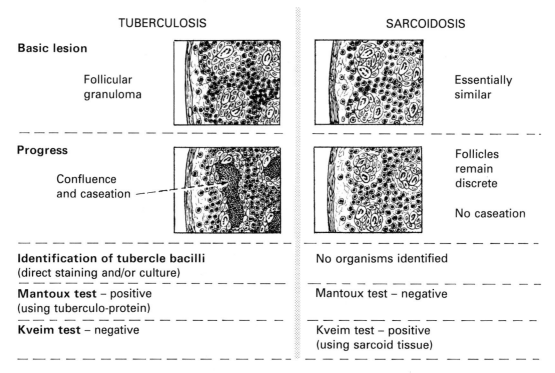

	TUBERCULOSIS	SARCOIDOSIS
Basic lesion	Follicular granuloma	Essentially similar
Progress	Confluence and caseation	Follicles remain discrete — No caseation
	Identification of tubercle bacilli (direct staining and/or culture)	No organisms identified
	Mantoux test – positive (using tuberculo-protein)	Mantoux test – negative
	Kveim test – negative	Kveim test – positive (using sarcoid tissue)

Somewhat similar follicular granulomata occur in other conditions, e.g. Crohn's disease, primary biliary cirrhosis, and other penetrating ulcerations of the alimentary tract.

CHRONIC LYMPH NODE ENLARGEMENT

Low grade infections (continued)

TOXOPLASMOSIS

In toxoplasmosis, a protozoal disease (*Toxoplasma gondii*) which may cause serious damage to the fetus or neonate and present with lymph node enlargement in the adult, the histological appearances in the node may indicate the aetiology. The diagnosis has to be confirmed by a serological dye test.

In addition to the usual reactive changes

↓

A scattering of small epithelioid granulomas — — — — — — —

↓

Numerous smaller monocytoid 'B' cells in the sinuses — — — — —

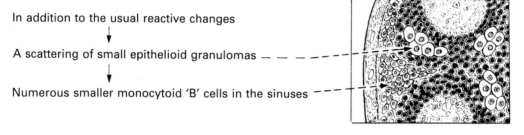

2. Enlargement due to filtration of surfaces and tissues – NON-INFECTIVE

In these conditions, particulate matter (and in some cases soluble material) of a non-infective nature is filtered and deposited in excess. In the majority of cases, there is a reactive hyperplasia and the enlargement is accentuated if the particles have an 'irritant' effect.

The source of particles may be:
Exogenous, e.g. exposure to environmental pollutant (lung hilar lymph nodes in SILICOSIS)
Endogenous, due to breakdown of tissues or abnormal metabolism,
e.g. (a) In **tumour necrosis**

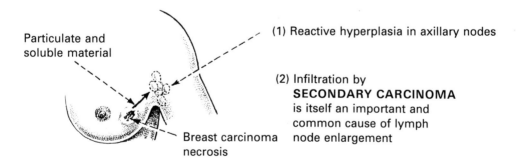

Particulate and soluble material

Breast carcinoma necrosis

(1) Reactive hyperplasia in axillary nodes

(2) Infiltration by **SECONDARY CARCINOMA** is itself an important and common cause of lymph node enlargement

In tumour cases, the distinction between these two causes of lymph node enlargement can only be made with certainty by histological examination.

CHRONIC LYMPH NODE ENLARGEMENT

Filtration – Non-infective (continued)

(b) In **chronic skin disease** with a considerable component of tissue damage.

In addition to the usual reactive hyperplasia the following may be seen lying free and in macrophages:
    Fat
    Melanin – from damaged skin
    Haemosiderin – from minor bleeding in skin

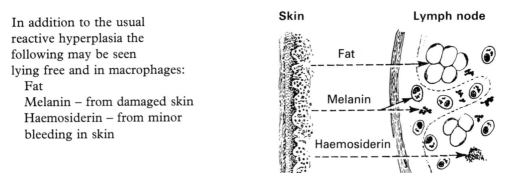

The identification of these substances in the node allows the diagnosis of **DERMATOPATHIC LYMPHADENOPATHY** (lipomelanic 'reticulosis').

In **metabolic diseases** such as haemachromatosis (p.30) and the storage diseases (p.20) the lymph nodes are enlarged due to the presence of large quantities of the abnormal deposit (e.g. iron, lipids). The contribution of reactive hyperplasia to the enlargement is usually small.

3. **Enlargement due to PRIMARY LYMPHOID NEOPLASMS** (see p.582)
    The main examples are:
      Hodgkin's disease and the non-Hodgkin's lymphomas particularly the follicular lymphomas in which lymph node enlargement may be considerable.
      There is an additional group of conditions involving a proliferation of macrophages, called histiocytosis-X in which lymph node enlargement is often a feature.

SPLEEN

The anatomy of the spleen reflects both its basic function, which is filtration of the blood, and sequential functions of phagocytosis and the immune response. Normal average weight – 150 g.

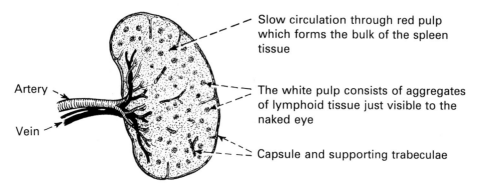

Slow circulation through red pulp which forms the bulk of the spleen tissue

Artery

Vein

The white pulp consists of aggregates of lymphoid tissue just visible to the naked eye

Capsule and supporting trabeculae

Microscopic appearance

Lymphoid aggregate – mediates IMMUNE RESPONSE.

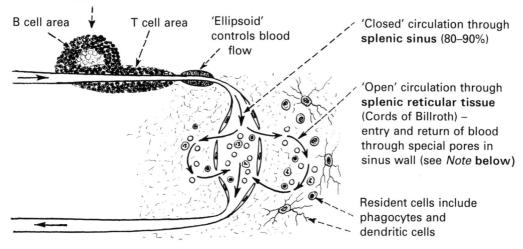

B cell area   T cell area   'Ellipsoid' controls blood flow

'Closed' circulation through **splenic sinus (80–90%)**

'Open' circulation through **splenic reticular tissue (Cords of Billroth)** – entry and return of blood through special pores in sinus wall (see *Note* below)

Resident cells include phagocytes and dendritic cells

The red pulp is the site of filtration and phagocytosis of the following:

1. Effete cells and cell debris – especially blood cells but also cell debris derived from the body generally

2. Microbes and their toxins

3. Abnormal or excess material derived from metabolic processes.

Note: The special pores allowing re-entry of RBCs to the circulation have a 2μ aperture: abnormal RBCs (e.g. spherocytes) cannot pass through and are trapped.

565

SPLENOMEGALY

Enlargement of the spleen is an important and common clinical sign. Increase in the red pulp due to increased numbers of phagocytes and/or increased numbers of blood cells is the major component; in chronic infections particularly, hyperplasia of the lymphoid tissue contributes.

An aetiological classification under 5 broad headings is convenient.

Enlargement associated with:

1. INFECTIONS
2. CIRCULATORY DISTURBANCES
3. STORAGE DISEASES and DEGENERATIONS
4. NEOPLASIA – primary and secondary
5. DISORDERS OF THE BLOOD.

1. INFECTIONS

In acute systemic bacterial infections the spleen shows slight to moderate enlargement (200–400 g).

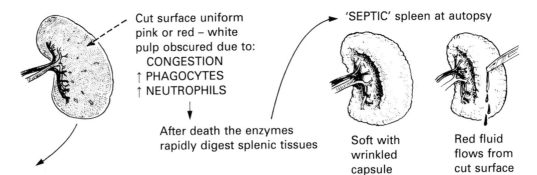

Cut surface uniform pink or red – white pulp obscured due to:
CONGESTION
↑ PHAGOCYTES
↑ NEUTROPHILS
↓
After death the enzymes rapidly digest splenic tissues

'SEPTIC' spleen at autopsy

Soft with wrinkled capsule

Red fluid flows from cut surface

Sequels

(a) Resolution as infection resolves.
(b) Occasionally spreads through capsule (perisplenitis) to adjacent tissues, with or without abscess formation.
(c) Only extremely rarely does abscess formation occur within the spleen.

In non-pyogenic and chronic infections, there may be moderate enlargement.

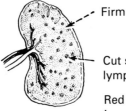

Firm

Cut surface shows lymphoid aggregates

Red pulp contains increased PHAGOCYTES often PLASMA CELLS

Examples: Subacute bacterial endocarditis
Tuberculosis
Typhoid fever
Infectious mononucleosis
Brucellosis
Malaria ⎱ protozoal
Kala-azar ⎰ diseases
– often massive enlargement

SPLENOMEGALY

2. CIRCULATORY DISTURBANCES

Congestive splenomegaly occurs in two main conditions:

(1) Congestive cardiac failure

Systemic venous congestion

Dilated failing heart

Hepatic veins

Splenic vein

Portal vein increased pressure

Centrilobular congestion is reflected through the liver to the portal vein

(2) Hepatic cirrhosis

Normal systemic venous return

Normal heart

Splenic vein

Portal vein increased pressure

Obstruction to portal venous flow due to fibrosis in liver

SPLENIC ENLARGEMENT

Moderate – rarely exceeds 500 g

Consistency – firm to hard; so-called 'cricket ball' spleen

Cut surface purple; white pulp just visible

May be severe, *e.g.* 1000+ g
May be focal capsular thickening

Consistency – firm to hard
Cut surface – pink to purple depending on amount of fibrous tissue

Small lymphoid aggregate

May be flecked with small brown spots (Gandy-Gamma nodules) due to organisation of old haemorrhages

Permanently dilated sinuses

The type of splenomegaly associated with portal venous hypertension may have serious haematological effects (see Hypersplenism).

567

SPLENOMEGALY

3. STORAGE DISEASES AND DEGENERATIONS
The diseases associated with this type of enlargement are rare.

Examples are:

Amyloidosis (see pp.21–24)

Lipid storage diseases, (see p.20) including Gaucher's disease,
Neimann Pick disease and Tay-Sachs disease

Some disorders of glycogen storage.

4. NEOPLASIA

(a) PRIMARY – the spleen is rarely the seat of primary tumour growth.

(b) SECONDARY – the spleen is rarely affected by other types of secondary tumour, e.g. carcinoma and sarcoma, but it is commonly affected during the systematised spread of **lymphomas** and **leukaemias**.

Normal
spleen
150 g

Moderate
enlargement
500 g

Massive
enlargement
1500 g

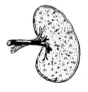

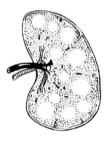

Nodules of white
lymphoma tissue
e.g. Hodgkin's disease

Uniform, beefy, cut surface
in chronic leukaemia

Splenic enlargement may be a feature of histiocytosis-X (see p.595).

SPLENOMEGALY

5. DISORDERS OF THE BLOOD
Splenic enlargement is associated with blood disorders in two main circumstances:

1. **Splenic enlargement causing blood disorders**

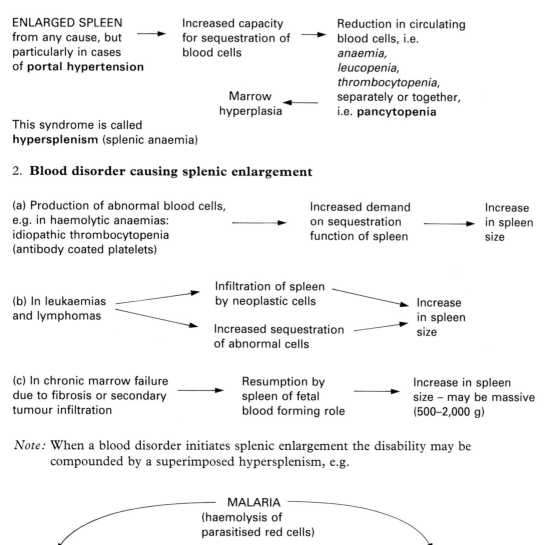

ENLARGED SPLEEN
from any cause, but
particularly in cases
of **portal hypertension** → Increased capacity
for sequestration of
blood cells → Reduction in circulating
blood cells, i.e.
anaemia,
leucopenia,
thrombocytopenia,
separately or together,
i.e. **pancytopenia**

Marrow ←
hyperplasia

This syndrome is called
hypersplenism (splenic anaemia)

2. **Blood disorder causing splenic enlargement**

(a) Production of abnormal blood cells,
e.g. in haemolytic anaemias:
idiopathic thrombocytopenia
(antibody coated platelets) → Increased demand
on sequestration
function of spleen → Increase
in spleen
size

(b) In leukaemias
and lymphomas → Infiltration of spleen
by neoplastic cells

Increased sequestration
of abnormal cells → Increase
in spleen
size

(c) In chronic marrow failure
due to fibrosis or secondary
tumour infiltration → Resumption by
spleen of fetal
blood forming role → Increase in spleen
size – may be massive
(500–2,000 g)

Note: When a blood disorder initiates splenic enlargement the disability may be
compounded by a superimposed hypersplenism, e.g.

MALARIA
(haemolysis of
parasitised red cells)

ANAEMIA

SPLENIC ENLARGEMENT

Anaemia
aggravated

INCREASED
SEQUESTRATION of RBCs

(HYPERSPLENISM)

569

DISEASES OF THE SPLEEN – MISCELLANEOUS

HYPOSPLENISM
Hyposplenism is not usually a cause of major disability. It occurs following splenectomy and in cases of splenic atrophy.

The effects are considered under two main headings:

1. **On the cells of the blood**

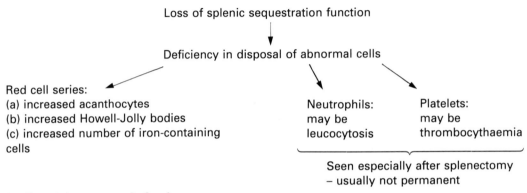

Loss of splenic sequestration function

↓

Deficiency in disposal of abnormal cells

Red cell series:
(a) increased acanthocytes
(b) increased Howell-Jolly bodies
(c) increased number of iron-containing cells

Neutrophils: may be leucocytosis

Platelets: may be thrombocythaemia

Seen especially after splenectomy – usually not permanent

2. **On resistance to infection**

Loss of filtration of bacteria from blood ⟶ Occasional cases of **septicaemia** – especially caused by *Streptococcus pneumoniae* – young children are particularly susceptible

CIRCULATORY AND VASCULAR CHANGES

(a) *Infarction*
(i) Embolism causing infarction is not uncommon but usually clinically unimportant.

(ii) Enlarged spleens are particularly susceptible to infarction without embolism.

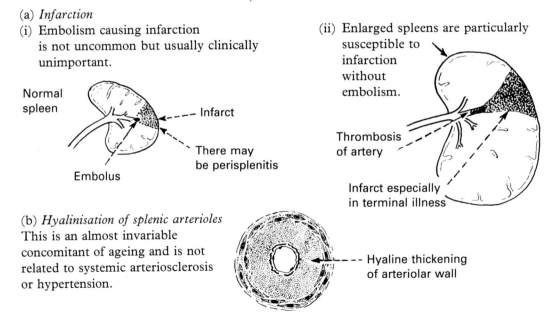

Normal spleen

Infarct

There may be perisplenitis

Embolus

Thrombosis of artery

Infarct especially in terminal illness

(b) *Hyalinisation of splenic arterioles*
This is an almost invariable concomitant of ageing and is not related to systemic arteriosclerosis or hypertension.

Hyaline thickening of arteriolar wall

THYMUS

This 'primary' lymphoid organ is concerned with the development and processing to maturation of the long-lived T lymphocytes which are then distributed to the lymphoid tissues and to the circulating pool of T lymphocytes.

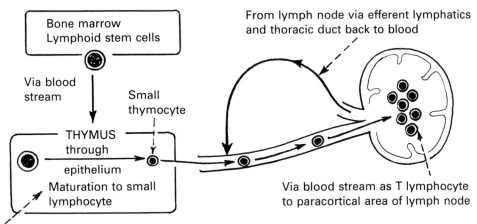

Mechanism – stimulation by hormones formed locally by thymic epithelial cells.

This activity is maximal in the fetal and childhood stages. Involution is rapid after puberty.

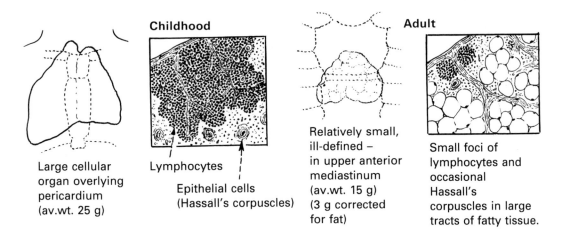

Large cellular organ overlying pericardium (av.wt. 25 g)

Childhood

Lymphocytes

Epithelial cells (Hassall's corpuscles)

Adult

Relatively small, ill-defined – in upper anterior mediastinum (av.wt. 15 g) (3 g corrected for fat)

Small foci of lymphocytes and occasional Hassall's corpuscles in large tracts of fatty tissue.

Congenital thymic aplasia or hypoplasia

The resulting T cell deficiency is associated with disordered cell-mediated immune response.

Note: Thymectomy in adult life has little pathological significance since the T lymphocytes produced in childhood are long enough lived to obviate serious immune deficiency.

571

THYMUS

Thymic hyperplasia

Assessment by weight alone is unsatisfactory due to the variability of the fat content in adult life. A weight over 35 g probably represents hyperplasia, but the appearance of lymphoid follicles with germinal centres is a more reliable indication of hyperplasia.

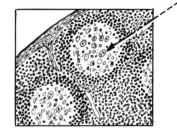

Associated conditions:
    Auto-immune disorders,
      e.g. Systemic lupus erythematosus
      Addison's disease
      Thyrotoxicosis
      Pancytopaenia
      and *NB* MYASTHENIA GRAVIS

Thymic tumours

Thymomas are rare tumours: they are essentially low-grade carcinomas with an admixture of lymphoid cells: they rarely metastasise. They may have an auto-immune component similar to thymic hyperplasia.

The sheer bulk of these lobulated and nodular tumours compresses adjacent mediastinal structures

(a) Compression of respiratory passages → dyspnoea and cough.

(b) Oesphagus → dysphagia.

(c) Great veins → cyanosis and suffusion of face.

Other primary tumours arising in the thymus are;
    (1) T cell lymphoblastic lymphomas (adolescent males).
    (2) Hodgkin's disease.
    (3) Germ cell tumours (e.g. teratoma).
    (4) Carcinoids.

The thymus in Myasthenia Gravis (MG)

MG is a disease of voluntary muscles in which weakness is the main feature. The association with the thymus is striking in that 4/5 of all cases of MG have either thymic hyperplasia or thymoma.

Follicular hyperplasia (80%) – seen especially in young females.
Thymoma (20%) – seen especially in middle aged males.
The results of thymectomy in MG patients are very unpredictable.

    The detailed pathological changes in MG and the mechanisms by which the thymus is linked with the disease are described on page 768.

LEUKAEMIA

Primary neoplasia of the bone marrow and lymphoreticular tissues

Since all these tissues are the sites of blood cell production or important staging posts in the complex circulation of the blood cells, it is convenient to consider their tumours together.

1. Neoplastic proliferation in the bone marrow usually leads to an increased number of circulating white blood cells – the condition is called LEUKAEMIA.

   In some cases there is no spill over into the blood, and the white cell count is low or normal – this condition is called ALEUKAEMIC LEUKAEMIA.

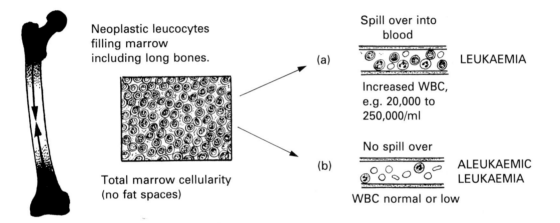

Neoplastic leucocytes filling marrow including long bones.

Total marrow cellularity (no fat spaces)

Spill over into blood

(a) LEUKAEMIA

Increased WBC, e.g. 20,000 to 250,000/ml

No spill over

(b) ALEUKAEMIC LEUKAEMIA

WBC normal or low

2. Neoplastic proliferation within the lymphoid tissues results in solid tumours – called LYMPHOMAS, but in some cases spill over into the blood occurs (leukaemic phase).

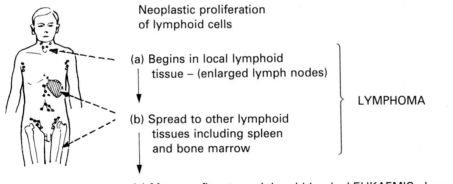

Neoplastic proliferation of lymphoid cells

(a) Begins in local lymphoid tissue – (enlarged lymph nodes)

(b) Spread to other lymphoid tissues including spleen and bone marrow

} LYMPHOMA

(c) May overflow to peripheral blood – LEUKAEMIC phase

573

LEUKAEMIA

In all leukaemias, the marrow is eventually over-run by functionally abnormal neoplastic cells.

CELL KINETICS

Cell longevity beyond the normal (due to failure of response to mechanisms controlling ageing and destruction) is as important as proliferative rates in increasing the marrow cell population.

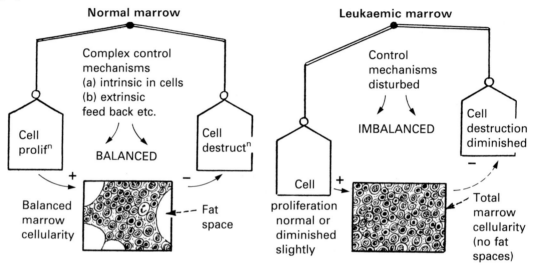

The rate at which marrow overcrowding occurs influences the rate of progress of the disease and allows classification into two broad groups: (1) the ACUTE and (2) the CHRONIC LEUKAEMIAS.

Cell differentiation

The ability of the leukaemic cells to differentiate also reflects the rate of progress.

Acute leukaemia
Numerous 'blast' cells.

Chronic leukaemia
Few blast cells – numerous cells on differentiation pathway to granulocytes or lymphocytes.

Considerations of cell kinetics and differentiations are important in treatment.

Further classification in two main groups depends on the neoplastic cell types.

(a) MYELOID LEUKAEMIA
– cells of the granulocytic series.

(b) LYMPHOCYTIC LEUKAEMIA
– cells of the lymphoid series.

Rarer leukaemias are of monocytic and plasma cell types. Similar proliferative conditions can affect red cells and megakaryocytes.

LEUKAEMIA

The marrow overcrowding and, more important, the functional abnormalities of the neoplastic cells lead to functional marrow failure and the complications which cause the major clinical signs.

Complications

(1) Deficiency of red cell production – **anaemia**
(2) Deficiency of platelet production – **thrombocytopenia** – bleeding tendency
(3) Deficiency of granulocyte phagocytic activity ⎫ FAILURE TO CONTROL
    Deficiency of lymphocytic immune response ⎭   INFECTION

   These complications occur rapidly and are lethal in acute leukaemia; in chronic leukaemia they may not develop for many years.

(4) Gout: the increased turnover of nuclear material leads to increased synthesis of uric acid and, in some cases, to clinical gout.

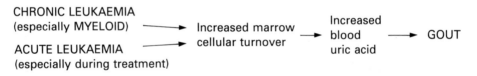

CHRONIC LEUKAEMIA
(especially MYELOID) ⟶   Increased marrow ⟶ Increased blood uric acid ⟶ GOUT
ACUTE LEUKAEMIA ⟶   cellular turnover
(especially during treatment)

Metastases

Since leukaemic cells have a natural tendency to circulate in the blood and/or lymph, it is theoretically possible for metastasis to occur anywhere in the body. Nodular deposits in the body generally are rare however.

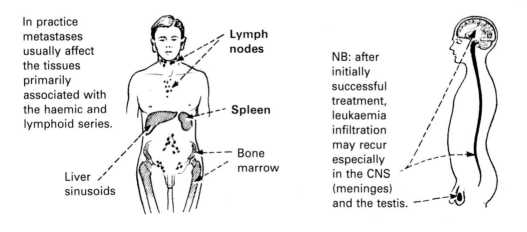

In practice metastases usually affect the tissues primarily associated with the haemic and lymphoid series.

Lymph nodes

Spleen

Bone marrow

Liver sinusoids

NB: after initially successful treatment, leukaemia infiltration may recur especially in the CNS (meninges) and the testis.

THE ACUTE LEUKAEMIAS

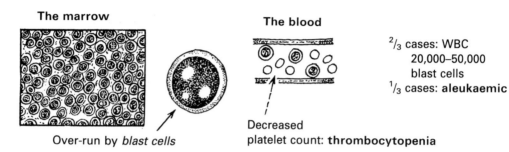

The marrow

Over-run by *blast cells*

The blood

Decreased
platelet count: **thrombocytopenia**

$^2/_3$ cases: WBC
20,000–50,000
blast cells
$^1/_3$ cases: **aleukaemic**

Other organs + splenomegaly + hepatomegaly + lymph node enlargement

Since modern chemotherapy is geared to the neoplastic cell type, it is important, if possible, to establish an accurate diagnosis. The most primitive blast cells are truly undifferentiated. However in most cases the cells go a short way towards differentiation. Cytochemical tests, particularly with enzyme markers, are used.

The modern classification (FAB) of the acute myeloid leukaemia includes the relatively rare monocytic or promyelocytic types.

Monocytic leukaemia

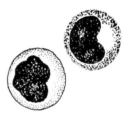

There are two morphological types:

1. The Naegeli (myelomonocytic) type –
   the cells have 'myeloid' features
2. The Schilling type –
   the cells closely resemble monocytes.

The serum contains an increased amount of lysozyme (muramidase) produced by the tumour cells.

Promyelocytic leukaemia

In this subtype maturation arrest occurs at the promyelocyte stage.

Primitive cell
with primary
myeloid
granules

 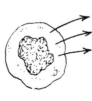

The destruction of effete cells releases
1. *Vit B$_{12}$ binding protein*
   High serum vit B$_{12}$
2. *Thromboplastic substances*

Coagulation and bleeding
complications (compounding
effects of thrombocytopenia)

THE ACUTE LEUKAEMIAS

The following table gives an indication of the methods used to differentiate the acute leukaemias.

	Acute myeloid (AML)	Acute lymphoblastic leukaemias (ALL)
Age	Adults mainly	Children mainly
Associated cells	May be recognisable granulocyte precursors	May be recognisable lymphocytic types
Blast cell: nucleoli	Multiple	Single
Cytoplasmic features PAS (glycogen)	+ Fine granules	++ Coarse granules
Peroxidase and Sudan Black B	++	–
Auer rods (crystalline – staining red)	+	–
Acid phosphatase	–	Lumps

In addition, monoclonal antibodies to surface antigens are very useful in differentiating the various types of acute leukaemia.

Surface Marker		
CD 19 (PanB)	NEGATIVE	POSITIVE in common ALL
CD 7 (PanT)	NEGATIVE	POSITIVE in T cell ALL
CD 13 or CD 33	POSITIVE	NEGATIVE

577

THE CHRONIC LEUKAEMIAS

These disorders occurring in middle and late adult life probably are present in latent form long before clinical presentation, and continue to evolve slowly over years. The basic pathological features are:

TOTAL MARROW CELLULARITY   ⟶   HIGH LEUCOCYTE COUNT
with differentiated cells   in BLOOD

INFILTRATION OF ORGANS
especially SPLENOMEGALY and HEPATOMEGALY
± lymph node enlargement

The two distinct types of chronic leukaemias – **myeloid** and **lymphocytic** will be described separately.

CHRONIC MYELOID LEUKAEMIA (CML)

Marrow

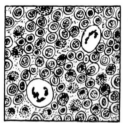

Total cellularity:
cells of granulocyte
series – late forms
numerous (including
eosinophil and
basophil types).

Often increase in
megakaryocytes;
may be increased fibrosis
Increased pressure in bones may cause
clinical tenderness and pain.

Blood
(a) WBC: 75,000–250,000/mm^3
Differential WBC
Blasts
Promyelocytes } <5%

Majority of cells are
late myelocytes and
mature granulocytes

(b) ANAEMIA

(c) THROMBOCYTOPENIA
(sometimes thrombocytosis)

Splenomegaly

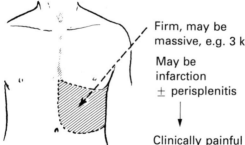

Firm, may be
massive, e.g. 3 kg

May be
infarction
± perisplenitis

↓

Clinically painful

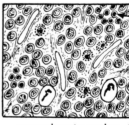

Lymphoid
follicles
inconspicuous

Red pulp
with cells of
granulocyte series ± megakaryocytes
± red cell precursors

Complications: 1. Bleeding and thrombotic tendency.   2. Gout.
Progress: 1. The majority of cases terminate in a '**blast cell crisis**' – the marrow is overrun by primitive myeloid cells and the course is that of acute leukaemia.
        2. A small minority end with marrow failure due to **FIBROSIS**.
Specific chromosomal abnormalities – the Philadelphia chromosome (Ph'):
     About 90% of cases show deletion of a short arm of chromosome 22 in the granulocyte precursors (red cell precursors and megakaryocytes are also affected).

CHRONIC LYMPHOCYTIC LEUKAEMIA (CLL)

This is the commonest leukaemia (30% of all cases); it is best considered as the leukaemic form of DIFFUSE LYMPHOMA – well differentiated lymphocytic type (see p.589).

The disease is found in late middle and old age and in many cases it has probably been present for many years before clinical symptoms appear: an increasing number of cases are discovered by blood examination during routine health checks.

The disease begins and spreads in the lymphoid tissues, and in the established case there is generalised moderate lymph node enlargement and splenomegaly.

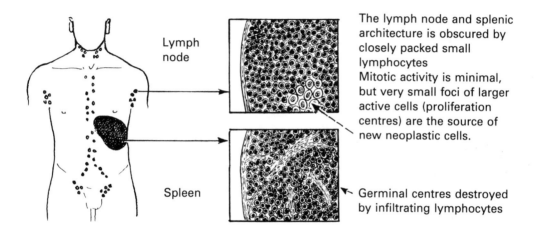

Lymph node

Spleen

The lymph node and splenic architecture is obscured by closely packed small lymphocytes
Mitotic activity is minimal, but very small foci of larger active cells (proliferation centres) are the source of new neoplastic cells.

Germinal centres destroyed by infiltrating lymphocytes

In some cases the lymphoid enlargement precedes the leukaemic phase.

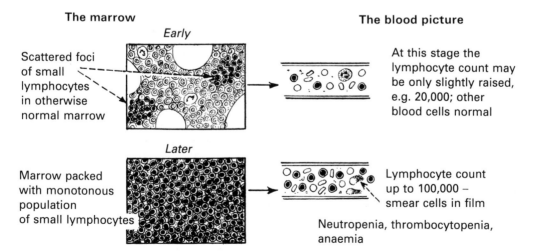

The marrow

Early

Scattered foci of small lymphocytes in otherwise normal marrow

Later

Marrow packed with monotonous population of small lymphocytes

The blood picture

At this stage the lymphocyte count may be only slightly raised, e.g. 20,000; other blood cells normal

Lymphocyte count up to 100,000 – smear cells in film

Neutropenia, thrombocytopenia, anaemia

CHRONIC LYMPHOCYTIC LEUKAEMIA (CLL)

The LYMPHOCYTE in CLL

The disease is usually the result of the very slow MONOCLONAL proliferation of B lymphocytes derived from the mantle zone of the node: they differentiate to the small LONG-LIVED type.

Although the cells can be recognised as B cells with typical surface markers (CD5+), they are usually functionally incompetent so that IMMUNOLOGICAL DEFICIENCY is an important complication.

The usual CLL is B cell type: the T cell type is very rare.

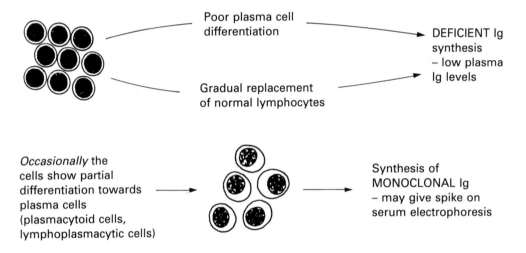

Poor plasma cell differentiation

DEFICIENT Ig synthesis – low plasma Ig levels

Gradual replacement of normal lymphocytes

Occasionally the cells show partial differentiation towards plasma cells (plasmacytoid cells, lymphoplasmacytic cells)

Synthesis of MONOCLONAL Ig – may give spike on serum electrophoresis

These features are dealt with in more detail on page 591.

The immunological deficiency allows opportunistic infections and occasionally *autoimmune haemolytic anaemia.*

Other complications are:
Hypersplenism – aggravating the anaemia,
                 neutropenia and
                 thrombocytopenia
                 mentioned on previous page
and
Skin rashes with pruritus.

LEUKAEMOID REACTIONS

Mimicking chronic myeloid leukaemia

In these rare reactions, the blood changes resemble leukaemia. CML may be mimicked by the reactive leucocytosis of pyogenic infections, in miliary tuberculosis and following treatment with folic acid in macrocytic anaemia of pregnancy.

The following points may be useful in diagnosis:

	CML	Leukaemoid reactions
Splenomegaly	+++	±
Blood film **shift to left** **myelocytes** **basophils**	+ + +	+ ± +
Alkaline Phosphatase **(in neutrophils)**	↓	↑
Serum vit. B$_{12}$	↑	Normal or ↓
Philadelphia **chromosome**	+	−

Mimicking lymphoid leukaemias

In childhood infections, e.g. whooping cough and chicken pox, and in glandular fever the peripheral blood picture with increased numbers of abnormal lymphocytes may cause diagnostic difficulty. The neoplastic lymphocytes are usually much more homogeneous in contrast to the range of morphological atypia seen in 'virocytes'.

THE LYMPHOMAS

These solid tumours which arise in the peripheral lymphoreticular tissues are divided into two main groups: (1) HODGKIN'S DISEASE (HD) and (2) The NON-HODGKIN LYMPHOMAS (NHL).

Paradoxically although the histogenesis of the neoplastic cell in HD is still not known, a histological classification of world-wide acceptance has been established and clearly linked with clinical progress and therapy. In contrast, the classification of NHL is confused due to differences in nomenclature and difficulty in relating the histological appearances to the rapidly growing knowledge of lymphocyte function.

HODGKIN'S DISEASE

Incidence

The disease, which is the commonest type of lymphoma, may occur at any age but there are two peaks of incidence.

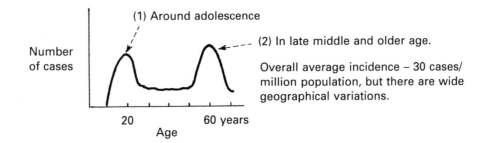

Natural course

1. The majority of cases evolve slowly – several years ⎫ Ultimately
2. A minority progress rapidly – months ⎭ fatal.

NB Modern therapy has completely changed the outcome in this disease – a majority of cases are now cured.

Presentation on spread

The disease begins in a single lymph node, followed by spread to adjacent nodes and then to other organs in a fairly consistent pattern. It often presents clinically as enlargement of accessible nodes (e.g. cervical) without other symptoms, but if the disease has begun in deep nodes considerable spread may have occurred and there are then clinical symptoms referrable to the complications.

HODGKIN'S DISEASE

Presentation and spread (continued)

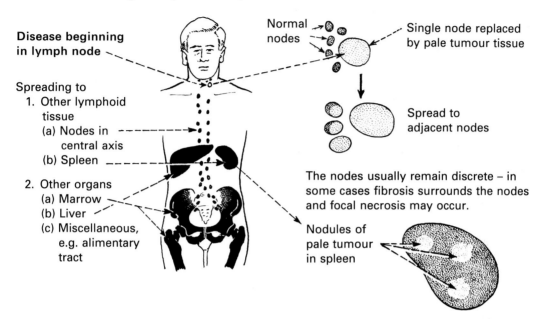

Disease beginning in lymph node

Spreading to
1. Other lymphoid tissue
   (a) Nodes in central axis
   (b) Spleen
2. Other organs
   (a) Marrow
   (b) Liver
   (c) Miscellaneous, e.g. alimentary tract

Normal nodes

Single node replaced by pale tumour tissue

Spread to adjacent nodes

The nodes usually remain discrete – in some cases fibrosis surrounds the nodes and focal necrosis may occur.

Nodules of pale tumour in spleen

The amount of spread which has already occurred at first clinical presentation influences prognosis and the therapeutic attack so that the 'staging' of the disease in the individual case is of great importance.

Staging

Stage I	Disease involving single node or group of nodes
Stage II	Disease in more than one site – all lesions either below or above the diaphragm
Stage III	Disease on both sides of diaphragm
Stage IV	Widespread involvement of extralymphoid sites ± lymph node involvement

The suffix (E) indicates localised **Extra-nodal** disease. (The spleen is considered a lymph node for staging purposes.) The absence (A) or presence (B) of systemic symptoms (see p.585) also relate to prognosis. E.g. Stage III EB means that disease is present in nodes on both sides of the diaphragm with minimal involvement of an extra-nodal site: systemic symptoms are present.

HODGKIN'S DISEASE

The diagnosis of Hodgkin's disease and the presence or absence of spread can only be made with certainty by microscopic examination of tissues.

The disease presents a considerable variety of histological patterns, but the one constant feature is the presence of Reed-Sternberg (RS) cells.

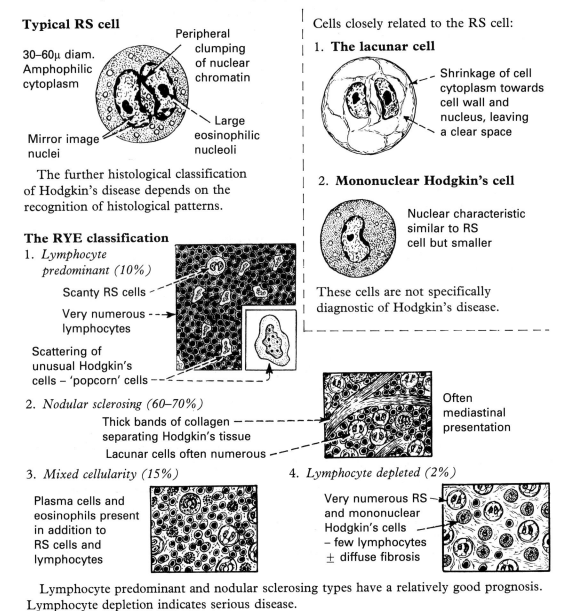

Typical RS cell

30–60μ diam.
Amphophilic
cytoplasm

Peripheral
clumping
of nuclear
chromatin

Large
eosinophilic
nucleoli

Mirror image
nuclei

The further histological classification of Hodgkin's disease depends on the recognition of histological patterns.

The RYE classification

1. *Lymphocyte predominant (10%)*

   Scanty RS cells

   Very numerous lymphocytes

   Scattering of unusual Hodgkin's cells – 'popcorn' cells

2. *Nodular sclerosing (60–70%)*

   Thick bands of collagen separating Hodgkin's tissue

   Lacunar cells often numerous

   Often mediastinal presentation

3. *Mixed cellularity (15%)*

   Plasma cells and eosinophils present in addition to RS cells and lymphocytes

Cells closely related to the RS cell:

1. **The lacunar cell**

   Shrinkage of cell cytoplasm towards cell wall and nucleus, leaving a clear space

2. **Mononuclear Hodgkin's cell**

   Nuclear characteristic similar to RS cell but smaller

These cells are not specifically diagnostic of Hodgkin's disease.

4. *Lymphocyte depleted (2%)*

   Very numerous RS and mononuclear Hodgkin's cells – few lymphocytes ± diffuse fibrosis

Lymphocyte predominant and nodular sclerosing types have a relatively good prognosis. Lymphocyte depletion indicates serious disease.

Note: Lymphocyte predominant HD may progress to a B cell lymphoma (large cell type): this and marker studies raise the possibility that it is an unusual type of B cell lymphoma.

HODGKIN'S DISEASE

Symptomatology and complications

The symptoms can be divided into two main groups:

1. Symptoms for which the mechanisms are obscure – include variable fatigue, weight loss, intermittent fever, night sweats and pruritus.

2. Symptoms associated with three broad groups of pathological complications.

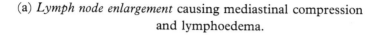

(a) *Lymph node enlargement* causing mediastinal compression and lymphoedema.

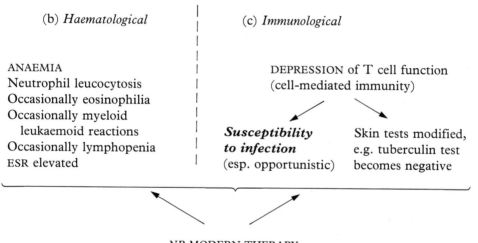

(b) *Haematological*

ANAEMIA
Neutrophil leucocytosis
Occasionally eosinophilia
Occasionally myeloid
   leukaemoid reactions
Occasionally lymphopenia
ESR elevated

(c) *Immunological*

DEPRESSION of T cell function
(cell-mediated immunity)

Susceptibility to infection
(esp. opportunistic)

Skin tests modified,
e.g. tuberculin test
becomes negative

NB MODERN THERAPY
may aggravate these complications

The nature of the disease

The essential nature is not clear – the aetiology is not known. The disease presents some of the features of a neoplasm, but inflammatory changes are also an intrinsic component.

The current, most widely held view is that it is a malignant neoplasm – the neoplastic cells being the Hodgkin's mononuclear cells of which the RS cells are a special type; the inflammatory and immunological changes are interpreted as being secondary to the neoplastic proliferation. There are tentative indications that the Hodgkin's cells are of 'B' lymphocyte lineage and that an infective agent (e.g. Epstein-Barr virus) is the carcinogen.

THE NON-HODGKIN LYMPHOMAS

The non-Hodgkin lymphomas are solid tumours arising in the peripheral lymphoreticular tissues, particularly of the LYMPH NODES but also of the oropharynx, the gut, skin and other sites.

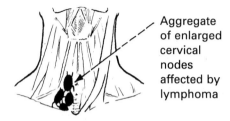

Aggregate of enlarged cervical nodes affected by lymphoma

By tradition the lymphoid neoplasms arising in the bone marrow and thymus are considered separately, but this separation is essentially artificial.

The relationship to leukaemia has also been referred to (see p.573).

Spread The spread reflects the natural circulation of lymphocytes.

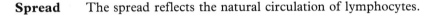

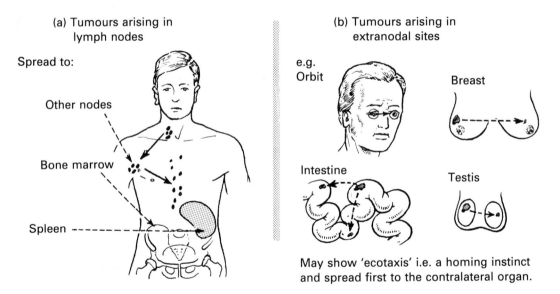

(a) Tumours arising in lymph nodes

Spread to:

Other nodes

Bone marrow

Spleen

(b) Tumours arising in extranodal sites

e.g. Orbit

Breast

Intestine

Testis

May show 'ecotaxis' i.e. a homing instinct and spread first to the contralateral organ.

Eventually spread can be generalised and many organs may be infiltrated, e.g. heart, CNS, kidney, liver and lungs.

CLASSIFICATION

The traditional classifications are purely morphological and were established when knowledge of the development and functional activities of lymphoid cells was minimal.

Modern classifications incorporating the new knowledge in various ways and using varying nomenclatures have been proposed and used by some authorities.

THE NON-HODGKIN LYMPHOMAS

CLASSIFICATION (continued)

Most modern classifications incorporate three basic components with varying emphasis on each: (1) morphological considerations, (2) degree of malignancy (.e. the rate of progress) and (3) functional cell types.

1. Morphological considerations

(a) *Architectural*

A striking architectural feature distinguishes two main groups:

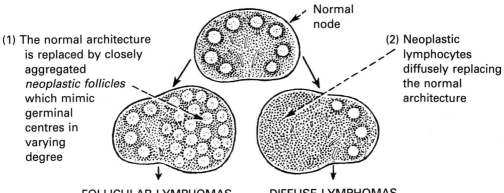

(1) The normal architecture is replaced by closely aggregated *neoplastic follicles* which mimic germinal centres in varying degree

Normal node

(2) Neoplastic lymphocytes diffusely replacing the normal architecture

FOLLICULAR LYMPHOMAS   DIFFUSE LYMPHOMAS

(b) *Cytological*

The cellular morphology of lymphomas can be related to some of the cell types seen in lymph nodes.

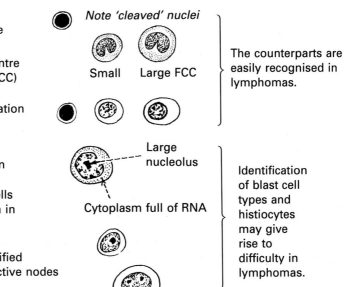

(1) Small round lymphocyte

(2) Cells of the germinal centre (follicular centre cells, FCC)

Note 'cleaved' nuclei

Small   Large FCC

The counterparts are easily recognised in lymphomas.

(3) Cells showing differentiation towards plasma cells. (lymphoplasmacytoid)

(4) Blast cells (rarely seen in normal nodes)
   (a) large transformed cells (immunoblasts) seen in reactive nodes
   (b) smaller blast cells (lymphoblasts) identified with difficulty in reactive nodes

Large nucleolus

Cytoplasm full of RNA

Identification of blast cell types and histiocytes may give rise to difficulty in lymphomas.

(5) Macrophages (histiocytes)

587

THE NON-HODGKIN LYMPHOMAS

DEGREE OF MALIGNANCY

The natural history tends to separate lymphomas into two main groups which have links with the morphological appearances.

1. *Low grade malignancy* associated with well differentiated relatively inactive cell types, – progress of years.

2. *High grade malignancy* associated with primitive actively proliferating cells, – progress over weeks or months.

FUNCTIONAL CELL TYPES

Using special techniques, the lymphomas can be classified in terms of the broad functional groups of normal lymphocytes (B, T and 'null' cell types), their precursors and of macrophages.

The older techniques using cumbersome procedures have now been replaced by methods using MONOCLONAL antibodies to identify specific cell markers. They particularly distinguish B and T cell types and cells of the mononuclear phagocytic system.

Antibodies to immunoglobulin light chains either on the surface of B cells or in their cytoplasm may also enable B cell proliferations to be identified as being MONOCLONAL and therefore NEOPLASTIC.

T cell monoclonality is recognised using the technique of gene rearrangement.

The great majority of lymphomas are of B cell type. They include all follicular and lymphoplasmacytoid types and most cases of chronic lymphocytic leukaemia (CLL).

The more primitive the cells the less likely are markers demonstrable, therefore many primitive tumours are of 'null' cell type.

The rapid advances which are now being made in the discrimination of lymphocyte subsets are superimposed on a basic morphological classification.

THE NON-HODGKIN LYMPHOMAS

CLASSIFICATION (continued)

In the meantime practical classifications have still to be based on the morphological appearances using light microscopy.

The Kiel classification is now widely used in Europe. The International Working Formulation (National Cancer Institute: USA) is designed for use by clinicians. It is important that the user consistently uses his chosen classification.

KIEL CLASSIFICATION		WORKING FORMULATION
B cell lymphomas	T cell lymphomas	
LOW-GRADE Lymphocytic: chronic lymphocytic and hairy cell leukaemia Lymphoplasmacytoid Plasmacytic: multiple myeloma Centroblastic/centrocytic follicular Centroblastic/centrocytic diffuse Centrocytic	Lymphocytic: chronic lymphocytic leukaemia Small cerebriform cell: mycosis fungoides and Sézary syndrome Angioimmunoblastic lymphadenopathy Lymphoepithelioid T zone lymphocytic Pleomorphic, small cell	**LOW-GRADE** Small lymphocytic: chronic lymphocytic leukaemia Plasmacytoid Follicular: predominantly small cleaved cell Follicular: mixed small cleaved and large cell
		INTERMEDIATE GRADE Follicular: predominantly large cell Diffuse: small cleaved cell Diffuse: small and large cell Diffuse: large cell
HIGH-GRADE Centroblastic Immunoblastic Anaplastic Lymphoblastic Burkitt's lymphoma	Immunoblastic Pleomorphic, medium or large cell (HTLV-1) Anaplastic Lymphoblastic	**HIGH-GRADE** Large cell: immunoblastic, plasmacytoid, clear cell, polymorphous Lymphoblastic: convoluted: non-convoluted Small non-cleaved cell: Burkitt's lymphoma

Note: Such morphological classifications do not imply that the tumour arises from the named cell: each tumour probably arises from a single stem cell with subsequent monoclonal proliferation and varying degrees of differentiation.

THE NON-HODGKIN LYMPHOMAS

Pathological complications

These are very similar to those of Hodgkin's disease.

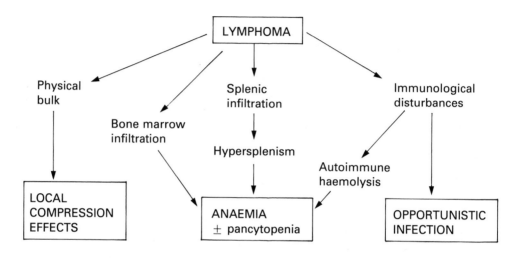

Progress of disease

Low grade malignancy

Often widespread especially to marrow → may be minimal clinical effects.

Follicular lymphomas particularly, may change at any time to blast cell type with serious deterioration.

High grade malignancy
Local nodes initially affected ⟶ to other nodes and extra-nodal sites

± leukaemia [lymphoblastic type: (ALL)]

Staging

Unlike Hodgkin's disease, there is no clear-cut relationship between the pathological staging and the clinical progress.

Five particular types of tumour are worthy of more detailed description since they present special features of interest.

1. The lymphoplasmacytic tumours
2. The plasma cell tumours
3. Lymphomas of the alimentary tract
4. Burkitt's lymphoma
5. Histiocytosis-X.

THE NON-HODGKIN LYMPHOMAS

The LYMPHOPLASMACYTIC TUMOURS

These low grade tumours, arising particularly in lymph nodes, but sometimes in the alimentary tract, synthesise and may secrete monoclonal immunoglobin (Ig) into the plasma.

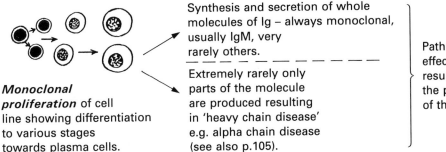

Monoclonal proliferation of cell line showing differentiation to various stages towards plasma cells.

Synthesis and secretion of whole molecules of Ig – always monoclonal, usually IgM, very rarely others.

Extremely rarely only parts of the molecule are produced resulting in 'heavy chain disease' e.g. alpha chain disease (see also p.105).

Pathological effects may result from the presence of these products

WALDENSTRÖM'S MACROGLOBULINAEMIA is the classic example. It affects the lymph nodes, marrow and spleen in the late middle aged and elderly, with a preponderance of males. In addition to the usual pathological complications of low-grade lymphomas, the production of IgM in large quantity produces special complications.

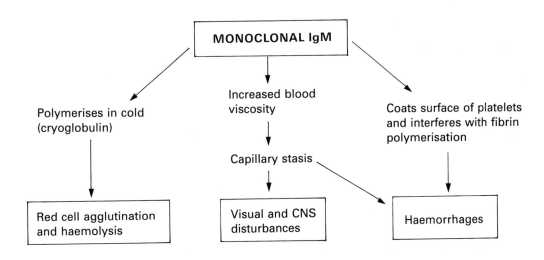

MONOCLONAL IgM

Polymerises in cold (cryoglobulin)

Increased blood viscosity

Coats surface of platelets and interferes with fibrin polymerisation

Capillary stasis

Red cell agglutination and haemolysis

Visual and CNS disturbances

Haemorrhages

591

PLASMA CELL TUMOURS

SOLITARY PLASMACYTOMA

A very small number of plasma cell tumours present as solitary growths, e.g. in the nasopharynx, a lymph node, alimentary tract or in a long bone. It is likely that these slow growing tumours have been present for long periods before they present clinically. In some cases, dissemination particularly to the bone marrow ensues. Elevation of the ESR or the presence of M proteins in the serum are indications of latent dissemination at the time of first clinical presentation.

MULTIPLE MYELOMA (MYELOMATOSIS)

The great majority of plasma cell tumours present as 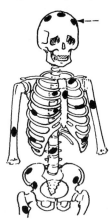 widespread deposits in the bone marrow. Classically the lesions are seen as punched out defects in the bones – the skull showing this appearance particularly well. These focal proliferations of plasma cells usually occur against a background of more diffuse infiltration throughout the marrow.

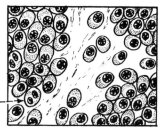

Binucleate cell - - - - →

The disease is not common, having an incidence similar to Hodgkin's disease, with an age peak in the 5th and 6th decades.

After initial presentation, the progress is usually fairly rapid leading to death in 2 to 4 years.

Pathological effects are considered under two main headings:

1. **Tumour growth and its effects**

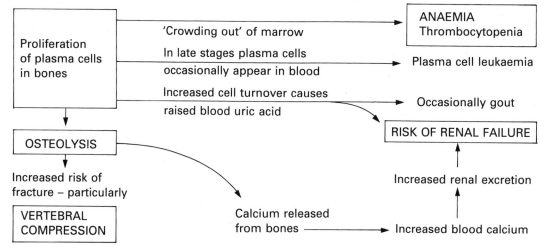

PLASMA CELL TUMOURS

Pathological effects (continued)

2. Synthesis of immunoglobulin and its effects

Myelomatosis, being a monoclonal tumour (see p.591), will produce a single Ig, but the type of Ig varies from case to case, unlike Waldenström's macroglobulinaemia where the immunoglobulin is always IgM. The common heavy chains are G (60%) and A (20%). Light chains of K type are encountered more frequently than λ reflecting the normal K: λ ratio, i.e. 65:35. Thus myeloma of IgGK is the most frequent.

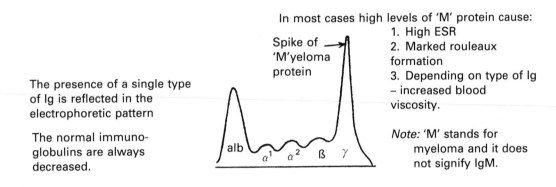

The presence of a single type of Ig is reflected in the electrophoretic pattern

The normal immuno-globulins are always decreased.

Spike of 'M'yeloma protein

In most cases high levels of 'M' protein cause:
1. High ESR
2. Marked rouleaux formation
3. Depending on type of Ig – increased blood viscosity.

Note: 'M' stands for myeloma and it does not signify IgM.

Release of light chains

In many myelomas, some of the Ig molecules are incompletely formed, and unattached light chains are released with important effects. Because of their low molecular weight the light chains:

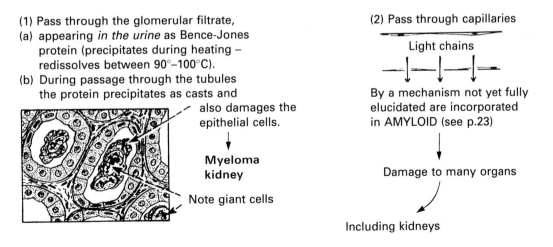

(1) Pass through the glomerular filtrate,
(a) appearing *in the urine* as Bence-Jones protein (precipitates during heating – redissolves between 90°–100°C).
(b) During passage through the tubules the protein precipitates as casts and also damages the epithelial cells.

Myeloma kidney

Note giant cells

(2) Pass through capillaries

Light chains

By a mechanism not yet fully elucidated are incorporated in AMYLOID (see p.23)

Damage to many organs

Including kidneys

Infections, often of opportunistic type, and particularly pneumonias are common since the immune response is deficient despite the high levels of 'M' protein.

LYMPHOMAS – MISCELLANEOUS

ALIMENTARY TRACT

Primary lymphomas of the alimentary tract are rare tumours (in the small intestine the incidence is about the same as that of adenocarcinoma). They are MALT (mucosa associated lymphoid tissue) tumours and may be solitary or multifocal. Histologically lymphomas of both B and T cell origin occur.

There are two main points of interest:

1. Solitary tumours of the small bowel may perforate early, ensuring detection and successful removal in some cases.
2. There is an increased incidence of lymphoma of the small intestine in cases of long-standing gluten enteropathy (coeliac disease). These are tumours arising from the intestinal epithelial lymphocytes (IEL) and are of T cell type.

BURKITT's LYMPOMA

This tumour is of particular interest because there are strong indications that environmental factors are of great importance in its aetiology. It is encountered in particular terrains with similar climatic characteristics in Equatorial Africa, Nigeria, New Guinea and South America where malaria is endemic; where malaria has been eradicated the incidence of the tumour falls. The relationship with the Epstein-Barr (EB) virus has already been described (pp.88, 160). Only very rare cases have been recorded in Europe and North America.

Chromosomal abnormalities are usual. The most common is a translocation between chromosomes 8 and 14: this may result in activation of an oncogene (c-myc).

The histological appearance is typical and striking.

Diffuse proliferation of lymphoblast-like B type cells (with surface Ig markers).

Cells medium-sized and uniform

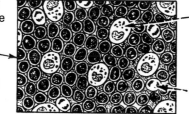

Scattering of macrophages containing debris derived from very rapid cell turnover – contributing 'starry sky' appearance.

Mitoses frequent

Progress: The disease usually first appears in the jaw (60%) or ovaries (retroperitoneal tissues in males) (30%), but grows extremely rapidly and spreads extensively, leading quickly to complications.

(a) The physical effects of sheer tumour bulk destroy and distort organs and tissues.
(b) The very rapid tumour cell turnover releases metabolites in excess, e.g. lactic acid → acidosis.
(c) A defective immune response due to T cell deficiency.

The tumour responds dramatically to treatment. *NB* sudden extensive necrosis may have serious effects, e.g. release of cellular potassium → hyperkalaemia.

MACROPHAGE TUMOURS

It is now known that most large cell lymphomas are either of T cell or B cell origin. Tumours of macrophage lineage within lymphoid tissues are extremely rare. In the connective tissue tumours considered to be of histiocytic origin are described. They range from benign neoplasms in the dermis (histiocytoma cutis) to aggressive sarcomas (malignant fibrous histiocytoma).

Histiocytosis-X

Antigen presenting cells (dendrite cells, see p. 101) are found in the tissues at many sites. The LANGERHANS cell is of particular interest. Although they are considered by some to be subsets of the macrophage series they have specific cell markers including S-100 protein. They are best recognised by electron microscopy which reveals diagnostic cytoplasmic 'Birbeck – – – – granules'.

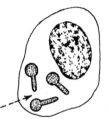

The term Histiocytosis-X encompasses a spectrum of diseases of unknown aetiology which have not been proved with certainty to be neoplastic but in all of which proliferation of LANGERHANS cells is an essential feature.

Benign end of spectrum

Eosinophilic granuloma of bone (*see p.807*)

(a) *Solitary*

Histology: Eosinophils   + + +
Mononuclear cells   + +
(Histiocytic) giant cells   +
Fibrosis   +

Progress: slow.

Hand-Schuller-Christian disease

(b) *Multifocal*→If skull bones affected there may be
- DIABETES INSIPIDUS
- EXOPHTHALMOS
- DEAFNESS

There may also be HEPATO-SPLENOMEGALY.

Age range: children usually; occasionally adults.

Malignant end of spectrum

Letterer-Siwe disease: An acute febrile illness with widespread organ and tissue involvement, particularly lymph nodes, spleen, liver, bones and skin.

Histology: Mononuclear cells (histiocytic)   + + +
           Lymphocytes and plasma cells   +
           Eosinophils   ±
           Neutrophils   +
           Necrosis   + +

Progress: Rapid → death.

Age: Infants only.

LYMPHOMAS – DIAGNOSIS

Lymph node enlargement is a common condition. Three broad groupings are considered.

Enlargement due to:

1. REACTIVE CHANGES–infection is the common cause .... Common
2. SECONDARY TUMOURS.. Common
3. PRIMARY LYMPH NODE NEOPLASIA .... Rare

Since the prognosis of group (1) is so different from (2) and (3), accurate diagnosis is essential. In the majority of cases, it is easily reached by a synthesis of all the clinical information. In a minority, laboratory tests are required.

Biopsy

The basis of an accurate diagnosis usually rests on LYMPH NODE BIOPSY.

The tissue has to be removed and processed with particular care since artefact can easily obscure the histological details so essential for accurate diagnosis.

Procedure: (1) A **whole** node is taken with minimal trauma.
(2) Preparation of routine and special histology.

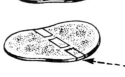

Using a sharp blade, two thin slices of the face of the cut surface are obtained.

(a) Fixation in 10% formalin – 48 hr., then routine processing.
(b) Frozen sections for surface markers – especially T cell identification.
(c) Imprints on slides. Special plastic section. Small blocks for EM (glutaraldehyde fixation).

Microscopic diagnosis

1. May be extremely easy, e.g. SECONDARY CARCINOMA stands out against the lymphoid tissues – but establishing the source of origin of the carcinoma from the histological appearances may be difficult.

2. Great difficulty may arise in distinguishing reactive conditions from primary neoplasia (e.g. follicular lymphoma).
   The recognition of a monoclonal cell population is important. Techniques demonstrating immunoglobulins and their components are useful in B cell tumours. In T cell tumours clonal rearrangement of T cell receptor genes can be detected.

Other laboratory tests may be useful e.g. to search for infecting organisms and to identify 'foreign' materials.
Full haematological examination, plasma protein analysis and assessment of the immune status may all make important contributions.

CHAPTER 13

GENITOURINARY SYSTEM

KIDNEY – ANATOMY AND PHYSIOLOGY

The kidney is essentially a lobulated organ and its blood supply is arranged in a regular pattern which frequently determines the extent of pathological lesions.

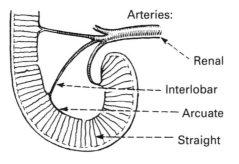

Blood supply

The renal artery divides into anterior and posterior branches which subdivide in a regular manner to supply the lobules.

From the straight arteries small branches (afferent arterioles) supply the functional unit of the kidney – the nephron.

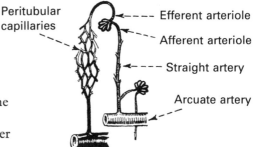

The arteries and afferent arterioles are end vessels.
Anastomoses unite the peritubular capillaries of one nephron unit with another, but where the blockage of the arteriolar supply occurs, these anastomoses are insufficient to maintain a proper circulation.

THE NEPHRON

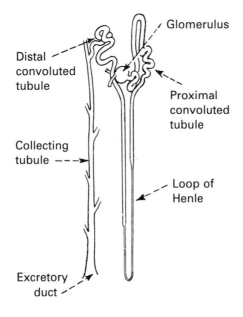

Each part of the nephron has its own special structure and function, its own peculiar blood supply and control mechanism – partly hormonal.

THE GLOMERULUS is a bulbous structure, the end of which is invaginated by a capillary network derived from the afferent arteriole.

The large surface area of the capillaries makes this an efficient filtration unit. The filtration is precisely controlled by the unique structure of the glomerulus.

KIDNEY – ANATOMY AND PHYSIOLOGY

Ultrastructure

The barrier separating blood from the lumen of the nephron consists of three layers:

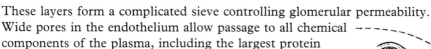

Mesangial matrix

Capillary

Mesangial nucleus

1. Endothelium (fenestrated)
2. Basement membrane
3. Epithelium

These layers form a complicated sieve controlling glomerular permeability. Wide pores in the endothelium allow passage to all chemical components of the plasma, including the largest protein molecules.

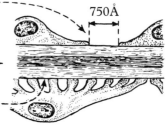

750Å

The basement membrane has a dense layer offering resistance to large molecules.

The epithelial cells are attached to the basement membrane by foot processes, leaving pores 300–400Å in width between. These pores are covered by a thin membrane which has slits 50 x 120Å in size, slightly smaller than a molecule of albumin (37 x 140Å).

The main barriers to filtration of large molecules are the lamina densa of the basement membrane and the slit diaphragm covering the epithelial pores.

Filtration

The glomerular filtrate is virtually protein free plasma. Its rate of production is dependent upon:

① Afferent arteriolar hydrostatic pressure

② Plasma protein osmotic pressure

③ Pressure within the renal tubule

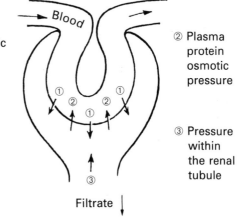

Blood

Filtrate

Variation in any of these factors affects the output of urine. Diminished urinary output results from a reduction in renal blood flow as in shock, from an increase in osmotic pressure as in haemoconcentration, or from obstruction to the outflow of urine.

599

KIDNEY – ANATOMY AND PHYSIOLOGY

Glomerular damage
The usual consequences of this are threefold:

      1. Reduction in urinary output

      2. Proteinuria

      3. Haematuria

The mechanism underlying these changes is probably as follows:

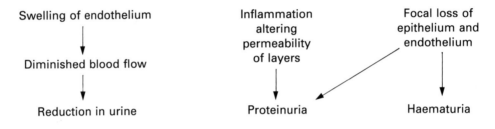

THE TUBULE
During passage along the tubule, the glomerular filtrate, initially isotonic and neutral, becomes hypertonic and quite strongly acid. Within 24 hours, 180 litres of filtrate are reduced to 1.5 litres of urine. The main functions of this process are:

(a) to get rid of waste products, particularly those of protein metabolism

(b) to aid in maintaining the normal acid-base balance

(c) to conserve fluid, electrolytes and other essential substances.

   Three mechanisms are involved:

1. Active absorption of substances from the filtrate by the tubular epithelium

2. Passive interchange between the filtrate and the interstitial tissues to maintain osmotic equilibrium

3. Secretion by the tubular epithelium.

KIDNEY – ANATOMY AND PHYSIOLOGY

PROXIMAL TUBULE

The main function is active reabsorption of sodium, potassium, glucose, amino acids, phosphate, calcium and uric acid.

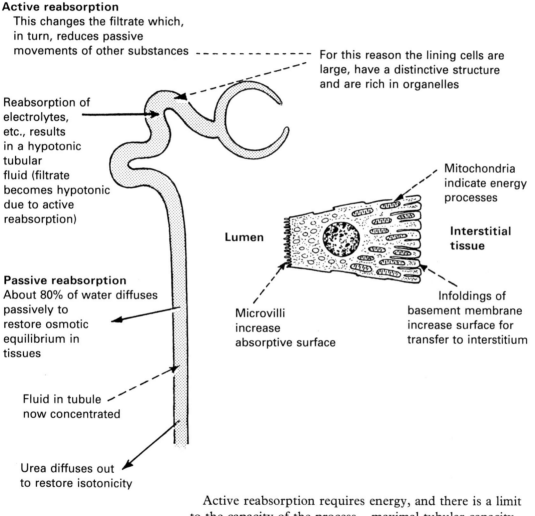

Active reabsorption
This changes the filtrate which, in turn, reduces passive movements of other substances - - - - - - - - - - - For this reason the lining cells are large, have a distinctive structure and are rich in organelles

Reabsorption of electrolytes, etc., results in a hypotonic tubular fluid (filtrate becomes hypotonic due to active reabsorption)

Mitochondria indicate energy processes

Interstitial tissue

Lumen

Passive reabsorption
About 80% of water diffuses passively to restore osmotic equilibrium in tissues

Microvilli increase absorptive surface

Infoldings of basement membrane increase surface for transfer to interstitium

Fluid in tubule now concentrated

Urea diffuses out to restore isotonicity

Active reabsorption requires energy, and there is a limit to the capacity of the process – maximal tubular capacity (Tm). When this is exceeded, the particular substance involved will appear in the urine. Glucose is an example. In diabetes, the amount of glucose in the filtrate far exceeds the absorptive capacity, and glycosuria results.

KIDNEY – ANATOMY AND PHYSIOLOGY

LOOP OF HENLE AND ASCENDING TUBULE

In this zone, there is active reabsorption of Na^+Cl^- and passive reabsorption of water. This is augmented by a counter current mechanism due to proximity of tubules and blood vessels. The changes are as follows:

Tubular mechanism

At A (ascending limb of Henle), a sodium 'pump' mechanism effected by aldosterone (see p.828) transfers the ion to the interstitium making it hypertonic. The descending tubule B is permeable to water which is attracted from it by the Na^+Cl^-. The urine therefore becomes hypertonic at C (Na^+Cl^- concentration high). This mechanism therefore exerts a multiplying effect.

Vascular mechanism

The multiplying mechanism would ultimately cause impossible tissue hypertonicity, but much of the reabsorbed Na^+Cl^- passes into the descending limb of the vasa recta (D). As the vessel turns and ascends (E), water is attracted into the blood. This helps to maintain the flow of water and sodium from the tubule into the tissues, and at the same time conserves them.

Urinary concentration

Water absorption occurs along the distal tubule and particularly in the collecting ducts under the influence of ADH. Some of the sodium from the hypertonic urine in the Henle's loop (C) moves passively into the medullary tissues. This attracts water (5%) from the collecting ducts to produce the final urinary concentration.

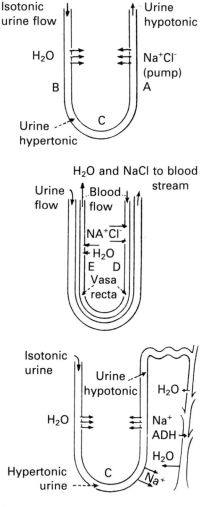

Urinary acidification

H ions, excreted by distal tubule, take part in three reactions:

1. $H^+ + HCO_3 = H_2CO_3$
2. $H^+ + NH_3Cl = NH_4Cl$
3. $H^+ + HPO_4 + Na = NaH_2PO_4$

} Urinary excretory products

KIDNEY – ANATOMY AND PHYSIOLOGY

Variations in nephrons

There are variations in the size of glomeruli, and therefore variation in the filtration surface, but the most striking difference is between the tubules of the cortical glomeruli and those of the juxtamedullary glomeruli.

The rate of blood flow through the medulla is only one-fifth of the cortical rate. This, together with the long loops of Henle of the juxtamedullary nephrons which allow reabsorption of large quantities of water, suggests a mechanism for conservation of fluid and electrolytes which may operate when the circulating volume of blood is low and cortical flow is reduced as in shock.

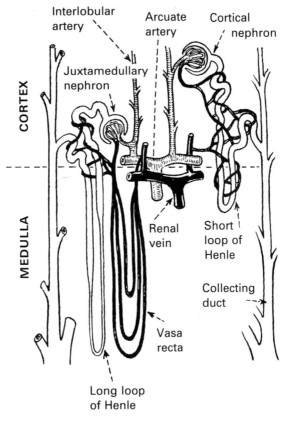

Effects of tubular damage

It is obvious that damage to the tubules will result in gross biochemical changes.

1. Loss of mechanisms controlling balance of electrolytes, water and urea.
2. Upset in acid-base balance.
3. Loss of substances in urine normally completely or almost completely reabsorbed – glucose, potassium, amino acids.
4. Proteinuria due to damage to associated capillaries.

It must also be apparent that glomerular lesions and pathological changes in the renal pelvis will upset tubular function by interfering with blood supply.

RENAL FUNCTION

INVESTIGATION

Numerous tests of renal function have been formulated, some simple, others sophisticated. It must be emphasised that the simple tests are, in their own context, important. Tests can be divided into three groups:

1. Simple diagnostic tests indicating renal damage

(a) Tests for the presence of protein, red cells, haemoglobin and neutrophils in the urine. Estimation of specific gravity and measurement of urinary output.

(b) Urinary casts. These are composed of foreign elements of various types which are moulded into cylindrical form by passage along tubules.

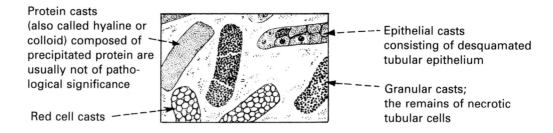

Protein casts (also called hyaline or colloid) composed of precipitated protein are usually not of pathological significance

Red cell casts

Epithelial casts consisting of desquamated tubular epithelium

Granular casts; the remains of necrotic tubular cells

In jaundice, casts of bile-stained debris are found.

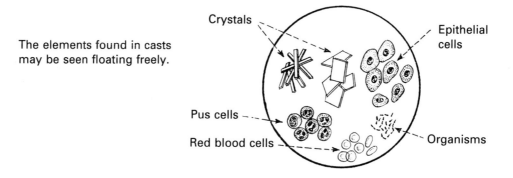

The elements found in casts may be seen floating freely.

Crystals

Epithelial cells

Pus cells

Red blood cells

Organisms

2. Blood chemistry

Many substances will show altered values in renal failure, but the following are always elevated and are commonly used in estimating the progress of the disease.

Urea —————————— normal range — — — — — 2.5–7.0 mmol/l
(20–40 mg/100 ml).

Creatinine ————————— normal range — — — — –50–100μmol/l
(0.6–1.2 mg/100 ml).

RENAL FUNCTION

3. Clearance tests

These are employed to determine the degree of renal damage and the residual function. The principle underlying all of these tests is similar – an estimation of the rate of extraction of a particular substance from the blood by the kidney in unit time. The simple formula UV/P is used to calculate the amount of blood so cleared.

U = the urinary concentration.

V = the volume of urine per minute.

P = the plasma concentration.

A loading dose of the test substance is administered intravenously followed by an infusion to sustain a constant blood level.

Glomerular filtration rate

Inulin is the ideal substance for this purpose. It is filtered at the glomerulus and is excreted unchanged in the urine. The amount appearing in the urine is proportional to the amount of blood being 'cleared' of inulin per unit time.

Following infusion of the inulin, a timed urine specimen is collected and a plasma sample is obtained halfway through the collection. The formula VU/P is applied to the values obtained. The normal filtration rate is around 125 ml/min.

Frequently in practice creatinine, which is a normal constituent of urine and blood and therefore eliminates the need for infusions, is used instead of inulin. It is also easier to estimate. The value obtained is not quite as accurate since creatinine is partly secreted by the renal tubules.

Renal plasma flow

Para-amino hippuric acid is both filtered at the glomerulus and secreted by the tubular epithelium so that 90% is extracted from the arterial blood. This gives an approximate idea of the renal plasma flow. The procedure is exactly the same as that employed for inulin. The same formula (UV/P) is used to calculate the clearance rate of PAH.

Average result is 630 ml/min. Since only 90% of PAH is cleared, the actual renal plasma flow will be:

$$\frac{\text{Clearance}}{\text{Extraction ratio}} = \frac{630}{0.9} = 700\text{ml/min}$$

Other substances, such as urea, can be used to give an indication of renal function. Since urea is normally present in the blood and urine, it eliminates the need for intravenous infusions.

NEPHRITIS

The pathological changes and clinical syndromes may be divided into 3 main groups, but two other less common and ill-defined conditions are described.

1. **Acute nephritis**
   This condition is characterised by moderate proteinuria, haematuria, oedema, oliguria and a degree of renal failure.

2. **Nephrotic syndrome**
   Affected individuals suffer a long continued illness with widespread oedema, effusions in serous cavities and susceptibility to infections. There is gross proteinuria and raised blood lipid. Nitrogen retention occurs late in the disease process, indicating renal failure.

3. **Serious renal failure**

   This may occur:
   - (a) ACUTE – within a few weeks or months. Uraemia is the main manifestation and it may end in death.
   - (b) CHRONIC – after several years. Hypertension develops and death may be due to vascular complications or uraemia.

Unfortunately, these syndromes are not disease entities. The aetiology of the three syndromes is very mixed, and the clinical features of all three may be exhibited at different times by the same patient. Different pathological processes may produce the same clinical condition. This is particularly true of the nephrotic syndrome. The clinical syndromes provide little indication of pathogenesis, nor are they a guide to prognosis. In addition, any one of these renal syndromes may be a manifestation of a number of systemic diseases.

It has been found that diagnosis and an estimate of prognosis are best achieved by a study of the histological changes using renal biopsies. In the following account, primary renal lesions will be described, beginning with the acute glomerulonephritic conditions. Subsequently, consideration will be given to renal dysfunction associated with systemic disease.

NEPHRITIS

ACUTE DIFFUSE PROLIFERATIVE GLOMERULONEPHRITIS

This condition in its classical form follows 2–3 weeks after an infection, usually a pharyngitis due to group A haemolytic streptococci. It is commonest in children and young adults.

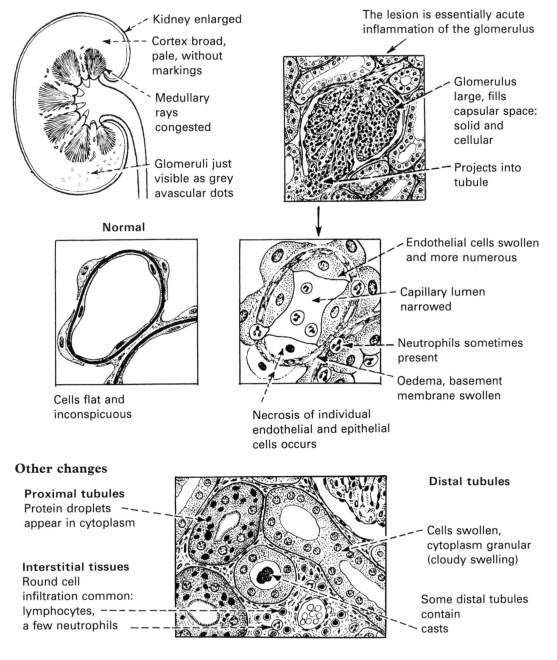

Kidney enlarged

Cortex broad, pale, without markings

Medullary rays congested

Glomeruli just visible as grey avascular dots

Normal

Cells flat and inconspicuous

The lesion is essentially acute inflammation of the glomerulus

Glomerulus large, fills capsular space: solid and cellular

Projects into tubule

Endothelial cells swollen and more numerous

Capillary lumen narrowed

Neutrophils sometimes present

Oedema, basement membrane swollen

Necrosis of individual endothelial and epithelial cells occurs

Other changes

Proximal tubules
Protein droplets appear in cytoplasm

Interstitial tissues
Round cell infiltration common: lymphocytes, a few neutrophils

Distal tubules

Cells swollen, cytoplasm granular (cloudy swelling)

Some distal tubules contain casts

607

NEPHRITIS

ACUTE DIFFUSE PROLIFERATIVE GLOMERULONEPHRITIS

Electron microscope studies
These studies reveal deposits of granular material in the glomerulus.

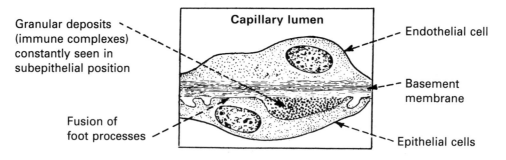

In addition to these deposits, the electron microscope shows focal fusion of the foot processes of the epithelial cells (podocytes).

Immunofluorescence staining reveals that the granular material in the subendothelial position consists of IgG, C3 factor of the complement complex and fibrin.

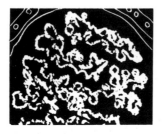

The proteins show as a granular, irregular deposit in the glomerular capillary walls. The white lines represent immunofluorescence staining.

Progress
This tends to vary with the age of the patient. Children almost always recover (95%) completely. Endothelial and epithelial changes are reversed. The protein deposits are either excreted in the urine or are phagocytosed by mesangial cells. Capillary patency is restored.

Complications arise in more than one third of adults.

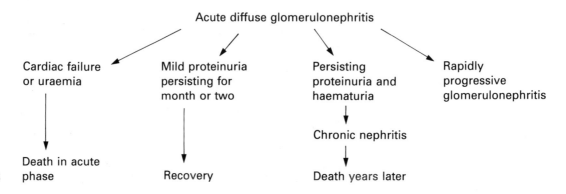

NEPHRITIS

ACUTE DIFFUSE PROLIFERATIVE GLOMERULONEPHRITIS (continued)
Clinical features

These may be relatively slight. Malaise with some facial oedema (periorbital), oliguria, the urine being smoky and dark, and a moderate increase in blood pressure are the most constant features. The relationship of clinical findings to pathological changes can be visualised as follows:

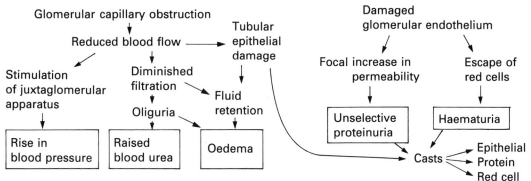

RAPIDLY PROGRESSIVE GLOMERULONEPHRITIS

Initially, this condition is clinically and pathologically indistinguishable from acute diffuse glomerulonephritis, but subsequently additional changes take place progressively over a few weeks. Crescent formation is the histological hall-mark.

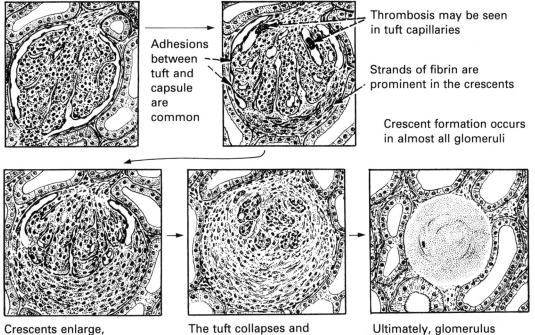

Adhesions between tuft and capsule are common

Thrombosis may be seen in tuft capillaries

Strands of fibrin are prominent in the crescents

Crescent formation occurs in almost all glomeruli

Crescents enlarge, compressing the tufts and obliterating capillaries.

The tuft collapses and collagen fibres appear in crescents and tuft.

Ultimately, glomerulus becomes a mass of hyaline fibrous tissue.

609

NEPHRITIS

RAPIDLY PROGRESSIVE GLOMERULONEPHRITIS

Electron microscope findings

Subendothelial and subepithelial granular deposits may be found in the tuft capillaries as in acute diffuse glomerulonephritis. In addition, as the lesion progresses, changes occur in the basement membrane.

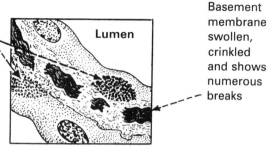

Lumen

Basement membrane swollen, crinkled and shows numerous breaks

Clinical features

These are similar to those found in acute diffuse proliferative glomerulonephritis but are much more evident and severe.

Aetiology

Rapidly progressive glomerulonephritis appears to arise mainly in two circumstances:

1. Primary

It may follow a streptococcal infection, and in the early stages is indistinguishable from acute diffuse glomerulonephritis (see p.607).

2. Secondary

Associated with lung disease. This usually takes the form of Goodpasture's syndrome, a condition almost exclusively confined to young adult males. There are repeated episodes of pulmonary haemorrhage causing severe anaemia. This is followed by renal changes. Death can be due to pulmonary or renal insufficiency. Autoantibodies to basement membranes are present in the blood and are thought to be responsible for the renal damage.

Vasculitis is also a frequently associated condition.

Immunofluorescence studies differentiate between these two aetiological forms of the nephritic process.

Post-streptococcal

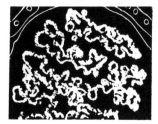

Granular deposits of IgG, IgM and C3

Goodpasture's syndrome

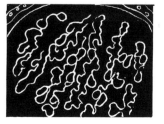

Linear deposits of IgG, IgM and C3 in the capillary basement membranes

NEPHRITIS

FOCAL GLOMERULONEPHRITIS

In this common condition the changes may occur in almost all glomeruli, or in only a small number. In addition, the lesion is usually only seen in one or two lobules of each affected glomerulus.

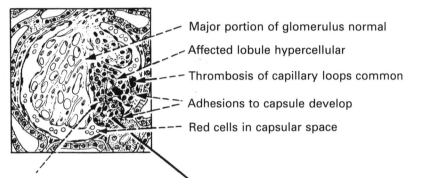

— Major portion of glomerulus normal

— Affected lobule hypercellular

— — Thrombosis of capillary loops common

— — Adhesions to capsule develop

— — — Red cells in capsular space

The hypercellularity is due to proliferation of mesangial cells. The capilliaries are often thrombosed and necrotic.

The reason for the focal nature appears to be due to the variation in size of the immune complexes. These reach all glomeruli, but the majority are small and pass through to the urinary space and are excreted. Others, larger, are held in the glomerular sieve and cause an acute reaction.

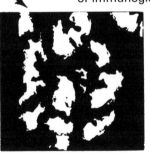

Immunofluorescence reveals deposits of immunoglobulins IgG and IgA in the ground substance (mesangium) of the affected lobule. The IgA molecule appears to be of particular significance.

No deposits in capillaries

Clinical features

Haematuria, sometimes severe, and proteinuria are the only signs. Usually they last only a few days and there is no sign of subsequent renal impairment, but the condition can recur repeatedly and may end in chronic renal failure.

Aetiology

1. A ***Primary Type*** is known as IgA Nephropathy or BERGER's DISEASE and is associated with the deposition of IgA in the glomerular mesangium. It is often preceded by ill-defined viral or bacterial infections.

2. The ***Secondary Type*** may be concomitant with Henoch-Schönlein purpura, infective endocarditis, polyarteritis nodosa and systemic lupus erythematosus (see p.619).

A similar lesion may be found as a complication in other diseases (see p.619).

NEPHROTIC SYNDROME

Renal lesions associated with nephrotic syndrome

In fatal cases, the kidneys may show striking
changes to the naked eye, but this gives little
indication of the pathological process involved.

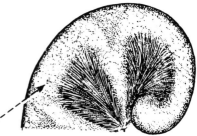

Enlargement and general pallor due to oedema

Yellow streaks of lipid

Histological changes

Several distinct conditions become apparent on microscopic examination:

MEMBRANOUS GLOMERULONEPHRITIS

In this form there are generalised changes in the glomerular capillary basement
membranes. Several stages can be recognised:

*Early
stage*

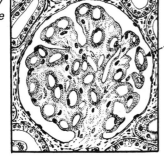

Tuft enlarges

Diffuse hyaline
thickening
of capillary

Glomeruli
not
hypercellular

Specific silver staining
of the basement membrane
shows a typical pattern.

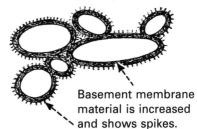

Basement membrane
material is increased
and shows spikes.

Immunofluorescence reveals
deposition of IgG and IgM
in the capillary walls.

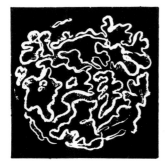

Electron microscope findings
explain this appearance.

Loss of foot
processes

Basement
membrane
material
between
deposit
≡ spikes

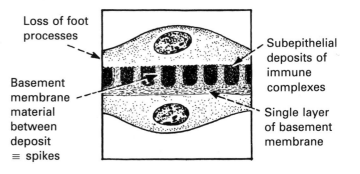

Subepithelial
deposits of
immune
complexes

Single layer
of basement
membrane

NEPHROTIC SYNDROME

Membranous Glomerulonephritis (continued)

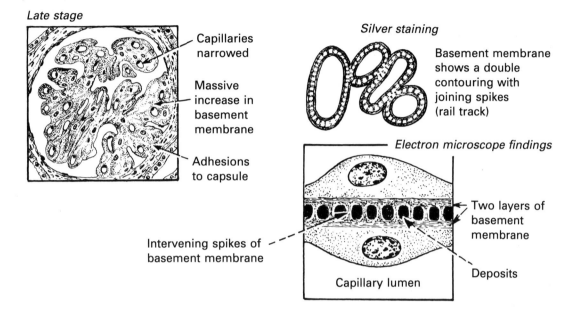

Late stage

Capillaries narrowed

Massive increase in basement membrane

Adhesions to capsule

Silver staining

Basement membrane shows a double contouring with joining spikes (rail track)

Electron microscope findings

Intervening spikes of basement membrane

Two layers of basement membrane

Deposits

Capillary lumen

Tubular changes

In the early stages, protein droplets and lipid globules appear in the tubular epithelium. Lipid is also found in the interstitial tissue. Foamy macrophages and giant cells form granulomas in association with cholesterol deposits. With progress of the disease, narrowing of the glomerular capillaries causes ischaemic atrophy of the tubules and interstitial fibrosis.

Clinical features

The disease is commonest in males and occurs more often in adults.

It presents with the usual features of the nephrotic syndrome – gross proteinuria and generalised oedema. Fluid accumulates in the serous cavities.

Biochemical changes include hypoproteinaemia due to loss of protein in the urine and hyperlipidaemia which accounts for the lipid deposits in the kidneys.

Serious infections can be troublesome. The disease is only slowly progressive and in about 50% of cases glomerular destruction ultimately leads to uraemia.

Aetiology

Most cases are idiopathic. In some there is an association with infections, the use of certain drugs (e.g. captopril and penicillamine) and malignant tumours.

The immune complexes contain IgG and complement. The antigens are not known.

613

NEPHROTIC SYNDROME

MINIMAL CHANGE GLOMERULONEPHRITIS

This occurs mainly in children but is occasionally seen in adults. It is the commonest cause of the nephrotic condition in children.

The macroscopic appearance of the kidneys is the same as that in all examples of the nephrotic syndrome, but the apparent lack of glomerular change gave rise to the term 'lipoid nephrosis'.

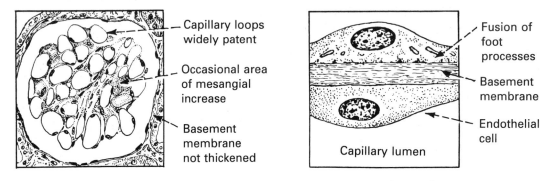

Capillary loops widely patent

Occasional area of mesangial increase

Basement membrane not thickened

Fusion of foot processes

Basement membrane

Endothelial cell

Capillary lumen

Immunofluorescence fails to demonstrate immunoglobulins or complement.

No evidence of deposits in or around basement membrane.

Tubular changes, common to all nephrotic states, consist of lipid and protein droplets in the epithelial cells.

Clinical features

These are the same as in any nephrotic process – gross oedema and proteinuria with hyperlipidaemia. The use of antibiotics has minimised the incidence of infections which once were a serious complication.

Glomerular filtration appears to be normal. The proteinuria is highly selective, only albumin being found in the urine, and is apparently due to increased permeability of the glomerular capillaries. Lipid-rich protein casts appear in the urine.

Aetiology and progress

This is unknown. Occasionally it may follow a respiratory infection but is not related to any particular type.

The condition in children responds to steroid therapy. It tends to recur, and the prognosis depends on the frequency of recurrence and the duration of the interval between attacks. The response to steroids suggests an immunological reaction. The lack of evidence of immunoglobulin in the glomerulus may be due to elimination.

In adults, the prognosis is not so clear and some patients may subsequently develop renal failure.

NEPHROTIC SYNDROME

FOCAL GLOMERULOSCLEROSIS (HYALINOSIS)

The clinical features of this condition are the same as those of minimal change glomerulonephritis, but the prognosis is quite different. In the early phase, the microscopic appearance of the glomeruli is almost the same as in the minimal change lesion, but it is a progressive lesion.

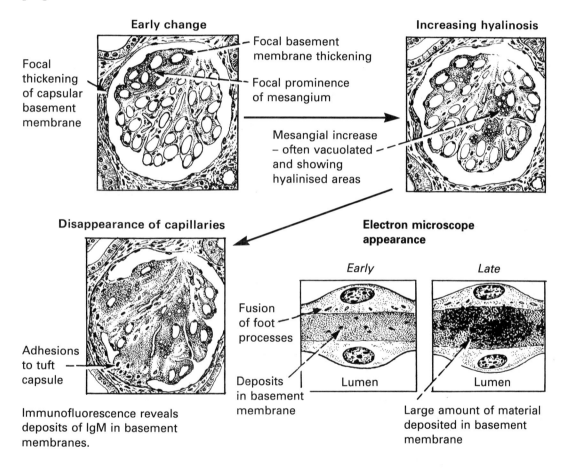

Early change

Focal thickening of capsular basement membrane

Focal basement membrane thickening

Focal prominence of mesangium

Mesangial increase – often vacuolated and showing hyalinised areas

Increasing hyalinosis

Disappearance of capillaries

Adhesions to tuft capsule

Immunofluorescence reveals deposits of IgM in basement membranes.

Electron microscope appearance

Early

Late

Fusion of foot processes

Deposits in basement membrane

Lumen

Lumen

Large amount of material deposited in basement membrane

Ultimately, the glomerulus becomes completely sclerosed. The process starts in juxtamedullary glomeruli but spreads peripherally to outer cortical glomeruli. Associated tubules undergo atrophy. Proteinuria is unselective and haematuria may occur. The condition is unresponsive to steroids and ends in renal failure.

Aetiology

The true aetiology is unknown. Historically it was thought to be a variant of minimal change glomerulonephritis but the focal glomerular lesions are similar only in the very early stages.

NEPHROTIC SYNDROME

MESANGIOCAPILLARY GLOMERULONEPHRITIS (Membranocapillary glomerulonephritis)

In many ways this lesion is a bridge between acute diffuse glomerulonephritis and membranous glomerulonephritis, showing some of the features of each of these conditions.

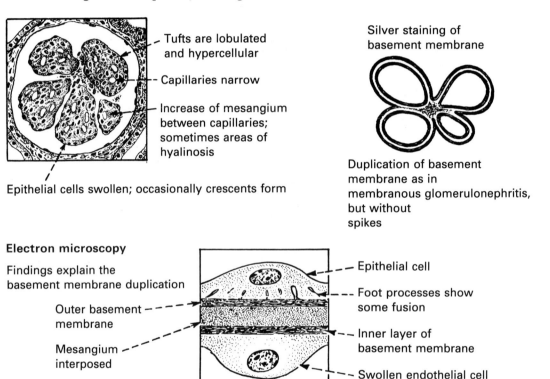

Tufts are lobulated and hypercellular

Capillaries narrow

Increase of mesangium between capillaries; sometimes areas of hyalinosis

Epithelial cells swollen; occasionally crescents form

Silver staining of basement membrane

Duplication of basement membrane as in membranous glomerulonephritis, but without spikes

Electron microscopy

Findings explain the basement membrane duplication

Outer basement membrane

Mesangium interposed

Epithelial cell

Foot processes show some fusion

Inner layer of basement membrane

Swollen endothelial cell

Subendothelial and mesangial deposits are found, and immunofluorescence shows that they are immunoglobulins IgG, IgA or IgM, C3 and granular fibrin.

The glomeruli usually show increasing hyalinisation until they are completely sclerosed. Tubules undergo atrophy with increasing interstitial fibrosis.

Clinical features

This condition usually affects older children. It may have an acute onset, but with no symptoms apart from proteinuria, progressing to a nephrotic syndrome. Some patients may recover, but most develop chronic renal failure. Hypertension may be a prominent feature. The blood level of C3 is always low.

Aetiology

This is unknown. In some cases there has been a preceding streptococcal infection, but other factors in the plasma, as yet not well defined, may activate the complement system in the glomerular tuft.

GLOMERULAR DISEASE MECHANISMS

Mechanisms of damage

The essential mechanism is the effect of immune complex deposition.

The glomerulus is the ideal site for the deposition of immune complexes because of its microstructure. The most important factor is the size of the complex, and this will vary with the stage and intensity of the immune reaction, e.g.:

(1) Antibody in low concentration (e.g. early in reaction)

(2) Antibody equivalent to antigen (immune reaction fully mounted)

(3) Intermediate amounts of antibody

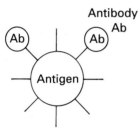

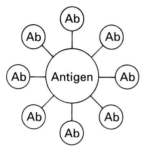

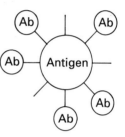

Very small soluble molecule – causes no trouble.

A very large insoluble molecule excites a macrophage reaction resulting in phagocytosis and digestion in the circulation, and causing no renal damage.

Molecules of intermediate size.

1. Deposition of circulating immune complex

The third type of molecule is important. All are able to pass through the fenestrations of the capillary endothelium. Thereafter their migration will depend mainly on their size and the degree of permeability of the basement membrane. The smallest molecules will reach a subepithelial position.

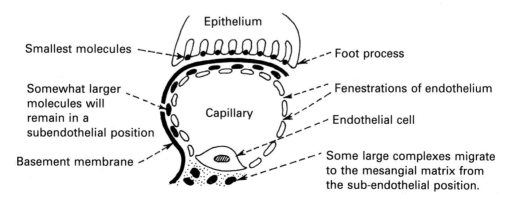

617

GLOMERULAR DISEASE MECHANISMS AND CHRONIC DISEASE

Subsequently, fixation of complement by these immune complexes takes place:

Complement fixation

Chemotaxis of neutrophils   Activation of complement factors

Release of enzymes   Formation of cell membrane damaging factors (anaphylotoxins)

Vascular damage

2. **In situ immune complexes** can form when circulating antibodies react with antigens in the glomerulus, e.g. in GOODPASTURE's SYNDROME there are circulating antibodies to glomerular basement membrane.

Factors modifying the pathological changes in the kidney

1. The amount of antigen and its persistence.
2. The intensity of the immune reaction and the rate of production of antibody; the type of antibody formed may also be important.
3. The availability of complement and the degree of its 'fixation'.

Factors (1) and (2) will determine the amount and rate of deposition of the immune complexes, and the interplay between all three factors can account for the variations in the pathological changes and clinical manifestations of glomerulonephritis, e.g. a short-lived infection (e.g. scarlet fever) may produce an acute nephritis, but the antigen disappears rapidly and the nephritis resolves. A more chronic condition with persisting antigens can result in a slower but ultimately more destructive process in the kidneys. Equally, a poor immunological reaction in a chronic disease can cause a similar picture.

CHRONIC GLOMERULONEPHRITIS is the final stage of glomerulonephritis when sclerosis has eliminated many glomeruli and their associated tubules.

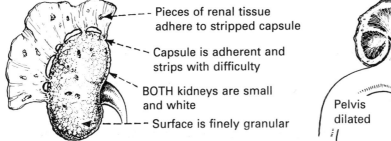

Pieces of renal tissue adhere to stripped capsule

Capsule is adherent and strips with difficulty

BOTH kidneys are small and white

Surface is finely granular

Cortex is narrow and irregular

Pelvis dilated

This is often the late result of membranous or membrano-proliferative glomerulonephritis, less commonly postinfectious acute nephritis. Many cases have a 'silent' onset and some may be of viral origin. At the end stage, it is difficult to determine the aetiology of the pathological lesion.

Uraemia is the main clinical feature, but hypertensive cardiac failure or cerebral haemorrhage may cause death.

RENAL MANIFESTATIONS OF SYSTEMIC DISEASE

In a number of diseases, the kidneys are sometimes severely affected, and the renal manifestations may dominate the clinical picture. According to their pathogenesis the renal lesions fall into two main groups.

GROUP A. Diseases associated with immune complex deposition.

Systemic lupus erythematosus. Two forms of renal disease may be found:

	EM and immuno-fluorescence	*Serum complement*	*Clinical features*
1. Membranous glomerulonephritis	Deposits of IgG, IgM and IgA	Low	Nephrotic syndrome
2. Glomerulonephritis, focal or general	Deposits of IgG, IgM, IgA, C1, C3	Low	Proteinuria, haematuria may proceed to nephrotic syndrome
Henoch-Schönlein purpura Glomerulonephritis, focal or general	Mesangial deposits of IgA, IgG, fibrin	Normal	Proteinuria, haematuria

GROUP B. Diseases associated with thrombotic phenomena.

Vasculitis of various forms e.g. periarteritis nodosa Glomerulonephritis, focal or general	Intracapillary fibrin and mesangial proliferation	Normal	Proteinuria, haematuria, azotaemia
Disseminated intravascular coagulation e.g. thrombocytopenic purpura, malignant hypertension	Capillary and subendothelial fibrin	Normal	Acute renal failure or progressive renal failure

This is by no means an exhaustive list. Many other systemic diseases can have signs of kidney damage, but in most instances the renal component is a minor manifestation of the clinical syndrome.

INTERCURRENT RENAL CONDITIONS

RENAL FUNCTION AND PREGNANCY

Four conditions affecting renal function may arise in pregnancy.

1. **Acute pyelonephritis** is relatively common, possibly due to (a) the effects of uterine pressure on the ureters and (b) relaxation of smooth muscle allowing uterine dilatation and reflux.

2. **Pre-eclampsia and eclampsia**. This is a syndrome characterised by hypertension, variable unselective proteinuria and oedema. The essential kidney lesion is glomerular; tubular changes are secondary.

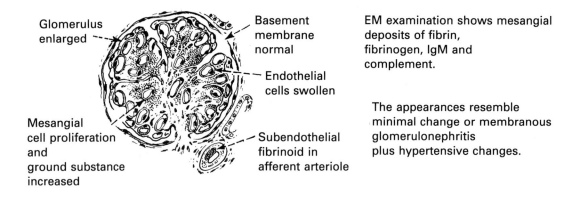

Glomerulus enlarged

Basement membrane normal

Endothelial cells swollen

Mesangial cell proliferation and ground substance increased

Subendothelial fibrinoid in afferent arteriole

EM examination shows mesangial deposits of fibrin, fibrinogen, IgM and complement.

The appearances resemble minimal change or membranous glomerulonephritis plus hypertensive changes.

The lesion appears to resolve rapidly after parturition. So far as kidney function is concerned, the danger of eclampsia lies in the occasional development of the third lesion.

3. **Acute tubular necrosis**. This is associated with complications of pregnancy causing SHOCK i.e. septic abortion, retroplacental haemorrhage and postpartum haemorrhage.

4. In more severe cases **bilateral cortical necrosis** may occur especially if disseminated intravascular coagulation (DIC) is superadded.

INTERCURRENT RENAL CONDITIONS

DIABETES

Renal complications are common in diabetes. Ten per cent of all diabetics die of renal failure. In juvenile diabetics, the figure is fifty per cent. In most cases the kidneys show typical changes.

The renal lesion is essentially a special form of the 'small vessel disease' seen systemically in insulin dependent diabetes e.g. diabetic retinopathy (see p.823).

Diabetic glomerulosclerosis   This takes one of two forms:

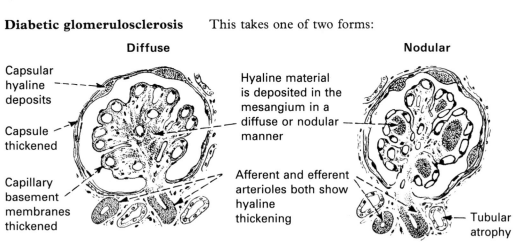

Diffuse

Capsular hyaline deposits

Capsule thickened

Capillary basement membranes thickened

Hyaline material is deposited in the mesangium in a diffuse or nodular manner

Afferent and efferent arterioles both show hyaline thickening

Nodular

Tubular atrophy

Deposited material is PAS-positive and resembles amyloid. The nodular form is often termed the Kimmelstiel-Wilson lesion. Progressive closure of capillaries can occur together with fibrous obliteration of the capsular space and the whole glomerulus. The changes in the afferent arterioles are an important factor in this process. Secondary tubular atrophy follows.

Clinical effects

Proteinuria is usually present and may produce a nephrotic syndrome. Chronic renal failure with uraemia and hypertension may ensue.

The cause is unknown, but poor control of diabetes and the development of antibodies to insulin may be contributory.

Pyelonephritis

This is common in diabetes and may be complicated by papillary necrosis.

Atheroma

This disease is uncommon in the renal arteries and their branches **except in diabetes**. It increases the renal ischaemia.

INTERCURRENT RENAL CONDITIONS

AMYLOID DISEASE

The general features of amyloidosis have already been described (p.22). Amyloid is deposited around the capillary basement membranes of the glomeruli.

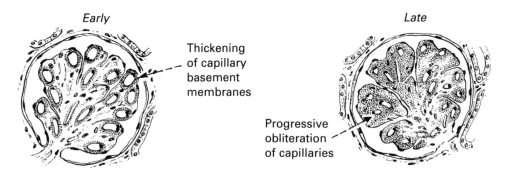

Early

Thickening of capillary basement membranes

Late

Progressive obliteration of capillaries

Gross proteinuria leading to a nephrotic syndrome is common. Interstitial fibrosis results from tubular degeneration and ischaemia due to glomerular and arteriolar lesions. Chronic renal failure results. Renal vein thrombosis can occur in amyloidosis causing acute renal failure.

DRUGS AND THE KIDNEYS

Three types of renal damage may be induced by drugs.

1. **Interstitial nephritis**. A hypersensitivity reaction induces a peritubular inflammation and tubular necrosis. Acute renal failure results.

2. **Acute tubular necrosis**. Mercurial diuretics and sulfonamide drugs can damage the tubular epithelium during concentration of the urine. The same mechanism may operate when using cytotoxic drugs and antibiotics, especially if renal function is already deficient.

3. **Chronic papillary necrosis**. This is the result of long-continued use of analgesics (aspirin, phenacetin) in large doses. The pathological picture is complicated by secondary changes.

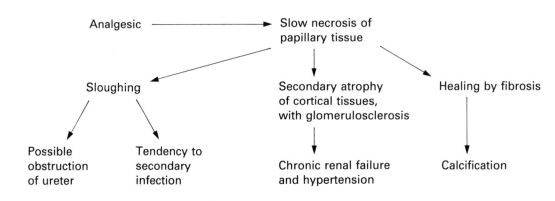

Analgesic ⟶ Slow necrosis of papillary tissue

Sloughing

Secondary atrophy of cortical tissues, with glomerulosclerosis

Healing by fibrosis

Possible obstruction of ureter

Tendency to secondary infection

Chronic renal failure and hypertension

Calcification

ACUTE TUBULAR NECROSIS

This arises in 2 circumstances:
1. During a state of shock, e.g. due to haemorrhage, burns, trauma, acute intestinal obstruction, incompatible transfusion and abdominal operations.
2. Following administration of toxic substances, e.g. carbon tetrachloride, trilene, ethylene glycol, compounds of mercury, uranium, chromic acid and various drugs.

The gross appearance of the kidneys is the same in both groups, although there is some difference in the type and distribution of the lesions.

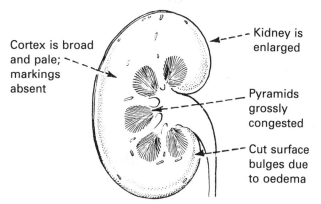

Cortex is broad and pale; markings absent

Kidney is enlarged

Pyramids grossly congested

Cut surface bulges due to oedema

Shock cases

The lesions are the result of ischaemia, and this determines the part of the kidney affected and the portion of the tubule damaged.

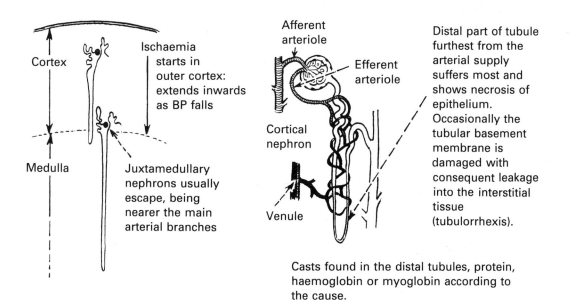

Cortex

Medulla

Ischaemia starts in outer cortex: extends inwards as BP falls

Juxtamedullary nephrons usually escape, being nearer the main arterial branches

Afferent arteriole

Efferent arteriole

Cortical nephron

Venule

Distal part of tubule furthest from the arterial supply suffers most and shows necrosis of epithelium. Occasionally the tubular basement membrane is damaged with consequent leakage into the interstitial tissue (tubulorrhexis).

Casts found in the distal tubules, protein, haemoglobin or myoglobin according to the cause.

623

ACUTE TUBULAR NECROSIS

Toxic cases

The lesions are evenly distributed, affecting all nephrons. They are maximal in the proximal tubules and are the direct result of the poison, the action of which is intensified by the concentrating activity of the tubule.

  The lesion is typified by carbon tetrachloride poisoning.

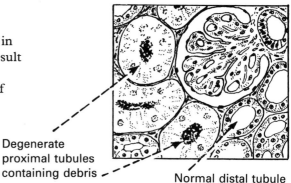

Degenerate proximal tubules containing debris

Normal distal tubule

Clinical effects

There are two clinical phases:

1. *Oliguria*

The glomerular filtration rate is greatly reduced. Unselective reabsorption of the filtrate occurs through the damaged tubule. The effects are:

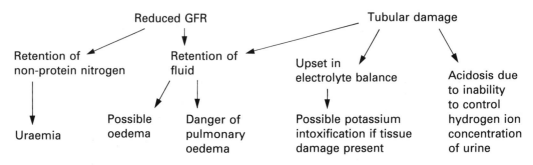

Reduced GFR   Tubular damage

Retention of non-protein nitrogen   Retention of fluid   Upset in electrolyte balance   Acidosis due to inability to control hydrogen ion concentration of urine

Uraemia   Possible oedema   Danger of pulmonary oedema   Possible potassium intoxification if tissue damage present

2. *Diuresis*

This occurs following healing of the lesions. The damaged tubular epithelium is replaced by a simple type which has not yet developed selective activities. Large volumes of dilute urine are passed. The clinical results are:

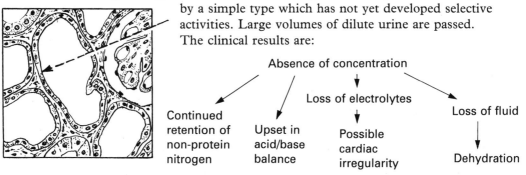

Absence of concentration

Loss of electrolytes   Loss of fluid

Continued retention of non-protein nitrogen   Upset in acid/base balance   Possible cardiac irregularity   Dehydration

Provided the patient can be maintained by countering the various biochemical upsets, the prognosis is good. The tubular epithelium has a great capacity for regeneration and ultimately regains its selective powers.

HAEMOLYTIC URAEMIC SYNDROME

This is a rare complication of many apparently dissimilar conditions. The mechanism appears to be as follows:

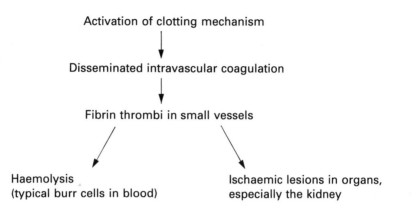

Activation of clotting mechanism

↓

Disseminated intravascular coagulation

↓

Fibrin thrombi in small vessels

Haemolysis
(typical burr cells in blood)

Ischaemic lesions in organs,
especially the kidney

The renal lesions are similar to those seen in malignant hypertension. There is fibrinoid necrosis of the afferent arterioles and capillaries of the glomeruli, and resulting areas of tubular necrosis. In the most extreme cases, bilateral cortical necrosis of the kidneys may occur. The underlying pathology is sometimes termed thrombotic microangiopathy. Clinical manifestations are varied. Renal failure, haemolytic anaemia, hypertension, and sometimes purpura with thrombocytopenia are the main features, but lesions in other organs and the symptoms of the initiating disease produce a complicated picture.

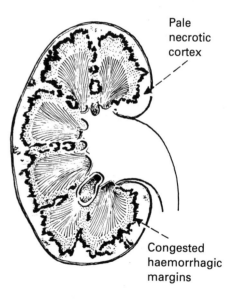

Pale
necrotic
cortex

Congested
haemorrhagic
margins

Aetiology

Activation of the clotting system can occur in many differing circumstances:

1. In children there is a close association with alimentary infections: particularly by *E.coli* 0157 which produces a verocystotoxin.

2. Shock conditions, e.g. following abruptio placentae in pregnancy, endotoxic shock.

3. Malignant hypertension. This can be a sequel to the syndrome and equally can predispose the patient to it.

625

TUBULAR LESIONS OF METABOLIC ORIGIN

This type of lesion is brought about by a metabolic defect which may arise outside the kidney (primary) or be the result of renal dysfunction (secondary).

The basic pathological mechanism is very similar in many of the conditions:

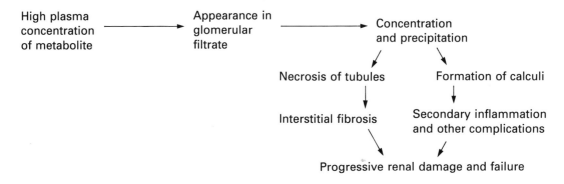

The following are some examples:

In **Renal Tubular Acidosis** the tubules are unable to produce an acid urine either due to an inherited defect or to damage by another renal disease. There may be hyperchloraemia and hypocalcaemia with hyperparathyroidism.

Hyperparathyroidism

Primary form. Hypersecretion of parathormone results in calcium deposition in and around the renal tubules.

Secondary form. Retention of phosphate due to renal failure causes parathyroid stimulation and withdrawal of calcium from bones. This causes a condition like osteitis fibrosa cystica and renal rickets in children. Renal deposition of calcium further affects the renal condition producing a vicious cycle.

Hypervitaminosis D

This rare condition, like hyperparathyroidism, produces a high plasma calcium with deposition in the kidney leading to fibrosis and calculus formation.

Gout

The deposition of urates in the renal pyramids causes tubular degeneration and interstitial inflammation progressing to fibrosis.

Fanconi syndrome

This is one example of a number of rare genetic defects causing aminoaciduria.

Cystinuria, glycosuria and phosphaturia are associated with acidosis resulting in renal deposition of calcium and cystine. Fibrosing interstitial nephritis follows, and the tubules show degeneration and cystic dilatations.

PYELONEPHRITIS

Pyelonephritis is the commonest type of renal disease and probably also the commonest single cause of renal failure. Two phases of the disease can be clearly defined, acute and chronic, but there is a spectrum of change and the division into phases is arbitrary.

ACUTE PYELONEPHRITIS

This is an acute pyogenic infection and the patient exhibits the usual general features of pyrexia, nausea, vomiting, headaches, rigors, etc., plus localising signs, e.g. frequency, dysuria, loin pain and sometimes haematuria.

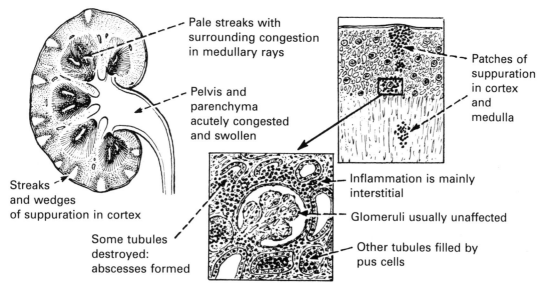

Pale streaks with surrounding congestion in medullary rays

Pelvis and parenchyma acutely congested and swollen

Streaks and wedges of suppuration in cortex

Some tubules destroyed: abscesses formed

Patches of suppuration in cortex and medulla

Inflammation is mainly interstitial

Glomeruli usually unaffected

Other tubules filled by pus cells

Urine

1. **Microscopy**

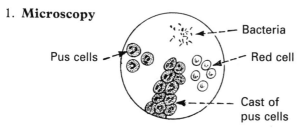

Bacteria

Pus cells

Red cell

Cast of pus cells

2. **Chemical** – protein, blood

3. Bacteriology

Large numbers of bacteria are found in the urine, several hundred thousand per ml in the acute phase.

The commonest infecting organism is *Escherichia coli*, but other faecal bacteria may also be found, e.g. pseudomonas, *Streptococcus faecalis*.

ACUTE PYELONEPHRITIS

Routes of infection

In the majority of cases, the condition is an ascending infection from the lower urinary tract, frequently associated with obstruction. Both sexes may be affected.

The condition is more common in females, possibly due to the short wide urethra, moist conditions in the perineum and proximity to the anus. In the male, obstruction is almost always present; in the female it may be absent. The condition occurs at an earlier age in the female.

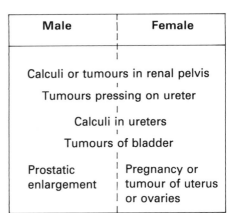

Male	Female
Calculi or tumours in renal pelvis	
Tumours pressing on ureter	
Calculi in ureters	
Tumours of bladder	
Prostatic enlargement	Pregnancy or tumour of uterus or ovaries

Influence of urinary tract obstruction

Obstruction of the urinary tract acts in 3 ways to promote infection:

1. The urine tends to stagnate and encourage growth of bacteria.
2. A tendency to vesicoureteral reflux during micturition develops especially when cystitis occurs.
3. Catheterisation is commonly carried out in these cases and can introduce infection. In this case the infection is likely to be mixed.

Progress The possibilities are as follows:

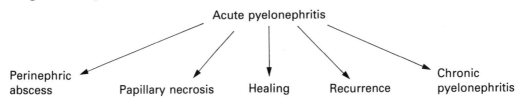

Acute pyelonephritis

Perinephric abscess   Papillary necrosis   Healing   Recurrence   Chronic pyelonephritis

Perinephric abscess and papillary necrosis are now rare due to specific antibiotic therapy.

Papillary necrosis (maximal at the kidney poles) is most apt to occur in cases associated with urinary obstruction.

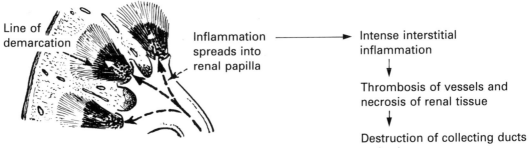

Line of demarcation

Inflammation spreads into renal papilla ——→ Intense interstitial inflammation

↓

Thrombosis of vessels and necrosis of renal tissue

↓

Destruction of collecting ducts and calyces

628   This can lead rapidly to renal failure.

ACUTE PYELONEPHRITIS

Healing stage

Involvement of the interstitial tissue and destruction of the tubules make resolution impossible and healing by a form of granulation tissue is inevitable.

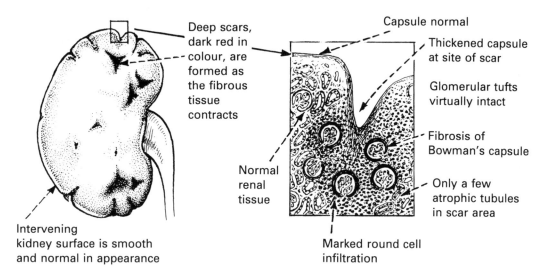

Deep scars, dark red in colour, are formed as the fibrous tissue contracts

Intervening kidney surface is smooth and normal in appearance

Normal renal tissue

Capsule normal

Thickened capsule at site of scar

Glomerular tufts virtually intact

Fibrosis of Bowman's capsule

Only a few atrophic tubules in scar area

Marked round cell infiltration

The lesions are very patchy, and the remaining kidney substance is normal. Eventually the whole area of the lesion is converted into fibrous tissue containing a few glomeruli showing progressive obliteration and sprinkling of round cells.

Danger lies in recurrence of infection, which is prone to happen especially in 'obstruction' cases. This causes a progressive destruction of the renal tissue leading to clinical chronic pyelonephritis.

Bacteriuria

Bacteria are commonly found in the urethra and are constantly flushed away by the urine. It becomes difficult therefore to assess the importance of their presence in a patient who may be ill and febrile but has no localising signs. It is now considered that a count of more than 100,000 bacteria per ml in a mid-stream specimen indicates urinary tract infection.

Significant bacterial counts may be found in patients with no signs or symptoms. This is not uncommon in female children and may account for those cases of chronic pyelonephritis where there has been no evidence of an acute phase.

CHRONIC PYELONEPHRITIS

Chronic pyelonephritis is essentially the result of repeated attacks of inflammation and healing. The process can be visualised as follows:

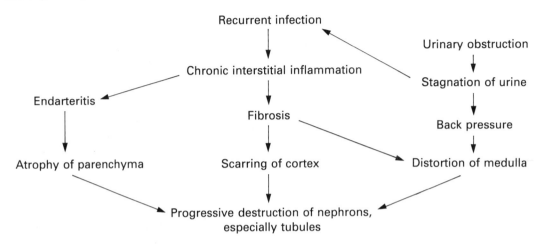

Kidney structure and function may be further prejudiced by the onset of hypertension. In cases with urinary obstruction, the external size of the kidney may remain normal or even be increased. Those with no underlying abnormality, commoner in the female, show progressive contraction of the kidney which becomes greyish white. The majority of cases are of this type.

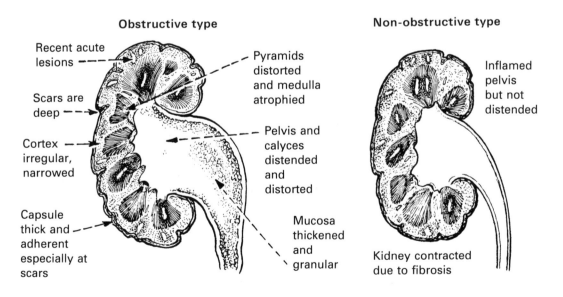

Depending on the cause, only one or both kidneys may be affected to variable degrees (c.f. chronic glomerulonephritis, p.618).

CHRONIC PYELONEPHRITIS

Microscopically, 3 types of lesion are seen in most cases:

1. Changes similar to those seen in the healing stage, but more advanced and extensive.

2. Occasionally acute suppurative lesions due to recent infection.

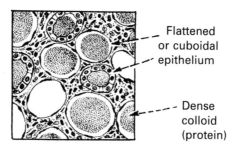

Periglomerular fibrosis

Heavy round cell infiltration
Absence of tubules

Endarteritis obliterans

3. Foci of dilated tubules in the cortex. This is due to destruction of the collecting tubules so that they end blindly. Upper tubules dilate, develop colloid casts and come to resemble thyroid tissue.

   The patchy inflammation results in fibrosis and atrophy irregularly distributed throughout the cortex and medulla.

Flattened or cuboidal epithelium

Dense colloid (protein)

Clinical effects

These are due to destruction of tubules and distortion of the anatomy of the renal medulla.

1. There is a progressive loss of the renal concentrating power.

2. The sodium pump effect of the counter-current mechanism is upset; base is lost thus causing acidosis. In children this can interfere with calcium metabolism.

   Renal failure with uraemia develops, although the patient may still be passing relatively large quantities of dilute urine. Chronic pyelonephritis is probably the commonest cause of fatal uraemia. Where unilateral obstruction is the cause only one kidney is affected and uraemia is not a feature.

3. Hypertension is common. Ninety per cent of patients are hypertensive when renal failure occurs. Equally striking, malignant hypertension develops in at least 15% of cases of severe chronic pyelonephritis. Where the inflammation is confined to one kidney, its removal has relieved the hypertension in some cases.

631

TUBERCULOUS PYELONEPHRITIS

This is now uncommon in many Western countries, due to population screening for tuberculosis and the effect of specific treatment. It is due to blood spread of infection from another site, e.g. the lungs. Alternatively, but much less commonly, there may be an ascending infection from some other part of the genitourinary system, e.g. epididymis or fallopian tubes. As usual, the tuberculous process develops slowly and lesions in the lungs which are the source of infection may have healed and disappeared by the time pyelonephritis is clinically apparent. The disease is commonly unilateral.

Stages

1. Tubercle bacilli settle in cortex

2. Caseous foci appear

3. Foci coalesce; spread via lymphatics and tubules

4. Process extends to medulla and ulcerates into pelvis

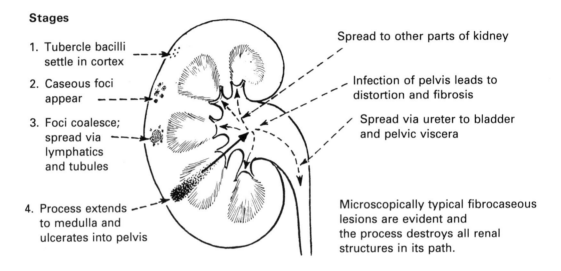

Spread to other parts of kidney

Infection of pelvis leads to distortion and fibrosis

Spread via ureter to bladder and pelvic viscera

Microscopically typical fibrocaseous lesions are evident and the process destroys all renal structures in its path.

Clinical features

There may be no localising features, the patient merely showing the general features of tuberculous infection – fever, night sweats and loss of weight. Lumbar discomfort or pain, dysuria and haematuria can develop. Secondary pyogenic infection is common leading to pyuria. Tubercle bacilli can usually be demonstrated in the urine either on direct microscopic examination or by culture. If, however, the ureter is blocked by caseous material, the urine, now coming solely from the uninfected kidney, may be sterile.

The danger is that infection may spread to the unaffected kidney and lead to renal failure.

THE KIDNEY AND ESSENTIAL HYPERTENSION

Two types of essential hypertension, benign and malignant, are recognised, and these have grossly different effects on the kidney function.

BENIGN ESSENTIAL HYPERTENSION

This is a chronic condition which may continue for 20–30 years. The anatomical changes in the kidney are due to progressive but patchy occlusion of the interlobular arteries and afferent arterioles.

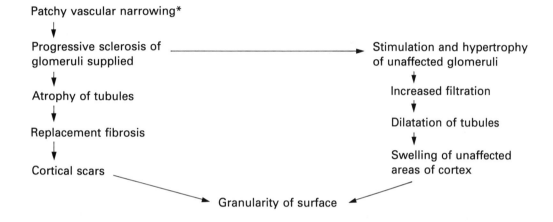

Patchy vascular narrowing*
↓
Progressive sclerosis of glomeruli supplied ⟶ Stimulation and hypertrophy of unaffected glomeruli
↓ ↓
Atrophy of tubules Increased filtration
↓ ↓
Replacement fibrosis Dilatation of tubules
↓ ↓
Cortical scars Swelling of unaffected areas of cortex
↘ ↙
Granularity of surface

*The renal ischaemia is also exacerbated by narrowing of the renal arterial orifices due to aortic atheroma.

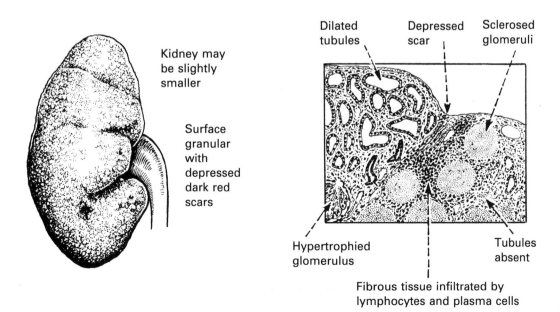

Kidney may be slightly smaller

Surface granular with depressed dark red scars

Dilated tubules

Depressed scar

Sclerosed glomeruli

Hypertrophied glomerulus

Tubules absent

Fibrous tissue infiltrated by lymphocytes and plasma cells

633

BENIGN ESSENTIAL HYPERTENSION

Where the changes are advanced, a contracted kidney is produced.
The vascular changes are of 2 types:

Interlobular arteries

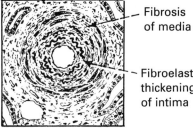

— Fibrosis of media

~ Fibroelastic thickening of intima

Afferent arterioles

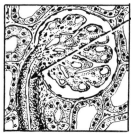

Intimal thickening due to plasmatic vasculosis

Hyaline material (fibrin) is deposited in subendothelial layer, reducing the lumen.

Various stages of atrophy can be recognised in the glomerular tufts as a result of these vascular changes.

Early

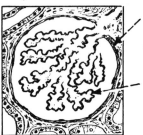

Fibrosis of Bowman's capsule

Wrinkling of capillary basement membrane

Intermediate

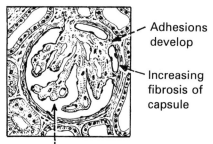

~ Adhesions develop

~ Increasing fibrosis of capsule

Capillaries collapse and disappear

Due to the patchy nature of the lesion, there is little clinical evidence of renal involvement and only rarely does renal failure develop in the uncomplicated case.

Usually patients die from one of three causes:

1. Cerebrovascular accident
2. Congestive cardiac failure
3. Coronary insufficiency.

Late

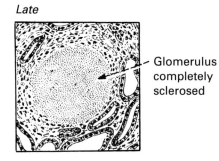

~ Glomerulus completely sclerosed

634

MALIGNANT HYPERTENSION

In this acute clinical condition, which ends in fatal uraemia in a matter of months if untreated, the blood pressure rises very rapidly to a high level. While the pathological lesions are patchy, they are rapidly progressive both in the degree of change in individual glomeruli and the number of glomeruli affected. As a primary condition, it is a disease of the 3rd and 4th decades in males. In most cases it is secondary to a pre-existing kidney lesion. The significant vascular lesions are to be seen in the afferent arterioles and interlobular arteries.

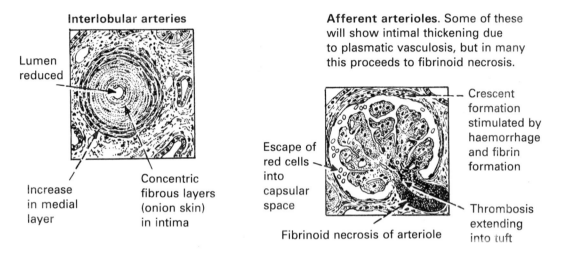

Interlobular arteries

Lumen reduced

Increase in medial layer

Concentric fibrous layers (onion skin) in intima

Afferent arterioles. Some of these will show intimal thickening due to plasmatic vasculosis, but in many this proceeds to fibrinoid necrosis.

Escape of red cells into capsular space

Crescent formation stimulated by haemorrhage and fibrin formation

Thrombosis extending into tuft

Fibrinoid necrosis of arteriole

Fibrinoid necrosis may also affect some of the interlobular arteries.

Related tubules of affected glomeruli show eosinophilic and red cell casts and necrosis of epithelium where the lesion is recent. This is followed by tubular atrophy. The gross appearance of the kidney is striking:

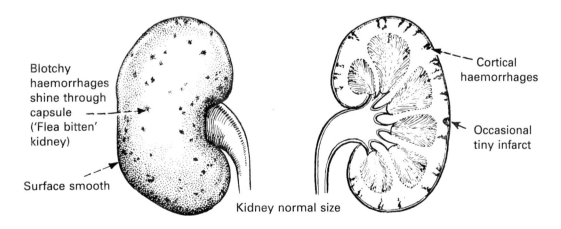

Blotchy haemorrhages shine through capsule ('Flea bitten' kidney)

Surface smooth

Kidney normal size

Cortical haemorrhages

Occasional tiny infarct

MALIGNANT HYPERTENSION

Clinical features

The main sign is high and rapidly increasing blood pressure. Proteinuria and haematuria are present intermittently. Oliguria eventually becomes progressive and symptoms and signs of uraemia supervene.

The same vascular changes occur in other viscera, e.g. intestines, and may cause symptoms. Headache is common and blurring of vision is caused by papilloedema and retinal haemorrhages, and the cerebral lesions of hypertensive encephalopathy may supervene.

HYPERTENSION AND THE KIDNEY

There is an obvious inter-relationship between renal disease and hypertension. Essential (primary) hypertension occasionally causes serious renal dysfunction, and the vascular changes are most marked in the kidneys. Primary renal disease on the other hand is almost always associated with hypertension (secondary). In cases of chronic renal failure, it is sometimes difficult to disentangle the factors involved. There is a spectrum of pathological change in which the contribution of each of the two factors – renal disease and hypertension – varies greatly. The causes of primary and secondary hypertension are unknown, but the opinion of many is that the kidney plays a central role in both and the search for a common factor continues. At the present moment, the following diagram provides a general idea of a possible mechanism.

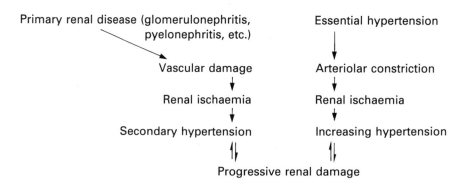

In this diagram the common factor is renal ischaemia, and it is thought that this stimulates the renin-hypertension mechanism. Experimentally, hypertension can be produced by restricting the blood flow to one kidney, and in the human situation hypertension has followed partial obstruction of one renal artery by atheroma or due to looping round a ureter. Removal of the affected kidney has allowed a return to normal blood pressure.

PROGRESSIVE RENAL FAILURE – END-STAGE KIDNEY

In any pathological condition in which there is significant loss of functioning renal tissue, compensating mechanisms are seen. The surviving nephrons show (1) COMPENSATORY HYPERTROPHY and are (2) CONTINUALLY ACTIVE with no 'down time'. (In the normal kidney, the nephrons do not all function simultaneously.)

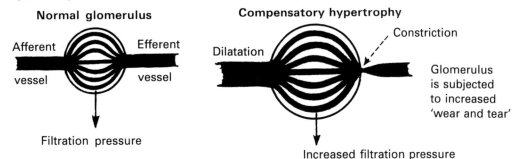

Wear and tear effects:

1. Endothelial cell damage → 2. Platelet thrombosis → 3. Hyalinisation → 4. Fibrosis (sclerosis)

The clinical state is eventually reached when the functional renal tissue has been reduced to a level where life cannot be maintained.

The major pathological causes are bilateral chronic pyelonephritis and less commonly chronic glomerulonephritis.

The progressive effects of this functional failure are uraemia and its complications.

URAEMIA

This is a syndrome encompassing a group of clinical and biochemical signs derived essentially from the retention of waste products and the failure to control fluid and electrolyte balance.

Classically, blood urea levels were measured to assess the degree of waste product retention; nowadays creatinine levels are more commonly measured. (Note that the retention of urea itself is not damaging.) The patient is lethargic. Anorexia, nausea and vomiting are usual, followed by mental confusion, muscle twitchings, convulsions and death if the condition is not alleviated. More commonly, a milder but inevitably progressive condition exists. An acute phase may be precipitated by intercurrent disease or further deterioration in the renal condition.

Since uraemia can be brought about by changes outwith the kidneys it is sometimes classified in three groups:

1. *Pre-renal.* Commonly due to conditions inducing shock, including haemorrhage, burns, severe infection, obstetric accidents, extensive surgery, etc.
2. *Renal.* Including glomerulonephritis, pyelonephritis, tubular necrosis due to poisons, toxins etc., transplant rejection.
3. *Post-renal.* Uraemia in this instance is due to obstructive lesions in the urinary tract, e.g. calculi, fibrosis, tumour, papillary necrosis and damage by trauma.

It is doubtful if such a classification is really useful, since in most cases the causes of a uraemic state are multiple. More important is to remember that the blood urea may rise in the absence of a renal lesion e.g. due to breakdown and absorption of the products of a large haematoma.

The following associations and complications are important (see p.638):

637

PROGRESSIVE RENAL FAILURE – END-STAGE KIDNEY

1. **Polyuria**. Despite the reduced glomerular filtration rate there is an increased volume of diluted urine. The mechanism is complicated but is presented in simplified form as follows:

	Normal kidney	End-stage kidney
Glomerular function	GFR – 125 ml/mm ≡ 180 litres/day	Many glomeruli sclerosed. ∴ GFR – say 10 ml/min ≡ 14 litres/day
Tubular function	99% reabsorption of water *Urine output:* 1 ml/min ≡ 1.4 litres/day	Many tubules damaged ∴ great reduction in reabsorption *Urine output:* 7 ml/min ≡ 10 litres/day

The inability to deal with water will lead to dehydration and rise in blood non-protein nitrogen if the intake is reduced.

If intake is increased it may cause water intoxication and rise in blood urea.

2. **Urine of fixed specific gravity** – usually 1010. This follows from the inability to concentrate the urine and the failure of the selective reabsorptive mechanisms, including the counter-current sodium pump. Urea, creatinine, uric acid, sulphate, chloride and phosphate are retained.

3. **Acidosis**. Difficulty in dealing with phosphates and the inability of the damaged tubules to form ammonia means that the hydrogen ion concentration of urine canot be varied to suit body needs, and retention acidosis results. Retention of phosphate causes a fall in plasma calcium leading to stimulation of the parathyroids. Bone lesions may result – renal osteo-dystrophy.

Complications

1. **Hypertension**. This is almost inevitable and several consequences are possible.

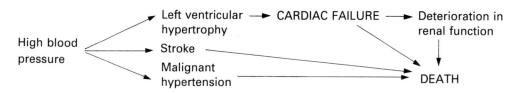

2. **Fibrinous exudates, e.g. fibrinous pericarditis, 'uraemic pneumonitis' with pleural exudate, uraemic colitis**.

3. **Haemorrhagic ulcers** of the gastro-intestinal tract.
   The lesions noted in 2 and 3 will cause further difficulty in maintaining biochemical equilibrium by causing changes in fluid balance and acid-base interchange.

4. **Anaemia**. This is due largely to depression of the bone marrow, due to deficient erythropoietin production by the kidney. Administration of genetically engineered erythropoietin alleviates the anaemia.

5. **Depression of immunological reaction**. Infections are common and will in turn affect renal function. Claims are made that the lack of reaction is beneficial in that there may be less likelihood of a renal transplant rejection.

PATHOLOGICAL COMPLICATIONS OF END-STAGE THERAPIES

The prognosis of end-stage renal failure has been greatly improved by (1) Dialysis and (2) Renal Transplantation. The following possible pathological complications are important:

Dialysis
(a) *Haemodialysis*
   (i) *Local* – infection and thrombosis at site of vessel access.
   (ii) *Systemic* – aluminium toxicity: historically, severe dementia was caused by using water containing excess aluminium. Aluminium and other impurities are now removed.

   In some cases of long-standing dialysis, small amounts of absorbed aluminium may be associated with mild mental deterioration.

   Amyloidosis affecting synovial tissues (e.g. carpal tunnel syndrome: joint stiffness) due to raised circulating B_2 microglobulin.
(b) *Continuous Ambulatory Peritoneal Dialysis (CAPD)* – peritonitis: obesity due to excessive glucose absorption.

Renal Transplantation
Rejection is the main complication. The mechanism is described on page 121.

Depending on the time after transplantation, rejection is classified as

(1) HYPERACUTE – within minutes/hours: (2) ACUTE – within a few weeks:
(3) CHRONIC – after months/years.

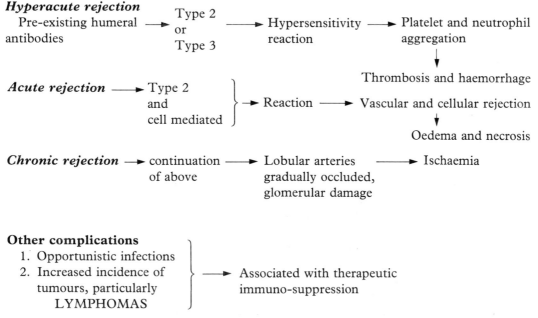

Hyperacute rejection
Pre-existing humeral antibodies ⟶ Type 2 or Type 3 ⟶ Hypersensitivity reaction ⟶ Platelet and neutrophil aggregation

Thrombosis and haemorrhage

Acute rejection ⟶ Type 2 and cell mediated } ⟶ Reaction ⟶ Vascular and cellular rejection

Oedema and necrosis

Chronic rejection ⟶ continuation of above ⟶ Lobular arteries gradually occluded, glomerular damage ⟶ Ischaemia

Other complications
   1. Opportunistic infections
   2. Increased incidence of tumours, particularly LYMPHOMAS } ⟶ Associated with therapeutic immuno-suppression

   3. Recurrence of original renal disease e.g. IgA nephritis in transplanted kidney.
Note: Similar complications occur in other transplant situations.

639

CONGENITAL DISORDERS

Malpositions and malformations of the kidney
are relatively common and the variations are numerous.
Some of the commoner are:

1. **Ectopic kidney (pelvic kidney)**
   One or both kidneys fail to reach the
   normal adult position. The condition causes
   difficulty:

   (a) During parturition
   (b) In differential diagnosis of pelvic neoplasms
   and infections
   (c) When the renal artery may originate at
   the normal level and the long vessel creates
   problems in arterial supply.

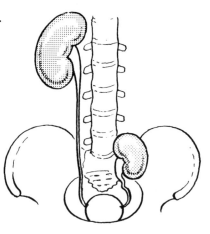

2. **Fusion of kidneys**

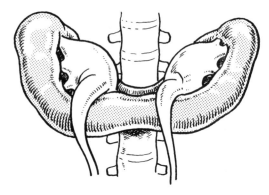

This is usually partial, producing
the so-called 'horse-shoe' kidney.
The ureters may be partially
obstructed leading to hydronephrosis,
infection and calculus formation.
Frequently the kidneys are also
ectopic, adding another hazard.

3. **Single kidney**
   This may be a form of fusion and there
   may be two ureters. In other cases, there is
   absence (agenesis) of one kidney, usually
   the left. There is no interference with
   renal function unless, of course, the single
   kidney becomes diseased.

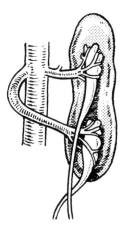

CONGENITAL CYSTIC DISEASE

This occurs in two main forms:

1. **Adult polycystic disease**

   This is relatively common, and varying degrees of the change may be seen from single cysts up to the classical type where the kidneys (rarely only one) are converted into a mass of cysts.

   It is an inherited autosomal dominant trait due to an abnormality on chromosome 16.

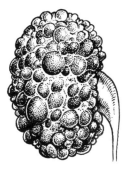

Kidney greatly enlarged:
(often exceeds 1 kg)

Cysts vary in size
(largest 5 or 6 cm)

Many are brownish
(fluid serous or mucoid)

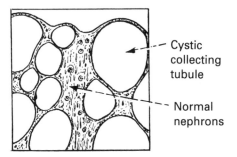

Cystic
collecting
tubule

Normal
nephrons

The defect is in the branching of some of the collecting tubules, causing a mixture of normal and abnormal nephrons. Cystic change develops after birth and is progressive, resulting in atrophy of normal nephrons by pressure. The cystic change may not be primarily due to obstruction, but opinion varies.

Intrahepatic cysts are often present but rarely numerous. Death from cerebral haemorrhage is more frequent than expected, partly due to the hypertension secondary to the kidney disorder and in some cases to aneurysms of cerebral arteries.

Clinical Findings

(a) Usually discovered during 3rd and 4th decades, rarely in childhood.

(b) Atrophy of the normal nephrons leads to chronic renal failure, uraemia and hypertension. Progress varies with the number of normal nephrons.

2. **Infantile polycystic disease (Polycystic kidney of the newborn: sponge kidney)**

   This is a rare condition.

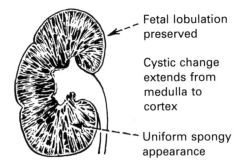

Fetal lobulation
preserved

Cystic change
extends from
medulla to
cortex

Uniform spongy
appearance

The nephrons are said to be normal in number and formation. Cystic dilatation is situated in the terminal branches of the collecting tubules. The disease is incompatible with life, and death occurs shortly after birth. It is due to an autosomal recessive trait. Small liver cysts and multiplication of the intrahepatic bile channels are often present.

TUMOURS OF THE KIDNEY

BENIGN GROWTHS

1. **Fibroma**. This is the commonest simple tumour arising from interstitial cells. It is found incidentally at autopsy in the medulla as a tiny round white nodule, usually less than 1 cm in diameter.

2. **Adenoma**. This is a relatively rare, small nodular proliferation of tubular type epithelium. Histologically they are similar to renal cell carcinomas (see below). It is arbitrarily stated that a tumour smaller than 3 cm in diameter is benign: larger than 3 cm may behave as a metastasising carcinoma.

MALIGNANT TUMOURS

Two are of importance: renal carcinoma and nephroblastoma.

Renal cell carcinoma (hypernephroma)
This is the commonest primary malignant renal tumour. It usually has a typical appearance.

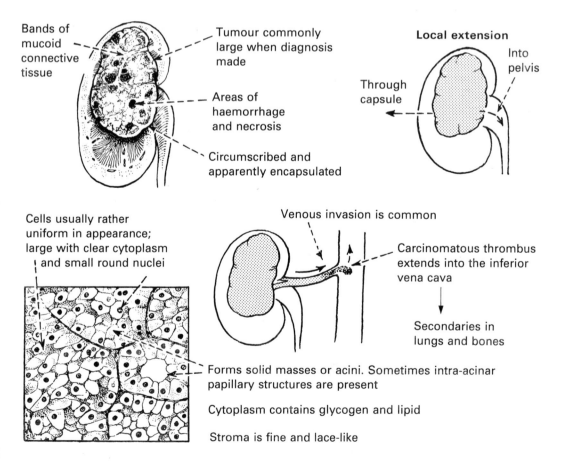

Bands of mucoid connective tissue

Tumour commonly large when diagnosis made

Areas of haemorrhage and necrosis

Circumscribed and apparently encapsulated

Local extension

Through capsule

Into pelvis

Cells usually rather uniform in appearance; large with clear cytoplasm and small round nuclei

Venous invasion is common

Carcinomatous thrombus extends into the inferior vena cava

Secondaries in lungs and bones

Forms solid masses or acini. Sometimes intra-acinar papillary structures are present

Cytoplasm contains glycogen and lipid

Stroma is fine and lace-like

TUMOURS OF THE KIDNEY

Malignant (continued)

Nephroblastoma (Wilm's tumour)
This is one of the commonest malignant tumours of childhood. It is an embryonic type of tumour derived from kidney rudiments, and forms a large well-circumscribed growth which rapidly invades blood vessels, giving rise to pulmonary secondaries. With modern therapy 90% long-term survival rates are achieved.

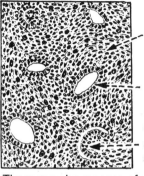

Much of the growth consists of spindle cells resembling sarcoma

This merges with tubules and acini

Occasionally there are primitive glomerular structures

There may be masses of striped muscle.

Secondary carcinoma
Secondary deposits of carcinoma are not common in the kidney.

DISEASES OF URINARY TRACT

The urinary tract is essentially a collecting and discharge system. There are 4 main pathological processes affecting its function: (1) obstruction, (2) infections, (3) calculus formation and (4) neoplastic disease.

Congenital anomalies, which are relatively rare, produce their effects by one or other of these processes.

Obstruction
Acute obstruction, if complete, causes rapid cessation of urine production. If both kidneys are involved, renal failure quickly follows. Chronic obstruction is more common and leads to anatomical changes, with sequels.

Hydronephrosis
This is a dilatation of the renal pelvis and calyces, due to chronic incomplete or intermittent obstruction.

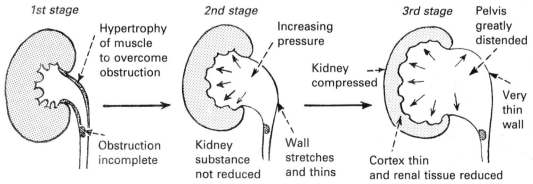

1st stage — Hypertrophy of muscle to overcome obstruction / Obstruction incomplete

2nd stage — Increasing pressure / Kidney substance not reduced / Wall stretches and thins

3rd stage — Pelvis greatly distended / Kidney compressed / Very thin wall / Cortex thin and renal tissue reduced

643

DISEASES OF URINARY TRACT

Hydronephrosis (continued)

Microscopically, the kidney shows atrophy of tubules in the third stage. This is followed by obliteration of glomeruli. Both changes are the result of pressure directly on the tubules and on the intrarenal vessles. Urine formation is upset and may eventually cease.

Sequels

1. **Infection**. This is almost inevitable and usually takes the form of a chronic pyelonephritis. It exacerbates the whole process and a vicious cycle is set up.

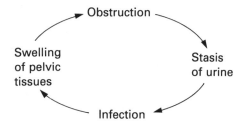

The effects on kidney function have already been considered (p.630 et seq).

2. **Calculus formation**. The combination of stasis and infection causes precipitation of phosphates and a stone is produced. The mechanism may be:

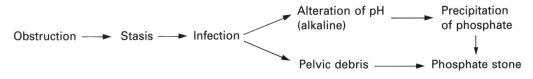

Aetiology
The condition may affect one or both kidneys. This is related to the site of obstruction.

Unilateral obstruction:
above the bladder

Common sites:
  1. Pelvi-ureteric junction.
  2. At pelvic brim.
  3. At entrance to bladder.

Causes:
1. Calculus.
2. Tumour growth.
3. Inflammatory stricture.
4. Congenital abnormality.

Gross hydronephrosis is more commonly unilateral.

Bilateral obstruction:
in or around bladder or urethra. The ureters are also affected and become dilated and tortuous.

Causes:
1. Prostatic enlargement.
2. Tumour of bladder.
3. Urethral stricture.
4. Pelvic neoplasm.

URINARY TRACT INFECTION

Pyelonephritis has already been considered. Inflammation of the ureters is due to extension upwards from an infection of the bladder and urethra.

Acute cystitis

The bladder shows the usual signs of inflammation. Small haemorrhages are common in the oedamatous mucosa. The following points are important:

1. It is common in females, especially frequent in pregnancy: and also associated with sexual intercourse.
2. In males it is usually secondary to obstruction, e.g. due to enlarged prostate or a urethral stricture.
3. Obstruction encourages infection, enhances its effects and prolongs the inflammatory process.
4. In non-obstructive cases, infection is usually due to *E. coli*. Mixed infections, proteus and staphylococcus, are common in obstructive cases.
5. Vesicoureteric reflux is very important allowing retrograde spread of infection to the kidneys. It occurs as a congenital defect in children but also may be secondary to cystitis.

Chronic cystitis

This is the result of repeated attacks of acute cystitis, but it is usually associated with obstruction of the urethra causing stasis of urine and is commonest in males.

Mixed infection including proteus is common and, together with urea-splitting organisms forming ammonia, result in an alkaline urine. Phosphates precipitate and can form crumbling whitish calculi.

Tuberculous cystitis

This is always secondary to a tuberculous infection elsewhere, usually in the kidney. Less commonly, the epididymis is the source of infection. Small tubercles form in the submucous layer, usually at the bladder base. These ulcerate and secondary infection is common.

Urethritis

Acute inflammation of the urethra is commonly due to the gonococcus, but another form is now more common in Western countries – non-specific urethritis. The actual cause is unknown: suggestions include virus, mycoplasma and allergy.

Urethritis may also occur in trichomonal infection and Reiter's disease in which arthritis and conjunctivitis are also present.

RENAL CALCULI

Three basic types of renal calculi are recognised.

 ← Surface is rough; colour brown, probably due to old blood pigment

(1) **Calcium oxalate**

← Smooth light brown colour

(2) **Uric acid and urates**

←-- Flaking surface, greyish white

(3) **Phosphate (calcium apatite)**

Commonly the stones are mixed.
1. Urate stones frequently have a rough covering of oxalate.
2. Both oxalate and urate stones tend to develop a covering of phosphates.

Sites of formation. Two suggestions have been made.

1. Precipitates form in the collecting tubules and pass into the renal pelvis where they enlarge.
2. Deposits are formed in the lymphatics of the renal papillae and are extruded into the renal pelvis.

Mode of formation. This is unknown, but the following is one modern theory:

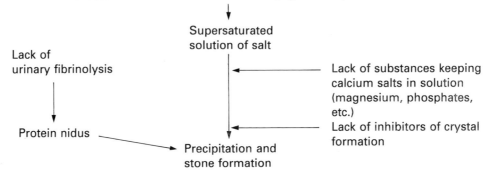

Excess excretion of stone substance (e.g. oxalate) + Calcium
↓
Supersaturated solution of salt

Lack of urinary fibrinolysis

Lack of substances keeping calcium salts in solution (magnesium, phosphates, etc.)

Lack of inhibitors of crystal formation

Protein nidus

Precipitation and stone formation

Predisposing factors
1. **Urinary pH**. Urate and oxalate stones form in an acid urine; phosphate stones in alkaline urine.
2. **Dehydration** – causing increased urinary concentration.
3. **Stasis**. Obstruction to urine flow encourages salt precipitation.
4. **Renal disease**. The pH of the urine is frequently disturbed, and the composition of the urine is always altered.
   (a) Renal infection is one of the most important factors. In many cases of renal sepsis, the urine becomes alkaline, favouring phosphate precipitation. Ischaemia causing degeneration and necrosis induces calcification in many chronic renal diseases, and this may lead to stone formation.
   (b) Renal tumours encourage stone formation. Areas of tumour necrosis may calcify, and tumours tend to cause urinary stasis.

RENAL CALCULI

Predisposing factors (continued)

5. **Metabolic factors**. These can operate by altering the pH of the urine and especially by increasing the output of substances e.g.:

   (a) Hypercalcuria and hyperphosphaturia. These may be caused by:
   Hyperparathyroidism, primary or secondary to renal failure
   Vitamin D overdosage
   Diet, e.g. excessive milk and alkalies over years in peptic ulcer cases
   Immobilisation leading to loss of calcium from bones.

   (b) Oxaluria. Due to:
   Congenital metabolic defect
   Poisoning by ethylene glycol.

   (c) Urate excess is found in:
   Gout
   Excess intake of purines
   Following ileostomy.

   (d) Rare stones, e.g. cystine, xanthine, are related to inborn metabolic defects.

Effects and complications

These are related to passage of the stone and develop in two situations.

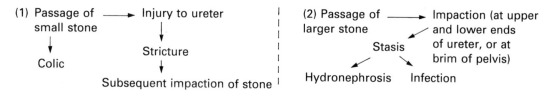

(1) Passage of small stone ⟶ Injury to ureter ↓ Stricture ↓ Subsequent impaction of stone
Colic

(2) Passage of larger stone ⟶ Impaction (at upper and lower ends of ureter, or at brim of pelvis)
Stasis
Hydronephrosis   Infection

With the development of stasis and infection, further stone formation is encourgaged. This can lead to some peculiar results, e.g:

Staghorn calculus

This large single stone is associated with suppuration and ulceration of the pelvis and calyces. It is composed mainly of phosphates.

Stones and infection in the pelvis can lead to squamous metaplasia of the epithelium. In a few instances this may develop into squamous carcinoma.

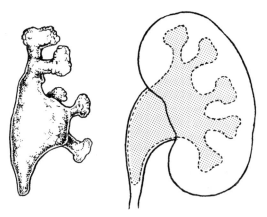

BLADDER CALCULI

These may have passed down the ureter. In the bladder they can increase greatly in size. Cystitis is common and the enlargement is due to deposit of phosphates. Stones may actually form in the bladder when there is urethral obstruction and chronic cystitis.

TUMOURS OF THE URINARY TRACT

These tumours occur in 2 main sites: (1) the renal pelvis and (2) the bladder (the commoner site). They arise from the stratified transitional epithelium lining the tract and are all considered to be CARCINOMAS but show a wide spectrum of malignant potential. They are graded I to IV as follows.

GRADE I – These are **Papillary Tumours**. Tumours at the benign end of the spectrum have a uniform, well-differentiated epithelial covering showing no mitotic activity. They have a slender stalk and delicate branching fronds. With this structure, and their fine vascular connective tissue, haemorrhage is common.

GRADE II – These also are **Papillary**. In malignant form, the stalk of the tumour is broader and the epithelial cells show mitoses and variability. Early stromal invasion may be present.

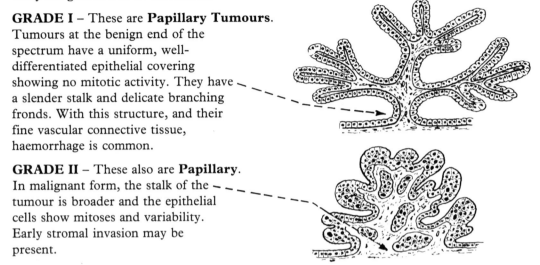

GRADES III and IV are **Solid Sessile Tumours**: They are distinguished by the degrees of cellular anaplasia, mitotic activity and aggressive growth. Infection with ulceration and necrosis is common: local penetration into the bladder muscle and lymphatic invasion are usual.

Squamous carcinoma and adenocarcinoma are rare tumours.

Note: (i) Urothelial tumours are often multiple and recurrence is common.
(ii) Progression from a low grade to higher grades is frequent.

Aetiology

Bladder tumours are an industrial hazard:
(a) in aniline dye manufacture due to beta-naphthylamine
(b) in the rubber industry
(c) in manufacturing processes involving benzidine.

SMOKING and CHRONIC ANALGESIC ABUSE are important associations. In the MIDDLE EAST chronic infestation by **Schistosoma haematobium** is an important association.

Mechanism

KIDNEY   ⟶   UROTHELIUM   ⟶   FIELD CHANGES
Excretion of carcinogen   chronic exposure
   (i) direct elimination   particularly in
or (ii) metabolite concen-   bladder
       tration in urine   **CARCINOMA**

FEMALE GENITAL TRACT – ANATOMY AND PHYSIOLOGY

The ovaries, fallopian tubes, uterus, vagina and vulva form an integrated system which is unique in that full function is limited to a period of roughly 40 years from puberty to menopause. A two-tier system of hormonal control operates. Secretion of steroids by the ovary prepares the uterus for pregnancy, and the ovarian secretion is controlled by the anterior pituitary and hypothalamus.

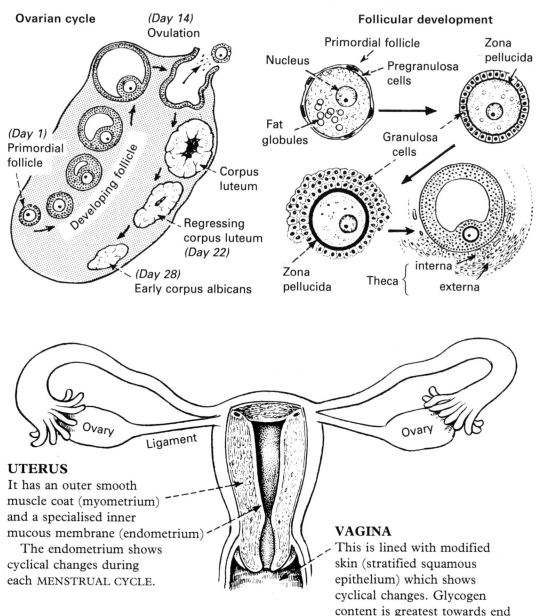

Ovarian cycle

(Day 14) Ovulation

(Day 1) Primordial follicle

Developing follicle

Corpus luteum

Regressing corpus luteum *(Day 22)*

(Day 28) Early corpus albicans

Follicular development

Primordial follicle

Nucleus

Pregranulosa cells

Zona pellucida

Fat globules

Granulosa cells

Zona pellucida

Theca { interna / externa

UTERUS
It has an outer smooth muscle coat (myometrium) and a specialised inner mucous membrane (endometrium).
 The endometrium shows cyclical changes during each MENSTRUAL CYCLE.

Ovary

Ligament

Ovary

VAGINA
This is lined with modified skin (stratified squamous epithelium) which shows cyclical changes. Glycogen content is greatest towards end of menstrual cycle.

649

CYCLICAL ENDOMETRIAL CHANGES

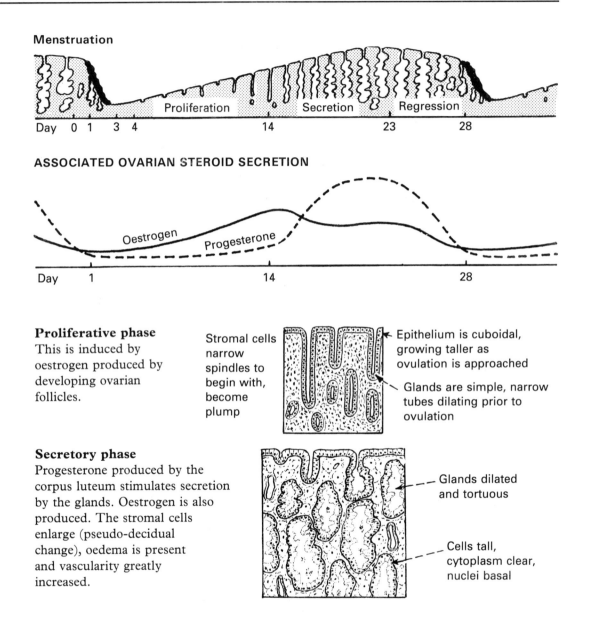

Menstruation

Proliferation   Secretion   Regression

Day 0 1 3 4   14   23   28

ASSOCIATED OVARIAN STEROID SECRETION

Oestrogen

Progesterone

Day   1   14   28

Proliferative phase
This is induced by oestrogen produced by developing ovarian follicles.

Stromal cells narrow spindles to begin with, become plump

Epithelium is cuboidal, growing taller as ovulation is approached

Glands are simple, narrow tubes dilating prior to ovulation

Secretory phase
Progesterone produced by the corpus luteum stimulates secretion by the glands. Oestrogen is also produced. The stromal cells enlarge (pseudo-decidual change), oedema is present and vascularity greatly increased.

Glands dilated and tortuous

Cells tall, cytoplasm clear, nuclei basal

Premenstrual regressive phase
Endometrial growth ceases 5–6 days before menstruation. Prior to menstruation, it shrinks due to decreased blood flow and discharge of secretion. This increases the tortuosity of glands and blood vessels.

CYCLICAL ENDOMETRIAL CHANGES

CONTROL MECHANISM
The control of these events
is two-way, involving both
steroids and gonadotrophins.
The time relationship between
these two classes of hormone
may be represented thus:

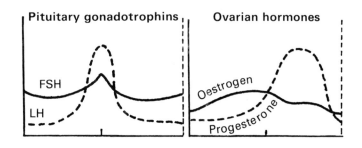

Feed back systems are involved in stimulating and controlling the hormones secreted.

1. At the end of a menstrual cycle,
the plasma oestrogen is low.
This is a signal to the pituitary
to secrete FSH (positive stimulation)
which stimulates follicular growth.

2. As follicles grow, they secrete
oestrogen which damps down the
secretion of FSH (negative feedback).
Only the larger follicles
possessing sufficient receptors for
FSH continue to grow.

3. The blood oestrogen goes on
rising as a result of secretion
from these large follicles. When
it reaches a sufficiently high
level, it stimulates the centre in
the median eminence which secretes
gonadotrophin releasing
factor (positive feedback). This
causes a surge of secretion of
FSH and LH which induce ovulation.

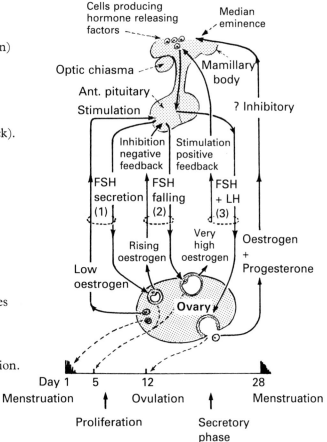

Morphological cyclical changes also take place in the fallopian tubes, cervix, vagina and
vulva.

651

DISEASES OF UTERINE BODY

CARCINOMA (continued)

Metastases

1. Via lymphatics

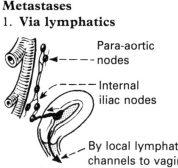

Para-aortic nodes

Internal iliac nodes

By local lymphatic channels to vagina

2. Via blood vessels
Secondary deposits in the vagina and ovaries may be due to this mode of spread

3. Via fallopian tube

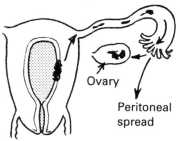

Ovary

Peritoneal spread

4. Distant metastases. At a late date, secondaries may appear in the liver, lungs and bones. These may be the result of lymphatic or blood spread.

Prognosis

The occurrence of bleeding early in the disease leads to early diagnosis. Lack of lymphatics in the endometrium limits extension for a considerable time. The prognosis is also related to the degree of differentiation but overall a 60% 5-year survival rate is to be expected.

Aetiology

Endometrial carcinoma is uncommon before the 5th decade. The most important factor is prolonged OESTROGENIC stimulation due to:

   (a) endogenous overproduction e.g. in cases of oestrogen-secreting ovarian tumours

   (b) exogenous – oestrogen therapy

   (c) in OBESITY: increased conversion of androstenedione (from adrenals) to oestrone

   (d) ATYPICAL HYPERPLASIA in an important precancerous stage.

ENDOMETRIAL SARCOMAS

These are rare tumours. They arise from stem cells which have the ability to differentiate into several different tissue types:

A pure homologous sarcoma differentiates to endometrial stroma only. This is a very rare tumour and is at the benign end of the spectrum of malignancy.

Tumours at the highly malignant end occur in elderly women and sometimes present as soft, lobulate grape-like masses projecting into the upper vagina from the cervical os.

(1) CARCINOSARCOMA
(mixed homologous)

   Endometrial adenosarcoma + sarcoma

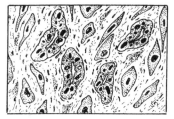

Stromal elements include malignant cartilage and striated muscle

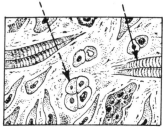

(2) MIXED MESODERMAL SARCOMA (mixed heterologous → or mixed MÜLLERIAN)

DISEASES OF UTERINE BODY

HYDATIDIFORM MOLE

This occurs in two forms:

1. **Complete**. This is a pregnancy lacking a fetus. It starts early in pregnancy and the uterus is filled by cysts of varying size.

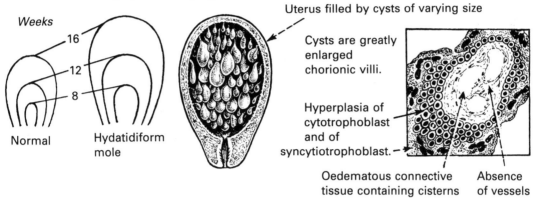

Uterus filled by cysts of varying size

Cysts are greatly enlarged chorionic villi.

Hyperplasia of cytotrophoblast and of syncytiotrophoblast.

Oedematous connective tissue containing cisterns

Absence of vessels

Blood and urine levels of chorionic gonadotrophin are high.

2. **Invasive**. Mole villi may penetrate the myometrium and invade blood vessels with pulmonary 'metastases'. There is usually complete regression after hysterectomy however.
3. **Partial**. Sometimes only part of the placenta shows hydatid change and a fetus, usually malformed, is present.

Prevalence: Uncommon in the West (1 in 2000 pregnancies) but common in the East (1 in 120 pregnancies).

Genetics: The genetic sex of the complete form is XX, but both chromosomes are paternal. It is thought that a single sperm penetrates a dead or dying ovum.

Progress: Abortion is the usual outcome: there is a 2–3% risk of CHORIOCARCINOMA developing.

CHORIOCARCINOMA

This is the malignant tumour of the trophoblast and is by definition of fetal origin.

It usually follows hydatid mole. Pleomorphic cytotrophoblast and syncytium, showing numerous mitoses, invade blood vessels causing haemorrhage and early lung metastases either as a single large 'cannon-ball' haemorrhagic mass or multiple small emboli ('snow-storm' lung). The high blood and urine concentrations of chorionic gonadotrophin are used to monitor progress and treatment.

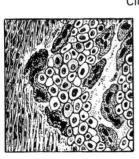
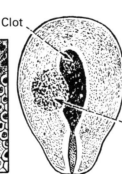

Clot

The myometrium is infiltrated by masses of malignant trophoblast and blood venous sinuses are eroded.

657

DISEASES OF UTERINE BODY

MYOMETRIUM

The myometrium is never a primary site of inflammation, acute or chronic. It is involved secondary to lesions in the endometrium or peritoneum. Tumours however are quite common.

LEIOMYOMA (Myoma, fibromyoma, fibroid)

This is a circumscribed growth derived from uterine muscle.

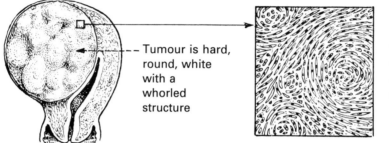

— Tumour is hard, round, white with a whorled structure

The cells are typical long spindle muscle cells, arranged in interlacing bundles

They vary in size from tiny (mm) growths to several cm in diameter and are frequently multiple. Apparent encapsulation is due to compression by adjacent muscle.

Fibroids may be found in any part of the uterus.

Tumours beneath the endometrium tend to bulge into the cavity and may eventually develop to form a fibroid polyp.

Similarly subserous polyps may form

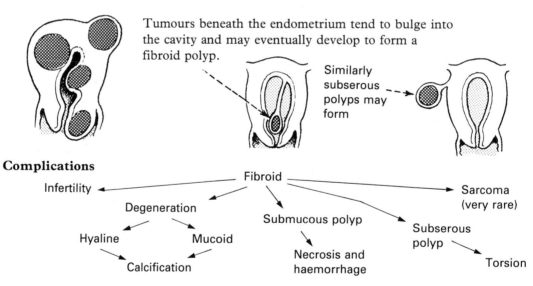

Complications

Leiomyoma is one of the commonest tumours, occurring in 15–20% of women over the age of 35. Growth ceases at the menopause.

SARCOMA

This is a rare tumour. It may arise from a preceding leiomyoma, but this is not certain. Usually it is extremely malignant.

DISEASES OF UTERINE BODY

ENDOMETRIOSIS

This consists of deposits of endometrium outside of the uterine cavity.

In almost all cases, the disease is confined to the pelvis and the genital tract.

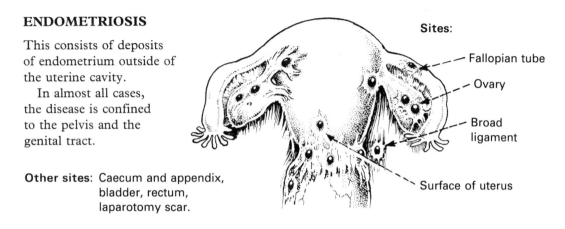

Sites:

— Fallopian tube

— Ovary

— Broad ligament

— Surface of uterus

Other sites: Caecum and appendix, bladder, rectum, laparotomy scar.

These deposits react to the stimulus of ovarian steroids and show cyclical changes. The result is haemorrhage into the local tissues at the time of menstruation. Adhesions develop.

Aetiology

In some instances deposits are formed in laparotomy scars after uterine operations, but in most cases there has been no surgical interference. Three theories have been proposed.

1. Retrograde spill of menstrual debris.
2. Metaplasia of tissues into Müllerian duct elements.
3. Lymphatic and blood borne emboli of endometrial tissue.

ADENOMYOSIS

This is a condition of ectopic endometrial deposits in the myometrium. There is an accompanying overgrowth of muscle and connective tissue. Two macroscopic forms occur:

1. **Diffuse**
   Deposits are confined to inner part of myometrium
   Foci of endometrium often brownish in colour

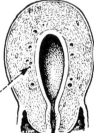

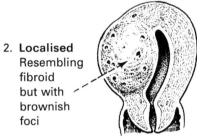

2. **Localised**
   Resembling fibroid but with brownish foci

The endometrial deposits are said to communicate with the uterine cavity, but despite this they often contain altered blood in the glands which become cystic. The diffuse type is commoner.

DISEASES OF CERVIX

The cervix constitutes the lower one third of the uterine body.

It is in two parts: endocervical and vaginal or ectocervical. The dividing line is quite sharp and is determined by the character of the lining epithelium.

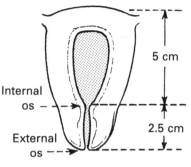

5 cm

Internal os —

2.5 cm

External os —

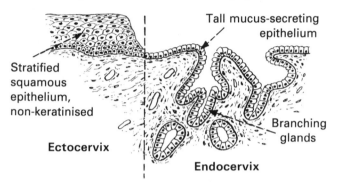

Tall mucus-secreting epithelium

Stratified squamous epithelium, non-keratinised

Branching glands

Ectocervix

Endocervix

The remainder of the cervical wall consists of circular smooth muscle lying in abundant fibroelastic tissue.

At the internal os, the structure gradually merges with that of the uterus proper, the branching glands giving place to the simple tubules of the endometrium, and the proportion of muscle increases greatly.

CERVICAL EROSION. This is a misnomer: it represents an unfolding and eversion of the distal ENDOCERVIX (columnar mucous epithelium) into an ECTOCERVICAL situation. The term CERVICAL ECTOPIA is preferred. Varying degrees of SQUAMOUS METAPLASIA follow and infection is common.

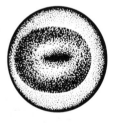

Red colour; soft velvety texture

Aetiology
1. Most cases are due to increased uterine bulk.
2. Common in pregnancy.
3. Related to hormonal stimulation (cyclical and contraceptive pill).

CERVICAL POLYP. This is a local proliferation of endocervical mucosa which becomes pedunculated and may protrude through the cervix.

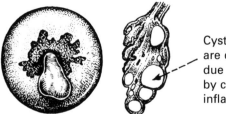

Cystic glands are common due to obstruction by chronic inflammation

660

DISEASES OF CERVIX

CERVICITIS

This is usually a mild, chronic condition and in most cases the bacterial flora is mixed, but in a small number of cases acute inflammation may result from gonococcal infection or infection with other pyogenic organisms particularly during childbirth with lacerations of cervix.

In chronic cervicitis, the mucus-secreting endocervical epithelium undergoes squamous metaplasia. This is a simple condition, the result of chronic irritation. In some instances, this squamous epithelium is 'restless', showing proliferative activity and cellular abnormalities, termed dysplasia. Dysplasia, intraepithelial carcinoma (carcinoma in situ) and invasive carcinoma are thought to be stages in a continuing process. Dysplasia was considered in three stages – mild, moderate and severe – but each stage merges with the next and the differentiation between severe dysplasia and carcinoma in situ is difficult. A new pragmatic classification has been adopted which provides a practical guide for the surgeon.

The **CERVICAL INTRAEPITHELIAL NEOPLASIA (CIN) Classification** provides a practical guide for the surgeon. It covers the whole spectrum of cervical premalignant change: there are 3 grades which relate to dysplasia and carcinoma in situ as follows:

Benign squamous metaplasia
Stratification well defined with:

Squames at
surface --->

Oval polygonal
cells form -- -->
several layers

Basal cells usually
a single layer
at right angles
to the surface.

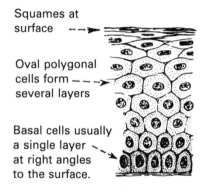

CIN 1 ≡ mild dysplasia

Upper two thirds
stratified - - - - >

Cells of basal third
have high nucleocytoplasmic
ratio; pleomorphic nuclei
at all levels

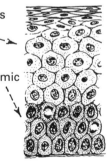
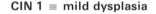

CIN 2 ≡ moderate dysplasia

Upper half of
epithelium shows
stratification and
maturation

Basal cells
occupy - - - - >
lower half

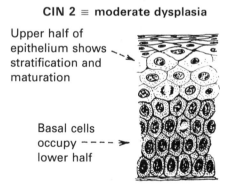

Although a clear distinction is made in these illustrations between CIN 1 and CIN 2, in practice all degrees of change are seen and the grading depends on the individual pathologist.

DISEASES OF CERVIX

Cervical intra-epithelial neoplasia (continued)

CIN 3: Severe dysplasia and carcinoma in situ are included in this grade. The differentiation between them is even more subjective. By adopting the CIN grading, this subjective problem is eliminated since no attempt is made to separate the two conditions, and the clinician understands that CIN is a dangerous lesion.

Examples are:

CIN 3 ≡ severe dysplasia or Ca in situ

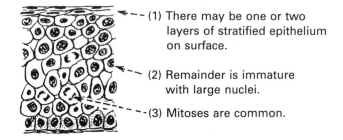

(1) There may be one or two layers of stratified epithelium on surface.

(2) Remainder is immature with large nuclei.

(3) Mitoses are common.

Classical Ca in situ

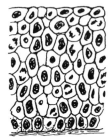

(1) Almost complete loss of stratification.
(2) Loss of polarity of the cells, the majority being at right angles to the surface; the remainder irregularly arranged.
(3) Variation in nuclear size with increase in nuclear/cytoplasmic ratio.
(4) Cells lose their squamous appearance.
(5) Mitotic figures found at all levels.

The lesion develops at the squamo-columnar junction, i.e. where endocervix and ectocervix meet. Less than 20% occur within the cervical canal. The epithelium is loosely attached to the underlying stroma, especially type 3 and may be removed by swabbing, thus leading to misdiagnosis.

This preinvasive stage may last for many years before invasion develops, but in many cases does not progress to the invasive stage. Most are diagnosed in the 4th decade but increasingly as early as the 2nd decade. Unfortunately, it is obviously impossible to say how soon invasion will occur.

DISEASES OF CERVIX

CARCINOMA

This is the most common malignant tumour of the female genital tract, even where there is a vigorous campaign for early diagnosis and eradication of carcinoma in situ. The growth is a squamous carcinoma in 70% of cases, a squamous carcinoma with an adenocarcinoma component (adeno-squamous carcinoma) in 20% and a pure adenocarcinoma in 5%. Most squamous carcinomas arise at the squamo-columnar junction: a minority (20%) and most adenocarcinomas arise within the endocervical canal.

The cervix becomes very indurated; necrosis and ulceration commonly follow quickly.

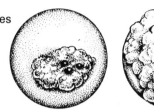 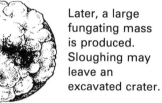

Later, a large fungating mass is produced. Sloughing may leave an excavated crater.

Spread

Until a very late stage, the disease is confined to the pelvic cavity. The patient commonly dies before distant metastases appear.

Local spread takes place in several directions:

1. **Downward extension**.

2. **Lateral extension**. The anatomy of this region is important.

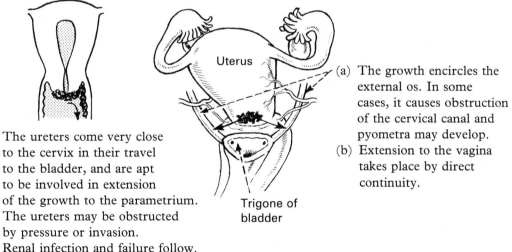

Uterus

Trigone of bladder

The ureters come very close to the cervix in their travel to the bladder, and are apt to be involved in extension of the growth to the parametrium. The ureters may be obstructed by pressure or invasion. Renal infection and failure follow.

(a) The growth encircles the external os. In some cases, it causes obstruction of the cervical canal and pyometra may develop.

(b) Extension to the vagina takes place by direct continuity.

DISEASES OF CERVIX

Spread of carcinoma (continued)

3. Anterior and posterior extension

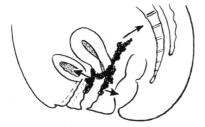

Direct invasion of the bladder or rectum results in fistulous communications. Spread along the uterosacral ligaments involves the sacral nerves, causing intractable pain.

4. Lymphatic spread

This occurs early and involves the chains of lymph nodes in the pelvis.

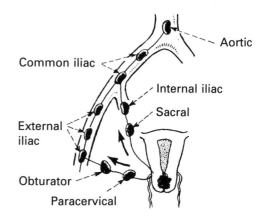

Histology

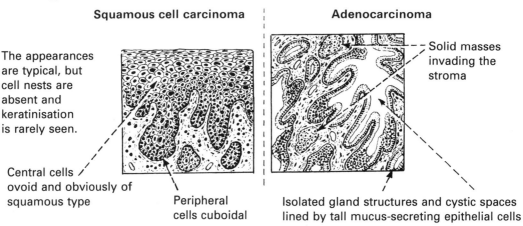

Squamous cell carcinoma

The appearances are typical, but cell nests are absent and keratinisation is rarely seen.

Central cells ovoid and obviously of squamous type

Peripheral cells cuboidal

Adenocarcinoma

Solid masses invading the stroma

Isolated gland structures and cystic spaces lined by tall mucus-secreting epithelial cells

Progress

With modern treatment there is an 80% 5-year cure rate when the disease is diagnosed early i.e. confined to the cervix: it falls significantly if spread to the pelvis has occurred.

Death is commonly due to a combination of renal failure and sepsis. Fatal haemorrhage from eroded vessels may occur.

DISEASES OF CERVIX

CARCINOMA (continued)

Aetiology

1. *Epidemiological facts*

(a) The disease is rare in virgins (in a community of nuns, no cases were seen) and the incidence is highest in prostitutes. The disease is rare in strictly orthodox Jewish women and significantly increased in less strict Jewish communities.

(b) Historically the disease was seen most commonly in the 4th and 5th decades. Nowadays, in Western Societies, dysplasia and carcinoma are seen in young women (2nd and 3rd decades) and the prevalence has greatly increaseed. These changes are statistically related to sexual promiscuity and early age of first coitus.

(c) The use of barrier methods of contraception are associated with a decreased incidence.

2. *Virus Infection*

In the great majority of cases HUMAN PAPILLOMA VIRUS (HPV) is associated with cervical carcinoma and is the postulated carcinogenic agent with male to female transmission.

Associations

HPV types 6 or 11	CIN I and II and condylomata
HPV types 16 or 18	CIN III and invasive carcinoma

3. Of other possible co-factors or mutagens ***Tobacco*** heads the list.

4. It seems likely that in many cases initiation of the progression to cancer begins at an early age before the cervical muco-squamous junction has stabilised.

CYTOLOGY and CERVICAL CANCER

Smears from the muco-squamous junction obtained by a specially designed wooden spatula are stained by Papanicolau's method. Various pathological processes can be identified by examination of the various cell types.

(1) Inflammatory and reactive processes – regular epithelial cells: pus cells.

(2) 'Benign' HPV infections (CIN I: condyloma) – superficial cells show KOILOCYTIC CHANGE. - - - - - ➤

(3) CIN II and III – over 90% of cases are identified and proceed to further colposcopic and punch biopsy investigation followed by cryo or laser ablation.

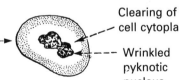

Clearing of cell cytoplasm

Wrinkled pyknotic nucleus

665

DISEASES OF VAGINA AND VULVA

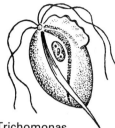

Trichomonas
vaginalis

Vaginal discharge is a common complaint especially in parous women. In many cases it is related to chronic cervicitis. There are however a number of inflammatory conditions which arise primarily in the vagina.

Gonococcal infection may produce an acute inflammation with purulent discharge but it is often asymptomatic.

Purulent discharge is also associated with infection by a protozoon, Trichomonas vaginalis. The discharge tends to be frothy. It is commonly transmitted during sexual intercourse. The male can also be infected.

Candida albicans infection is common in pregnancy and in patients undergoing antibiotic or immunosuppressive therapy.

Primary tumours of the vagina are rare. Squamous carcinoma occurs in the upper vagina of old women and leads to fistula formation between the vagina and the bladder and rectum.

Clear cell adenocarcinoma is sometimes found in adolescent girls. It has been traced to the effect on the fetus of administration of diethylstilboestrol to the patient's mother during early pregnancy.

Vulval inflammation is common in postmenopausal women. It is related to atrophy of the skin, which has very thin epithelial covering at this phase of life and is easily abraded. Inflammation at other periods of life frequently involves Bartholin's gland.

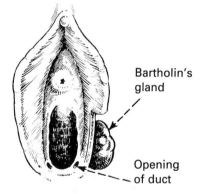

Bartholin's
gland

Opening
of duct

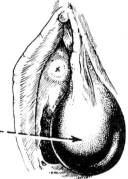

The duct which opens into the vagina in front of the hymen is apt to become blocked. If the inflammation subsides a simple cyst of the duct arises but an abscess may form.

Two conditions which mainly occur in the tropics and are seen only very occasionally in temperate countries are:

1. **Lymphogranuloma venereum**. This is a chlamydial infection which starts as an ulcer on the vulva or in the vagina. It heals in a short time, only to be followed by a chronic suppurative reaction in the inguinal and sometimes pelvic lymph nodes. This leads to extensive scarring and sometimes fistulous openings in the pelvic viscera.

2. **Granuloma inguinale**. This begins as a papule on the vulva, perineum or vagina. It ulcerates and can spread widely, causing extensive destruction of tissue. Histologically, it is a granuloma and the infecting organism (Donovan bodies) can be seen in macrophages.

DISEASES OF VAGINA AND VULVA

LEUKOPLAKIA AND PREMALIGNANCY

Leukoplakia is a descriptive term meaning white patches. These are common on the vulval and perineal regions in almost any chronic inflammatory skin condition due to the local moist conditions, e.g. neurodermatitis, fungal infection and in atrophic lesions, e.g. senile keratosis and lichen sclerosis et atrophicus.

There is however one type of lesion appearing as white patches in this region which shows epithelial dysplasia and is premalignant.

Hyperkeratosis and Parakeratosis
Epithelial hyperplasia with mitotic activity and abnormal cells

Chronic inflammatory reaction

Hyalinisation of superficial dermis

The degree of dysplasia varies, amounting to carcinoma in situ in some cases.

These changes are now numerically graded VIN I, II and III, i.e. Vulvar Intraepithelial Neoplasia (analogous to CIN) – see p.661.

TUMOURS OF THE VULVA

Simple tumours are common. CONDYLOMATA ACUMINATA are papillary proliferations due to infection by Human Papilloma Virus (HPV) types 6 or 11. Koilocytosis (see p.665) in the superficial keratinocytes are the histological marker.

Sweat gland tumours (hidradenomas) may also occur.

Carcinoma of vulva

This is a rare condition found in women in the 6th and 7th decades of life.

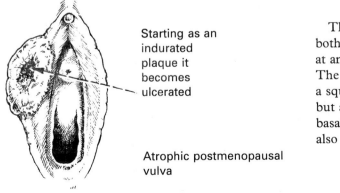

Starting as an indurated plaque it becomes ulcerated

Atrophic postmenopausal vulva

The inguinal glands on both sides are invaded at an early date.
The growth is usually a squamous carcinoma but adenocarcinoma and basal cell carcinoma also occur.

DISEASES OF FALLOPIAN TUBE

Acute Salpingitis

The inflammation is the result of ascending infection from the endometrium: some cases follow abortion and puerperal infection. In addition to the infecting organisms causing acute endometritis (see p.659) members of the Chlamydia and Mycoplasma species are now known to cause acute salpingitis.

The inflammation is usually bilateral and primarily involves the tubal plicae which are congested and oedematous: there is a purulent exudate.

If resolution of the acute inflammation does not occur (antibiotic therapy is important) chronic salpingitis and its possible complications are established.

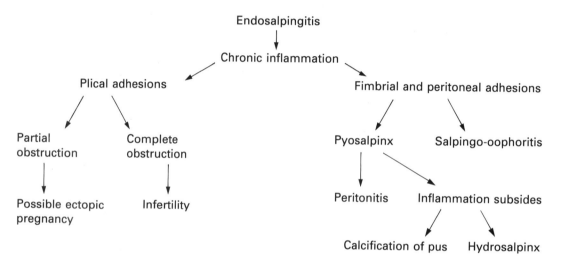

Tuberculous salpingitis

Tuberculous infection of the female genital tract, for some unexplained reason, almost always starts in the fallopian tube. It is usually due to blood spread from some other site: only very occasionally it is secondary to tuberculous peritonitis.

The complications are these expected of a chronic salpingitis with the added element of caseation.

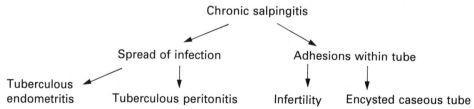

Tumours of the fallopian tube

Benign tumours such as fibroma and myoma occasionally occur. Small cysts of congenital origin are common around the fimbrial ends of the tubes.

Carcinoma, usually a papillary adenocarcinoma, is extremely rare. There may be a profuse watery secretion which appears as a vaginal discharge.

ECTOPIC PREGNANCY

This means implantation of the fertilised ovum outside the uterine cavity.

Sites of implantation

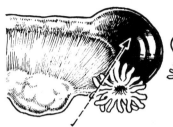

Ampullary implantation
This is the commonest.

Interstitial implantation (rare)

Lumen of tube

Broad ligament

Ovum implants in tubal wall

There is minimal decidua and it burrows into the muscular wall.

Uterine changes

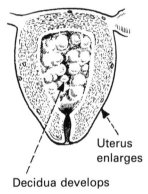

Uterus enlarges

Decidua develops

Erosion of the tubal tissues by the ovum results in **rupture**. This is the commonest finding. The direction of rupture varies:

(1)

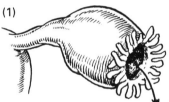

Rupture into the lumen of the tube and leakage into peritoneal cavity.

(2)

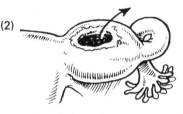

Rupture directly into the peritoneal cavity. If the implantation is interstitial, there may be a further complication – damage to the uterine arteries with **arterial bleeding**.

(3)

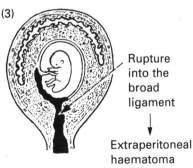

Rupture into the broad ligament

↓

Extraperitoneal haematoma

Exceedingly rarely the whole pregnancy – ovum and placental tissue – aborts into the peritoneal cavity where it reimplants. Usually development is limited and the fetus dies, but continuation of the pregnancy almost to term has been reported.

Aetiology. Most commonly the tube has been previously damaged by salpingitis, leading to partial blockage of the tube. There has been an increased incidence of ectopic pregnancy in women fitted with intrauterine contraceptive devices.

DISEASES OF OVARIES

Oophoritis

Inflammation of the ovaries is always secondary to disease of the fallopian tubes or peritoneum. In the case of the tube, the inflamed fimbrial end becomes adherent to the ovary and direct spread of infection occurs. Extensive changes take place despite treatment.

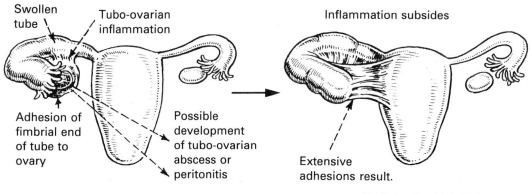

Swollen tube

Tubo-ovarian inflammation

Adhesion of fimbrial end of tube to ovary

Possible development of tubo-ovarian abscess or peritonitis

Inflammation subsides

Extensive adhesions result.

If bilateral, which is frequent, sterility results.

The ovary may be similarly involved in tuberculous salpingitis, and caseating lesions can occur.

Ovarian changes of functional origin

The control mechanisms of ovarian function frequently develop faults resulting in abnormalities of structure:

Follicular cysts

These may be single or multiple. The maximum diameter of a normal Graafian follicle is 1.5–2 cm. Single follicular cysts may be several centimetres in diameter. Amenorrhoea is common in such instances. Multiple follicular cysts, usually small, are associated with endometrial hyperplasia.

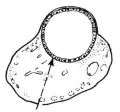

Granulosa cells lining cyst

Theca lutein cysts

These are cysts from which the granulosa cells have disappeared, leaving cysts surrounded by luteinised thecal tissue. Bilateral, multiple small cysts of this nature occur in polycystic ovarian disease and are associated with obesity, hirsutes and oligomenorrhoea (Stein-Leventhal syndrome).

DISEASES OF OVARIES

A multiplicity of types of ovarian tumours exist. Various classifications have been suggested; none are completely satisfactory. The following is a simple working classification:

1. Epithelial tumours (derived from surface epithelium).
2. Sex cord/stromal tumours.
3. Germ cell tumours.
4. Secondary (metastatic) tumours.

1. COMMON EPITHELIAL TUMOURS

These comprise 60% of all ovarian tumours and 90% of malignant tumours and are found in adult life, very rarely in children.

Histogenesis: The ovarian surface epithelium and the various mature Müllerian structures have a common origin in EMBRYONAL COELOMIC epithelium. The ovarian surface epithelial stem cells retain the ability to differentiate along different pathways: this explains the histological appearance of these tumours.

EMBRYONAL COELOMIC EPITHELIUM → MATURE OVARIAN SURFACE EPITHELIUM

STEM CELLS

	Mature Müllerian tissues	*analogous TUMOURS*
e.g.	1. Tubal epithelium	SEROUS
	2. Endocervical epithelium	MUCINOUS
	3. Endometrial epithelium	ENDOMETRIOID
	4. Transitional epithelium	BRENNER

The histological features relate to a spectrum of behaviour:

(1) Benign   (2) Borderline   (3) Malignant.

Serous cystadenoma

Twenty-five per cent of all ovarian tumours are of this variety. In a third of cases they are bilateral, but they almost never reach the large size of the mucinous growths.

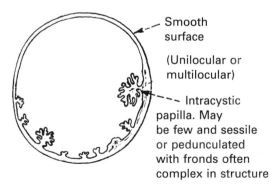

Smooth surface

(Unilocular or multilocular)

Intracystic papilla. May be few and sessile or pedunculated with fronds often complex in structure

Some tumours have small loculi with papillary formations making them appear solid.

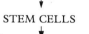

Epithelium cuboidal with central nuclei. Fluid is watery.

Torsion may occur as in the mucinous type.

Complications

1. Torsion may occur as in the mucinous variety of cyst.
2. Malignant transformation is common and 30% of malignant tumours are bilateral.

671

DISEASES OF OVARIES

Common epithelial tumours (continued)

Mucinous cystadenoma

This accounts for 20% of all ovarian tumours. It can reach a very large size and is typically multilocular. Twenty three per cent are bilateral.

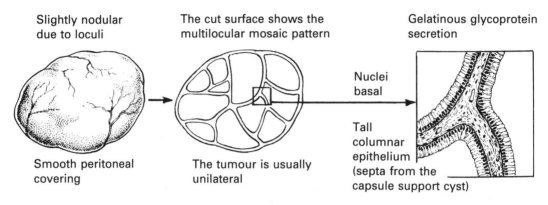

Slightly nodular due to loculi

Smooth peritoneal covering

The cut surface shows the multilocular mosaic pattern

The tumour is usually unilateral

Gelatinous glycoprotein secretion

Nuclei basal

Tall columnar epithelium (septa from the capsule support cyst)

Complications

1. **Torsion of the pedicle**. This is not uncommon with a large ovarian tumour of any type.
2. **Rupture**. This may lead to seeding of the mucin-secreting epithelium on the peritoneum. It continues to secrete, leading to the condition 'pseudomyxoma peritonei', with a peritoneal cavity filled with mucin.
3. **Malignant transformation** (Borderline tumour) Cells large, with large irregular nuclei. Mitoses common. Slight secretion present. Stroma minimal.

Congestion, often infarction due to interruption of blood flow

DISEASES OF OVARIES

Common epithelial tumours (continued)

Mucinous cystadenocarcinoma

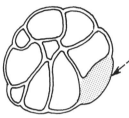

This accounts for 20% of all cases of primary carcinoma of the ovary. It almost always arises as a malignant transformation of a benign cystadenoma.

Areas of solid growth appear in the cyst wall.

Frequently in the malignant areas, florid papillary structures are formed and where the change is widespread it may be difficult to differentiate it from the malignant f)rm of papillary cystadenoma.

Papillary (serous) cystadenocarcinoma

This is the commonest malignant tumour of the ovary – responsible for 60% of the total. Usually it takes the form of exuberant papillomatous growths extending over the surface and obliterating the ovarian structure.

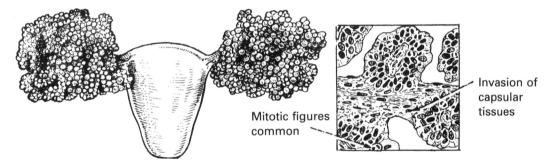

Mitotic figures common

Invasion of capsular tissues

Endometrioid carcinoma

In a considerable number of cases, ovarian carcinoma has a solid or semi-solid appearance and as such starts off as a growth smaller than either of the cystic tumours. Microscopically, they are frequently anaplastic, but sometimes they show differentiation towards an endometrial pattern and are termed 'endometrioid'. There is no 'benign' equivalent.

Progress in ovarian carcinoma

Spread of ovarian cancer in the early stages is by direct extension to the pelvic peritoneum.

The papillary serous cancer seeds widely in the peritoneal cavity and only later are lymphatics invaded and metastases appear.

The mucinous variety rarely spreads by lymphatics.

The overall 5-year survival rate for ovarian cancer is only 30% and death often takes place within 2–3 years due to cachexia and interference with intestinal and renal function.

Brenner tumours

These are essentially *benign* and show islands of transitional epithelium in a fibrous stroma.

673

DISEASES OF OVARIES

2. SEX CORD and STROMAL TUMOURS

These may be divided into two broad groups:

1. Those tending to produce excess oestrogen: granulosa cell tumours and thecomas.
2. Those producing androgens and virilisation: Sertoli-Leydig cell tumours, hilus cell tumours and lipid cell tumours.

Granulosa cell tumour

This is composed of cells resembling the granulosa cells lining Graafian follicles. They vary in size from a few mm to large cystic structures. Commonly, the smaller varieties are found deep in the ovarian substance.

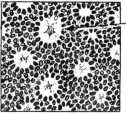

Rosettes of cells with nuclei radially arranged are common (Call-Exner bodies)

   This tumour may be found at any age: 5% occur in children; 60% in the child-bearing years; 30% postmenopausally.

   Occasionally these tumours recur – sometimes many years after removal.

Thecoma

This is a growth consisting of spindle cells and often resembles a fibroma. It has been suggested that fibromas found in ovaries are thecomas which have undergone fibrous degeneration. They are found mainly during the 3rd, 4th and 5th decades of life. They are of simple nature and rarely recur.

   Function of these tumours varies widely. Oestrogen manifestations consist of:

1. Precocious puberty in children
2. Hyperplasia of endometrium. This may be atypical and carcinoma is said to develop in 14%
3. Enlargement of breasts.

Sertoli-Leydig cell tumours (androblastoma, arrhenoblastoma)

Tubules lined by SERTOLI cells, sometimes pyramidal with clear cytoplasm.

LEYDIG cells occasionally with Reinke crystalloids in their cytoplasm

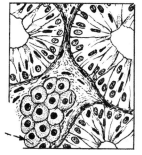

This typifies the virilising tumour group. It is a rare tumour. The degree of virilisation varies. Usually a small yellow tumour within the ovarian substance, it has a characteristic microscopical structure.

   Some of these tumours are malignant and consist of poorly differentiated spindle cells with occasional tubule formations.

The androgens, if secreted, result in:

1. Atrophy of breasts and external genitalia
2. Deepening of voice, temporal recession of hair
3. Growth of facial and body hair
4. Enlargement of clitoris.

DISEASES OF OVARIES

3. GERM CELL TUMOURS

These arise from primitive germ cells capable of differentiating in many ways. The following diagram indicates the main varieties of tumour produced.

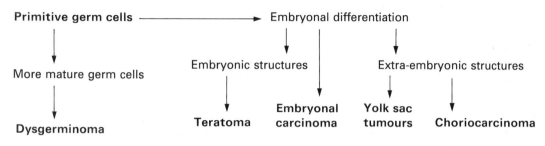

Dysgerminoma

This is a solid tumour of characteristic appearance. It is usually ovoid with a smooth capsule, greyish colour and rubbery consistence. Like all germ cell tumours it is commoner in younger age groups and is often bilateral. Some cases are found in association with intersex.

Microscopically, it consists of large clear round cells with large nuclei resembling germ cells. These are arranged in alveoli separated by fine connective tissue infiltrated by lymphocytes. These histological appearances are similar to those of seminoma of the testis.

Lymphocytes

Dysgerminomas are malignant tumours spreading to para-aortic lymph nodes. They are radio-sensitive and also respond to chemotherapy.

Teratomas

These are of two main varieties: (1) cystic and (2) solid.

Cystic teratoma *(dermoid)*

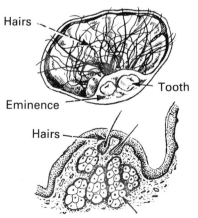

Hairs

Eminence

Tooth

Hairs

Sebaceous glands

This is one of the commonest ovarian tumours and it occurs at all ages.

It is unilocular with an eminence on one aspect from which hairs grow. Teeth may be present on this eminence. It is lined by stratified squamous epithelium. Sebaceous glands, nervous tissue, respiratory, intestinal epithelium and thyroid tissue may also be present.

Very occasionally the squamous epithelium may undergo malignant change.

675

DISEASES OF OVARIES

Teratomas (continued)

Solid teratoma

This consists of a mixture of all types of tissue arranged in no set order. The variation in histological appearance is so great, no adequate description can be given. This type of tumour is more common in younger age groups, and one or more of the tissue components usually shows malignant change.

Solid tumours are occasionally seen consisting only of thyroid tissue (struma ovarii) or carcinoid tumour cells.

Extra-embryonic tumours (embryonal carcinoma, yolk sac tumour, choriocarcinoma)

These are very rare. The main feature in all of them is their extreme malignancy, but modern chemotherapy has revolutionised the outlook.

4. SECONDARY TUMOURS

The ovaries are often the site of metastatic growths from the breast, lung, intestinal system, etc. They are commonest during the child-bearing years.

Krukenberg tumour

This is a very characteristic secondary tumour due to metastatic deposits from an undiscovered stomach carcinoma in a pre-menopausal woman. Both ovaries are involved. They are firm and fibrous, of equal size, smooth and slightly lobulated. No adhesions are present.

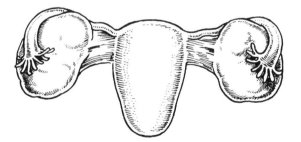 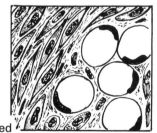

Histologically they may be mistaken for a spindle cell sarcoma, but among the undifferentiated cells are large cells with eccentric nuclei and clear cytoplasm containing mucin (signet ring cells).

Other tumours

Fibromas are not uncommon: a rare complication is an association with peritoneal and pleural effusions (Meig's syndrome).

BENIGN DISEASES OF THE BREAST

Acute inflammation
Clinically, two forms of breast inflammation are recognised:

1. **Associated with lactation**. This appears to be due to failure to establish lactation and may be hormonal in origin. Although there is congestion, oedema and frequently pyrexia, there appears to be no infection.
2. **Pyogenic mastitis**. This also occurs most frequently in the lactating breast. Fissures or abrasions of the nipple predispose to the condition. Infection is transmitted by the suckling neonate who is carrying hospital staphylococci. Abscesses may form in the lobules of the breast leading to scarring during healing.

Granulomatous mastitis: Duct ectasia (plasma cell mastitis)
This generally follows acute mastitis and is a localised granulomatous reaction.

Another chronic inflammatory reaction is associated with ectasia of the ducts (cystic dilatation).

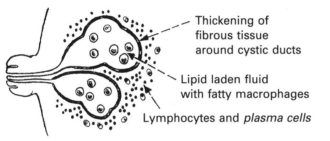

Thickening of fibrous tissue around cystic ducts

Lipid laden fluid with fatty macrophages

Lymphocytes and *plasma cells*

Infection of the dilated ducts allows escape of contents into the tissues resulting in *granulomatous* reaction. Clinically it may raise suspicion of duct carcinoma.

Traumatic Fat Necrosis occurs in obese pendulous breasts and results in an irregular granulomatous fibrous reaction which may mimic carcinoma.

In some cases of **Silicone Implant**, continuing granulomatous inflammation with fibrosis occurs in the 'capsule' due to leakage of silicone.

Fibrocystic change (Non-neoplastic hyperplasia of the breast)
In this condition there are four characteristic features, and the form which the disease takes varies according to the relative proportions of these features:

1. **Fibrosis**. This is mainly an increase in the amount of collagen rather than a true growth of fibrous tissue.
2. **Cyst formation**. Obstruction of ducts leads to dilatation of the ducts and acini. The lining epithelium may show apocrine metaplasia.
3. (a) **Adenosis**. This is an increase in the number of lobules and in the size of existing lobules.

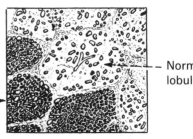

Hyperplastic lobules

Normal lobule

   (b) **Sclerosing adenosis**
   This is a localised condition which may simulate carcinoma. There is proliferation of acini and stroma, and mitotic activity can be marked but there is no danger of malignancy.

677

BENIGN DISEASES OF THE BREAST

Fibrocystic change (continued)

4. **Epithelial hyperplasia** is the most important component because it forms a link between simple proliferation and malignant change.

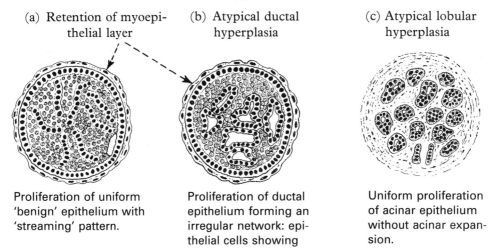

(a) Retention of myoepi-
thelial layer

(b) Atypical ductal
hyperplasia

(c) Atypical lobular
hyperplasia

Proliferation of uniform
'benign' epithelium with
'streaming' pattern.

Proliferation of ductal
epithelium forming an
irregular network: epi-
thelial cells showing
mild atypia.

Uniform proliferation
of acinar epithelium
without acinar expan-
sion.

Fibrocystic change is very common, and the various changes are ascribed to abnormal and exaggerated responses of the breast tissues to the cyclical physiological menstrual hormonal stimuli; they are essentially benign, but a link with carcinoma has been established when the epithelial component shows ATYPICAL CELLULARITY (DYSPLASIA). In these circumstances, particularly if the changes are widespread, the risks of carcinoma are increased (see p.682).

Lesions related to Fibrocystic change

1. **Fibroadenoma**

This is a benign nodular proliferation, now considered to be a component of fibrocystic change and not a true neoplasm. It is usually single, occurring in young women. It presents clinically as a small, firm, mobile lump.

Gross appearance
Well circumscribed,
rounded and elastic
in consistency:
glistening,
greyish cut
surface
1–3 cm
diam.)

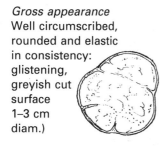

Small acinar
and duct
structures
resembling
normal breast

Fibrous tissue
arranged
around acini

Microscopic appearance

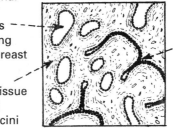

Epithelium
forms clefts:
these are due
to pressure
from the
projecting
fibrous tissue

2. **Radial scar**

This small (up to 1 cm diam.), firm lesion shows a central dense fibrous core with radiating fingers of fibrosis entrapping and distorting glandular elements. It is benign but can be confused with carcinoma even on histological examination.

BENIGN BREAST TUMOURS AND IN SITU CARCINOMA

Duct papilloma

This tumour may develop in any part of the duct system of the breast, but is most common in the lacteal sinuses at the nipple. Two forms exist:

1. **Solitary papilloma.** These are almost always near the nipple.

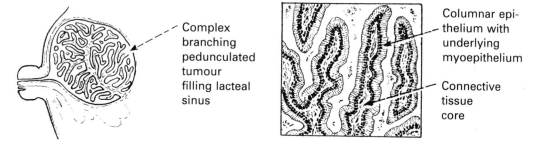

Complex branching pedunculated tumour filling lacteal sinus

Columnar epithelium with underlying myoepithelium

Connective tissue core

Prominent myoepithelium gives a double layer of cells covering the fronds.

2. Multiple papillomata

These may be distributed throughout the duct system. In this form, multicentric carcinoma occasionally develops.

In both forms, there may be a discharge from the nipple which may be haemorrhagic. Examination of the discharge will reveal the tumour epithelial cells which are benign. Other benign breast tumours are extremely rare.

Intra-duct carcinoma

This is a carcinoma in situ of the ducts. It may be visible as greyish-white material filling the dilated ducts, and central necrotic debris may be squeezed out of the ducts (comedocarcinoma).

Solid or cribriform cylinders of cells show the usual features of malignancy – variation in size and shape of both cell and nucleus, relatively greater size of nuclei, mitotic figures, etc. The condition has to be differentiated from atypical ductal hyperplasia.

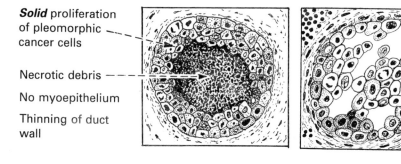

Solid proliferation of pleomorphic cancer cells

Necrotic debris

No myoepithelium

Thinning of duct wall

Cribriform pattern with rigid 'Roman bridges'

Lobular carcinoma in situ: This lesion is usually multifocal and *bilateral*. The breast acini of affected lobules are distended by fairly uniform carcinoma cells which grow into the duct system or break through basement to become infiltrative lobular carcinoma.

679

CARCINOMA OF THE BREAST

This is the commonest form of malignancy in the female. It may be found in any part of the breast but most frequently it is in the upper outer quadrant.

INFILTRATING DUCTAL CARCINOMA

This, the commonest form, presents as a firm to hard lump. The following illustrations show a large carcinoma with significant local spread. It is emphasised that modern screening methods aim to detect the disease at a much earlier stage (see p.682).

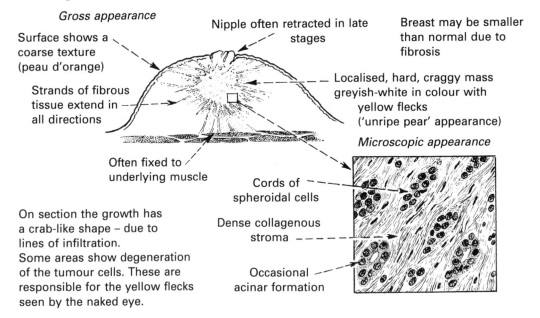

Gross appearance

Surface shows a coarse texture (peau d'orange)

Nipple often retracted in late stages

Breast may be smaller than normal due to fibrosis

Strands of fibrous tissue extend in all directions

Localised, hard, craggy mass greyish-white in colour with yellow flecks ('unripe pear' appearance)

Microscopic appearance

Often fixed to underlying muscle

Cords of spheroidal cells

Dense collagenous stroma

Occasional acinar formation

On section the growth has a crab-like shape – due to lines of infiltration.
Some areas show degeneration of the tumour cells. These are responsible for the yellow flecks seen by the naked eye.

INFILTRATING LOBULAR CARCINOMA

Ten per cent of breast cancers are of this type. Based on distribution of the 'in situ' precursor, this tumour may be multicentric within the breast and there is a 30% chance of a similar tumour arising in the contralateral breast. Microscopically the tumour infiltrates the tissues as single files of malignant cells.

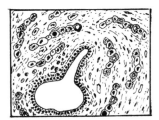

Infiltrating lobular carcinoma

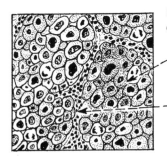

Medullary carcinoma

Large spheroidal cells

Fine stroma often heavily infiltrated by lymphocytes

More rare forms of breast cancer are TUBULAR CARCINOMA – showing well differentiated cells often with intra-tubular calcification: MEDULLARY CARCINOMA – a highly cellular tumour with a florid lymphocytic infiltrate, and MUCOID CARCINOMA where the malignant cells lie in pools of mucin.

680

CARCINOMA OF THE BREAST

Local Spread: Breast cancers are usually slow growing: tumour size is proportional to duration. In late stages local infiltration causes skin ulceration and there may be direct penetration of the chest wall. In addition, intra-epithelial spread occurs. The classical example is **PAGET'S DISEASE OF THE NIPPLE.**

Spread via duct epithelium to skin surface

Infiltrating cancer

Nipple is red, swollen and inflamed with crusts on the surface.

Fluid exudes from surface

Microscopic examination reveals:

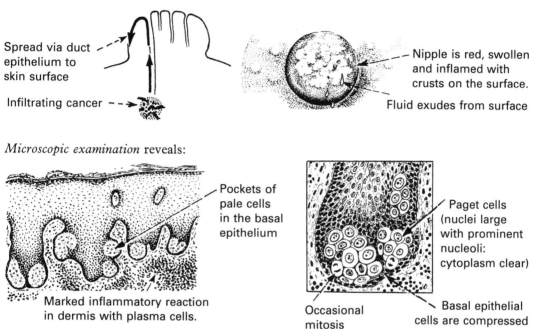

Pockets of pale cells in the basal epithelium

Marked inflammatory reaction in dermis with plasma cells.

Paget cells (nuclei large with prominent nucleoli: cytoplasm clear)

Occasional mitosis

Basal epithelial cells are compressed and atrophic

Metastatic Spread: This is by lymphatic and blood streams.

Early
(When the tumour is still small)

2 ← 1

via LYMPHATICS
1. To axillary nodes from all sites of breast.
2. Through internal mammary lymphatics to thorax (esp. in cancers sited medially).

via BLOOD STREAM
? to bone marrow where cells can lie dormant for long periods.

Late   Local spread via skin lymphatics causing:
  (a) Widespread lesion – skin becomes stiff and board-like: 'cancer-en-cuirasse'.
  (b) Blockage of dermal lymphatics: oedema of skin except at anchorage points, giving a fine mamillated appearance: 'peau d'orange' (see p.190).

Secondaries appear in many viscera, particularly liver, lung and BONE (spinal column).

681

CARCINOMA OF THE BREAST

Prognosis

Crude mortality rates are 40% at 5 years: 60% at 10 years and 75% at 25 years. Important factors which influence these crude rates are: 1. Age of detection – older age: improved prognosis. 2. Tumour size (reflects duration). 3. Differentiation of tumour (Graded 1, 2, 3). 4. Degree of lymph node involvement.

Aetiology

Breast cancer is uncommon below the age of 30 years. The risk increases with age, the maximal incidence being in the later decades.

The important risk factors are:

1. *Genetic:*

   There is a strong familial association. Abnormalities in chromosomes 11 and 17 involving amplification of oncogenes and deletion of tumour suppressor genes have been identified (deletion of suppressor gene p53 is common).

2. *Sex hormone associations:*

   (a) Commoner in nulliparous women.

   (b) Early menarche and late menopause increase risk – ? prolonged cyclical exposure to sex hormones.

   (c) Breast feeding reduces risk.

   Note: Some breast carcinomas are hormone (oestrogen) dependent and slowing of the growth can be achieved by minimising oestrogenic stimulation. The cells of such tumours show surface oestrogen receptors.

3. *Virus infection:*

   No virus has yet been incriminated, although possible virus material has been identified in a few breast cancers.

Screening for Breast cancer

The aim of screening is to detect either pre-malignant conditions or cancer at an early stage and is very important where there is a family history of cancer. Mammography is capable of detecting intra-duct carcinoma and pre-cancerous lesions. Focal calcification is an important indicator but is not diagnostic of malignancy because it also occurs in benign tumours. Whatever method of screening is used the diagnosis must be established on morphological evidence using fine needle aspiration, trochar biopsy and, even occasionally, open biopsy.

Other rare tumours of the breast include PHYLLODES TUMOUR – large and usually benign, affecting elderly women: occasionally sarcoma of the stroma is present. Soft tissue sarcomas and primary lymphoma are exceedingly rare.

THE MALE BREAST

The breast is seldom the seat of disease in males. Abnormal enlargement – gynaecomastia – may occur in a temporary form at puberty or as a permanent feature in intersex states, e.g. Klinefelter's syndrome (XXY). Oestrogen metabolic upsets (e.g. in liver disease) or excess intake (e.g. treatment of prostatic cancer) are other causes. All tumours are rare.

DISEASES OF MALE GENITALIA

The male genital tract consists of a number of structures connected by ducts opening into one another. These interconnections are important in the spread of infection.

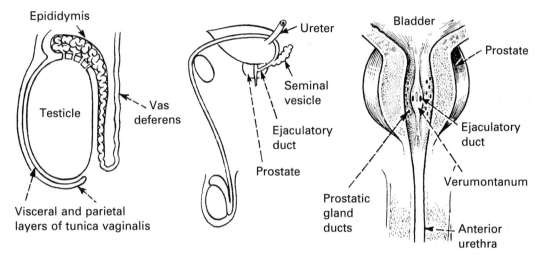

Inflammation of the genital tract in most cases starts in the posterior urethra and spreads to other structures.

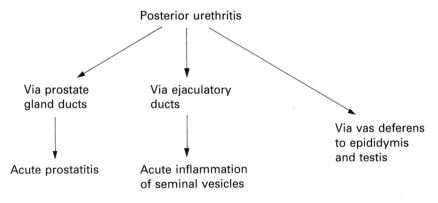

The condition in these instances is secondary to urinary infection associated with urethral obstruction caused by an enlarged prostate or urethral stricture. This is indicated by the fact that in 80% of cases of prostatitis, the infecting bacterium is *E.coli*. In the remaining 20%, various organisms may be isolated – staphylococci, streptococci, pseudomonas and proteus. Frequent catheterisation is an aetiological factor.

Anterior urethritis is almost always a sexually transmitted disease. Gonococci, trichomonads, mycoplasma and chlamydia are the usual agents. In the case of gonorrhoea, infection may spread back to the posterior urethra and thence to other structures.

683

DISEASES OF MALE GENITALIA

GONORRHOEA

This has been relatively uncommon in Western countries in recent years but is now becoming somewhat more prevalent due to the emergence of drug resistant strains of *Neisseria gonorrhoea*.

Gonorrhoeal infection is important because of the complications which may arise:

1. Chronic urethritis → urethral stricture
2. Prostatitis, acute and chronic
3. Occasionally epididymitis and orchitis
4. Blood spread leading to arthritis, endocarditis, etc
5. Infection of sexual partner ———→ endometritis and sterility
   ———→ gonorrhoeal ophthalmitis of newborn.

PROSTATITIS

The prostate consists of five ill-defined lobes:

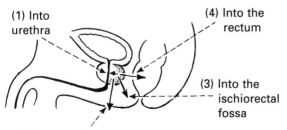

Anterior — Median

Posterior

Lateral (two)

Main glands

Its internal structure is a series of branching glands in a fibromuscular stroma.

Urethra

Periurethral glands

Inflammation of the prostate always involves the posterior urethra and seminal vesicles. The usual congestion, exudation and neutrophil infiltration take place and may proceed to abscess formation. These abscesses are usually small, but if they coalesce and extend they may rupture in several directions.

(1) Into urethra

(4) Into the rectum

(3) Into the ischiorectal fossa

(2) Through the perineum

Chronic prostatitis may follow an acute episode, but it is often of insidious onset. Subsequent fibrosis may cause urethral obstruction.

Abscesses may also form in the seminal vesicles. These can extend to the ischiorectal fossa.

DISEASES OF MALE GENITALIA

EPIDIDYMITIS AND ORCHITIS

Acute inflammations due to bacteria are less common in these organs, but spread via the vas deferens does occasionally take place and may result in destructive suppuration.

In 20% of adult cases of mumps, the epididymis and testes become acutely inflamed. The condition is usually unilateral, but if bilateral there is a distinct danger of subsequent infertility.

Acute inflammation of the testis may be confused with torsion. Torsion generally occurs within the tunica vaginalis and leads to obstruction of the testicular vessels. Infarction results, with destruction of the tissue. Recurrent minor degrees of torsion can cause atrophy.

Chronic inflammations are important, although rare, in this region.

Chronic granulomatous orchitis

This is a condition of unknown origin. The testis is infiltrated by macrophages, plasma cells and lymphocytes. Atrophy of the germinal epithelium occurs and the testis becomes fibrotic.

TUBERCULOSIS

In this disease, the epididymis is usually the first part of the genital tract to be affected.

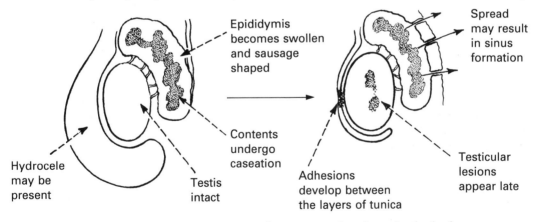

Epididymis becomes swollen and sausage shaped

Spread may result in sinus formation

Contents undergo caseation

Hydrocele may be present

Testis intact

Adhesions develop between the layers of tunica

Testicular lesions appear late

Infection is almost always haematogenous from some other focus in the body. Subsequently the process may spread along the vas deferens to the seminal vesicles, prostate and bladder. In rare cases the infection is in the opposite direction – kidney → bladder → prostate → vas → epididymis.

SYPHILIS

The penis is the usual site of the primary chancre (see p.82). In the tertiary stage ORCHITIS is a common condition with gummatous or granulomatous destruction of the testis.

685

DISEASES OF MALE GENITALIA

SYPHILIS

Apart from the primary sore which appears on the penis, the only other site of syphilitic lesions is the testis. These are common in the tertiary stage, their incidence being only second to those in the aorta at this phase. Two types of lesion are found:

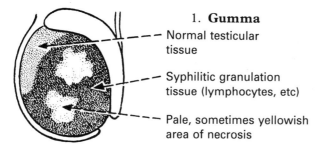

1. **Gumma**
   — Normal testicular tissue
   — Syphilitic granulation tissue (lymphocytes, etc)
   — Pale, sometimes yellowish area of necrosis

2. **Granulomatous lesion** leading to scar formation with destruction of seminiferous tubules.

The primary lesion of lymphogranuloma venereum (see p.666) appears on the penis and, as in the female, it spreads and causes chronic suppuration in the inguinal lymph nodes. But late complications are less drastic in their effects.

BENIGN PROSTATIC HYPERPLASIA

Several different forms are described:

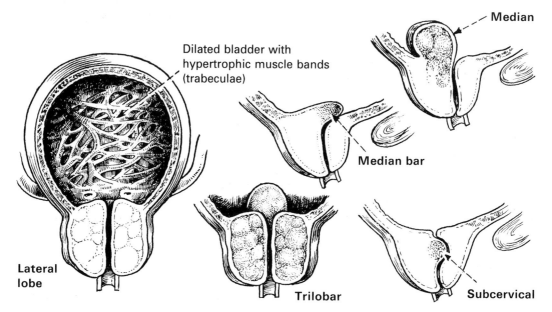

Dilated bladder with hypertrophic muscle bands (trabeculae)

Median

Median bar

Lateral lobe

Trilobar

Subcervical

DISEASES OF MALE GENITALIA

Benign prostatic hyperplasia (continued)

In practice, the appearances are very variable and can include two or more of the forms illustrated on previous page.

There is a hyperplasia of both the glandular tissue and fibromuscular stroma, the relative proportions varying greatly. Secretion of the prostate reveals:

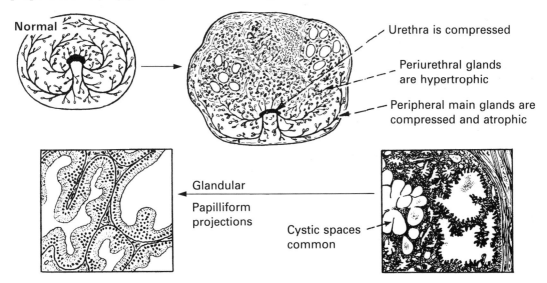

Normal

Urethra is compressed

Periurethral glands are hypertrophic

Peripheral main glands are compressed and atrophic

Glandular

Papilliform projections

Cystic spaces common

The atrophic compressed peripheral tissue forms a false capsule from which the hypertrophied mass can be shelled out.

Aetiology

This is obscure. It is a disease of the elderly and there is often asymptomatic prostatic enlargement in old age. The periurethral glands are said to predominate at this period and hyperplasia may be an exaggeration of this process. It has also been claimed that the central glands are sensitive to oestrogen and hence the hyperplasia may be related to the normal drop in androgens in old age, leaving the action of oestrogen, normally present, unopposed. On the other hand, it has been noted that prostatic enlargement is never seen after castration and does not occur in patients suffering from hepatic cirrhosis (oestrogens are not inactivated).

Complications

1. Chronic retention of urine.
2. Attacks of acute retention are common, usually due to oedema and congestion of the prostatic urethra.
3. Cystitis and pyelonephritis.
4. Hydronephrosis.
5. Bladder stone.
6. Bladder diverticulum.

DISEASES OF MALE GENITALIA

CARCINOMA OF THE PROSTATE

This is a common cancer and is the fifth most common cause of male death.

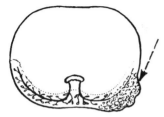

It takes origin from the subcapsular region, i.e. where the main glands are found. Often the prostate also shows benign hyperplasia, but this is coincidental and not causally related. It is almost always an adenocarcinoma.

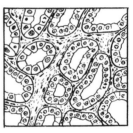

Closely set small irregular acini lined by a single layer of epithelium

Histological grading:

The GLEASON system (Grades 2 through 10) indicates the degree of differentiation from (2) very well differentiated to (10) aggressive anaplastic tumours.

Spread

1. Direct spread occurs throughout the prostate and outwards to the pelviprostatic tissue.

2. Lymphatic spread is the main mode of extension. There is a rich lymphatic plexus and the perineural lymphatics are particularly affected. The pelvic nodes are invaded and subsequently the abdominal chain.

3. Bone metastases tend to be common, especially in the vertebrae. This is due to retrograde spread from the prostatic venous plexus to the vertebral veins. These secondaries are often characterised by the formation of new dense bone around them (osteosclerosis).

Biochemical tests

1. These tumours produce *acid phosphatase* and, *when metastases are present*, an increased level may be found in the blood. When bones are invaded, blood alkaline phosphatase may also rise.

2. Prostatic specific antigen (PSA) measured in the blood using an immuno-histochemical technique is a useful diagnostic marker.

Latent carcinoma

Small subcapsular foci with the histological features of very well differentiated carcinoma may be found in a prostate showing benign hyperplasia. They are discovered incidentally at autopsy in cases dying from causes unconnected with prostate disease. The incidence increases with age and reaches 90% at age 80. Although invasion of local peri-neural spaces may be seen there is never any metastatic growth.

DISEASES OF MALE GENITALIA

TUMOURS of the PENIS

Papillomatous proliferations (condylomata acuminata), sometimes sessile but often florid, usually arise in the coronal sulcus or glans. They are due to sexually transmitted infection by Human Papilloma Virus (HPV) Types 6 and 11, and are analogous to similar lesions in the female genitalia (see p.667).
Peyronie's disease is a cellular fibromatosis related to Dupuytren's contracture.

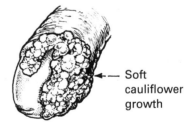

Precancerous lesions

Leukoplakia and Bowen's disease are occasionally found on the penis. Another condition involving epithelial hyperplasia is Queyrat's erythroplasia. The histological appearances vary in these lesions, but all show epithelial dysplasia and usually amount to *carcinoma in situ*.

Carcinoma of the Penis

Accounts for less than 2% of all male malignancy. The site of growth is always in the preputial area, often in the coronal sulcus, but it extends to involve the glans penis. Two forms of growth occur:

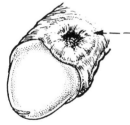

— — Ulcer with sloughing base and hard rolled edges; usually it is adherent to the underlying tissues

— Soft cauliflower growth

The growth spreads by the lymphatics to the regional nodes. Distant metastases occur late. The prognosis is reasonably good, the 5-year survival rate being greater than 50%.

Aetiology

1. Early circumcision virtually confers immunity against carcinoma; the risk is greatly increased in the presence of poor penile hygiene.
2. Human Papilloma Virus (HPV) Types 16 and 18 are the initiating carcinogens. Inspissated smegma trapped behind the foreskin may be an important promoter (co-factor).

CANCER of the SCROTUM

This is a lesion which is rarely seen nowadays. Previously it was an occupational disease due to exposure to carcinogenic agents, e.g. soot, industrial oils, arsenic, etc.

DISEASES OF MALE GENITALIA

GERM CELL TUMOURS of the TESTICLE

These are rare, the incidence being 2–3 per 100,000 males in Western countries. Their importance is related to the fact that most are malignant and they occur in young adults. In this group of the population they account for 1/7th of all cancer deaths. Tumours are more common in undescended testicles.

The 2 main tumour types are SEMINOMA and TERATOMA.

Seminoma This corresponds to the dysgerminoma in the female. It is rare before puberty and has its peak incidence in adults in their 30's. It accounts for 50% of all testicular tumours.

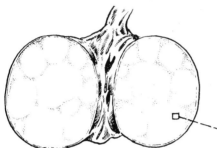

The testis is uniformly enlarged; the surface is smooth.
On section it has a faint lobular appearance and is often described as the 'potato' tumour because of its white solid appearance.

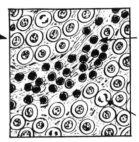

Spread is principally via the lymphatics along the spermatic cord.

The prognosis is good, probably because of early diagnosis. It appears to be better if lymphocytic reaction in the tumour is strong.

Fine stroma infiltrated by lymphocytes

Large germ cells sometimes in mitosis

The growth is extremely radiosensitive. Orchidectomy and abdominal radiotherapy gives a 95% cure rate.

Malignant Teratoma This type of growth is found in 35% of testicular growths. It takes origin from totipotent germ cells capable of differentiating into derivatives of ectoderm, endoderm and mesoderm. It is customary to classify them according to the degree and type of differentiation exhibited. The lack of differentiation indicates the malignancy of the tumour.

The tumours form a spectrum of well differentiated to anaplastic highly malignant growths and are classified as follows:

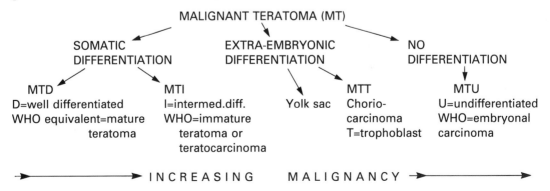

MALIGNANT TERATOMA (MT)

SOMATIC DIFFERENTIATION — EXTRA-EMBRYONIC DIFFERENTIATION — NO DIFFERENTIATION

MTD
D=well differentiated
WHO equivalent=mature teratoma

MTI
I=intermed.diff.
WHO=immature teratoma or teratocarcinoma

Yolk sac

MTT
Chorio-carcinoma
T=trophoblast

MTU
U=undifferentiated
WHO=embryonal carcinoma

→ INCREASING MALIGNANCY →

DISEASES OF MALE GENITALIA

Malignant Teratoma (continued)

These tumours, unlike seminoma, are usually irregular in shape and show focal haemorrhage and necrosis: in the better differentiated tumours small cysts are common.

Differentiated teratoma

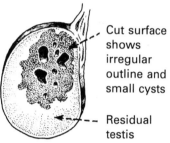

Cut surface shows irregular outline and small cysts

Residual testis

1. **MTD** – In this tumour organoid differentiation is easily recognisable (e.g. formation of intestinal glands, squamous epithelium, cartilage etc.): it is unlike its ovarian counterpart in important respects, however (a) it is very rare and (b) although apparently histologically benign, metastases may occur.

2. **MTI** – In addition to mature organised tissue this tumour contains varying amounts of clearly malignant tissue (e.g. adenocarcinoma, sarcoma).

3. **MTU** – These tumours are almost completely anaplastic showing only focal areas of poor attempts at differentiation.

4. **Yolk sac and Trophoblastic elements** occur commonly in malignant teratomas: pure forms are very rare. α-fetoprotein (from yolk sac elements) and chorionic gonadotrophins (from trophoblastic elements) are used in diagnosis and monitoring process.

5. **Combined Germ-Cell Tumours** – Between 10 and 15% of germ-cell tumours consist of a mixture of seminomatous and teratomatous elements.

Spread: Vascular invasion with lung metastasis is the usual mode of spread.
Prognosis: Modern therapy has greatly improved the overall prognosis.

MISCELLANEOUS TUMOURS

The following tumours are rare: Sertoli cell tumours,
Leydig cell tumours,
Lymphoma.

INFERTILITY

The causes of infertility are multiple and can affect both male and female. The main pathological findings may be grouped in the following manner, but the list does not indicate any form of priority or incidence.

A. Lack of germ cells – due to failure of fetal germ cell migration to the genital ridge. It may be associated with chromosomal abnormalities.

B. Chromosomal defects
1. *Klinefelter's syndrome*. Phenotype male. Genotype XXY or XXXY. No germ cells are present. Testes become atrophic. Usually mental retardation.
2. *Turner's syndrome*. Phenotype female. XO genotype. Genitalia are infantile. The ovaries, lacking germ cells, consist of fibrous tissue.
3. *Super-female*. Extra X chromosome present, e.g. XXX. Fertility reduced.
4. *True hermaphroditism*. XX and XY cells are present. Phenotype usually male. Internally there is a testis and epididymis on one side and an ovary, fallopian tube and uterus on the other.

C. Hormonal abnormalities
1. *Prolactinoma*. The presence of a pituitary adenoma (see p.812).
2. *Adrenogenital syndrome*. This is due to an enzyme defect in cortisol production. Androgens are produced instead, causing virilisation in female infants.
3. *Testicular feminisation*. An abnormality in androgen activity prevents descent of testes with complete feminisation. It is due to a defective gene on the X chromosome transmitted by a female carrier.
4. Administration of oestrogen or its accumulation due to liver disease causes defective testicular function.

D. Anatomical abnormalities. Maldescent of the testes is the most common. Abnormal external genitalia are an obvious cause of infertility.

E. Infections, X-irradiation, tumours and poisons interfere with fertility. Venereal disease and tuberculosis affect both sexes. Septic abortion in the female and mumps in the male are other causes.

F. Functional defects. In a number of cases, no physical cause for infertility can be found. In the female, alterations in pituitary function upset the normal cyclical ovulation rhythm. In the male, oligospermia and abnormal sperm may be found.

CHAPTER 14

NERVOUS SYSTEM

NERVOUS SYSTEM – ANATOMY AND PHYSIOLOGY

Considerations of anatomy and physiology have important applications to diseases of the central nervous system (CNS), particularly their effects and spread.

The anatomy of the various coverings is important.

The skull and vertebrae form a rigid compartment protecting the delicate CNS tissues.

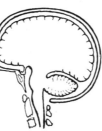

This rigidity has serious disadvantages when pressure inside the skull increases, e.g. an expanding lesion soon takes up the small reserves of space available and the delicate brain tissues are progressively compressed, with very serious results.

Meninges and cerebrospinal fluid (CSF)

The CSF circulating freely in the subarachnoid space over the whole CNS surface and in the ventricular system acts as a protective water bath.

Diseases (particularly infections) at this site are usually *widespread* over the whole brain and cord surfaces, e.g. meningitis. Impediment to the flow of CSF causes serious effects – hydrocephalus.

The detailed arrangement of the meninges is important.

The thick **dura**, closely applied to the skull, acts as the periosteum – its rigid reflections (falx cerebri and tentorium cerebelli) complicate the effects of increased intracranial pressure.

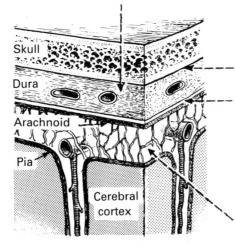

Skull
Dura
Arachnoid
Pia
Cerebral cortex

Extradural lesions tend to be localised; they have to strip the dura from the bone.

Subdural lesions remain local but can spread more widely since the arachnoid and dura are loosely attached.

The **arachnoid**, a delicate membrane, is loosely attached to the dura and sends trabeculae across the subarachnoid space which contains the cerebral blood vessels and the CSF.

Disease in the **subarachnoid** space can spread widely over the whole surface of the brain and spinal cord but is prevented from penetrating into the brain tissue by the **pia**.

NERVOUS SYSTEM – ANATOMY AND PHYSIOLOGY

The **pia** is invaginated into the brain substance along with the small penetrating vessels.

The dura, arachnoid and pia act as barriers which selectively separate the CSF and the blood from the CNS tissues.

It is important to understand that, although the CSF is very similar in composition to the extracellular fluid of the brain, changes in the CSF only very indirectly reflect changes in the CNS in disease.

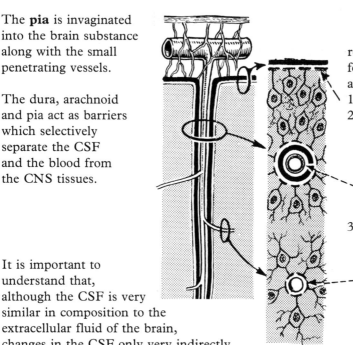

The Pia's barrier function is reinforced by the membrane formed by the foot processes of astrocytes:
1. on the brain surface
2. around the penetrating vessels. The potential space between the vessel wall and the pia is called the Virchow Robin space and is analogous to the subarachnoid space
3. at capillary level the pia is not present, but the foot processes along with the capillary endothelium and basement membrane form a specialised and selective 'blood-brain barrier'.

Thus the PIA and the membrane formed by the foot processes of the astrocytes separate types of tissue derived from two embryological layers.

(1) **Neuroectodermal**
i.e. CNS tissue paper consisting of
Neurones
Neuroglia ⎯ Ependyma
Astroglia
Oligodendroglia

Pia

(2) **Mesodermal**
i.e. Blood vessels, meninges (fibrous tissues)

and

MICROGLIA (most are resident round blood vessels) ⟵ MACROPHAGES

During embryological development these enter the CNS tissues proper and become microglia

These SPECIALISED tissues are subject to INJURY and DEGENERATIVE processes.

These tissues behave similarly to mesodermal tissues elsewhere in the body, e.g. INFLAMMATORY RESPONSE.

NEURONAL DAMAGE

NEURONES are sensitive to damage by a wide variety of agents including anoxia, hypoglycaemia, virus infections and intracellular metabolic disturbances (e.g. associated with vitamin B deficiencies).

There are two main types, depending on the rapidity of the changes.

1. *Rapid NECROSIS* – associated with acute failure of function.

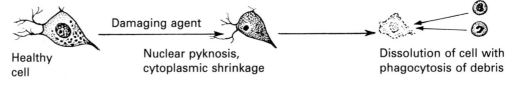

Healthy cell — Damaging agent → Nuclear pyknosis, cytoplasmic shrinkage → Dissolution of cell with phagocytosis of debris

2. *Slow ATROPHIC CHANGES* – associated with gradual loss of function.

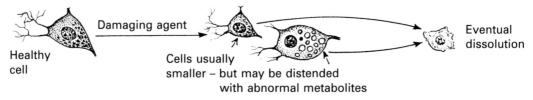

Healthy cell — Damaging agent → Cells usually smaller – but may be distended with abnormal metabolites → Eventual dissolution

The process of ageing involves cumulative atrophy and disappearance of neurones; in some individuals the process is speeded up resulting in **presenile dementia**.

NB There is *no* regeneration of destroyed neurones. A large group of disorders of cerebral function seen in psychiatric practice have (as yet) no morphological evidence of nerve cell damage. They are probably caused by disturbances of poorly understood biochemical control mechanisms within the brain.

In addition to the PRIMARY degenerations described above, neurones are subject to SECONDARY degeneration in certain circumstances.

1. **Retrograde degeneration** – when the main axon is damaged there is degeneration of the neurone as well as the classical distal degeneration of the axon.

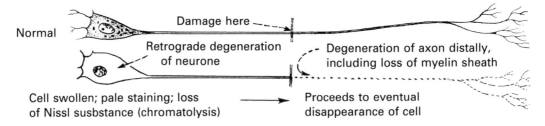

Normal — Damage here

Retrograde degeneration of neurone — Degeneration of axon distally, including loss of myelin sheath

Cell swollen; pale staining; loss of Nissl susbstance (chromatolysis) → Proceeds to eventual disappearance of cell

2. **Trans-synaptic degeneration** – in closely integrated neurone systems, neurone loss may be followed by degeneration of associated neurones across synapses.

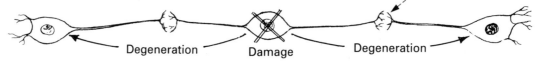

Degeneration — Damage — Degeneration

GLIAL REACTIONS

The glial cells react vigorously in many diseases of the CNS.

1. The **NEUROGLIAL** cells have supportive and nutritive functions.

   (a) The **astrocytes** with their numerous fibrillary processes give structural support. They are less susceptible to damage than neurones.

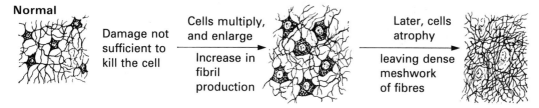

This process is called GLIOSIS. It is a feature of many diseases and is analogous to scar tissue. These cells and fibres contain Glial Fibrillary Acidic Protein (GFAP), recognition of which, using antibodies, is useful in histological sections.

Note: Collagenous scar tissue is only formed in the CNS when mesodermal structures such as large blood vessels and their sheaths are damaged.

   (b) The **oligodendrocytes** – small cells with short processes – have a nutritive function in respect of neurones and especially myelin. This reaction is best seen when neurones are damaged.

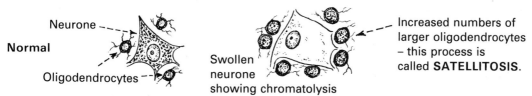

2. The **MICROGLIAL** cells are members of the mononuclear-phagocytic system. Reaction is best seen when there is necrosis of tissues.

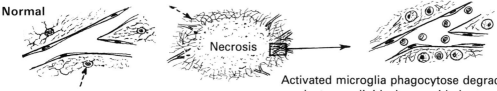

Microglial cells are well seen in and around infarcts; the activated cells which have ingested lipids are strikingly different from the small inactive microglia.

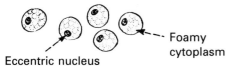

These cells have been given a variety of names: e.g. 'gitter' cells, or lipophages.

697

DEMYELINATION

Loss of the myelin sheath may occur in two main circumstances:

1. **Primary** specific destruction of myelin. Demyelination precedes any axon damage. It is usually not related to specific nerve tracts.

   The mechanism is not clear; it may be autoimmune reaction or virus infection, or both.

   This type, although rare, occurs in an important group of diseases – the DEMYELINATING DISEASES (p.729).

2. **Secondary** loss following nerve cell and axon destruction. This type usually affects nerve tracts in an anatomically predictable way.

   The mechanism is similar to that described in peripheral nerves (Wallerian degeneration, p.61).

   This type occurs in many disease processes, e.g. the nerve tract degeneration following regional infarction (p.739).

The pathological sequels which are influenced by time factors are similar in both types.

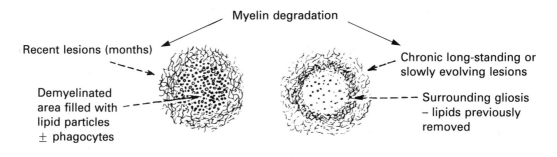

Myelin degradation

Recent lesions (months)

Demyelinated area filled with lipid particles ± phagocytes

Chronic long-standing or slowly evolving lesions

Surrounding gliosis – lipids previously removed

Demonstration of demyelination

Because routine histological stains are unsuitable, special methods are required. The following example showing descending degeneration (and demyelination) of the corticospinal tract in the cord following infarction of the internal capsule in the brain illustrates the two main methods.

1. '*POSITIVE*' method used in **recent** (months) lesions. The lipid particles are stained, e.g. Marchi's method or Sudan black stain.

2. '*NEGATIVE*' method – used in lesions of **any duration**. Absence of staining using stains for normal myelin, e.g. Weigert-Pal or Loyez methods.

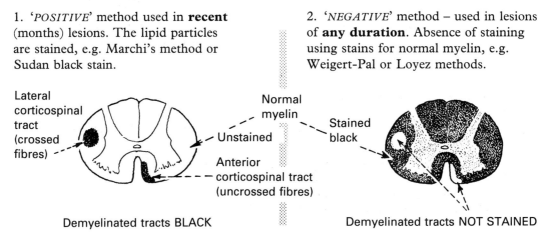

Lateral corticospinal tract (crossed fibres)

Normal myelin

Unstained

Stained black

Anterior corticospinal tract (uncrossed fibres)

Demyelinated tracts BLACK

Demyelinated tracts NOT STAINED

CEREBRAL OEDEMA

Swelling of the brain, of which oedema is the major component, is an important complication of many brain diseases because the enlargement either initiates or aggravates increased intracranial pressure.

The process may be localised or generalised depending on the type of initiating disorder.

Localised conditions

Examples:
  Infarcts, and local ischaemia
  Haematomas (due to vessel rupture
      and injury)
  Tumours

Generalised conditions

Examples: Intoxications
  Metabolic disturbances, e.g. hypoglycaemia
  Generalised hypoxia
  Severe head trauma
  Malignant hypertension

The pathological mechanism is as follows:

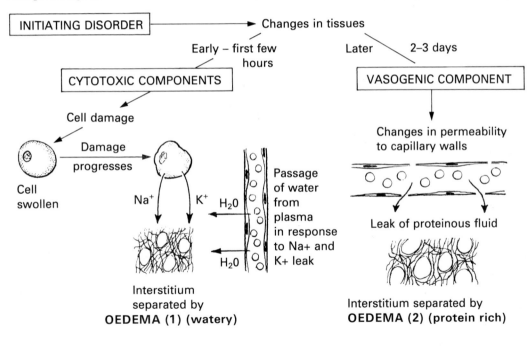

Interstitium
separated by
OEDEMA (1) (watery)

Interstitium separated by
OEDEMA (2) (protein rich)

Notes

(a) Components (1) and (2) overlap.

(b) The oedema fluid tends to spread in the white matter.

(c) The severity of oedema formation is very variable and unpredictable clinically.

(d) In clinical practice, therapy has two aspects:

 1. Treatment of the initiating disorder by any appropriate means.

 2. Minimising the formation of oedema by the use of
   (i) osmotic agents, e.g. urea or mannitol
   (ii) steroids (the mechanism is not known).

INCREASED INTRACRANIAL PRESSURE

INCREASED INTRACRANIAL PRESSURE occurs in two main circumstances:
1. Due to the presence of an EXPANDING LESION
2. Due to obstruction of the free flow of the CSF – this causes hydrocephalus and is dealt with on page 748.

INTRACRANIAL EXPANDING LESIONS
These lesions may occur within the brain substance or in the meninges. Important examples are:

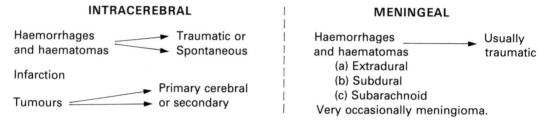

The situation is often aggravated by cerebral OEDEMA.
The severity of the effects is modified by two important factors:
(1) the size of the lesion and (2) the rapidity of expansion.
There are three stages in the progress of increased intracranial pressure ICP.

(1) The stage of **Compensation**

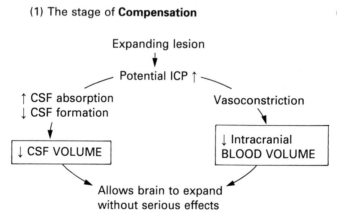

(2) The stage of **Decompensation**

At this stage there are herniations and distortions of the brain with their associated complications. The systemic blood pressure is raised and the pulse slow ('Cushing' effect).

(3) A vicious circle is established leading to the stage of **vasomotor paralysis**.

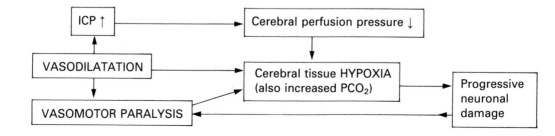

INCREASED INTRACRANIAL PRESSURE

Effects

DISTORTIONS and DISLOCATIONS of the brain substance

These are to some extent dependent on the site of the initiating lesion; the effects of a unilateral expanding lesion are illustrated.

(1) Flattened cerebral convolutions (diminished subarachnoid space)

(2) Herniation of cingulate gyrus under the falx (Supracallosal hernia)

(3) Movement of interventricular septum across the mid-line with distortion of ventricles

(4) Herniation of parahippocampal gyrus past the free edge of the tentorium cerebelli (tentorial hernia)

(5) Midbrain pushed against tentorium of opposite side (Kernohan notch); may give rise to paradoxical signs

(6) Cerebellar tonsils and medulla pushed down into foramen magnum

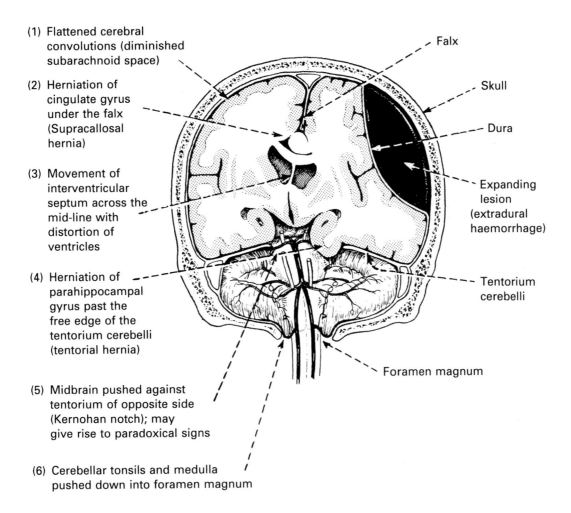

Falx

Skull

Dura

Expanding lesion (extradural haemorrhage)

Tentorium cerebelli

Foramen magnum

NB The sudden removal of even small amounts of CSF by **LUMBAR PUNCTURE** may precipitate medullary 'coning' with fatal results due to damage to the 'vital centres'.

INCREASED INTRACRANIAL PRESSURE

SECONDARY COMPLICATIONS

1. **Vascular damage**
   (a) Compression of the
   central retinal vein
   causes PAPILLOEDEMA,
   an important clinical
   sign of raised ICP.

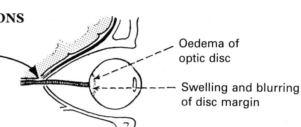

Oedema of
optic disc

Swelling and blurring
of disc margin

   (b) Stretching and compression of blood vessels may cause haemorrhage and infarction
   quite remote from the initiating lesion – secondary midbrain and calcarine infarction
   and haemorrhage are common.

2. **Intracranial nerve damage**
   Oculomotor (III) and abducens (VI) nerves
   are particularly prone to damage, giving rise
   to paralysis of ocular movements in varying
   combinations.

   The VIth nerve is specially vulnerable due
   to its long subarachnoid course. It is often
   the nerve on the side opposite the lesion
   which is stretched giving rise to paradoxical
   signs.

Vessels compressed

III

3. **Obstruction of flow of CSF**

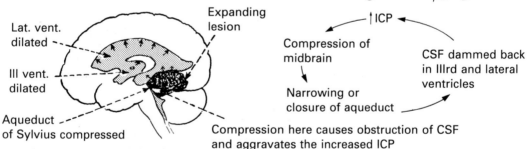

Lat. vent.
dilated

III vent.
dilated

Aqueduct
of Sylvius compressed

Expanding
lesion

↑ICP

Compression of
midbrain

Narrowing or
closure of aqueduct

CSF dammed back
in IIIrd and lateral
ventricles

Compression here causes obstruction of CSF
and aggravates the increased ICP

4. **Changes in the skull bones**
   Long continued ICP causes bone erosion and thinning visible on X-ray.
   (a) Erosion of posterior clinoid processes of sphenoid bone.
   (b) In children, before the skull is fully ossified, the inner table is thinned at the sites of
   convolutional pressure giving a striking X-ray appearance.

CIRCULATORY DISTURBANCES

(1) Hypoxia and ischaemia and (2) Intracranial haemorrhage are the important and common mechanisms causing brain damage.

ACUTE HYPOXIC DISORDERS

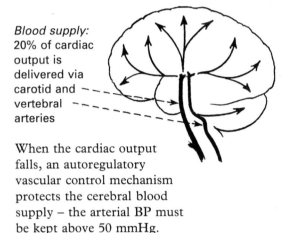

Blood supply: 20% of cardiac output is delivered via carotid and vertebral arteries

When the cardiac output falls, an autoregulatory vascular control mechanism protects the cerebral blood supply – the arterial BP must be kept above 50 mmHg.

Neuronal aerobic metabolism of glucose

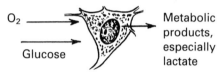

O_2 ⟶ [neuron] ⟶ Metabolic products, especially lactate

Glucose ⟶

There are no reserves of O_2 or glucose in the brain, therefore a constant delivery via arterial blood is necessary.

Neurones are very susceptible to hypoxia and (hypoglycaemia); with complete O_2 deprivation neronal **necrosis** occurs in 5–7 minutes (at normal temperatures).

The following flow diagram illustrates the factors which influence availability of O_2 and the conditions giving rise to hypoxia.

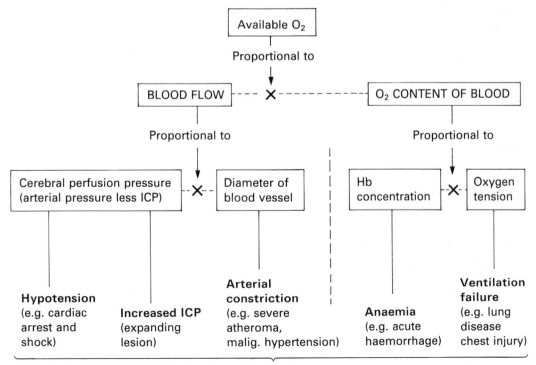

These conditions, singly or together, can be responsible for cerebral hypoxia.

HYPOXIA

GENERALISED (diffuse) brain damage results when delivery of oxygen to the brain as a whole is severely deficient, e.g. in cardiac arrest. *Note:* A similar type of neuronal damage occurs in severe acute hypoglycaemia, acute carbon monoxide and barbiturate poisoning.

LOCALISED (focal) damage occurs in less severe O_2 deficiency and under the influence of modifying factors.

(a) **Anatomical arterial distribution –** Watershed infarcts occur at sites of arterial boundary zones (see p.201)

(b) **Selective anatomical sites –** where neurones are particularly sensitive to hypoxia, e.g. the hippocampus, layers III, V and VI of the cortex, in the sulci, the Purkinje cells of the cerebellum.

(c) **Pre-existing pathological changes –** in the cerebral arterial system, e.g. the random distribution of atheroma.

These focal lesions are to some extent predictable.

These lesions are not predictable.

The variable operation of these three factors potentiates very variable severity and distribution of damage from case to case.

Pathological appearances

Modern ventilators allow maintenance of respiratory and circulatory functions in the presence of total brain necrosis – in such cases there is liquefaction of the whole brain with no vital reaction.

In cases of focal brain damage, the duration of survival after the damage modifies the pathological appearances.

	Up to 12 hours	Over 12 hours	2–7 days	Weeks
Gross	No changes seen	May be cerebral oedema	Focal softenings	Shrinking and scarring of brain
Microscopic	Early neuronal damage seen	Neuronal damage obvious	Loss of cells in selective areas, e.g. Purkinje cells; reactive changes	Reactive gliosis established

CEREBRAL INFARCTION (SOFTENING)

This common condition, one of the two main types of stroke (the other is spontaneous intracerebral haemorrhage), is caused by failure of the supply of oxygen (and glucose) to maintain the viability of the tissues in the territory of a cerebral arterial branch. This is not always due to simple local arterial occlusion, and very often a component of central circulatory deficiency is contributory. The lesion is essentially necrosis of all the tissues in the affected territory.

Mechanism

Precipitating condition→Perfusion failure→INFARCTION (ischaemic necrosis)

LOCAL ARTERIAL DISEASE (particularly ATHEROMA) and its complications, are the most common.

1. Arterial occlusions

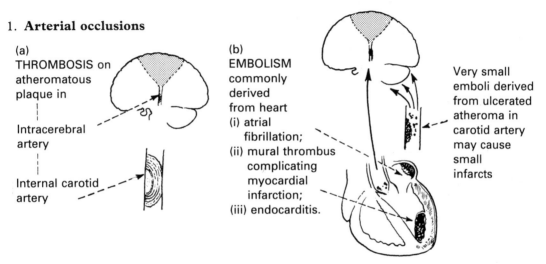

(a)
THROMBOSIS on atheromatous plaque in

Intracerebral artery

Internal carotid artery

(b)
EMBOLISM commonly derived from heart
(i) atrial fibrillation;
(ii) mural thrombus complicating myocardial infarction;
(iii) endocarditis.

Very small emboli derived from ulcerated atheroma in carotid artery may cause small infarcts

2. Arterial stenosis

ATHEROMA – the widespread loss of arterial lumen potentiates cerebral perfusion deficiency in two ways: (1) by distributing the normal arterial flow and (2) by prejudicing anastomotic communications.

Atheromatous stenosis alone is not usually a cause of infarction, but when central circulatory deficiency is added, infarction is common, e.g. this may vary from the slight fall in BP during sleep to the severe hypotension of shock or myocardial infarction.

Other rarer causes of arterial stenosis are dissecting aneurysm and arteritis. Arterial spasm is a rare cause.

CEREBRAL INFARCTION

SITES

While infarcts may occur anywhere in the brain, depending on the vagaries of the precipitating arterial lesions, certain sites are more commonly affected.

1. In cases of local arterial occlusion, **internal structures supplied by 'end' arterial branches** are particularly vulnerable. The cortex is often protected in variable degree by anastomoses of other cerebral arteries. This is illustrated in the territory of the middle cerebral artery.

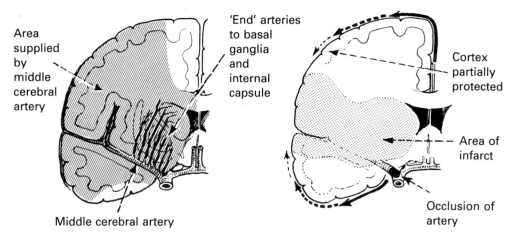

Area supplied by middle cerebral artery

'End' arteries to basal ganglia and internal capsule

Middle cerebral artery

Cortex partially protected

Area of infarct

Occlusion of artery

2. **Boundary zones** (see p.201)

The cortex is damaged particularly in boundary zone infarction. In these cases, central circulatory deficiency is an important component, e.g. hypotension.

3. **Ischaemic (arteriopathic) cerebral atrophy**

In cases of widespread severe atheroma of the cerebral arteries, a diffuse form of cerebral atrophy with neuronal loss and reactive gliosis occurs. There may be microinfarction, and the changes seen in the ageing brain may also be present. In Western societies, this type of cerebral atrophy is one of the causes of senile dementia.

CEREBRAL INFARCTION

The diagram below illustrates the evolution of an infarct, e.g. in the territory of the middle cerebral artery. Up to 24 hours there is virtually no visible change.

18–24 hr	After 24 hours	After a few days	After weeks/months

Gross appearances

Less difficult to see | Line of demarcation seen | Demolition + scarring

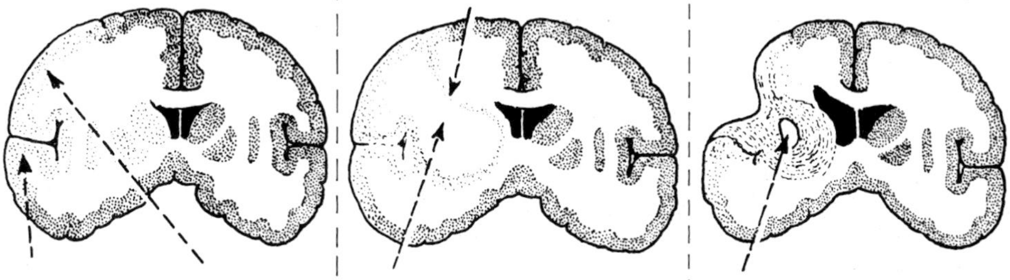

Very difficult to see

Slight swelling | Blurring of white/grey junction | Necrotic tissue. Soft to touch; usually pale but may be congested if blood has permeated in | Cyst with pale or yellowish fluid | Shrinkage of scarred area: compensatory dilatation of ventricle

Microscopic appearances

Early neuronal damage | Early neuronal damage ↓ Necrosis of neurones | Organisation of infarct begins Macrophages appear; capillary sprouting; oedema diminishing | Organisation well established; neurones disappear; numerous macrophages; gliosis

Clinical associations

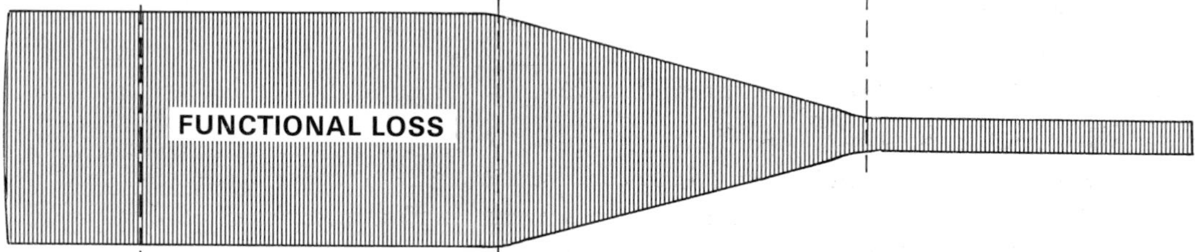

FUNCTIONAL LOSS

Effects are maximal in the early stages when oedema and circulatory disturbance in the adjacent tissues augment the functional loss caused by infarct. Larger infarcts may be associated with loss of consciousness.

The prognostic assessment of final functional loss cannot be made until the changes have subsided and any possible functional compensations have been established. This may take several weeks.
Complete clinical recovery may follow small infarcts.

INTRACRANIAL HAEMORRHAGE

Spontaneous intracranial bleeding is the second main type of stroke. In the great majority of cases there is localised arterial disease aggravated by hypertension. A small number are associated with cerebral tumours, systemic bleeding diathesis or arteriovenous malformations.

Haemorrhages are divided into two main anatomical groups: (1) **intracerebral** and (2) **subarachnoid**.

INTRACEREBRAL HAEMORRHAGE

In most hypertensives over middle age, **microaneurysms** are found in the very small cerebral arteries. It is believed that rupture of one of these aneurysms is the immediate cause of intracerebral haemorrhage.

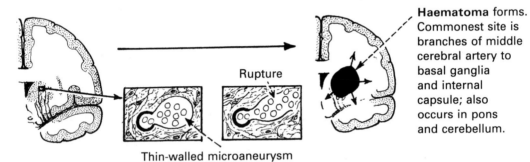

Rupture

Haematoma forms. Commonest site is branches of middle cerebral artery to basal ganglia and internal capsule; also occurs in pons and cerebellum.

Thin-walled microaneurysm

Progress

The onset is usually sudden with headache and, because of the high blood pressure, progress is rapid and the haemorrhage large.

↓

Associated raised ICP effects

↓

Death in many cases

When the bleeding is limited, there is survival with varying residual paralysis.

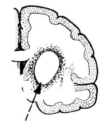

Final outcome
Cystic space containing yellow-brown fluid walled off by gliosis.

Apoplectic cyst

NB Intracerebral bleeding may track irregularly and often reaches the subarachnoid space and ventricles.

INTRACRANIAL HAEMORRHAGE

SUBARACHNOID HAEMORRHAGE

This is commonly but not exclusively the result of rupture of a 'berry' aneurysm at or near the circle of Willis. The basic abnormality is a congenital weakness of the elastic tissues in the arterial wall; only rarely is an aneurysm present at birth, and while subarachnoid haemorrhage does occur in young people, the incidence increases with age.

Sites
Often multiple, near arterial junctions.

Circle of Willis

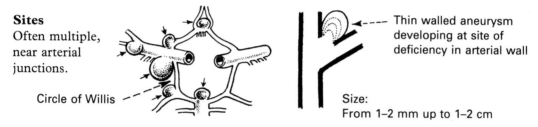

Thin walled aneurysm developing at site of deficiency in arterial wall

Size:
From 1–2 mm up to 1–2 cm

Not all aneurysms rupture; they are found incidentally at autopsy.
Massive haemorrhage may be preceded by one or more small leaks – marked by headache and no functional loss.

Progress

Haemorrhage spreading throughout subarachnoid space — generalised ICP increased; blood-stained CSF.

Local infarction may be a complication

Irritant effect of haemorrhage causes local arterial spasm

NB The aneurysm may rupture directly into the brain and mimic an intracerebral haemorrhage.

CSF findings

1–24 hours — blood stained; blood content constant in sequential samples
    (distinguishes blood derived from a traumatic tap)
    — centrifuge supernatant – may be pink due to haemolysis.
24 hours onwards — supernatant shows xanthochromia (yellow colour due to
     presence of blood degradation products).

Other causes of cerebral haemorrhage of either type are vascular malformations and coagulation disorders.

HYPERTENSION

The incidence of strokes in hypertensive subjects is very significantly increased.

1. Intracranial haemorrhage

Mechanism

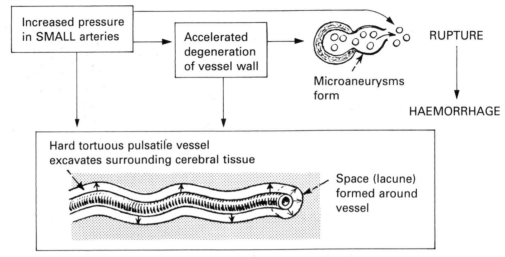

2. **Cerebral infarction** – risk increased indirectly.

Mechanism

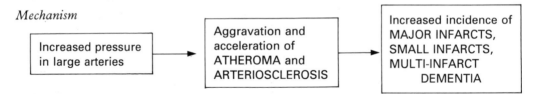

In MALIGNANT HYPERTENSION, an additional dimension, HYPERTENSIVE ENCEPHALOPHATHY, is added.

Mechanism

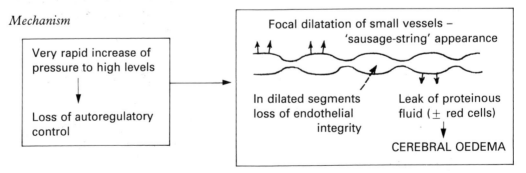

Clinically, signs of cerebral 'irritation' including convulsions progress through stupor to coma. Papilloedema, evidence of increased intracranial pressure, is always present.

HEAD INJURY

Head injuries of varying severity are common nowadays, particularly as a consequence of road traffic accidents. Immediate damage is caused by two main mechanisms which overcome the protection of the vulnerable cerebral tissues provided by the skull and the CSF 'water cushion'.

1. **Direct blows to the head**

   usually cause injury to the soft tissues of the scalp and often fracture of the skull with contusion or laceration of the underlying brain.

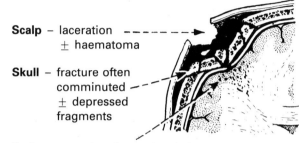

Scalp – laceration ± haematoma

Skull – fracture often comminuted ± depressed fragments

Brain – contusion, laceration or haematoma

2. Since the head is usually freely moveable on the neck, the sudden application of forces derived from **acceleration, deceleration** and, particularly, **rotation** of the head often cause serious injury.

   (a) **Acceleration/deceleration**

   Sudden deceleration

   (i) *Skull damage*

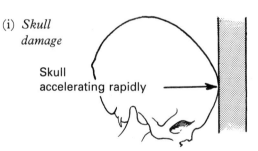

Skull accelerating rapidly

Sudden deceleration due to impact against a hard flat surface.

Severe distortion and bursting effect causes linear fractures of both vertex and base

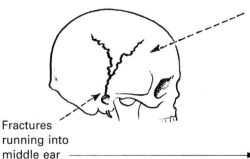

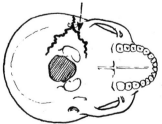

Fractures running into middle ear ⟶ Continuing into skull base

HEAD INJURY

Acceleration/deceleration injury (continued)

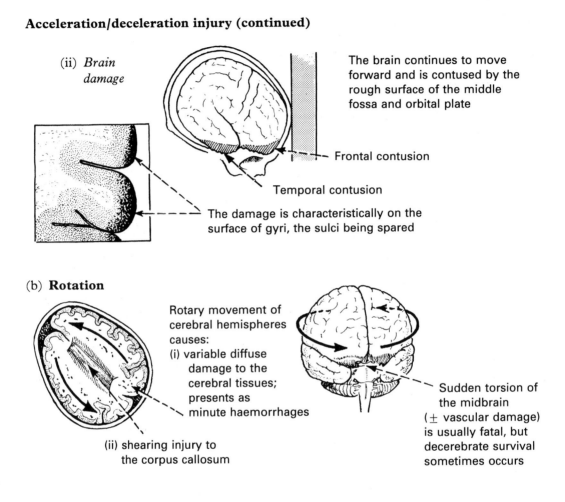

(ii) *Brain damage*

The brain continues to move forward and is contused by the rough surface of the middle fossa and orbital plate

— Frontal contusion

Temporal contusion

The damage is characteristically on the surface of gyri, the sulci being spared

(b) **Rotation**

Rotary movement of cerebral hemispheres causes:
(i) variable diffuse damage to the cerebral tissues; presents as minute haemorrhages

(ii) shearing injury to the corpus callosum

Sudden torsion of the midbrain ($\pm$ vascular damage) is usually fatal, but decerebrate survival sometimes occurs

Notes:

1. **CONCUSSION** is the clinical state of transient loss of consciousness due to temporal neuronal dysfunction following relatively slight impact. The damage is not permanent and full recovery usually ensues.
2. It will be appreciated that more serious cerebral damage is the result of interaction of complex physical forces and anatomical features. An understanding of these mechanisms explains why serious cerebral injury is not uncommon in the absence of damage to the scalp or fracture of the skull, and also why brain damage may be remote from the site of impact: so-called 'contre-coup' injury is sustained when the brain tissue opposite the site of impact is contused.

HEAD INJURY

DELAYED COMPLICATIONS

In addition to damage sustained immediately at the time of impact, certain serious complications may supervene over the next hours or few days.

1. **Haemorrhages**
   (a) **Extradural haematoma**

      This type of haemorrhage classically occurs as a complication of linear fracture of the skull vault when the middle meningeal artery is torn.

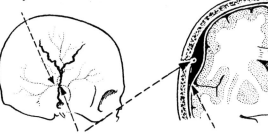
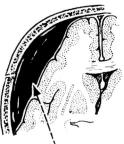

| Artery torn at site of fracture | Haemorrhage gradually strips dura from bone | A large, saucer-shaped haematoma forms |

The classical clinical association is a direct blow to the head from which recovery is rapid. After a lucid interval of varying duration up to several hours, signs of increased intracranial pressure supervene. This chain of events is explained by the time taken for the haemorrhage to accumulate by stripping the dura from the skull.

(b) **Subdural haematoma**. This may occur at any site and is often extensive because of the loose attachment of the dura and arachnoid membranes. It is usually due to rupture of small bridging veins.

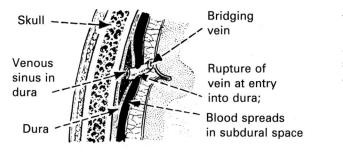

Skull

Venous sinus in dura

Dura

Bridging vein

Rupture of vein at entry into dura;

Blood spreads in subdural space

These acute subdural haematomas are often associated with subarachnoid haemorrhage and cerebral contusions.

(c) **Intracerebral haematomas** occur in association with the cortical contusions particularly in the temporal and frontal lobes, but also at random deep within the hemispheres due to shearing at the time of impact. Large haematomas are uncommon.

713

HEAD INJURY

Delayed complications (continued)

2. **Cerebral oedema** is an important complication.

   ↓

   Increased intracranial pressure→Cerebral hypoxia.

3. **External leakage of CSF** (and blood) from the ear and nose may complicate fractures of the skull base. This complication may be of long duration and is always a potential entry for infection.

4. **Local infection** may complicate compound fractures and proceed to meningitis.

LATE COMPLICATIONS

1. **Scarring and Epilepsy**

   During the healing process, resorption of necrotic tissues and blood degradation products is gradually effected, leaving pigmented scars. These may act as trigger foci for epilepsy, particularly if the meninges are adherent to the underlying brain.

2. **Chronic subdural haematoma**

   This occurs in the elderly and alcoholics. A thick layer of fluid and partially clotted blood gradually accumulates between the dura and arachnoid membranes which show considerable reactive thickening.

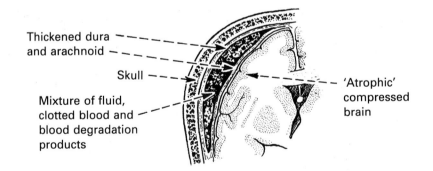

Thickened dura and arachnoid

Skull

Mixture of fluid, clotted blood and blood degradation products

'Atrophic' compressed brain

The precise cause is not known; most cases occur in alcoholics or in elderly people already suffering from cerebral atrophy, and it is possible that the small bridging veins are unduly stretched and become more susceptible to damage.

The clinical signs are usually insidious in onset and progressive, and in nearly all cases there is a history of either no or only very trivial injury.

AGEING AND ATROPHY

It has long been established that progressive atrophy of the brain begins in the 3rd decade and definite morphological changes are associated with simple ageing.

The mean loss of cerebral volume is at the rate of 2–3% per decade from age 20 years and the mean loss of brain weight in old age is 100 g from the weight in the 3rd decade.

However it is very important to understand that these figures are means derived from individual measurements covering a wide range and that the individual variation in respect of rate and degree of ageing change is very wide indeed, as is the maintenance of mental and intellectual capacities in old age. Also our ability to link functional loss with morphological change is limited at the present time.

Nevertheless, where dementia occurs in the elderly it is usually associated with obvious degenerative or atrophic changes in the brain.

Changes in old age
1. **Gross** as seen naked-eye at autopsy

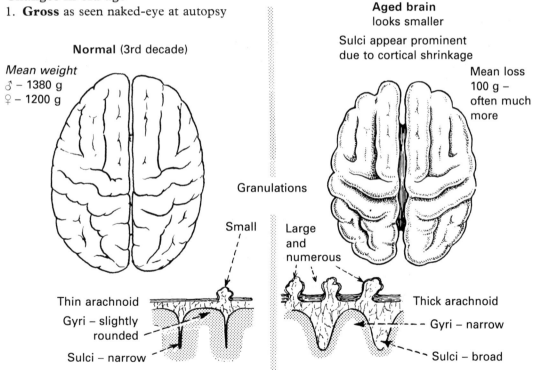

Normal (3rd decade)

Mean weight
♂ – 1380 g
♀ – 1200 g

Aged brain
looks smaller

Sulci appear prominent
due to cortical shrinkage

Mean loss
100 g –
often much
more

Granulations

Small

Large
and
numerous

Thin arachnoid
Gyri – slightly
rounded
Sulci – narrow

Thick arachnoid
Gyri – narrow
Sulci – broad

There is compensatory enlargement of the lateral ventricles.

2. **Microscopic changes**
In normal ageing, degenerative changes in both neuronal and glial tissues are mild as is the associated memory and intellectual impairment.

In SENILE DEMENTIA and ALZHEIMER's pre-senile dementia (i.e. onset before 60 years) there are marked microscopic changes and serious functional defects.

715

SENILE AND ALZHEIMER'S DEMENTIAS

The most important change is degeneration and loss of neurones particularly in the neocortex, the Purkinje layer of the cerebellum and the motor cells in the spinal cord. This loss is accompanied by the following lesions:

Associated with neurones

(1) *Senile plaques*
(Silver stain)

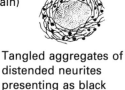

Tangled aggregates of distended neurites presenting as black dots and rods with a centre core of amyloid

(2) *Alzheimer's neurofibrillary degeneration*

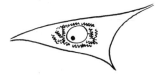

Helical strands of neuroprotein form around the nuclei of neurones.

(3) *Lipofuscin deposition*
(Light microscopy)

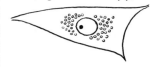

Aggregation of yellow wear-tear pigment not of pathological significance

Associated with supporting tissues

(1) *Gliosis*

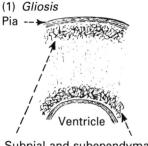

Subpial and subependymal

(2) *Corpora amylacea*

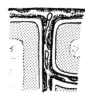

Spherules containing glycogen develop in astrocyte processes (also occurs in other pathological conditions)

(3) *Amyloid*

Deposited in meninges and blood vessel walls

Clinical associations: These reflect the progressive pathological changes and may be very rapid. There is loss of mental functions, particularly memory and the ability to deal with numbers. This progresses inexorably into confusion and inability to perform everyday functions. Death is due to malnutrition, dehydration, heart failure or infection.

Aetiology: The great variability of these 'ageing' changes indicates that they are not related solely to the passage of time and that there is a multifactorial aetiology including genetics, environmental factors and ageing.

> *Genetics* – There are associations with the following chromosomes:
>> (i) Chromosome 21 – note the early onset of dementia in Down's syndrome.
>> (ii) Chromosome 19 – a defective gene is present in 60% of late onset dementia.
>> (iii) Chromosome 14 – the theory is that an abnormal gene causes excess production of apolipoprotein-4 which is associated with loss of intra-cellular neuronal stability leading to degeneration.

> *Other factors* – In Western countries the high incidence of arterial degenerative disease (which itself is age-related) may contribute significantly to the loss of brain tissue (see p.706).

INFECTIONS

Compared with the high incidence of infection generally, infection of the central nervous system is uncommon. The pathological effects may be slight and wholly recoverable as in some virus infections, or severe, leading to permanent damage or death.

Anatomically, infections fall into two main groups which tend to remain separated due to the intervention of the **pial** barrier (see p.695).

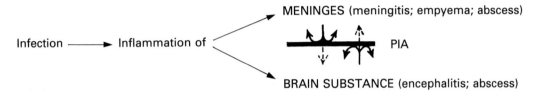

Infections will be considered in three broad aetiological groups:
(1) Bacterial, (2) Viral and (3) Miscellaneous types.

BACTERIAL INFECTIONS
1. **Most commonly by the blood stream**

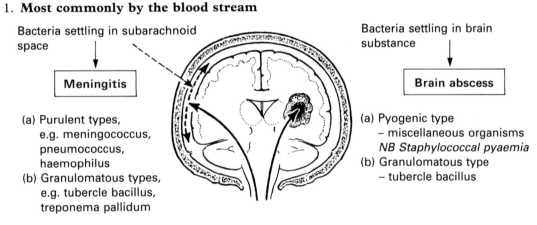

Bacteria settling in subarachnoid space

| **Meningitis** |

(a) Purulent types,
 e.g. meningococcus,
 pneumococcus,
 haemophilus
(b) Granulomatous types,
 e.g. tubercle bacillus,
 treponema pallidum

Bacteria settling in brain substance

| **Brain abscess** |

(a) Pyogenic type
 – miscellaneous organisms
 NB Staphylococcal pyaemia
(b) Granulomatous type
 – tubercle bacillus

2. **From an adjacent local infected site** – these are pyogenic infections.

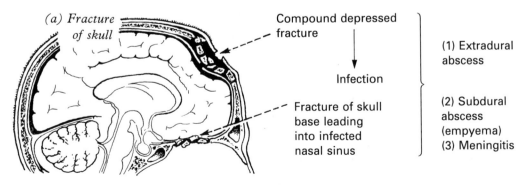

(a) Fracture of skull

Compound depressed fracture

↓

Infection

Fracture of skull base leading into infected nasal sinus

(1) Extradural abscess

(2) Subdural abscess (empyema)
(3) Meningitis

BACTERIAL INFECTION

Bacterial infections from an adjacent local infected site (continued)

(b) *Middle ear and mastoid disease*

In untreated purulent otitis media, three serious complications may arise from spread of the inflammation.

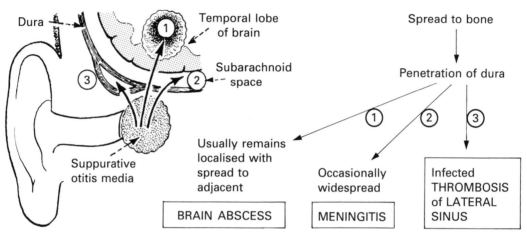

PURULENT MENINGITIS

The whole subarachnoid space contains purulent exudate which is maximal in sulci and around the brain base cisternae.

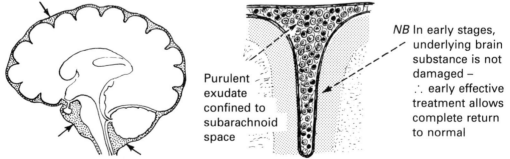

In untreated or ineffectively treated cases which survive, complications include cranial nerve damage, hydrocephalus and variable actual brain damage.

The CSF in the acute stage contains neutrophils and the infecting organism can usually be demonstrated.

BACTERIAL INFECTION

PURULENT BRAIN ABSCESS
The abscesses resulting from direct spread of adjacent infection or by blood borne infection – as seen particularly in bronchiectasis – are often well circumscribed by a pyogenic membrane.

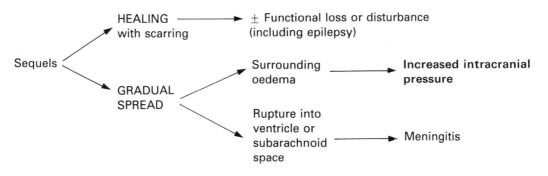

Clinical note: An abscess is often silent early in its evolution, and the infection at the site of entry may have healed before the onset of serious complications causes clinical signs.

Multiple small abscesses occur in staphylococcal pyaemia and microabscesses may complicate bacterial endocarditis. The cerebral pathology in these circumstances is only one facet of serious systemic infection.

TUBERCULOSIS
Meningitis is the result of blood borne spread, usually from a primary complex and is often the important component of generalised miliary tuberculosis (see p.79). Although the incidence has fallen sharply in Western countries, it is emerging as a serious complication of AIDS. It remains prevalent in many parts of the world.

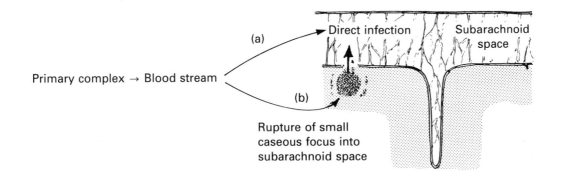

TUBERCULOUS MENINGITIS

Evolution

Before the advent of antibiotic and chemotherapy, tuberculous meningitis was invariably fatal after an illness lasting from several days to a few weeks.

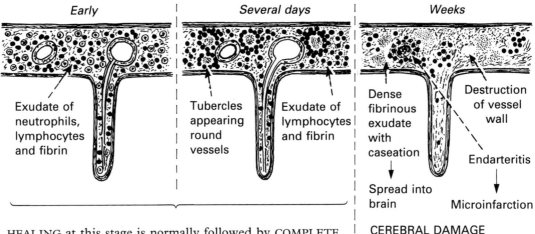

Early	Several days	Weeks

Exudate of neutrophils, lymphocytes and fibrin

Tubercles appearing round vessels

Exudate of lymphocytes and fibrin

Dense fibrinous exudate with caseation

Destruction of vessel wall

Endarteritis

Spread into brain

Microinfarction

HEALING at this stage is normally followed by COMPLETE RECOVERY.

The CSF characteristically contains lymphocytes and fibrinogen which forms a delicate fibrin web on standing. Tubercle bacilli can be demonstrated or cultured.

CEREBRAL DAMAGE
Complete recovery prevented by
(a) permanent meningeal adhesions
(b) focal cortical scarring

At autopsy, the brain usually shows a diagnostic appearance:

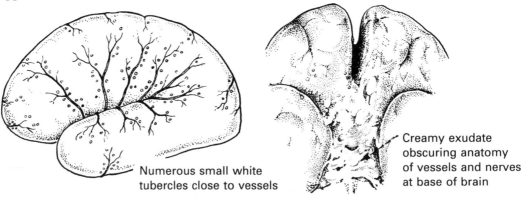

Numerous small white tubercles close to vessels

Creamy exudate obscuring anatomy of vessels and nerves at base of brain

TUBERCULOMA: These localised tuberculous cerebral abscesses are now very rare.

SYPHILIS: Neurological syphilis is rare nowadays. The main pathological lesions are described on page 84.

VIRUS INFECTIONS

Compared with the incidence of virus infections in general, affection of the central nervous system is rare, even with viruses having an affinity for the CNS –

NEUROTROPIC VIRUSES

There are three broad groups:-

1. **Acute**

   Cell lysis occurs towards the end of the viraemic phase of infection. This is the common type of disease.

2. **Persistent**

   Viruses which usually cause damage outside the CNS behave uncharacteristically and cause continuing and active disease of the CNS over a long period (months – years).

3. **Slow**

   In these diseases the agents have not yet been fully categorised. After a very long (years) incubation period, unremitting and fatal disease ensues.

   Latent virus infection is seen in herpes zoster and possibly plays a role in the demyelinating diseases.

   Virus infection also has a possible role in oncogenesis within the CNS.

Routes of infection

Most viruses arrive at the CNS via the blood, but the factors which potentiate the establishment of disease within the CNS are poorly understood.

Primary portal of entry

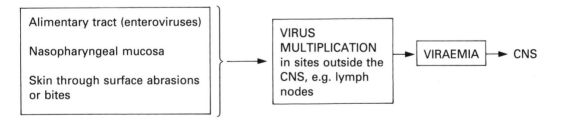

In rabies, the virus travels from the wound up the peripheral nerves to the CNS.

VIRUS INFECTIONS

BASIC PATHOLOGICAL EFFECTS

(a) Commonly the disease is mild and only the meninges are affected – **ASEPTIC MENINGITIS**. Recovery is usually complete.

(b) In more severe cases, the brain substance is also damaged in varying degree – **ENCEPHALITIS** (meningoencephalitis).

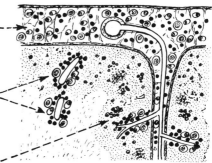

The meninges (CSF) contain increased protein, normal sugar and a mononuclear cellular infiltrate (particularly **lymphocytes**, plasma cells and large mononuclears).

In the brain the characteristic changes are:

1. PERIVASCULAR CUFFING (same infiltrate as meninges)
2. ACUTE NEURONAL DAMAGE up to complete lysis with accompanying neuronophagia and inflammatory changes. In some conditions, surviving neurones contain cytoplasmic and/or nuclear inclusions.

To these basic changes, damage to myelin and glial tissue may be added, and small focal haemorrhages may be seen. The damage is effected in two ways:

1. **Certainly** by the direct effects of virus on cells
2. **Possibly** in some cases indirectly due to virus-antibody complexes initiating a vascular inflammatory response.

Diagnosis

Examination of the CSF is helpful in establishing a diagnosis of aseptic meningitis or meningoencephalitis (see p.762).

NB The findings in tuberculous meningitis are very similar except that in tubercular meningitis the CSF **sugar is low**.

The specific virus aetiology is more difficult to establish and in severe cases brain biopsy may be required.

Clinical associations and progress

In aseptic meningitis, the illness is mild with fever, headache and neck stiffness the main signs. Recovery is almost always complete.

In meningoencephalitis, signs of cerebral 'irritation' and neuronal damage are seen, e.g. mental confusion, delusion, stupor, convulsions and coma, and there may be localising signs. In mild cases, recovery is complete, but in more severe cases, residual paralyses and other signs indicative of permanent brain damage may follow. Death in coma with respiratory failure occurs in very severe cases.

VIRUS INFECTIONS

ENTEROVIRUSES

These are small RNA viruses (picornavirus group) and include POLIOVIRUSES, COXSACKIE VIRUSES and ECHOVIRUSES.

Infection is acquired by ingestion of faecally contaminated material followed by proliferation in the intestine. In only a small minority of infected cases does the virus pass the blood-brain barrier and cause disease of the CNS.

In addition to aseptic meningitis, the POLIOVIRUSES (and very occasionally Coxsackie and Echo viruses) cause the classical paralytic disease, **ANTERIOR POLIOMYELITIS**.

Pathological changes

The pathological changes are reflected in three clinical stages: (1) acute, (2) recovery and (3) permanent residual disability.

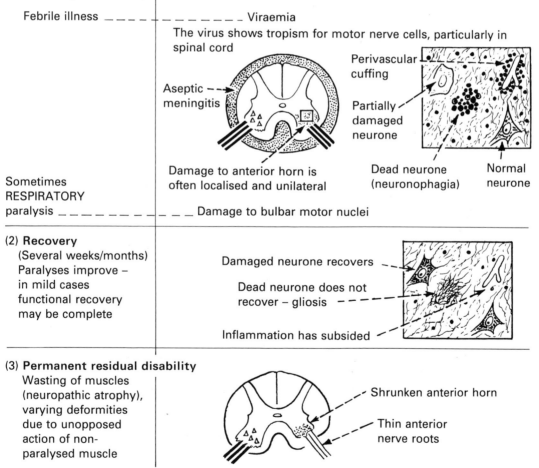

(1) **Acute** (up to 2 weeks)

Febrile illness _ _ _ _ _ _ _ _ _ _ _ Viraemia

The virus shows tropism for motor nerve cells, particularly in spinal cord

Aseptic -- → meningitis

Perivascular cuffing

Partially damaged neurone

Damage to anterior horn is often localised and unilateral

Dead neurone (neuronophagia)

Normal neurone

Sometimes RESPIRATORY paralysis _ _ _ _ _ _ _ _ _ _ Damage to bulbar motor nuclei

(2) **Recovery**
(Several weeks/months)
Paralyses improve –
in mild cases
functional recovery
may be complete

Damaged neurone recovers

Dead neurone does not recover – gliosis

Inflammation has subsided

(3) **Permanent residual disability**
Wasting of muscles (neuropathic atrophy), varying deformities due to unopposed action of non-paralysed muscle

Shrunken anterior horn

Thin anterior nerve roots

VIRUS INFECTIONS

HERPES ZOSTER (See also p.87)

This is a disease of adults, presenting as a painful vesicular rash, usually unilateral and affecting one or a few adjacent dermatomes only. It is due to recurrence of a latent varicella (chickenpox) infection.

Mechanism   Virus lying latent from infection in childhood

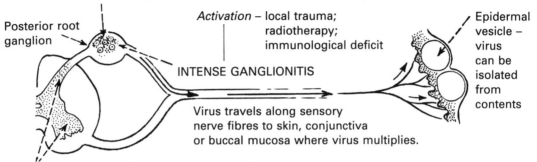

Posterior root ganglion

Activation – local trauma; radiotherapy; immunological deficit

INTENSE GANGLIONITIS

Virus travels along sensory nerve fibres to skin, conjunctiva or buccal mucosa where virus multiplies.

Epidermal vesicle – virus can be isolated from contents

Minor secondary degenerative changes in cord

Sequels   1. An occasional sequel is intense pain with varying paraesthesia and anaesthesia long after the acute phase has healed.
2. In cases of Vth nerve herpes, serious damage to the eye may result.

HERPES SIMPLEX

In addition to encephalitis seen in infants suffering from disseminated herpes simplex infection and cases of mild aseptic meningitis, herpes simplex virus on rare occasions causes a severe ACUTE NECROTISING ENCEPHALITIS affecting particularly the temporal lobes. A few cases arise against a background of immune deficit, but the majority are unexplained.

RABIES

The rabies virus shows marked neurotropism and can infect most mammals. Various wild carnivores (fox, jackal, skunk, vampire bats) are the natural reservoir. Many human cases are contracted from dogs.

Mechanism

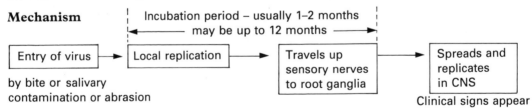

Incubation period – usually 1–2 months
may be up to 12 months

| Entry of virus | Local replication | Travels up sensory nerves to root ganglia | Spreads and replicates in CNS |

by bite or salivary contamination or abrasion

Clinical signs appear

An unremitting encephalitis particularly affecting the grey matter is established. Diagnostic Negri bodies (virus inclusions) are found at autopsy in the pyramidal cells of the hippocampus and the Purkinje cells of the cerebellum.

Clinically, the encephalitis presents with extreme excitation of the sensory system. The classical hydrophobia (fear of water) is due to serious disturbance of the swallowing mechanism with muscular spasm. Death invariably occurs and is due to respiratory muscle spasm or paralysis.

VIRUS INFECTIONS

AIDS and the NERVOUS SYSTEM

Serious pathological changes are associated with Human Immunodeficiency Virus (HIV) infection.

They arise in 2 ways:
1. By direct invasion of the CNS cells by the virus causing:
   (a) dementia, myelopathy and peripheral neuropathy
   (b) microglial proliferation
   (c) glial tumours.
2. The results of opportunistic infections
   e.g. Fungi, Toxoplasma, cryptococcus, cytomegalovirus (CMV).

SLOW VIRUS INFECTION

Spongiform encephalopathies: PRION disease

These rare diseases are not strictly virus diseases but are due to a transmittable agent and occur in man and various animal species.

Kuru is an example of a subacute spongiform encephalopathy. It occurs in the eastern highlands of New Guinea and is associated with cannibalism. The disease presents as a progressive cerebellar ataxia and is invariably fatal. There is a prolonged incubation period (often many years) with a rapidly progressive course following the first symptoms.

The pathological changes are neuronal degeneration and loss with astroglial proliferation presenting as small cystic areas in the grey matter (spongiosis). It is noteworthy that there is no inflammation.

Creutzfeld-Jacob disease in man, **Scrapie** in sheep and, more recently, **bovine spongiform encephalopathy** (BSE) ('Mad cow disease') belong to this group.

In these diseases an abnormal form PRION PROTEIN (PrP), a membrane glycoprotein, is present in high concentration in neurones and viscera but not in muscles. In certain cases of familial dementia there is evidence that the PrP gene is abnormal.

The TRANSMISSIBLE AGENT differs from viruses in showing resistance to heat and other sterilization procedures: it contains no nucleic acid and does not evoke an immune response or interferon production.

Transmission: It is thought that cattle contracted the disease from commercially concentrated food-stuff containing infected (scrapie) sheep offal. The chances of transmission to man by eating meat (muscle) are insignificant.

ARTHROPOD BORNE VIRUSES (ARBOVIRUSES)

These cause encephalitis in many parts of the world. Biting insects transmit the viruses from animal reservoirs.

PERSISTENT VIRUS INFECTION

An example is subacute sclerosing panencephalitis, a rare invariably fatal disease which affects children and young adults. There is progressive widespread destruction of neurones with reactive inflammatory changes giving the white matter a firm consistency.

The infecting agent is thought to be a reactivated but modified measles virus: high titres of measles antibodies are present in the blood.

MISCELLANEOUS INFECTIONS AND INFESTATIONS

1. FUNGAL INFECTIONS

(a) **Primary infections**. In healthy adults, fungal infections are rare. Occasionally in the presence of heavy exposure to fungus, localised infection, often clinically insignificant, may occur and in very rare cases, CNS infection is a complication. In CRYPTOCOCCOSIS (*C. neoformans*), the fungus exhibits neurotropism and occasionally causes meningitis in otherwise healthy subjects.

(b) **Opportunistic infections** are becoming more common nowadays due to the use of immunosuppressive therapy and the increasing prevalence of AIDS. Various fungi including *Candida, Aspergillus nocardia* may cause serious cerebral damage.

2. PROTOZOAL INFECTIONS

(a) CEREBRAL MALARIA

Cerebral complications may occur in the severe acute malaria (falciparum type) which affects non-immune adults. Clinically, coma rapidly proceeds to death.

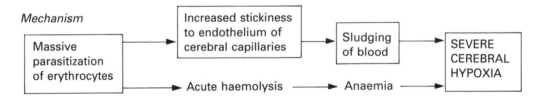

At autopsy the brain is swollen (oedema) and there may be petechial haemorrhages. Histologically, the capillaries are congested and malarial parasites and pigment easily seen.

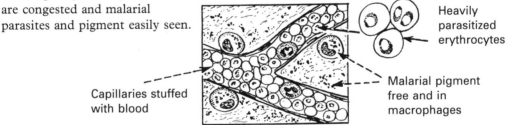

MISCELLANEOUS INFECTIONS AND INFESTATIONS

Protozoal infections (continued)
(b) TOXOPLASMOSIS

Although infection by *T.gondii* is common, serious nervous tissue damage is rare and is seen in two main circumstances. In both, it occurs as part of a systemic infection.

(i) In **congenital toxoplasmosis**, the infection is acquired by the fetus during a primary maternal infection.

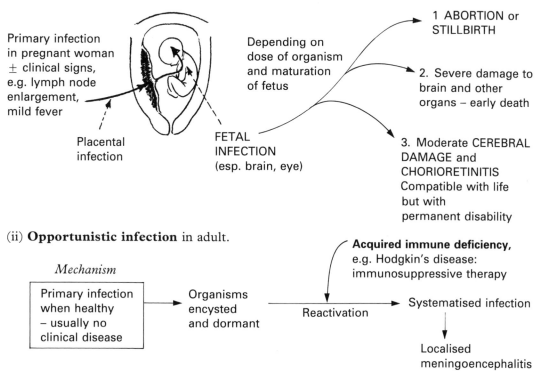

Primary infection in pregnant woman ± clinical signs, e.g. lymph node enlargement, mild fever

Placental infection

FETAL INFECTION (esp. brain, eye)

Depending on dose of organism and maturation of fetus

1 ABORTION or STILLBIRTH

2. Severe damage to brain and other organs – early death

3. Moderate CEREBRAL DAMAGE and CHORIORETINITIS Compatible with life but with permanent disability

(ii) **Opportunistic infection** in adult.

Mechanism

Primary infection when healthy – usually no clinical disease → Organisms encysted and dormant —— Reactivation ——→ Systematised infection

Acquired immune deficiency, e.g. Hodgkin's disease: immunosuppressive therapy

Localised meningoencephalitis

(c) TRYPANOSOMIASIS (AFRICAN SLEEPING SICKNESS)

T.brucei infection is transmitted to man from animal reservoirs by the Tsetse fly. The organism is neurotropic and a meningoencephalitis results. The infection is associated with excessive IgM production. The 'cuffing' infiltrate has a high component of plasma cells and also 'Mott' cells – plasma cells distended by eosinophilic globules (denatured Ig).

Mott cell

Cerebral capillary

Lymphocytes and plasma cells

3. METAZOAL INFESTATION
CRYTICERCOSIS

The larvae of *Taenia solium* may encyst in the brain and can be the cause of epilepsy.

HYDATID CYST – also occurs in the brain (see p.462).

DEMYELINATING DISEASES

ACUTE DISSEMINATED ENCEPHALOMYELITIS

An acute encephalitis in which demyelination is a prominent and characteristic feature is a very rare sequel to many natural viral diseases and to vaccination, particularly against smallpox and rabies.

Clinically, there is fever, headache, vomiting and drowsiness followed by coma. There may be clinical evidence of focal neurological damage. Pathological changes are widespread in the brain and cord and rapidly progressive.

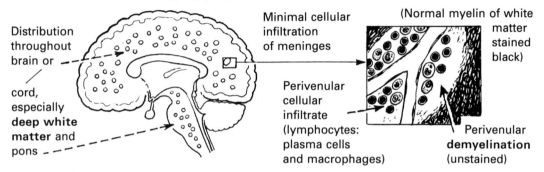

Distribution throughout brain or cord, especially **deep white matter** and pons

Minimal cellular infiltration of meninges

Perivenular cellular infiltrate (lymphocytes: plasma cells and macrophages)

(Normal myelin of white matter stained black)

Perivenular **demyelination** (unstained)

In **ACUTE HAEMORRHAGIC LEUKOENCEPHALITIS,** to these are added actual petechial haemorrhages from damaged vessels, particularly in the white matter; not all cases follow virus infection.

Mechanism. It is thought that in these disorders (particularly encephalitis following anti-rabies inoculation) the damage to the myelin is not the result of direct virus attack but is an *autoimmune* reaction in which the antigen is a component of myelin and the virus in some unknown way acts as a trigger.

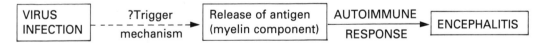

VIRUS INFECTION — ?Trigger mechanism → Release of antigen (myelin component) — AUTOIMMUNE RESPONSE → ENCEPHALITIS

Experimental allergic encephalomyelitis (EAE) in animals closely mimics the human disease.

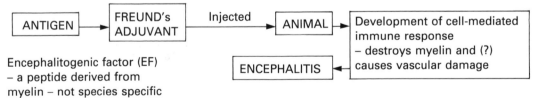

ANTIGEN → FREUND's ADJUVANT — Injected → ANIMAL → Development of cell-mediated immune response – destroys myelin and (?) causes vascular damage → ENCEPHALITIS

Encephalitogenic factor (EF) – a peptide derived from myelin – not species specific

The importance of these rare diseases is that they form a link between virus infections and the chronic DEMYELINATING DISEASES.

DEMYELINATING DISEASES

In the demyelinating diseases, the breakdown of myelin occurs as an almost random patchy process in the white matter; at the same time, neurones and axons usually remain healthy. There are two main types:

1. The '**myelinoclastic**' type.
   The myelin is apparently normal until adult life and then breaks down.

2. The '**dysmyelinative**' type.
   The myelin is structurally abnormal usually from an early age.

1. MULTIPLE SCLEROSIS (MS)
This is a chronic disease of young adults.

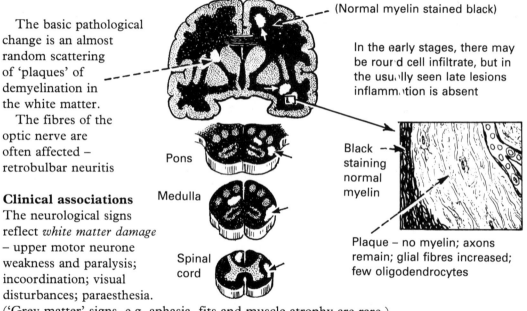

The basic pathological change is an almost random scattering of 'plaques' of demyelination in the white matter.

The fibres of the optic nerve are often affected – retrobulbar neuritis

(Normal myelin stained black)

In the early stages, there may be round cell infiltrate, but in the usually seen late lesions inflammation is absent

Pons

Medulla

Black staining normal myelin

Spinal cord

Plaque – no myelin; axons remain; glial fibres increased; few oligodendrocytes

Clinical associations
The neurological signs reflect *white matter damage* – upper motor neurone weakness and paralysis; incoordination; visual disturbances; paraesthesia.
('Grey matter' signs, e.g. aphasia, fits and muscle atrophy are rare.)

Course of Disease

Onset
Often acute;
may be unnoticed.

Progress over many years
Remission . . . Relapse . . . Remission →
Incremental deterioration → Death

Variants are: 1. acute severe disease – rapid progress to death
2. chronic progression without remission
3. minimal signs with very long remissions.

DEMYELINATING DISEASES

MULTIPLE SCLEROSIS (continued)
Aetiology

The cause remains unknown and the basic mechanisms poorly defined.

1. The geographical pattern is of interest, but does not as yet contribute to our understanding of the aetiology. The disease is common (60 cases per 100,000 population) throughout temperate Europe and North America and small pockets of much higher incidence do occur. The incidence is low in the tropics.
2. The three most plausible current theories which are not mutually exclusive are based on as yet inconclusive evidence:

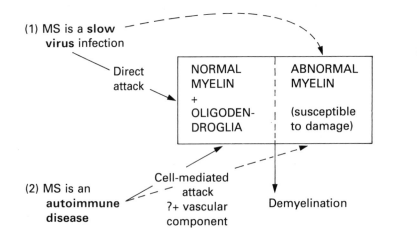

(1) MS is a **slow virus** infection

Direct attack

NORMAL MYELIN + OLIGODEN-DROGLIA

ABNORMAL MYELIN

(susceptible to damage)

(2) MS is an **autoimmune disease**

Cell-mediated attack ?+ vascular component

Demyelination

(3) The apparently normal myelin of MS is really abnormal and contains less unsaturated fatty acids (UFA). It is not known whether this condition is genetic or acquired.

2. DYSMELINATING DISEASES

In this group of 'leukodystrophies', the molecular structure of myelin is abnormal due usually to abnormal or deficient enzyme action. Most cases are genetically determined, present in early life and progress fairly rapidly.

Abnormal metabolites which can be specifically identified accumulate in macrophages, glial cells and sometimes neurones.

> e.g. 1. In **metachromatic leukodystrophy,** the accumulation of a *sulphatide* gives a metachromatic staining reaction and characteristic EM appearance.
>
> 2. In **Krabbe's disease** there are typical multinucleated histocytes (called globoid cells) containing *cerebroside*.

In some disorders, when the loss of myelin is associated with marked gliosis, the name 'diffuse cerebral sclerosis' is applied.

MISCELLANEOUS DISORDERS

NUTRITIONAL, TOXIC AND METABOLIC DISORDERS (ENCEPHALOPATHIES)

In the last analysis, all disorders in this group are mediated by disturbed neuronal metabolism, so that exact classification may present some difficulty. However, it is convenient to consider them in three broad groups.

1. NUTRITIONAL DEFICIENCY

The vitamins of the B group are important coenzymes in several intracellular oxidative pathways. Deficiency, which may arise from primary malnutrition but more commonly in association with alcohol abuse, is the cause of degenerations of the brain, spinal cord and peripheral nerves.

Wernicke's encephalopathy

Clinically, this condition presents with disturbances of consciousness, ataxia and visual disturbances, and without prompt treatment progresses to death in coma.

In Western countries, chronic alcoholism is usually present; often a particularly heavy bout of drinking precipitates the condition.

Chronic alcoholism ⟶ Poor diet ⟶ NUTRITIONAL DEFICIENCY of vit B complex, esp. THIAMIN.

Bout of heavy drinking ⟶ Vomiting ⟶ *Accentuates*

The blood PYRUVATE level is raised.

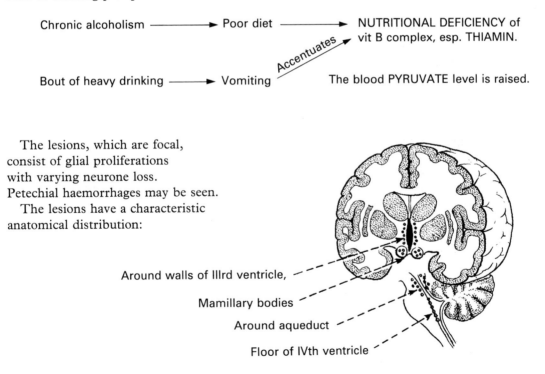

The lesions, which are focal, consist of glial proliferations with varying neurone loss. Petechial haemorrhages may be seen.

The lesions have a characteristic anatomical distribution:

Around walls of IIIrd ventricle,

Mamillary bodies

Around aqueduct

Floor of IVth ventricle

Prompt treatment with thiamin minimises the damage, but if treatment is omitted or delayed, permanent damage results. At autopsy, there is visible shrinkage of the mamillary bodies.

731

MISCELLANEOUS DISORDERS

2. EXOGENOUS TOXIC DISORDERS

The nervous system is affected by a wide range of poisons, many of which are used in medical treatment, including particularly hypnotics and narcotics.

In many acute cases, neuronal metabolism is seriously depressed and may result in death. Very often the effects of cerebral hypoxia as well as the metabolic disturbances caused by damage to other organs are superimposed so that it may be difficult to define neurological damage specifically caused by the poison.

The diagram shows the effects of acute poisoning.

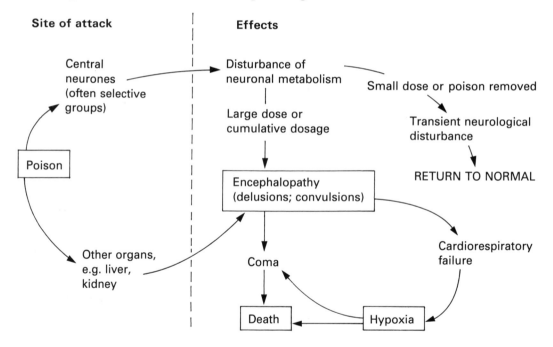

These disorders are the result of biochemical changes in the first place and minimal or no morphological damage is caused. However, at autopsy there are non-specific oedematous and hypoxic changes: specific toxic effects are usually not identifiable.

In some cases, the peripheral nerves are damaged – neuropathy.

Chronic alcoholic intoxication exemplifies this scheme. Specific toxic effects on neurones are difficult to identify, but the brain is damaged by nutritional deficits and as a result of liver disturbance.

Metallic poisons

In the case of heavy metals and arsenic, there is a build up of the poison within the nervous system and encephalopathy with morphological damage results.

MISCELLANEOUS DISORDERS

3. METABOLIC DISORDERS

A. Disorders due to inborn errors of metabolism

These are often due to lysozomal enzyme deficiency.

(a) The *dysmyelinating diseases* (leukodystrophies) in which abnormal central nervous cellular metabolism, especially in glial cells, produces abnormal myelin have already been mentioned.

(b) In the *neuronal storage diseases*, which usually present during the first decade, deficiency of lysozomal enzymes leads to accumulation of intermediate metabolites in the neurones. The diagnosis of the condition often depends on the identification of the abnormal metabolite by histochemistry or EM.

Tay-Sach's disease (amaurotic familial idiocy) is an illustrative example.

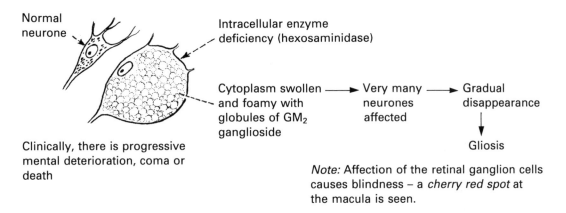

Normal neurone

Intracellular enzyme deficiency (hexosaminidase)

Cytoplasm swollen and foamy with globules of GM_2 ganglioside ⟶ Very many neurones affected ⟶ Gradual disappearance ↓ Gliosis

Clinically, there is progressive mental deterioration, coma or death

Note: Affection of the retinal ganglion cells causes blindness – a *cherry red spot* at the macula is seen.

In these disorders, other organs may be mildly affected by the enzyme defect but the neurological effects are predominant.

(c) In the following examples, the metabolic defect causes neurological disorder, but in addition, other organs are seriously disturbed.

(i) *Aminoacidopathies*

A wide variety of hepatic enzyme defects in the complex metabolism of amino acids have now been described. When neurological damage occurs, it is essentially non-specific and developing in the immediate postnatal period, a critical time in the development of the brain which leads to *mental retardation*.

Phenylketonuria is an example.

The importance of this disease is that the effects can be prevented by dietary restriction of phenylalanine-containing substances, provided the treatment is begun within 60 days of birth.

MISCELLANEOUS DISORDERS

Phenylketonuria (continued)

Mechanism

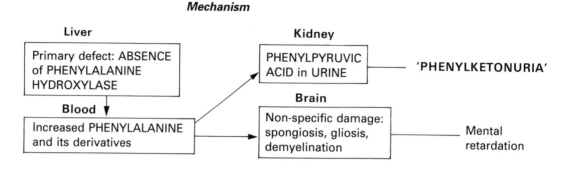

Liver	**Kidney**	
Primary defect: ABSENCE of PHENYLALANINE HYDROXYLASE	PHENYLPYRUVIC ACID in URINE	—— 'PHENYLKETONURIA'
Blood ↓	**Brain**	
Increased PHENYLALANINE and its derivatives	Non-specific damage: spongiosis, gliosis, demyelination	Mental retardation

(ii) *Hepatolenticular degeneration (Wilson's disease)*

In this rare inherited disorder (autosomal recessive: parental consanguinity in one third of cases) accumulation of COPPER causes serious toxic effects.

The primary lysozomal defect is in the liver cells: in many cases there are also low levels of caeruloplasmin (glycoprotein which normally transports Cu).

Basic mechanism

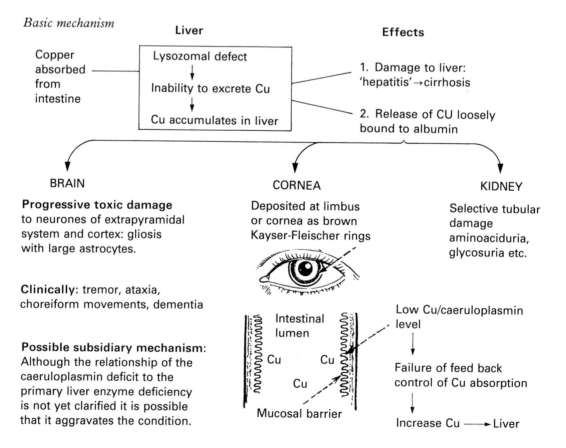

Liver   **Effects**

Copper absorbed from intestine —— Lysozomal defect ↓ Inability to excrete Cu ↓ Cu accumulates in liver

1. Damage to liver: 'hepatitis' → cirrhosis

2. Release of CU loosely bound to albumin

BRAIN

Progressive toxic damage to neurones of extrapyramidal system and cortex: gliosis with large astrocytes.

Clinically: tremor, ataxia, choreiform movements, dementia

Possible subsidiary mechanism: Although the relationship of the caeruloplasmin deficit to the primary liver enzyme deficiency is not yet clarified it is possible that it aggravates the condition.

CORNEA

Deposited at limbus or cornea as brown Kayser-Fleischer rings

Intestinal lumen

Cu   Cu

Cu

Mucosal barrier

KIDNEY

Selective tubular damage aminoaciduria, glycosuria etc.

Low Cu/caeruloplasmin level

↓

Failure of feed back control of Cu absorption

↓

Increase Cu —→ Liver

MISCELLANEOUS DISORDERS

METABOLIC (continued)

B. Secondary

The metabolism of the nervous system may be seriously affected by disease elsewhere in the body.

Acute hypoxia and **hypoglycaemia**
cause disturbance of the basic neuronal metabolism and serious damage results if these conditions are not corrected quickly.

In many other disorders, the neuronal disturbances are usually reversible even in cases of fairly long duration, and permanent damage is seen only in late or severe disease.

Clinically, the condition progresses from delirium through the stuporose state to coma and death.

The mechanisms are complex, often indirect and not certainly defined. They include particularly:

1. disturbances of water and electrolyte (especially Na^+ and K^+) balance, and also pH affecting neuronal environment.

2. the activity of abnormal 'toxic' metabolites, e.g. ketones; organic acids (including amino acids) directly affecting neuronal metabolism.

3. (1) and (2) combined influence chemical transmission

The following common and important disorders are illustrative:

(a) Diabetes mellitus – the important derangements which act in various combinations are: hypovolaemia (due to dehydration); hyperosmolarity (due to hyperglycaemia); Na^+ and K^+ depletion; ketonaemia and lactic acidosis.

(b) Liver failure – complex disturbances of NH_3 and amino acid metabolism (see p.456).

(c) Renal failure (uraemia) – complex disturbances involving water, electrolyte and nitrogenous waste products (see p.637).

In addition, in some cases of renal failure, malignant hypertension contributes to the neurological disturbance (see p.710).

EXTRAPYRAMIDAL DISORDERS

The extrapyramidal system is interposed between the higher motor centres (cortical) and the effector motor cells of the anterior horn of the spinal cord.

It consists of the basal ganglia nuclei in the midbrain and pons, and complex interconnections between the nuclei and other parts of the cerebrum, cerebellum and cord.

Its function, which is to integrate motor and sensory impulses so that muscle tone reflexes and movements are smooth and coordinated, is finally effected by facilitation and restraint of anterior horn neurone activity.

Important neurotransmitters within the system are DOPAMINE (also catecholamines and 5-hydroxytryptamine), acetylcholine and γ-aminobutyric acid (GABA).

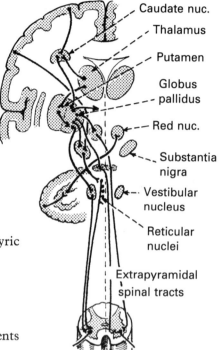

Caudate nuc.
Thalamus
Putamen
Globus pallidus
Red nuc.
Substantia nigra
Vestibular nucleus
Reticular nuclei
Extrapyramidal spinal tracts

Disorders of the system result in:
1. muscular rigidity
2. tremors
3. incoordinated and abnormal muscle movements
4. disturbances of postural reflexes.

Theoretically, damage to any part of the system may be associated with all or any of these derangements.

The following two disorders are illustrative:

1. PARKINSONISM (Paralysis agitans)

Aetiology: The disease occurs in two main circumstances:

(a) *Idiopathic*: occuring in people over 50; nowadays not infrequent in an ageing population.

(b) *Secondary*: 1. **Postencephalitic**, i.e. as a sequel to encephalitis lethargica which occurred in epidemic form in the 1920s. The number of such cases now surviving is rapidly diminishing.

2. **Drug induced**. The use of neuroleptic drugs may induce the syndrome temporarily (occasionally permanently), presumably by disturbing the balance of the chemical transmitters.

3. **Arteriopathy**.

4. **Heavy metal poisoning**.

EXTRAPYRAMIDAL DISORDERS

Clinically, **Parkinsonism** illustrates the classical features of extrapyramidal damage.

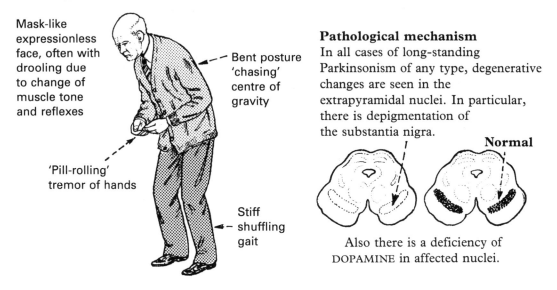

Mask-like expressionless face, often with drooling due to change of muscle tone and reflexes

Bent posture 'chasing' centre of gravity

'Pill-rolling' tremor of hands

Stiff shuffling gait

Pathological mechanism
In all cases of long-standing Parkinsonism of any type, degenerative changes are seen in the extrapyramidal nuclei. In particular, there is depigmentation of the substantia nigra.

Normal

Also there is a deficiency of DOPAMINE in affected nuclei.

In the idiopathic type, it is possible that the dopamine deficiency is an acquired metabolic disorder which leads to the neuronal degeneration, but this has not yet been established.

2. THE CHOREAS

These are extrapyramidal disorders in which the presenting sign is involuntary incoordinate movements. There are 2 main types which, apart from both presenting with choreiform movements, differ in many respects.

	INFECTIOUS	HUNTINGTON'S
Age of onset	Childhood	35–50 years
Progress	Recovery – complete (may be recurrences)	Deterioration and cerebral cortical degeneration (dementia)
Pathogenesis	Associated with infections, esp. rheumatic fever. *NB* often associated with endocarditis	Hereditary (autosomal dominant: defect in chromosome 4) – associated with reduction of neurotransmitter GABA
Pathology	Essentially inflammatory: mild encephalitis (? arteritis) affecting basal ganglia	Essentially neuronal degeneration in caudate nucleus, putamen and cortex

DISEASES OF SPINAL CORD

In purely spinal lesions, basic disease processes have important anatomical and functional implications. Lack of space for expansion produces important compression effects. Examples are:

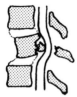

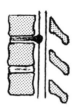

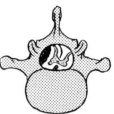

Fracture/
dislocation
of vertebra

Tumour (usually
secondary) in vertebrae
growing into canal

Prolapse of
intervertebral
disc

Tumour of
meninges or
nerve sheath

Effects

Normal

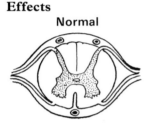

Compression

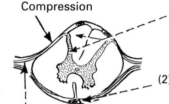

(1) *Damage to neurones and nerve tracts*
May be focal but is often transverse and complete

(2) *Vascular compression*
Impairment of circulation may be actual infarction; this is important particularly in traumatic cases

Cord, nerve roots and
blood vessels loosely
suspended in CSF
'water bath'

(3) *Damage to nerve roots* (radiculitis); a common complication of spondylosis

At the level of the lesion, there is loss of the sensory and motor connections which constitute the spinal reflex.

In addition, severance of the longitudinal tracts cuts off the cerebral connections to all parts below the lesion.

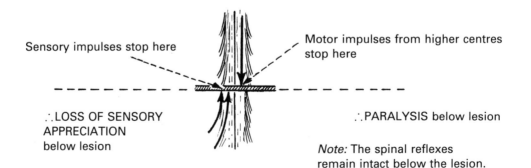

Sensory impulses stop here

Motor impulses from higher centres stop here

∴LOSS OF SENSORY
APPRECIATION
below lesion

∴PARALYSIS below lesion

Note: The spinal reflexes remain intact below the lesion.

DISEASES OF SPINAL CORD

ASCENDING AND DESCENDING DEGENERATIONS

The long tract fibres which are cut off from their neurones progressively degenerate.

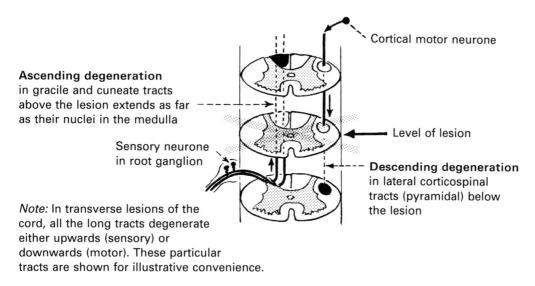

Cortical motor neurone

Ascending degeneration
in gracile and cuneate tracts
above the lesion extends as far
as their nuclei in the medulla

Level of lesion

Sensory neurone
in root ganglion

Descending degeneration
in lateral corticospinal
tracts (pyramidal) below
the lesion

Note: In transverse lesions of the
cord, all the long tracts degenerate
either upwards (sensory) or
downwards (motor). These particular
tracts are shown for illustrative convenience.

The commonest example of **descending degeneration** is seen following cerebral infarction involving the internal capsule; the degeneration extends from the lesion along the corticospinal axons to their terminations in the anterior horn.

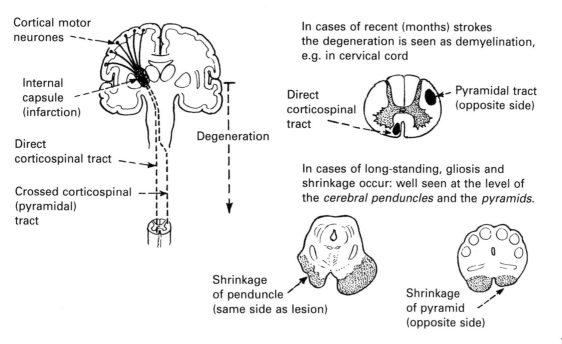

Cortical motor
neurones

In cases of recent (months) strokes
the degeneration is seen as demyelination,
e.g. in cervical cord

Internal
capsule
(infarction)

Direct
corticospinal
tract

Pyramidal tract
(opposite side)

Direct
corticospinal tract

Degeneration

Crossed corticospinal
(pyramidal)
tract

In cases of long-standing, gliosis and
shrinkage occur: well seen at the level of
the *cerebral peduncles* and the *pyramids*.

Shrinkage
of peduncle
(same side as lesion)

Shrinkage
of pyramid
(opposite side)

DISORDERS OF MOTOR PATHWAYS

The concept of upper and lower motor neuronal activity, based on anatomical and physiological evidence, has great clinical value in diagnosis.

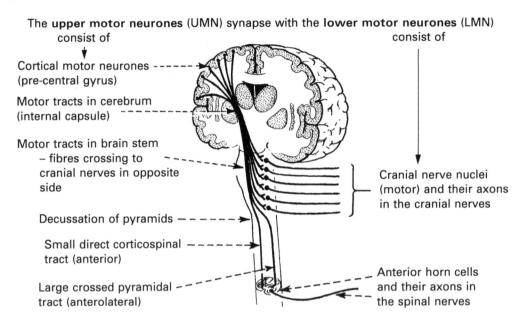

The **upper motor neurones** (UMN) consist of

Cortical motor neurones (pre-central gyrus)

Motor tracts in cerebrum (internal capsule)

Motor tracts in brain stem – fibres crossing to cranial nerves in opposite side

Decussation of pyramids

Small direct corticospinal tract (anterior)

Large crossed pyramidal tract (anterolateral)

synapse with the **lower motor neurones** (LMN) consist of

Cranial nerve nuclei (motor) and their axons in the cranial nerves

Anterior horn cells and their axons in the spinal nerves

It will be appreciated that in its long course from the cerebral cortex to the anterior horn, the upper motor neurone is susceptible to damage from a variety of disease processes acting at various sites. The lower motor neurone may be damaged in the cord or in the peripheral nerve. Important illustrative examples are:

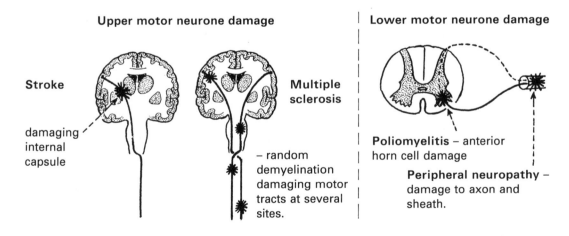

Upper motor neurone damage

Lower motor neurone damage

Stroke

damaging internal capsule

Multiple sclerosis

– random demyelination damaging motor tracts at several sites.

Poliomyelitis – anterior horn cell damage

Peripheral neuropathy – damage to axon and sheath.

DISORDERS OF MOTOR PATHWAYS

Clinical points

PARALYSIS occurs in disorders of both systems but the reflexes show important differences.

Upper motor neurone damage

↓

Lower motor neurone
released from cortical control
∴ muscle tone increased,
tendon jerks (and other
spinal reflexes) increased,
plantar reflex extensor

Lower motor neurone damage

↓

Loss of final effector mechanism
∴ reflexes absent,
also muscle atrophy

MOTOR NEURONE DISEASE

In contrast to these motor disorders, secondary to known diseases, motor neurone disease is of unknown aetiology occurring in adults with a predominant incidence in males.

The basic lesion is a specific progressive degeneration of both cortical and spinal motor neurones with its accompanying pathological effects. There are variations depending on the relative involvement of the upper and lower motor neurone components and the sites of initial damage. Even in the early stages when differentiating features are best seen, there may be considerable overlap and usually in the later stages the distinctions are blurred due to the inexorable progression with severe and widespread motor neuronal degeneration.

1. In **progressive muscular atrophy,** as the name implies, the main signs are of neurogenic atrophy due to degeneration of the anterior horn cells (LMN).

Predilection for
cervical cord

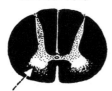

Gradual (several years)
degeneration of anterior
horn cells
↓
Gliosis
↓
Shrinkage

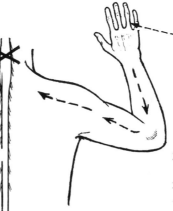

Sites particularly affected are:

1. Small muscles of hand –
   wasting ('Simian hand')
   Note: While degeneration of
   neurones is proceeding
   spontaneous
   irregular discharges
   cause muscle twitching –
   FASCICULATION
2. Muscles of arm and shoulder
   girdle.
3. Spread towards medulla.
4. Later leg weakness and paralysis
   reflect both LMN and UMN damage.

741

DISORDERS OF MOTOR PATHWAYS

MOTOR NEURONE DISEASE (continued)

2. In **Amyotrophic lateral sclerosis** the main damage is in the UMN: 'lateral sclerosis' indicates the degeneration of the pyramidal tracts.

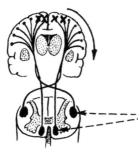

The degeneration affects the *cortical motor cells* – particularly those supplying the lower limbs but spreading over a few years to involve the neck and head centres. Voluntary movements of the face, jaw and tongue muscles are defective.
Corticospinal tracts showing degeneration and, later, gliosis.

The lesions are very rarely pure UMN type even initially, and with progression, the LMN lesions increase.

3. **Progressive bulbar palsy and pseudobulbar palsy**
In a few cases, the disease begins with signs of cranial nerve dysfunction – swallowing and facial movements are impaired.

In progressive bulbar palsy, the LMN is affected (cranial nerve nuclei); muscle atrophy and fasciculation occur.

In pseudobulbar palsy the lesion is in the UMN and no muscle atrophy is seen.

Overlap of varying amount is again not unusual.

The following diagram illustrates the overlap of UMN and LMN components in motor neurone disease.

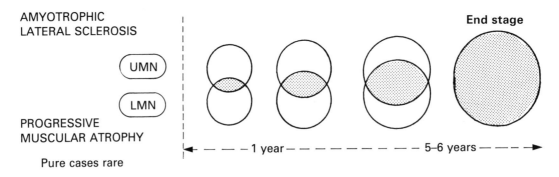

AMYOTROPHIC
LATERAL SCLEROSIS

UMN

LMN

PROGRESSIVE
MUSCULAR ATROPHY

Pure cases rare

End stage

←— — — 1 year — — — — — — — — 5–6 years — — — →

Progress
In motor neurone disease after a long progressive illness, the stage is reached when the bulbar degeneration is severe enough to prevent elimination of secretions from the respiratory tract. Death is usually due to aspiration bronchopneumonia but occasionally to acute asphyxia.

DISORDERS OF SENSORY PATHWAYS

In **HERPES ZOSTER**, where there is inflammation of the posterior root ganglia in one or two spinal segments on one side only, the damage is not sufficient to affect the ascending spinal tracts.

In **TABES DORSALIS**, a tertiary manifestation of syphilis in which the lumbar cord is commonly affected, there is degeneration of the posterior nerve roots and columns.

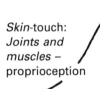
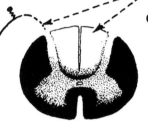

Skin-touch:
Joints and muscles –
proprioception

Clinically
Loss of vibration sense and reflexes
Ataxia
Trophic skin ulcers
Severe joint derangement (Charcot)

Additional features
Cranial and sympathetic nerve involvement – disturbance of pupillary reflex

Painful visceral crises

MIXED MOTOR AND SENSORY DISORDERS

SUBACUTE COMBINED DEGENERATION OF CORD
Due specifically to vit B_{12} deficiency. If replacement therapy is begun early enough, there is restoration to normal.

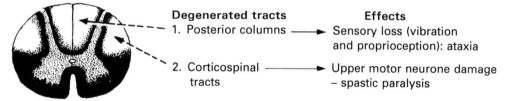

Degenerated tracts
1. Posterior columns ⟶
2. Corticospinal tracts ⟶

Effects
Sensory loss (vibration and proprioception): ataxia

Upper motor neurone damage – spastic paralysis

SYRINGOMYELIA
In this condition, a glial-lined cystic space gradually expands within the cord, usually in the cervical region. The pathogenesis is not certain, but it is suggested that the lesion is essentially an expansion of the central canal associated with a mild developmental abnormality of the distal end of the IVth ventricle.

Effects
Damage to sensory fibres decussating in the cord. Loss of temperature and touch in local segments **(dissociated anaesthesia)**.

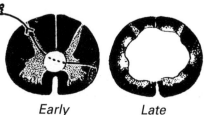

Early   *Late*

Destruction of grey matter and gradual affection of long tracts. Loss of local reflexes. Severe sensory loss. Spastic paralysis.

743

MIXED MOTOR AND SENSORY DISORDERS

Friedreich's ataxia

In this disease, which has a strong familial basis, there is progressive degeneration of sensory (spinocerebellar tracts and posterior columns) and motor tracts. It begins in childhood and progresses to death in a few years. Postural and skeletal deformities complicate the progressive ataxia and paralysis. In some cases there is a cardiomyopathy with arrhythmia.

This disease is mentioned to illustrate the **spinocerebellar degenerations**, a large group of related disorders, usually familial, in which there is neuronal and tract degeneration particularly affecting gait, posture, equilibrium and movement. There is sometimes optic nerve and retinal damage and intellectual disturbance.

THE PERIPHERAL NERVES

The nerves are a mixture of different types of fibre, myelinated and non-myelinated of varying thickness and length, subserving sensory and motor functions. In most disorders, both functions are disturbed, but in the early stages, selective damage to particular fibre types is often seen.

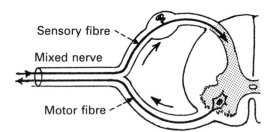

In affection of one or other nerve roots pure motor or sensory disturbance may be seen separately.

THE NEUROPATHIES

The term neuropathy is preferred to neuritis since most disorders are not essentially inflammatory.

There are two broad groups:

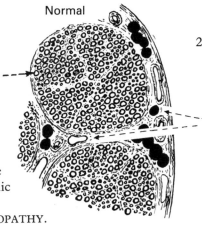

1. *Parenchymatous*
   The axon and its closely associated Schwann cells and myelin sheath are affected primarily; note that myelin is produced and maintained by Schwann cells.
   Most disorders of this type are due to toxic or metabolic disturbances and affect many nerves – POLYNEUROPATHY.

2. *Interstitial*
   The damage is primarily in the blood vessels or supporting tissues (epi-, peri- and endoneurium). In this type, single nerves or several nerves may be affected, depending on the nature of the interstitial damage.

THE NEUROPATHIES

The **POLYNEUROPATHIES** occur in a wide range of conditions.

Toxic – diphtheria; lead; arsenic; drugs used in medicine.
Deficiency states – particularly vit B complex deficiency causing Beri-Beri.
Metabolic disorders – diabetes mellitus, porphyria, metachromatic leukodystrophy, associated with malignant tumours, in uraemia treated by dialysis.

There are two main mechanisms of degeneration.

1. Degeneration of the axon with concomitant demyelination. This is closely allied to Wallerian degeneration following nerve transection.

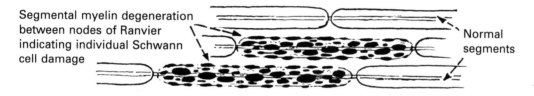

Ovoids of lipid indicating degenerating myelin

Degenerate axons

2. Primary degeneration occurs patchily in Schwann cells; axon degeneration follows slowly.

Segmental myelin degeneration between nodes of Ranvier indicating individual Schwann cell damage

Normal segments

Since in many polyneuropathies the long large fibres degenerate first, the early clinical effects are referable to the distal ends of the nerves. Also damage may affect particular nerves and nerve groups selectively.

INTERSTITIAL NEUROPATHY

Mononeuropathy

Single nerves are subject to damage by compression. The nerve structures may be damaged directly or more usually as a result of ischaemia.

Examples are the carpal tunnel syndrome in which the median nerve is compressed between the carpal bones and ligaments, and following drunken stupor where abnormal postures have compressed nerves. The cranial nerves within the skull are subject to such distortions leading to degeneration where intracranial pressure is increased.

Prolapsed Intervertebral Disc (slipped disc) is a common cause of compression damage to nerve roots in the lumbar region particularly.

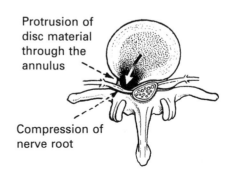

Protrusion of disc material through the annulus

Compression of nerve root

THE NEUROPATHIES

Ischaemic neuropathy
Nerve degeneration may be seen in cases of acute arteritis.

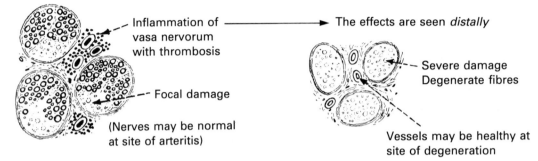

Inflammation of ⟶ The effects are seen *distally*
vasa nervorum
with thrombosis

Severe damage
Degenerate fibres

Focal damage

(Nerves may be normal
at site of arteritis)

Vessels may be healthy at
site of degeneration

Since the vascular lesions are usually patchy and random, several individual nerves are variously damaged – the condition is called mononeuritis multiplex.

NEURITIS
Nerve damage due to inflammation occurs in three main circumstances.

1. The Landry-Guillain-Barré and related syndromes. The onset is acute, often following 7–21 days after a mild non-specific febrile illness. There are peripheral neurological signs with usually a motor (LMN) deficit predominant, beginning in the lumbar nerves and ascending fairly rapidly (ascending paralysis) so that respiratory failure, requiring supportive treatment, is a serious complication.

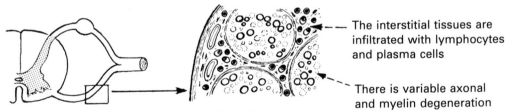

The interstitial tissues are
infiltrated with lymphocytes
and plasma cells

There is variable axonal
and myelin degeneration

The nerve roots are predominantly affected.

The CSF usually contains excessive protein but few cells.

The disease probably has an immunological basis and is allied to experimental allergic encephalitis (see p.728).

Progress: usually recovery is complete.

2. In **leprosy**, a low grade chronic inflammation of the nerve sheaths is associated with fibrosis and fibre degeneration.

3. Peripheral nerves may be damaged by direct spread of inflammation from adjacent tissues.

THE NEUROPATHIES

1. Bell's palsy

This is a unilateral facial weakness of sudden onset. The cause is not known with certainty, but some cases are associated with draughts and chilling.

The mechanism is thought to be inflammation with swelling and compression of the facial nerve in its course in the bone adjacent to the internal auditory meatus.

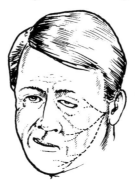

Note drooping and loss of facial expression on paralysed side. Facial muscles pull across the mid line — mouth is distorted.

Progress in 75% of cases, there is recovery in about 4–8 weeks.

2. **Distal neuropathy** may occur in long-standing cases of lower limb ischaemia→nerve sheath fibrosis→nerve degeneration.
This mechanism is a component of . . . . .
3. **Diabetic neuropathy** where there is narrowing of the small vessels, but a metabolic component with consequent segmental Schwann cell degeneration also contributes.
4. In **amyloid disease** of the hereditary type particularly, neuropathy due to compression of nerve fibres by amyloid material may occur.
5. **Segmental neuropathy** is exemplified in diphtheria and lead poisoning. Because the functional effects in particular paralyses are essentially due to demyelination without axon degeneration, recovery is usually more rapid than in many other neuropathies.

PORPHYRIAS

These are diseases due to partial deficiencies of liver or marrow enzymes engaged in haem synthesis. The individual is usually healthy; precipitating factors aggravate the defects and increase porphyrin precursors causing symptoms. Two forms exist:

1. **Acute** porphyrias with abdominal pain, neuropathies, psychotic symptoms and often hypertension. Respiratory paralysis may occur. All are due to an autosomal dominant hepatic enzyme defect.

2. **Chronic** porphyrias cause skin blistering and scarring. Most are due to autosomal recessive or dominant marrow enzyme defects. Precipitating factors in both: alcohol, barbiturates, analgesics, tranquillisers, oral contraceptives, hepatic poisons. Ultraviolet light is important in chronic forms.

HYDROCEPHALUS

In hydrocephalus, the volume of the CSF is increased and the ventricles are dilated. In the majority of cases, there is an increase in intracranial pressure. Three possible theoretical **mechanisms** are considered.

1. **Overproduction of CSF**
   The choroid plexus will secrete more CSF to compensate for any external leak, but overproduction is *not* a cause of hydrocephalus.
2. **Obstruction to the flow of CSF** is the **common** mechanism.

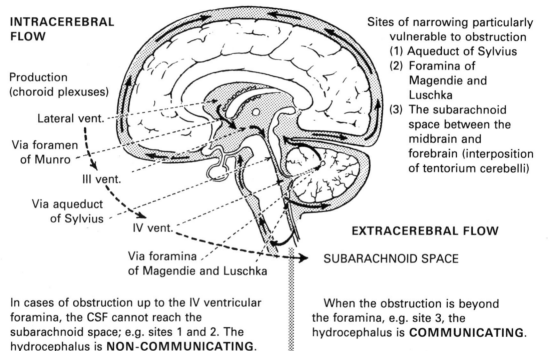

INTRACEREBRAL FLOW

Production (choroid plexuses)

Lateral vent.

Via foramen of Munro

III vent.

Via aqueduct of Sylvius

IV vent.

Via foramina of Magendie and Luschka

Sites of narrowing particularly vulnerable to obstruction
(1) Aqueduct of Sylvius
(2) Foramina of Magendie and Luschka
(3) The subarachnoid space between the midbrain and forebrain (interposition of tentorium cerebelli)

EXTRACEREBRAL FLOW

SUBARACHNOID SPACE

In cases of obstruction up to the IV ventricular foramina, the CSF cannot reach the subarachnoid space; e.g. sites 1 and 2. The hydrocephalus is **NON-COMMUNICATING**.

When the obstruction is beyond the foramina, e.g. site 3, the hydrocephalus is **COMMUNICATING**.

3. **Defective absorption of CSF** is a rare mechanism.

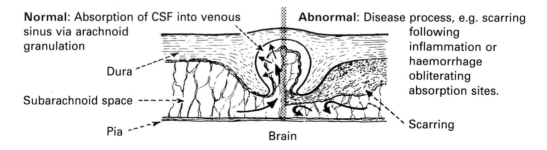

Normal: Absorption of CSF into venous sinus via arachnoid granulation

Dura

Subarachnoid space

Pia

Brain

Abnormal: Disease process, e.g. scarring following inflammation or haemorrhage obliterating absorption sites.

Scarring

HYDROCEPHALUS

CAUSES

The diseases causing hydrocephalus fall into two groups:

1. **Congenital (developmental) abnormalities**

   The common conditions are:

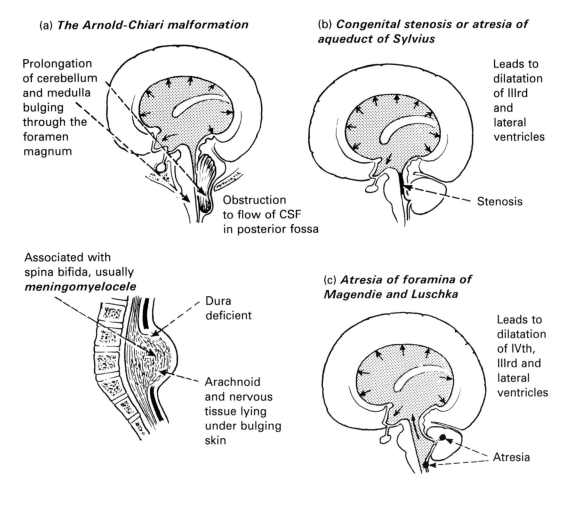

(a) *The Arnold-Chiari malformation*

Prolongation of cerebellum and medulla bulging through the foramen magnum

Obstruction to flow of CSF in posterior fossa

Associated with spina bifida, usually *meningomyelocele*

Dura deficient

Arachnoid and nervous tissue lying under bulging skin

(b) *Congenital stenosis or atresia of aqueduct of Sylvius*

Leads to dilatation of IIIrd and lateral ventricles

Stenosis

(c) *Atresia of foramina of Magendie and Luschka*

Leads to dilatation of IVth, IIIrd and lateral ventricles

Atresia

2. Acquired hydrocephalus

Of the many possible conditions causing hydrocephalus, the following are most common: (a) cerebral tumour (primary or secondary) and (b) scarring of the meninges following meningitis or subarachnoid haemorrhage.

As already explained, whether any particular disease produces hydrocephalus depends largely on the site affected.

HYDROCEPHALUS

EFFECTS

In **the infant and young child**, the pliable skull expands to accommodate the enlarging brain.

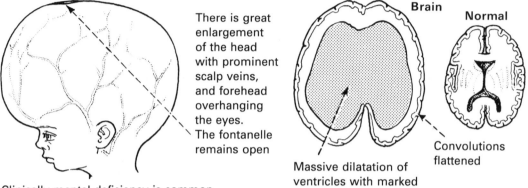

There is great enlargement of the head with prominent scalp veins, and forehead overhanging the eyes. The fontanelle remains open

Clinically mental deficiency is common

Brain

Normal

Massive dilatation of ventricles with marked thinning and stretching of brain

Convolutions flattened

In **the older child and adult**, enlargement of the brain is prevented by the inability of the skull to expand. The main change is dilatation of the ventricles associated with the effects on the brain of increased intracranial pressure.

SPECIAL TYPES OF HYDROCEPHALUS

1. In cases of generalised cerebral atrophy, the ventricular system enlarges to compensate for the loss of cerebral tissue. This also happens locally when cerebral tissue is lost, e.g. following infarction.

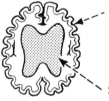

Primary atrophy of brain (deepened sulci, thinned convolutions)

Secondary dilatation

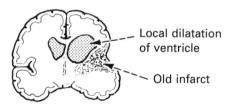

Local dilatation of ventricle

Old infarct

No increase in pressure is involved and the pathological and clinical effects wholly reflect the primary loss of cerebral tissue. The condition is sometimes called **secondary hydrocephalus**.

2. **Normal pressure hydrocephalus**

In this rare condition, progressive mental deterioration (dementia) and disturbances of gait and micturition are associated with ventricular dilatation. Random sampling often shows normal CSF pressures but continuous monitoring shows significant intermittent increases. (Some prefer the title Intermittent Hydrocephalus.) The diagnosis has assumed importance because in some cases CSF shunt procedures have arrested the progress. The aetiology is obscure.

DEVELOPMENTAL ABNORMALITIES

Developmental abnormalities of the brain and cranium are relatively common, varying from virtually complete absence of cerebral substance (anencephaly), with associated failure of formation of the cranial meninges and the skull, to minor local malformations, e.g. meningocele and encephalocele. Often they are associated with congenital defects in other parts of the body.

SPINA BIFIDA

In the lumbosacral and cervical regions particularly, local defects in the development and closure of the neutral tube and vertebral arches result in spina bifida.

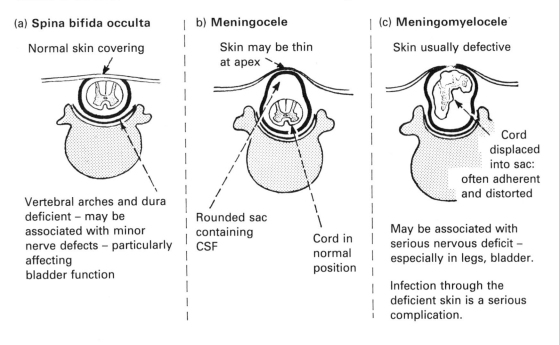

(a) Spina bifida occulta

Normal skin covering

Vertebral arches and dura deficient – may be associated with minor nerve defects – particularly affecting bladder function

b) Meningocele

Skin may be thin at apex

Rounded sac containing CSF

Cord in normal position

(c) Meningomyelocele

Skin usually defective

Cord displaced into sac: often adherent and distorted

May be associated with serious nervous deficit – especially in legs, bladder.

Infection through the deficient skin is a serious complication.

The cause of these defects is not yet known. In some cases there are heredito-familial influences; in others, teratogens are possibly involved and, recently, circumstantial evidence implicates nutritional deficiency (particularly of FOLIC ACID) as a cause.

Diagnosis in utero

α-fetoprotein leaks through the defective skin covering and increased amounts are found in the amniotic fluid. Ultrasonography may also reveal the defect.

Complications

In addition to severe neurological deficits which are aggravated by infection, an important complication even in minor defects is **HYDROCEPHALUS**.

TUMOURS OF THE NERVOUS SYSTEM

The following scheme illustrates the various non-specific clinicopathological effects of a tumour within the skull.

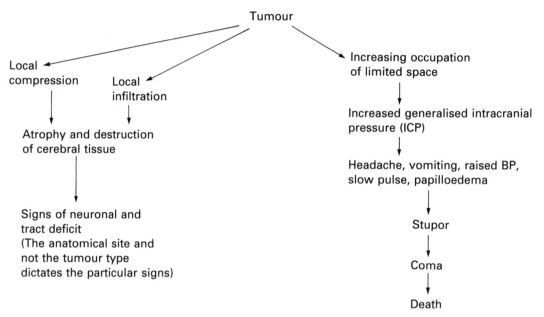

An important factor which materially influences the relative importance of each of these effects is the rate of tumour growth.

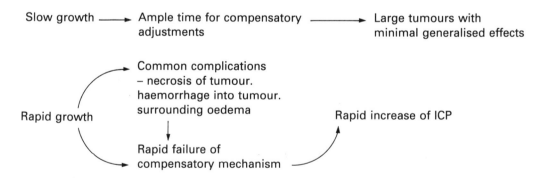

Tumours will be considered in more detail under the following broad headings:

1 Neoplasms of neuroectodermal origin.

2 Neoplasms arising in supporting tissue (mesodermal).

3 Neoplasms and swellings of developmental origin.

4 Neoplasms of nerve sheaths.

5 Secondary neoplasms.

TUMOURS OF THE NERVOUS SYSTEM

1. GLIOMAS

Derived from astrocytes, these are the commonest primary neurological tumours. They vary in growth rate and differentiation over a wide spectrum.

Astrocytoma, at the benign end, is slow growing and the cells well differentiated forming many fibres.

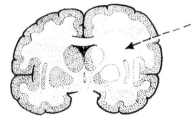

The tumour which has ill-defined margins grows irregularly into the surrounding brain tissues and only latterly causes increased ICP

Note enlargement of hemisphere by ill defined growth.

Glioblastoma multiforme, in contrast, is highly malignant. The cells are pleomorphic, unlike astrocytes, rapidly growing and showing poor fibre formation.

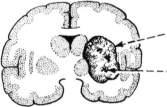

Tumour looks well defined, contrasting with the compressed adjacent cerebral tissue

Necrosis and haemorrhage are common

Tumours derived from oligodendroglia and ependyma occur rarely.

Note: Since none of these tumours ever metastasise outside the nervous system, the terms 'benign' and 'malignant' are relative. Tumours are malignant in respect of their rapid growth and progress to death. Because they often have ill-defined margins, 'benign' tumours are difficult to eradicate and slowly but inexorably they grow and eventually cause death.

2. TUMOURS of NEURONE TYPE CELLS

Fully differentiated neurones can neither multiply nor give rise to neoplasms. Tumours of this type, derived from primitive nerve precursors (blast cells), are seen in infancy and childhood before completion of differentiation.

TUMOURS OF THE NERVOUS SYSTEM

TUMOURS OF NEURONE TYPE CELLS (continued)
They display a basic histological pattern.

Closely aggregated small cells with hyperchromatic round or oval nuclei and ‑ ‑ ‑ scanty cytoplasm

Rosettes, the centres of which are formed by rudimentary ‑ ‑ nerve fibres, are often seen and represent a step towards differentiation

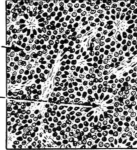

Depending on the site of origin, specific names are given:

Cerebellum:
MEDULLOBLASTOMA

Retina:
RETINOBLASTOMA

Sympathetic ganglia (including adrenal medulla):
NEUROBLASTOMA and GANGLIONEUROMA

Medulloblastoma
This highly malignant tumour arises in and spreads over the surface of the cerebellum, often invading the IVth ventricle. Diffuse tumour nodules may develop on surfaces bathed by CSF.

Retinoblastoma
These tumours, which arise in the retina and cause blindness, spread into the optic nerves. Some cases are clearly seen as a hereditary disease and are bilateral: others arise sporadically due to a genetic mutation after conception and are usually unilateral. The genetic mechanism is now known to be a defective (or missing) tumour suppressor gene [the Retinoblastoma (RB) gene] on chromosome 13.

Neuroblastoma
These are not tumours of the CNS but are derived from the precursor cells of the autonomic system; the majority occur in the adrenal medulla. They grow rapidly to become large, soft, haemorrhagic and necrotic retroperitoneal masses soon metastasising to lymph nodes, liver and bones (esp. skull).

Ganglioneuroma
In some cases, neuronal differentiation proceeds, and mature ganglion cells appear and nerve fibres are formed. In some instances, differentiation is complete; such tumours are found in adult life particularly in the mediastinum where they may grow slowly, eventually causing signs due to their size, but never metastasising. Poorly differentiated forms are termed ganglioblastoma, while with intermediate degrees of differentiation the name ganglioneuroblastoma is used.

The chemical neurotransmitters noradrenaline and dopamine, which are secreted in varying amounts by these tumours, are useful diagnostic markers as are their urinary degradation products, including vanillyl mandelic acid (VMA) and homovanillic acid respectively.

TUMOURS OF THE NERVOUS SYSTEM

Meningiomas

These are thought to arise from arachnoid granulations and so are found most commonly adjacent to venous sinuses. They are slow growing and essentially 'benign'.

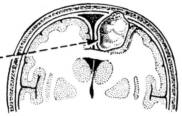

A smooth firm lobulated tumour arising from a broad base adjacent to the sagittal sinus

The effects are due to local compression of nervous tissues.

The skull may be eroded.

Growth to large size is usually slow so that the compensating mechanisms prevent increased intracranial pressure.

The histological appearances are variable depending on the relative amounts of cells and collagen, and they mimic in varying degree the arachnoid granulations.

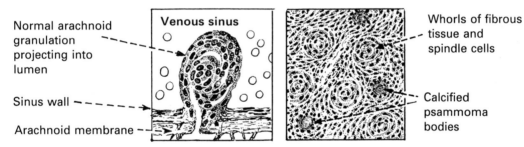

Normal arachnoid granulation projecting into lumen

Venous sinus

Sinus wall

Arachnoid membrane

Whorls of fibrous tissue and spindle cells

Calcified psammoma bodies

Other mesodermal tumours

True vascular neoplasms are rare, but vascular HAMARTOMAS are fairly common and are a cause of intracranial haemorrhage and epilepsy. These lesions show great variation in site, size and complexity.

Occasionally such tumours as lipomas and osteomas cause compression effects.

Primary microglial and lymphoid tumours are rare; the latter may be intrinsic to the CNS or be metastatic from a primary tumour outside the CNS. Primary lymphomas are an important complication of AIDS.

The incidence of CNS lymphomas is apparently increasing. This may be due to better diagnosis and/or to the more common use of therapeutic immunosuppression.

TUMOURS OF THE NERVOUS SYSTEM

The fairly common vascular hamartomas and the several developmental defects involving closure of the skull, spinal arches and meninges have already been mentioned.

Small vestigial foci of misplaced epithelial cells are not uncommon around the skull base, particularly in relation to the pituitary. Rarely these give rise to slowly enlarging cysts or tumours which cause compression effects.

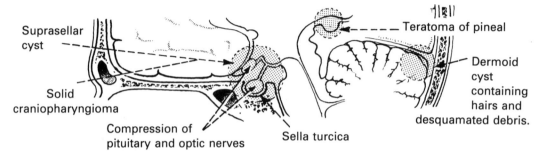

TUMOURS OF PERIPHERAL NERVES

These are essentially collagenous tumours arising in nerve roots within the skull and spine, or in the peripheral nerves. Nomenclature is based on the tissue of origin.

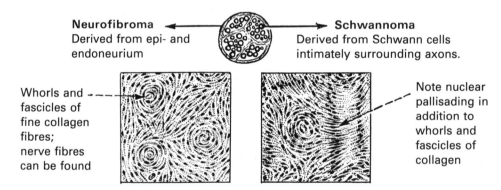

Neurofibroma
Derived from epi- and endoneurium

Schwannoma
Derived from Schwann cells intimately surrounding axons.

Whorls and fascicles of fine collagen fibres; nerve fibres can be found

Note nuclear pallisading in addition to whorls and fascicles of collagen

Note: 1. In many cases, histological distinctions are blurred and are not of importance in diagnostic histology.
2. Since neurones do not give rise to neoplasm, the term neuroma is not used. Traumatic neuroma indicates proliferating nerve endings following injury and is not a true neoplasm (see p.62).

Nerve sheath tumours may be single or multiple; their effects are due to compression of adjacent nervous tissue and are seen best within the skull or spinal cord.

TUMOURS OF PERIPHERAL NERVES

Single tumours

Accoustic Schwannoma is a good example of the single type.

This tumour arises from the VIIIth nerve in the cerebellopontine angle. Although this tumour is 'benign', it grows around adjacent structures and has an irregular surface so that it may be difficult to remove.

The tumour exerts its effects by compression – distortion of the VIIIth nerve (tinnitus→ deafness) and adjacent nerves. Pressure on IVth ventricle→ hydrocephalus→increased intracranial pressure.

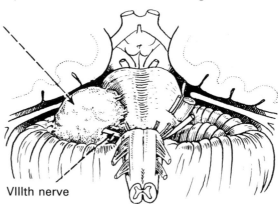

VIIIth nerve

Multiple tumours

These may affect peripheral nerves over a wide area or occupy a single group of nerves. They either form rounded nodules or fusiform swellings and may be cosmetically disfiguring.

These conditions occupy the borderland between neoplasms and hamartomas; very occasionally true neoplasia is superimposed with the development of neurofibrosarcoma.

In **Von Recklinghausen's disease** (neurofibromatosis), small nodules which may be very numerous form particularly in subcutaneous nerves.

In **plexiform neurofibroma**, the proliferation slowly proceeds along a group of nerves forming complex thickenings. Growth within the spinal canal causes serious complications.

Pigmentation

The presence of melanin in some of these tumours and the occurrence of skin pigmentation (café au lait spots) in some cases of Von Recklinghausen's disease is a reminder of the common neuroectodermal origin of nerve sheath cells and melanocytes.

Aetiology

About half the cases of neurofibromatosis show a family history with an autosomal dominant pedigree. The others are due to sporadic mutations. The defective gene is on chromosome 17 and has tumour suppressor functions.

SECONDARY TUMOURS

In the general population the incidence of metastatic cerebral tumour is higher than that of primary cerebral neoplasm. The two most common primary sites are lung and breast, but any malignant tumour can metastasise to the brain.

The common presentation is in the form of multiple, well-delineated spherical nodules, randomly distributed

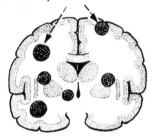

Only occasionally is there a single nodule.

A less common distribution is by permeation of the subarachnoid space – **meningeal carcinomatosis**.

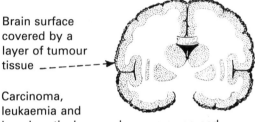

Brain surface covered by a layer of tumour tissue _ _ _ _ _ _ →

Carcinoma, leukaemia and lymphoreticular neoplasms may spread in this way (malignant cells may be seen in the CSF).

Secondary tumours may cause serious spinal damage by destroying the integrity of the vertebrae. The prostate and cervix, in addition to lung, breast and kidney, are usual primary sites.

In contrast to tumours causing neurological damage by their physical presence and growth, less commonly *non-metastatic effects of cancer* are seen.

The tumours cover a wide range of disorders which are conveniently divided into two groups:

1. Neurological disorders in which the mechanism and association with cancer are known:

Examples	*Mechanism caused by cancer*
Opportunistic infections ———————	Immune depression
Metabolic and hormonal ——————— imbalance	Destruction of organs, e.g. liver, kidney Inappropriate secretion
Vascular accidents ———————	Coagulation disorders

2. A group of conditions in which the mechanism is not known. This includes dementia, encephalopathy, cerebellar degeneration, neuropathies and a syndrome mimicking myasthenia gravis.

HEADACHE

The symptom of headache can be caused by a wide variety of pathological conditions of which only a minority are intracranial.

Intracranial

Only certain tissues are 'pain sensitive' – particularly to stretching.

Extracranial

All tissues are pain sensitive and pain referred to the head via these nerves is very common.

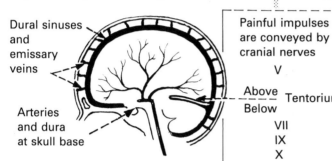

Dural sinuses and emissary veins

Arteries and dura at skull base

Painful impulses are conveyed by cranial nerves

V

Above ----- Tentorium -
Below

VII
IX
X
and C1, 2, 3

Pathological conditions in distribution of these nerves.

1. Any inflammatory disease, e.g. sinuses, teeth, ears, eyes.

2. Prolonged muscle contraction – particularly back of neck and jaws.

Pathological conditions

1. Conditions distorting and stretching pain sensitive areas, e.g. brain tumour.
2. Conditions associated with arterial dilatation, e.g. in fevers, intoxications, ? hypertension.
3. Meningeal inflammation and haemorrhage.

3. Vascular distension, e.g. migraine – the extracranial arteries in the neck and head show episodic constriction followed by dilatation due to an as yet unknown mechanism

COMA

Coma is a clinical state in which there is loss of consciousness and unresponsiveness to stimuli. Various pathological conditions have been seen to proceed to coma.

Basic mechanisms

Consciousness depends on the integrity of the interplay between the cortex and brain stem nuclei on both sides.

Pathological conditions:

which destroy these connections:

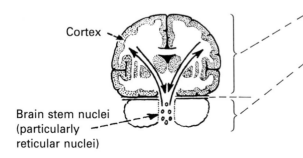

Cortex

Brain stem nuclei (particularly reticular nuclei)

(1) **Supratentorial lesions** e.g. large haemorrhage, tumours.

(2) **Subtentorial lesions** e.g. haemorrhage, infarct, tumour, abscess.

(3) **Metabolic and diffuse lesions** e.g. anoxia, hypoglycaemia, drugs, poisons, meningitis, concussion.

EPILEPSY

Organic brain disease is a significant factor in only a proportion of epilepsies which are essentially disorders of cerebral function associated with recurrent episodic excessive and abnormal neuronal discharges. The classical signs of generalised convulsions and loss of consciousness are not seen in all epilepsies.

Note: The common single seizures associated with febrile illnesses in children are not epilepsy, although the basic mechanism is similar.

Incidence: Epilepsy occurs in about 1% of the population.

Mechanism

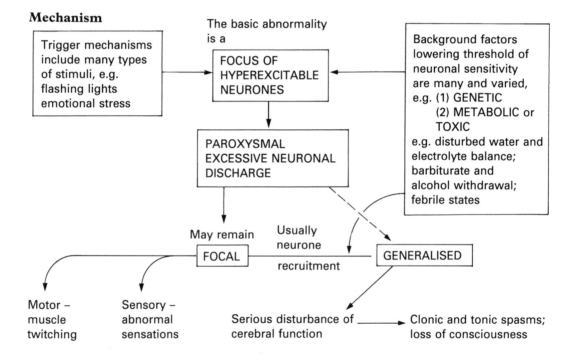

The neurones of the motor cortex, limbic system and the temporal lobe are particularly epileptogenic.

Aetiology

Acquired epilepsy. About 25% of cases are associated with known disease. The hyperexcitable neuronal focus may be due to established brain disease of which congenital abnormalities, post-traumatic scarring and ischaemic change are the most common.

Idiopathic epilepsy. In the remaining 75% of cases, although there is no known cause, genetic influences are important. A hyperexcitable focus is often present deep in the brain substance associated with the reticular system.

CEREBROSPINAL FLUID

Although the CSF and extracellular fluid of the central nervous system are essentially similar in composition, changes in the CSF are not reliable indicators of disease within the brain parenchyma.

However, since the CSF reflects conditions in the subarachnoid space, in clinical practice detailed examination and analysis are important and are mandatory in suspected meningitis. The important observations using CSF obtained by lumbar puncture are grouped under headings as follows.

NORMAL	Meningitis		Virus infection	Miscellaneous
	Pyogenic	Tuberculous	Meningo-encephalitis	
Pressure 60 – 180 mm H_2O	↑Over 200	↑Over 200	↑	↓ Below spinal block
Appearance Crystal clear *(for blood staining see below)	Turbid	Opalescent: may be fine fibrin web	Opalescent	–
Cell content 0–4 mononuclears/µl	+ + + > 1000 Neutrophils	+ + + Lymphocytes	± + Lymphocytes	–
Biochemistry Protein 0.2–0.4 g/l	↑1 – 10 g/l	↑1 – 3 g/l	↑ 0.5 – 2 g/l	↓ Very high in spinal block
Glucose 50–80 mg/100 ml (2.8–4.4 mmol/l)	↓ greatly or absent	Low 20–30 mg	Normal	Normal

IN DISEASE

*When the CSF is blood-stained, it is important to distinguish between contamination due to trauma caused by the tap and true intracranial haemorrhage.

	Contamination	True haemorrhage
Supernatant after centrifugation	Clear	Yellow due to bilirubin (red cell degeneration)
Cell count – leucocyte/RBC ratio	Normal	Increased

Microbiology. Identification of organisms is very important.

(1) Deposit and/or fibrin web – stained —— Gram – pyogenic bacteria and fungi
                                          ZN   – tubercle bacilli

(2) Culture: virus isolation

(3) Tests for microbial antigens —— Wassermann reaction for syphilis
                                          Immunoelectrophoresis for other antigens

MUSCULO-SKELETAL SYSTEM

SKELETAL MUSCLE

It is useful to consider the anatomy at various levels of magnification.

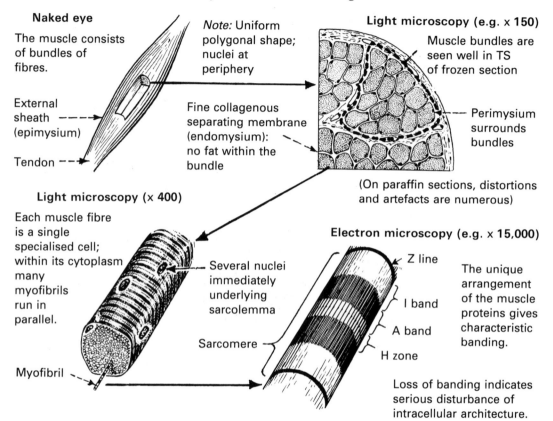

Naked eye

The muscle consists of bundles of fibres.

External sheath (epimysium) – – –

Tendon – –

Note: Uniform polygonal shape; nuclei at periphery

Fine collagenous separating membrane (endomysium): no fat within the bundle

Light microscopy (e.g. x 150)

Muscle bundles are seen well in TS of frozen section

Perimysium surrounds bundles

(On paraffin sections, distortions and artefacts are numerous)

Light microscopy (x 400)

Each muscle fibre is a single specialised cell; within its cytoplasm many myofibrils run in parallel.

Myofibril –

Several nuclei immediately underlying sarcolemma

Sarcomere

Electron microscopy (e.g. x 15,000)

Z line

I band

A band

H zone

The unique arrangement of the muscle proteins gives characteristic banding.

Loss of banding indicates serious disturbance of intracellular architecture.

MUSCLE CONTRACTION

Within each muscle cell the basic mechanism by which energy is mobilised and released is as follows:

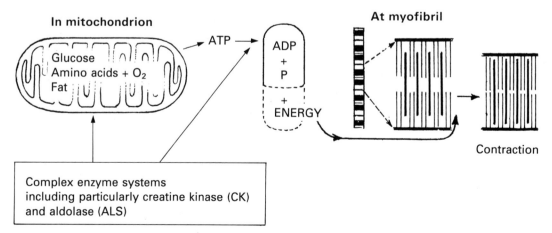

In mitochondrion

Glucose
Amino acids + O_2
Fat

ATP

ADP + P + ENERGY

At myofibril

Contraction

Complex enzyme systems including particularly creatine kinase (CK) and aldolase (ALS)

SKELETAL MUSCLE

The existence of two types of muscle fibre is related to differences in functional activity.

	Mito-chondria	Oxidative enzymes	ATPase	Myoglobin and lipid	Glycogen	Type of contraction
Type I **(red muscle)**	+++	+++	+	+++ ·	+	SLOW Sustained
Type II **(white muscle)**	+	+	+++	+	+++	FAST short duration

In sections, the two fibre types, which are indistinguishable by routine stains, can be identified using histochemical methods.

Normal muscle stained H & E

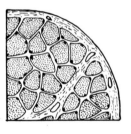

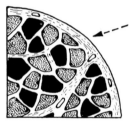

Normal muscle – stained for oxidative enzyme

Type I fibres stain black

Note: random mosaic of two types.

It is of interest that the muscle fibre function is not intrinsic but is conditioned by its type of nerve supply: any single anterior horn cell innervates fibres only of one or other type.

MUSCLE INNERVATION
The **motor unit** consists of:

a single lower motor neurone and —— the muscle fibres it supplies.
 (LMN)

Disease in any part of the LMN leads to **atrophy** of the fibres supplied.

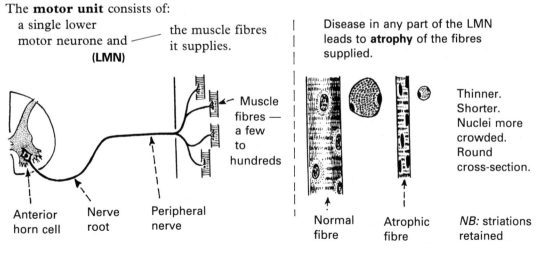

Muscle fibres — a few to hundreds

Anterior horn cell | Nerve root | Peripheral nerve

Normal fibre | Atrophic fibre

Thinner. Shorter. Nuclei more crowded. Round cross-section.

NB: striations retained

765

NEUROGENIC ATROPHY

The distribution of nerve fibres within the muscle is important and is represented diagrammatically in respect of two motor units: A and B.

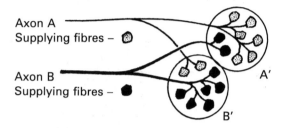

Axon A
Supplying fibres –

Axon B
Supplying fibres –

A'

B'

Note that while A and B respectively innervate the majority of fibres in bundles A' and B', there is overlap between bundles. Since many axons supply a muscle the overlap is considerable

Apart from complete traumatic section of a peripheral nerve, it is unusual for all motor fibres to a muscle to be destroyed. Both the basic pattern of innervation and the variations in nerve fibre damage are reflected in the histological appearances in the denervated muscle.

1. **Pattern of atrophy**

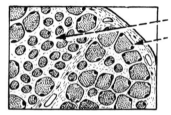

Groups of atrophic denervated fibres with adjacent groups of normal fibres.

Note the overlap – atrophic fibres among normal, and vice versa.

This is the striking basic pattern seen in most diseases of the LMN.

2. **Re-innervation**
In an area of denervation, the terminal axonal branches of intact neurones sprout and can re-innervate the atrophic fibres.

(i) **Normal**

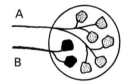

A

B

This muscle bundle is predominantly innervated by axon A, but axon B is also represented

(ii) **Denervation of A**

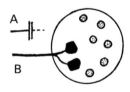

A

B

Fibres supplied by A atrophy

Fibres supplied by B remain normal.

(iii) **Re-innervation**

(a)

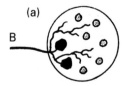

B

(b)

B

Terminal filaments sprout and make contact with atrophic fibres.

(iv) **Restoration of fibre size**

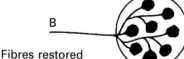

B

Fibres restored to normal – terminal filaments of B now innervate several fibres.

NEUROGENIC ATROPHY

3. Change in muscle type

Since the type (fast or slow) of each muscle fibre is conditioned by its nerve supply, the pattern of distribution of fast and slow fibres within a muscle may be changed by re-innervation.

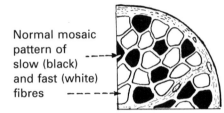

Normal mosaic pattern of slow (black) and fast (white) fibres ------

Following re-innervation by a 'slow' type neurone 'slow' fibres now ---- predominate
Mosaic pattern is lost

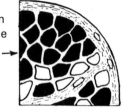

Thus, although a muscle may be restored to normal in terms of routine histological assessment, slight changes in functional activity may be present.

MUSCLE SPINDLES AND INNERVATION

The crude muscle contraction effected by the motor unit is controlled and refined by neurological connections through the muscle spindles which are situated in the middle of the muscle. Each spindle consists of a delicate, cigar-shaped envelope containing 2–15 specialised muscle cells which are intimately connected to a complex of motor and sensory nerve filaments.

The spindles are connected to the cord by a special nervous circuit; the diagram shows how the cerebellum influences function of the LMN via the muscle spindle.

Because the muscle spindles have a separate innervation, in motor neurone disease they may be spared.

Note: surviving normal spindles. There is a spurious impression of increased numbers owing to the severe atrophy of the surrounding muscle fibres.

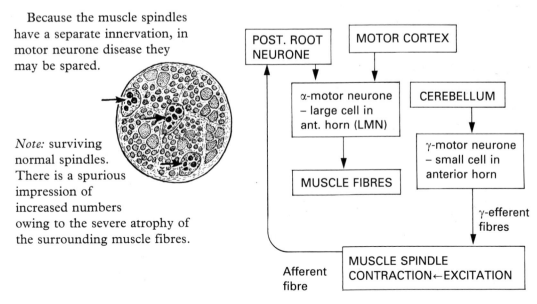

MYASTHENIA GRAVIS

The **MOTOR END-PLATE** is the specialised neuromuscular junction situated at the middle of each muscle fibre.

The nervous impulse causes release of **ACETYLCHOLINE** at the specialised nerve endings – depolarisation at this site is the stimulus to contraction. The sarcolemma at this site contains abundant **CHOLINESTERASE**.

In MYASTHENIA GRAVIS, the essential disorder is at the motor end-plate where there is a defect in the production or release of acetylcholine. This rare disease occurs mainly in young females, the important clinical features being muscle weakness and early fatigue of the ocular and head and neck muscles particularly.

Aetiology and mechanism

This is essentially an auto-immune disease (see p.119).

1. Antibodies to ACETYLCHOLINE RECEPTORS are present in 90% of cases.
2. There is a strong association with THYMIC abnormalities. In young women this is usually *thymic germinal centre hyperplasia*: in middle aged males a *thymoma* (mixed lymphoid or epithelial type) may be present.
3. There is an association with hyperthyroidism (this has an autoimmune basis).

In the affected muscles, aggregates of lymphocytes with occasional single necrotic fibres may be seen.

ATROPHY AND HYPERTROPHY

Generalised disuse atrophy occurs as a result of prolonged immobilisation in bed. Local atrophy follows immobilisation due to joint disease or often bone fractures.

Hypertrophy of muscle tissue in response to increased work load is well seen in heavy event athletes. Localised hypertrophy can compensate for damage to adjacent muscular tissues.

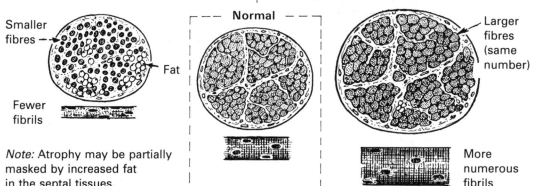

Smaller fibres

Fat

Fewer fibrils

Normal

Larger fibres (same number)

More numerous fibrils

Note: Atrophy may be partially masked by increased fat in the septal tissues.

MUSCLE DAMAGE

Having dealt with the effects on muscle of denervation and of motor end-plate disorder, muscle disease will be dealt with further under two main headings:

1. Muscle damage which is clearly secondary
2. Disorders in which the abnormality is in the muscle fibres – the myopathies.

1. DISORDERS SECONDARY to TRAUMA, ISCHAEMIA and INFLAMMATION and INFECTION

(a) Trauma and ischaemia

In severe cases where trauma and ischaemia combine to cause necrosis of a considerable mass of muscle, the effects may be serious.

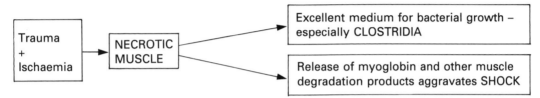

The latter situation is well exemplified in the CRUSH SYNDROME – classically seen in building collapse.

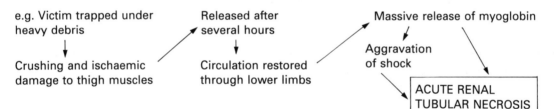

Repair of massive muscle damage

The basic inflammatory response is followed by organisation with removal of the dead muscle.

There are two possible results:

(i) If the gap is not too great, regeneration effects restoration to normal.

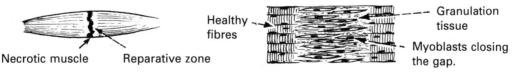

(ii) If the gap is too great, scar tissue prevents the regeneration.

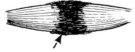

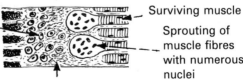

769

MUSCLE DAMAGE

SECONDARY MUSCLE DISORDERS (continued)
(b) Inflammation

In most inflammatory processes, including the common pyogenic infections, the intermuscular fascial planes are involved and muscle damage is negligible and superficial, consisting of degeneration and necrosis of individual fibres.

Abscess formation may follow intramuscular injections.

Viral myositis

A true myositis with focal necrosis of fibres, lymphocyte and macrophage infiltration can be caused by the *Coxsackie group* of viruses. The muscles of the upper thorax are particularly affected.

Parasitic myositis

In trichinosis, the parasitic larvae encyst in the interstitial tissues within muscles. The adjacent muscle fibres become necrotic; focal calcification is often a late sequel.

Repair of focal muscle damage

In cases of mild trauma and inflammation where there is only focal muscle fibre damage, and particularly when the endomysium remains intact, complete restoration to normal is effected by muscle cell regeneration.

2. THE MYOPATHIES

In this broad group of disorders, the abnormalities, which are essentially disturbances of muscle metabolism, are within the muscle fibres and are reflected in a limited, non-specific range of morphological changes.

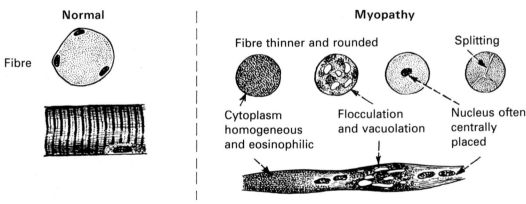

Normal — Fibre

Myopathy — Fibre thinner and rounded — Splitting

Cytoplasm homogeneous and eosinophilic — Flocculation and vacuolation — Nucleus often centrally placed

Loss of striations

MYOPATHIES

Normal

MYOPATHIES

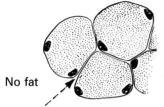

No fat

Endomysium very thin

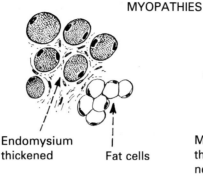

Endomysium thickened

Fat cells

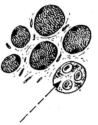

Macrophages invading the endomysium of a necrotic fibre

In some disorders, the fat may mask the muscle atrophy and there may even be pseudohypertrophy.

Note: Inflammation is not a feature of most myopathies: there may be a mild inflammatory response to actual muscle necrosis.

A case of **Duchenne dystrophy**:
Prominent winging of scapulae and scoliosis due to muscle weakness
Pseudohypertrophy of calves due to fatty infiltration

In some disorders, occasional muscle fibres show hypertrophy alongside atrophic fibres, and regenerating fibres may also be seen. Since these basic changes vary in their incidence within muscles and in their rate of progress, a cross-section of affected muscle need not be expected to show them all at one time.

Biopsy of:
Moderately affected muscle

Late stage muscle

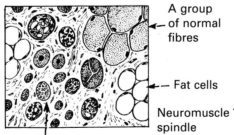

A group of normal fibres

Fat cells

Neuromuscle spindle

Fibres showing various degrees of atrophy

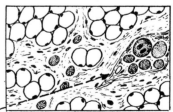

Almost complete replacement of muscle by fat; only a few atrophic fibres remain.

INHERITED MYOPATHIES

The myopathies will be considered further under two main headings:
The abnormality is (1) GENERALLY determined, or (2) ACQUIRED.

1. The INHERITED MYOPATHIES

Muscular dystrophies

In this group, the nature of the abnormality within the fibre is unknown. Various disorders are separated and identified by their particular type of inheritance, clinical differences including age of onset, rate of progression and particular groups of muscle affected.

Three dystrophies are described:

1. ***The Duchenne type*** (pseudohypertrophic muscular dystrophy)

    Inheritance – X-linked recessive. Affects boys exclusively (apart from a few cases recorded in Turner's syndrome).

    The muscle changes are present *in utero*, but usually the first clinical disability presenting as lower limb weakness appears in childhood; progress is relentless with involvement later of the shoulder muscles. Death often occurs in the teens due to bronchopneumonia or cardiac failure.

    The pathological mechanism is a lack of DYSTROPHIN and its associated proteins in the SARCOLEMMA with consequent intra-myocyte metabolic disturbance which may proceed to necrosis of individual fibres.

    The gene (Duchenne Muscular Dystrophy gene) coding for DYSTROPHIN is on the short arm of chromosome X.

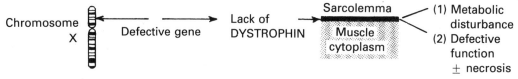

2. ***Facioscapulohumeral dystrophy***

    Inheritance – autosomal dominant. Affects both male and female.

    Age of onset variable – if in childhood, progress is often fairly rapid.
               – if in adult life, progress may be very slow.

    Muscle changes begin in facial and shoulder muscles and are often asymmetrical; lower limb muscles may be affected late in the disease.

3. The myotonic disorders in which voluntary muscle movement, particularly in the cold, is slower to initiate and lasts longer than normal, is exemplified by:

Myotonic dystrophy

Inheritance – autosomal dominant. Affects both male and female. Age of onset – usually in adult life.

The facial and tongue muscles are affected first, followed by the distal limb muscles; progress is slow but inexorable.

This dystrophy is usually associated with abnormalities in other systems, e.g. gonadal atrophy, cataracts, cardiac conduction defects, defective androgen production or abnormal insulin response may be present.

The disease shows genetic linkage with the secretor ABH system so that its diagnosis *in utero* can be inferred from genotyping using the presence of ABH antigen in amniotic fluid.

INHERITED MYOPATHIES

The inherited myopathies (continued)

Specific metabolic defects

An enlarging group of genetic myopathies with specific biochemical or morphological abnormalities is emerging due to the application of modern biochemical, histochemical and morphological (e.g. EM) techniques.

In some, the specific inborn error of metabolism is generalised and includes muscle; in others it is confined to the muscle fibre. Some examples will be given under broad headings:

(1) Glycogen storage	(2) Lipid metabolism	(3) Periodic paralyses
Type 2 – deficiency of (Pompe) acid maltase Type 5 – muscle (McArdle) phosphorylase Type 7 – phosphofructo-kinase (PEK)	Defect in free fatty acid transport into and utilisation within fibre. (a) carnitine palmityl transferase (CPT) (b) and muscle carnitine deficiency	Associated with hypo- and hyperkalaemia – the muscle defect is a vacuolar degen-eration of the sarcolemma

(4) Morphological abnormalities
(a) *Mitochondrial*   (b) *Others*

Large or increased numbers of mitochondria – abnormal oxidative processes	(i) Central core myopathy Central area is abnormal (ii) Rod body myopathy (nemaline) Rods of tropomysin under sarcolemma	(iii) Centronuclear myopathy Nucleus in middle of cell (iv) Disporportion of fibre types I and II

These various myopathies exhibit a wide range in respect of age of onset, clinical presentation and prognosis.

A further rare but interesting autosomal dominant genetic abnormality of muscle is malignant hyperpyrexia. In this condition the administration of general anaesthetic precipitates acute muscle damage. Clinically, there is very high fever, muscle stiffness, cyanosis and acidosis very often resulting in death.

ACQUIRED MYOPATHIES

2. The ACQUIRED MYOPATHIES

Cachectic myopathy

In any wasting disease, loss of muscle with weakness is seen.

Primary condition

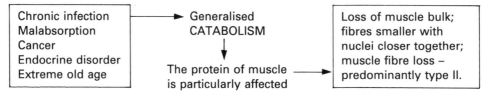

| Chronic infection
Malabsorption
Cancer
Endocrine disorder
Extreme old age | → | Generalised
CATABOLISM
↓
The protein of muscle
is particularly affected | → | Loss of muscle bulk;
fibres smaller with
nuclei closer together;
muscle fibre loss –
predominantly type II. |

Endocrine, toxic and nutritional myopathies

(a) Myopathy is seen in acromegaly, hyperthyroidism, hypothyroidism, hyperaldosteronism (due to hypokalaemia), hyperparathyroidism and in corticosteroid excess.

(b) In alcohol and a variety of drugs in addition to corticosteroids, e.g. chloroquine, vincristine; and in vitamin D deficiency.

Polymyositis

This important condition links the myopathies with the inflammatory disorders of muscle. There is very strong evidence that it is an ***autoimmune*** disorder in which lymphocytes sensitised to muscle constituents cause destruction of muscle fibres, mimicking myopathy.

The onset is in middle life with a preponderance in women. Progress is variable; deterioration may be rapid or very slow, remissions are not uncommon and recovery is possible.

In a proportion of cases when the disorder also affect the skin, the term **dermatomyositis** is applied.

Pathology

A mixture of chronic inflammatory infiltrate and muscle fibre damage ranging from necrosis to atrophy.

Aetiology

In 2/3 cases the disorder appears to be idiopathic but in some cases COXSACKIE VIRUS material has been identified in muscles. Antibodies cross-reacting with muscle constituents are a possible explanation of the auto-immunity.

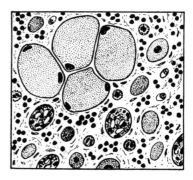

In 1/3 cases there is an associated disease which falls into one of 2 main groups:

1. *Cancer* – the tumour may be clinically latent at the time of the presentation of the myositis.
2. *Generalised collagen or vascular disease* e.g. systemic lupus erythematosis, polyarteritis, rheumatoid arthritis.

MYOPATHY – DIAGNOSIS

In clinical practice, although in only a few conditions is curative therapy available, accurate diagnosis of cases of muscular weakness and atrophy is important since there is considerable variation in prognosis and management of these diverse disorders.

A diagnosis is usually reached from a synthesis of the information obtained from investigations under three main headings:

1. **General clinical considerations are fundamental**. Of particular importance are *family history, age of onset, distribution of muscle weakness* and *rate of progress*. To these are added clinical neurological assessment.

2. **Special investigation of neuromuscular electrical activity**. The rate of motor and sensory nerve conduction can be measured electrically.

   The ELECTROMYOGRAM records the activity of groups of muscle fibres and even of individual fibres (usually fine needle electrodes). The broad basic pathological changes already described are reflected in variations of the electrical potential within the muscle during various types of activity.

   These methods are particularly useful in distinguishing primary myopathies, including myotonias, from denervation atrophy.

3. **Laboratory tests**

   (a) *MUSCLE BIOPSY*. The motor unit area of a moderately weak muscle is chosen (end-stage muscle should not be taken). Special precautions must be taken to minimise artefacts. Routine histological examination will usually distinguish the broad groups of disorders and identify the occasional rare myopathy with specific morphological features.

   Histochemical and EM examination and biochemical analysis may identify specific disorders.

   (b) *SERUM ENZYMES*. In the myopathies where actual muscle fibre destruction is proceeding, increased levels of creatine kinase (CK) and aldolase (ALS) are found.

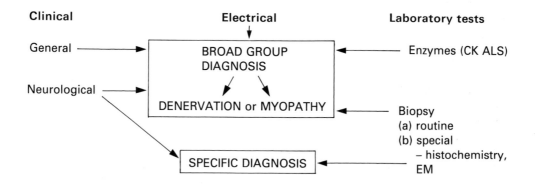

775

POST-VIRAL FATIGUE SYNDROME

This syndrome has recently come to prominence due to an increased prevalence, both in sporadic cases and in small epidemics. For many years, post-viral depression (e.g. after influenza) and fatigue (e.g. after glandular fever) have been recognised and are self-limiting usually after only a few weeks; the pathological mechanisms remain obscure.

The syndrome now so prevalent is associated particularly with **enterovirus infection** (e.g. Cocksaxic viruses) and there may be severe functional deficits which are often long-lasting (years). Alternative names for the syndrome are **myalgic encephalomyelitis (ME)** or **chronic fatigue syndrome** (U.S.A.).

The clinical signs and symptoms are protean, but the major complaint is extreme fatigue after minimal exercise. For many years the condition was considered to be psychologically induced and was labelled a form of hysteria.

It is now clear that there is a firm organic basis, but the mechanisms are not yet established with certainty.

The flow diagram illustrates possible mechanisms:

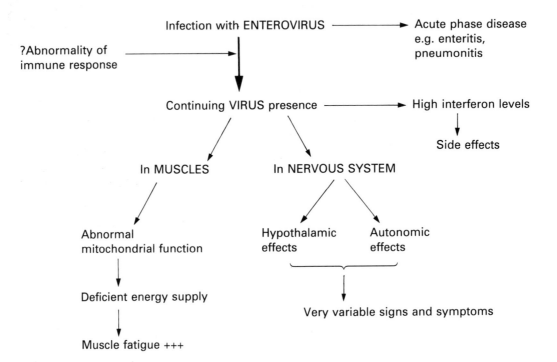

BONE

A bone shows two gross anatomical forms in varying proportions, depending on the particular type of supportive function required of it.

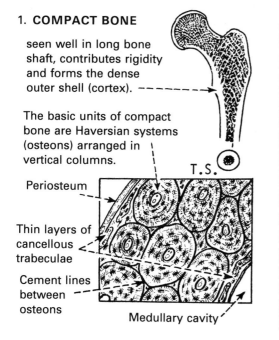

1. COMPACT BONE

seen well in long bone shaft, contributes rigidity and forms the dense outer shell (cortex). – – – – – – →

The basic units of compact bone are Haversian systems (osteons) arranged in vertical columns.

T.S.

Periosteum

Thin layers of cancellous trabeculae

Cement lines between osteons

Medullary cavity

2. CANCELLOUS BONE

(along with marrow) occupies the medullary cavities. This arrangement as exemplified in a vertebral body contributes some compressibility and pliability.

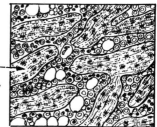

The basic unit of cancellous bone is the trabecula, arranged less regularly but not randomly.

In both types of bone, there is a basic **lamellar** structure.

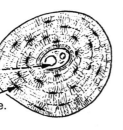

A single Haversian system showing central canal with capillaries, concentric laminae and osteocytes in lacunae.

A single trabecula showing:

Capillaries in marrow tissue

parallel lamellae, osteocytes in lacunae;

occasional osteoblasts on surface.

Bone GROWTH

In **endochondrial ossification**, seen at the metaphyseal ends of long bones, the cartilage dies and is invaded by osteoblasts which lay down bone to replace it.

In **membranous ossification**, seen in certain flat bones, the osteoblasts appear in an immature connective tissue matrix. This type is rarely seen in pathological processes.

BONE

Bone DEPOSITION

Haversian system

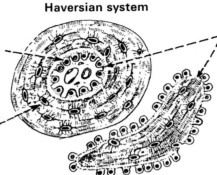

Rows of plump osteoblasts laying down lamellar collagen matrix. They are incorporated into the bone and housed in small lacunae as *osteocytes*.

Note the newly formed non-calcified *osteoid* in the centre of the osteon and on the surface of the trabecula. Normally calcification very quickly follows.

Note: During osteoblastic activity, **alkaline phosphatase** is liberated into the local tissue fluids and thence to the blood. In bone disorders, a raised serum alkaline phosphatase indicates increased osteoblastic activity.

Bone RESORPTION

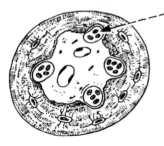

Osteoclasts – multinucleated phagocytes removing bone. The indentations formed are called Howship's lacunae.

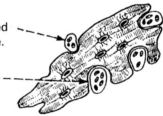

Note that all the constituents of the bone including calcium are removed. This process is called **OSTEOCLASIS**.

The *osteocytes* lying in the bone lacunae have long branching processes which permeate fine channels in the bone. Their function is to control and maintain the integrity of the bone matrix, including the crystalline calcium content. One activity is to release calcium into the blood without disruption of the matrix. This process is called **OSTEOLYSIS**.

In **bone NECROSIS** the osteocytes are dead and the lacunae empty. The lamellar structure of the matrix is retained for long periods and on histological section the bone appears normal except for the loss of cells.

BONE

WOVEN BONE (non-lamellar), a primitive form laid down in fetal development.

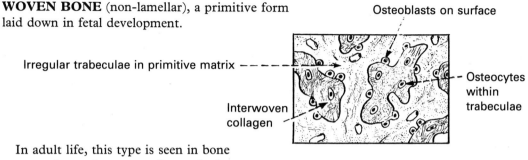

Osteoblasts on surface

Irregular trabeculae in primitive matrix

Interwoven collagen

Osteocytes within trabeculae

In adult life, this type is seen in bone regeneration and tumours. It may be later replaced by lamellar bone.

BONE and CALCIUM

(a) Calcification of bone

Exactly how precipitation of calcium phosphate occurs in osteoid is not known.

In a solution containing Ca^{++} and PO_4^{3-}, when the product of Ca^{++} and PO_4^{3-} exceeds a critical level, precipitation occurs. Where plasma calcium is low, usually due to inadequate absorption, bone calcification is defective and the diseases rickets and osteomalacia result (see p.805).

(b) Bone and calcium haemostasis

The bony skeleton acts as a reservoir for calcium and responds to the need to maintain plasma levels within a fairly narrow range (9.2 – 10.4 mg/dl or 2.3 – 2.6 mmol/l – these figures are for total plasma calcium and are used in clinical practice). This response is controlled mainly by a direct action of parathormone on bone as shown below.

(i) Response to low blood calcium

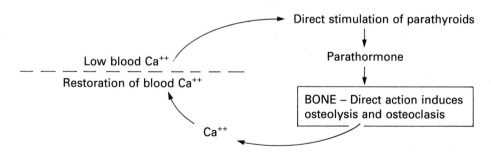

Direct stimulation of parathyroids

Low blood Ca^{++}

Restoration of blood Ca^{++}

Parathormone

BONE – Direct action induces osteolysis and osteoclasis

Ca^{++}

In parathyroid hyperplasia or neoplasia, this process occurs in excess, causing hypercalcaemia and pathological bone resorption.

(ii) When the blood calcium is high, parathormone is not secreted and bone resorption is in abeyance.

Calcitonin antagonises the action of parathormone, but its role in health and disease has not yet been fully assessed.

779

OSTEOPOROSIS

OSTEOPOROSIS (bone atrophy) is defined as a reduction in the amount of bone tissue; the tissue remaining is normally calcified.

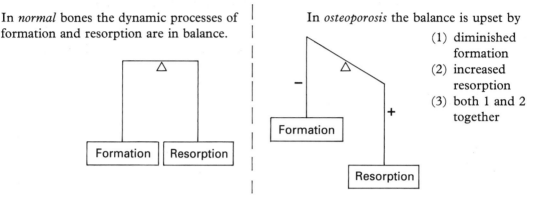

In *normal* bones the dynamic processes of formation and resorption are in balance.

In *osteoporosis* the balance is upset by
(1) diminished formation
(2) increased resorption
(3) both 1 and 2 together

This imbalance may be continuous with progressive loss of bone substance, or sometimes the balance is temporarily or permanently restored with arrest of the process.

The bone loss is most obvious in cancellous bone with rapid turnover, but the changes eventually are recognisable even in the cortical haversian systems.

The following changes in vertebral bodies are illustrative.

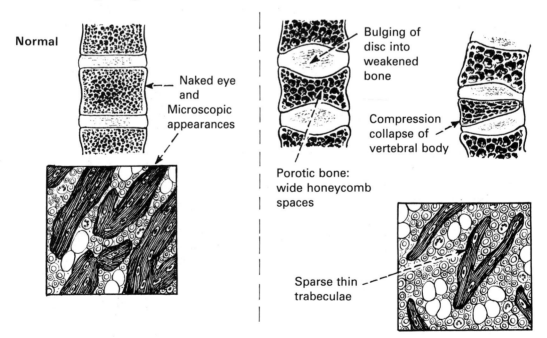

Normal

Naked eye and Microscopic appearances

Bulging of disc into weakened bone

Compression collapse of vertebral body

Porotic bone: wide honeycomb spaces

Sparse thin trabeculae

Note: The atrophied trabeculae have a normal calcium content, but because the total trabecular mass is reduced, the total bone calcium is also reduced.

OSTEOPOROSIS

Osteoporosis may be localised or general.

Localised osteoporosis is commonly due to disuse and is seen as a complication of other disorders, e.g. local IMMOBILISATION following fracture; limb paralysis and adjacent to severe joint disease with limitation of movement.

This process can be acute with active osteoclasis, but when function is resumed, normal bone structure is often restored.

General IMMOBILISATION, particularly if prolonged, leads to –

General osteoporosis. Renal calculus is an important complication.

Mechanism:

General $\longrightarrow$ General $\longrightarrow$ Ca^{++} mobilised $\rightarrow$ Hypercalcaemia $\rightarrow$ Hypercalcuria $\rightarrow$ Renal
immobilisation osteoporosis from bones   calculus

IDIOPATHIC GENERALISED OSTEOPOROSIS

This is the most common disorder of bone. From middle age onward there is progressive atrophy of bone with changes similar to those seen in osteoporosis, and some consider that generalised osteoporosis is an accelerated form of ageing atrophy. The dividing line between the conditions is ill-defined. Although the disease is generalised, weakness at particular sites leads to important complications:

1. Compression fracture (collapse) of vertebral bodies (usually preceded by gradual loss of height and kyphosis); often associated with sudden pain on weight lifting

2. Fracture of neck of femur or other long bones

3. In the elderly, during manual cardiac massage, fracture of the ribs or sternum may be sustained.

Note: In this type of osteoporosis, the routine serum biochemical tests – particularly the calcium levels – are within the normal range.

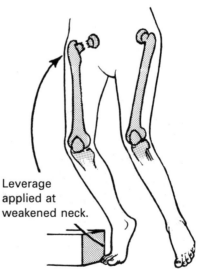

Leverage applied at weakened neck.

OSTEOPOROSIS

Aetiology and mechanisms

Although the majority of cases are idiopathic, there are some pointers to indicate a multifactorial aetiology.

1. **Hormonal influences**
   (a) Incidence: female > male.
      Progressive after the menopause; rate of bone loss is greater in female than in male.
   (b) A severe type of osteoporosis is seen in Cushing's syndrome (glucocorticoid excess) and complicating prolonged steroid therapy.
      This suggests that the balance between anabolic steroids (androgens and oestrogens) and antianabolic steroids (cortisol, etc.) is important.
   (c) Other hormones have an influence – untreated thyrotoxicosis may be complicated by osteoporosis, and parathyroid overactivity has already been dealt with.
   It is possible that disturbances of various hormones influence the cellular activities of bone and upset the balance of formation and resorption.

2. **Calcium haemostasis**
   Although there is no evidence that calcium metabolism at the bone trabecular level is abnormal, over the years there is a net total calcium loss and it is suggested that a mildly deficient calcium absorption may contribute. In these circumstances, the action of parathormone assumes importance.

3. **The initial bulk of skeleton** has an important theoretical bearing on whether osteoporosis will be severe enough to cause complications in old age. The following diagram illustrates the possible relationships:

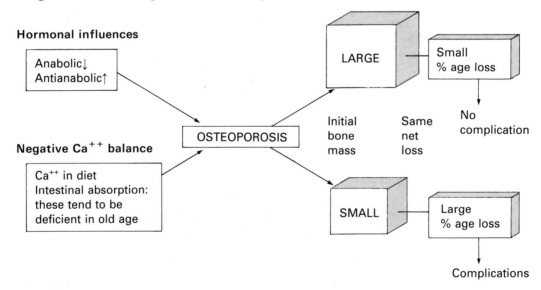

It is important in the treatment of osteoporosis that mobility and activity be maintained.
The superimposed effects of disuse atrophy can be very serious.

OSTEOMALACIA AND RICKETS

Osteomalacia and rickets are disorders of bone in which the essential defect is failure of calcification in newly formed osteoid, caused by vitamin D deficiency.

Osteomalacia occurs in adult life and affects the osteoid which is being continually laid down in the normal remodelling of bone.

Rickets affects the growing child, and serious additional disturbances are seen at the growing ends of long bones. Clinically there is pain, weakness of bones with a tendency to distortion and even fracture. Looser's zones, seen in X-ray, are linear partial fractures of long bones which have failed to calcify.

The mechanisms by which vitamin D deficiency prevents calcification are complex and not completely elucidated. The following simplified diagram indicates the important sites of activity.

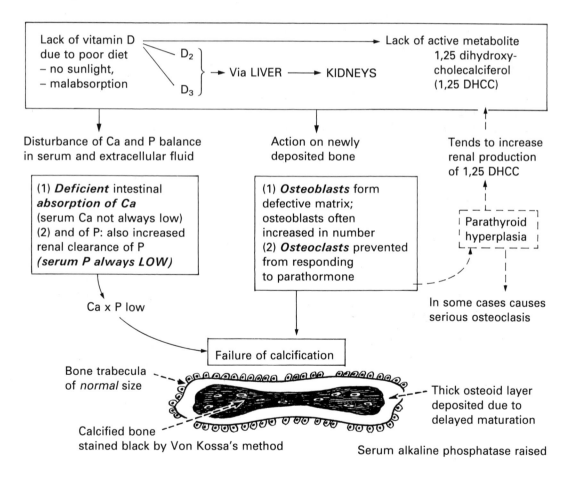

Bone trabecula of *normal* size

Calcified bone stained black by Von Kossa's method

Thick osteoid layer deposited due to delayed maturation

Serum alkaline phosphatase raised

Note:
1. In many cases the serum calcium may not be low.
2. Parathyroid activity may cause bone resorption.

OSTEOMALACIA AND RICKETS

In **rickets** there are important changes at the growing ends of long bones.

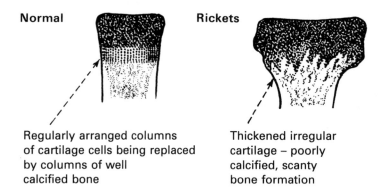

Normal

Rickets

This results in stunting of growth and bowing of the lower limbs.
In females permanent deformities of the pelvis can cause serious difficulty during childbirth

Regularly arranged columns of cartilage cells being replaced by columns of well calcified bone

Thickened irregular cartilage – poorly calcified, scanty bone formation

Since osteomalacia can be treated by vitamin D, it is important to distinguish it from osteoporosis: bone biopsy and biochemical tests are useful.

	Osteomalacia	Osteoporosis
Biopsy – appearance of trabeculae	Size – normal Thick uncalcified osteoid seams	Thin and small Normal calcification
Osteoblasts	Often increased	Normal numbers
Serum biochemistry Alkaline phosphatase	Raised	Normal
Phosphate	Low	Normal
Calcium	May be low	Normal

In cases of malabsorption occurring after middle age, in women particularly, osteomalacia and osteoporosis occur together.

Renal osteodystrophy (renal rickets)

In any renal disease associated with uraemia, abnormalities of bone occur. They are the result of abnormal calcium/phosphate balance, causing an osteomalacia-like disorder. The essential factors are failure of kidneys to produce 1,25 DHCC, the active metabolite of vitamin D, and the failure of the kidneys to eliminate phosphate. These lead to important secondary effects:

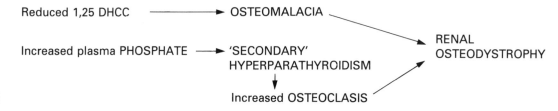

Reduced 1,25 DHCC ⟶ OSTEOMALACIA

Increased plasma PHOSPHATE ⟶ 'SECONDARY' HYPERPARATHYROIDISM

↓

Increased OSTEOCLASIS

RENAL OSTEODYSTROPHY

BONE – MISCELLANEOUS

HYPERPARATHYROIDISM

In about 20% of cases of primary hyperparathyroidism, due either to adenoma or idiopathic hyperplasia, bone changes are marked (see also p.824).

The essential change is increased bone resorption due to greatly increased osteoclastic activity; usually osteoblastic activity is also increased but cannot cope with the resorption.

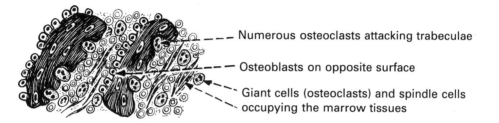

\- \- \- Numerous osteoclasts attacking trabeculae

\- \- Osteoblasts on opposite surface

\- Giant cells (osteoclasts) and spindle cells occupying the marrow tissues

These changes, although generalised, may be locally severe causing cystic spaces – the fully developed disorder is called **osteitis fibrosa cystica**. In some cases giant cell tumour of bone may be mimicked.

The biochemical changes are (1) RAISED blood CALCIUM – due to mobilisation from bones and increased activity of 1,25 DHCC and (2) RAISED alkaline PHOSPHATASE due to increased osteoblast activity.

HYPERTROPHY OF BONE

In **acromegaly** the enlargement of the jaws, hands and feet is due to subperiosteal osteoblastic proliferation and the re-establishment of endochondrial bone formation under the influence of pituitary growth hormone.

Hypertrophic osteoarthropathy (including finger clubbing) affects the digits, distal ends of long bones and the distal joints.

Oedema and increase of vascular connective tissues under nail bed

Periosteal new bone formation

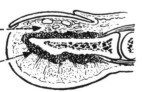

The mechanism is unknown, but the condition is associated with chronic lung disease, cyanotic heart disease and chronic intestinal inflammatory conditions.

Its importance is as an indicator of serious disease elsewhere, and it is of interest that if the primary disease can be cured, the osteoarthropathy may resolve.

785

BONE – MISCELLANEOUS

FIBROUS DYSPLASIA OF BONE

This disorder of unknown
aetiology may affect a single (monostotic)
or several bones (polyostotic). The lesion is a
well demarcated fibrous tissue containing small
abnormal bone trabeculae. The normal bone is
gradually replaced; small cysts may be present.

Complications

Fracture or deformity of the weakened bone.

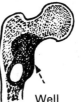

Well
circumscribed
lesion – partly cystic

Lobster claw
trabeculae

PAGET'S DISEASE OF BONE

This disease of unknown aetiology usually presents after the age of 50 years and affects
males predominantly. It is fairly common (3% of autopsies), but only in its more severe
forms are there clinical symptoms. The disorder is focal but tends to spread slowly but
progressively. The bones particularly affected are the pelvis, lower vertebrae, skull and
lower limbs.

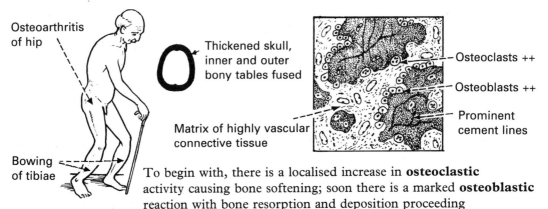

Osteoarthritis
of hip

Thickened skull,
inner and outer
bony tables fused

Osteoclasts ++

Osteoblasts ++

Prominent
cement lines

Matrix of highly vascular
connective tissue

Bowing
of tibiae

To begin with, there is a localised increase in **osteoclastic**
activity causing bone softening; soon there is a marked **osteoblastic**
reaction with bone resorption and deposition proceeding
chaotically, so that a mosaic of defective irregularly calcified bone trabeculae is formed.
The bone may be thickened, but its structure is defective and weak. **Biochemical** changes
reflect the cellular activity at trabecular level:

Alkaline phosphatase ↑ (osteoblastic); *urinary hydroxyproline* ↑ (collagen destruction).

The important **complications** are:

1. **Fracture** of weakened bones (including partial long bone fracture and vertebral
   compression).
2. **Osteoarthritis** of joints due to abnormal stresses caused by bony deformity.
3. An increased risk ($\times 30$) of the development of **bone sarcoma**.
4. The increased circulatory load through the vascular stroma may cause high output
   cardiac failure.

The use of **Calcitonin**, the physiological antagonist of parathormone, and
diphosphanates offer effective therapy in many cases.

BONE – MISCELLANEOUS

AVASCULAR BONE NECROSIS

(a) The usual processes involved in fracture healing have been dealt with (p.63). Due to details of vascular anatomy at particular sites, fractures may be complicated by severance of the blood supply to one of the bone fragments. This results in a high incidence of **avascular (aseptic) bone necrosis**. Fractures of the femoral neck and scaphoid bone are good examples.

(b) In other cases of aseptic bone necrosis, trauma is not obviously an aetiological factor. In some, but not all of a miscellany of conditions, (which includes working at increased atmospheric pressure (caisson disease), hyperlipidaemia, Gaucher's disease, gout, sickle cell anaemia and prolonged corticosteroid therapy), local ischaemia may be due to sludging of blood in end arteries to bone.

Bone necrosis of this type has important effects when it occurs at an articular surface: serious degenerative arthritis may ensue.

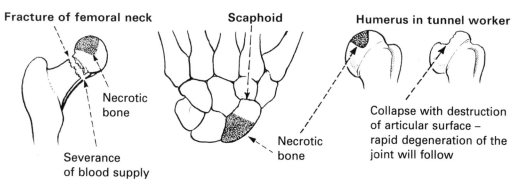

Note: These areas of necrotic bone may be relatively radiodense due to disuse osteoporosis of the adjacent living bone.

(c) In children and adolescents osteonecrosis occurs at several epiphyseal sites for no known cause (repeated minor trauma may be operative in some cases). The general name for this condition is osteochondritis juvenalis, and various eponymous terms are applied depending on the site affected. The commonest is Perthes' disease in which necrosis of one or both femoral heads occurs in children aged 4–10 years: (male: female = 5:1).

SUBPERIOSTEAL HAEMATOMA

In scurvy, the lack of vitamin C is the cause of abnormal collagen synthesis and there is a bleeding tendency due to capillary fragility.

In very young children, large haematomas may form under the periosteum in response to relatively minor trauma. The osteoblasts on the undersurface proceed to form irregular bone and considerable time is required for remodelling to occur. Similar haematomas with ossification may be seen on radiographs of the bones of 'battered babies'.

INFECTIONS OF BONE

The following basic pathological processes occur in all bone infections.

1. Destruction of bone due to necrosis.   2. Reactive and reparative processes.

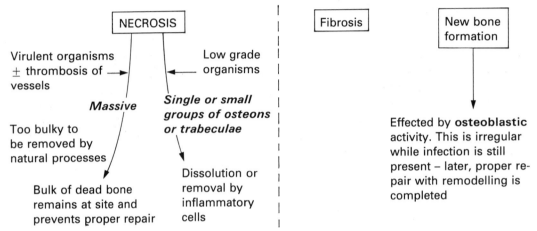

As the infection progresses, the balance between the various components changes. In chronic infections, fibrosis and reparative new bone growth may be very striking.

In addition to the usual accompaniments of inflammation, other important complications are: (1) weakening of bone resulting in deformity or fracture and (2) local complications of the inflammation, particularly abscess and sinus formation.

The following bone infections are illustrative:

ACUTE OSTEOMYELITIS

Classically caused by the *Staphylococcus aureus* and affects the growing ends of the metaphyses of long bones in children. Nowadays the incidence has been greatly reduced by the use of antibiotics. The organisms are blood borne and settle in the cancellous bone of the metaphysis. The effects are dramatic and rapidly progressive.

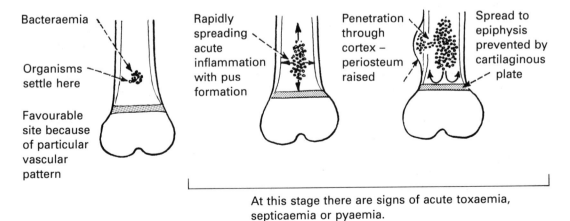

At this stage there are signs of acute toxaemia, septicaemia or pyaemia.

INFECTIONS OF BONE

Acute Osteomyelitis (continued)

Unless treatment is started promptly, the expanding inflammatory process within the rigid bone is seriously complicated.

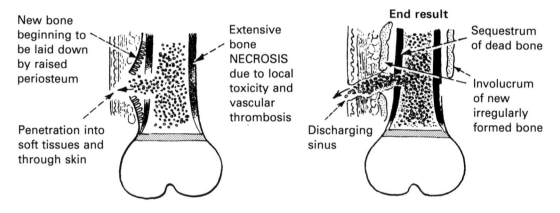

New bone beginning to be laid down by raised periosteum

Extensive bone NECROSIS due to local toxicity and vascular thrombosis

Penetration into soft tissues and through skin

End result

Sequestrum of dead bone

Involucrum of new irregularly formed bone

Discharging sinus

The presence of necrotic bone ensures that the inflammation and sinus discharge continue. With large sequestra, the usual natural methods of removal of dead tissue are inadequate so that surgical treatment is necessary.

At a late chronic stage, in addition to the local disability and disturbance of bone growth, **AMYLOID** disease may supervene and occasionally squamous carcinoma arises in a sinus.

Other pyogenic bacteria can cause osteitis – the salmonella group (esp. *S.typhi*) and brucella, the latter often causing a low grade osteitis of the spine.

With inadequate antibiotic treatment, acute inflammatory processes may be converted into low grade osteitis. Staphylococcal infection of the spine may present in adults in this way.

TUBERCULOSIS

The incidence of bone and joint infection parallels the incidence of the more common pulmonary and intestinal infections. It is therefore very low in developed countries but still significant elsewhere.

The spine and growing ends of long bones including the epiphyses are commonly affected by blood borne spread and, because of the proximity of joints, tuberculous arthritis is a frequent concomitant.

The basic pathological process is destruction of bone and replacement with tuberculous granulation tissue. Caseous necrosis is common and tracking and spread into adjacent tissues, particularly in relation to spinal tuberculosis, leads to cold abscess formation.

Although the progress is much less rapid than in acute osteomyelitis, without adequate treatment serious damage to bones and joints occurs.

DEVELOPMENTAL ABNORMALITIES

Local abnormalities are fairly common and include cleft palate, spina bifida and many structural variations of limb development. In the majority the aetiology is uncertain: the presence of teratogens (e.g. thalidomide) is suspected in many and, in a few, genetic inheritance has been established.

Generalised abnormalities are rare and usually inherited.

1. **ACHONDROPLASIA** causes a particularly striking dwarfism.
   Short, deformed limbs cause a waddling gait. The bones at the skull base are underdeveloped.
   The basic abnormality is defective, irregular development of cartilage cells, particularly at the growing metaphyseal plate. This results in stunted long bones.

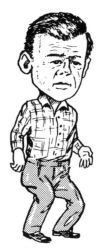

2. In **OSTEOGENESIS IMPERFECTA,** if there is survival beyond infancy, the thin brittle bones fracture easily and a history of multiple fractures with minimal cause is the usual presentation.
   The basic defect is in the osteoblasts which fail to synthesise lamellar collagen properly. The defects are due to mutations affecting genes controlling collagen synthesis on chromosomes 7 and 17.

A long bone showing three fractures.

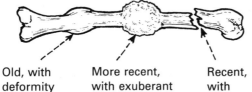

| Old, with deformity | More recent, with exuberant callus | Recent, with displacement |

Associated conditions due to the same defect are:
(a) very thin sclerae which appear blue
(b) abnormal tooth development due to defective dentine formation.

3. **OSTEOPETROSIS** (Marble bone disease of Albers-Schönberg) is a disorder in which osteoclasts are absent or defective. This results in failure of bone remodelling and abnormal conversion of cartilage to bone. The whole skeleton becomes dense and the bones thickened.
   Complications are: (a) anaemia due to marrow replacement
   (b) fractures
   (c) cranial nerve compression.

Replacement of osteoclasts by marrow transfusion has been done with success.

CYSTIC LESIONS IN BONE

True, simple cysts in bone are not uncommon. They have a well defined collagenous capsule and occur in the proximal humeral and femoral metaphyses in children. As they expand, the risk of fracture increases and this is the most usual presenting sign.

In contrast, cyst-like spaces occur in many bone disorders and even fairly solid non-calcified lesions may appear cystic on radiological examination. Examples of such disorders are cystic degeneration adjacent to osteoarthritic joints, giant cell tumour of bone, aneurysmal bone cyst, hyperparathyroidism, histiocytosis X, localised developmental defects involving fibrous tissue or cartilage and, most commonly, metastatic tumour in bone. Because of the very different prognostic implications, in clinical practice accurate histological diagnosis is essential.

Contains clear watery fluid

Capsule

There is no distortion of bone shape

Eosinophilic granuloma (at the benign end of the spectrum of histiocytosis X, see p.595) usually presents as single osteolytic radiolucent lesions of bone in children. The effects may be serious if skull bones are destroyed, otherwise resolution is to be expected. The histological appearances are typical.

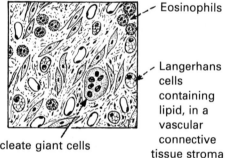

Eosinophils

Langerhans cells containing lipid, in a vascular connective tissue stroma

Multinucleate giant cells

TUMOURS IN BONE

Simple tumours present as proliferations of a variety of tissues, varying from rounded excrescences of cartilage and hard bone (simple exostoses and osteomas) through multiple irregular nodules of cartilage (endochondromas) to areas of replacement of bone by fibrous or myxomatous tissue. In the field of simple bone tumours, the borderland between true neoplasia and developmental defect is ill-defined.

The importance of simple bone tumours is that:

1. They may cause cosmetic and slight functional defects.
2. Pathological fracture may occur.
3. In some conditions (e.g. multiple enchondromatosis and giant cell tumour), there is a tendency to malignant transformation.

TUMOURS IN BONE

OSTEOID OSTEOMA

Although rare, this is worthy of particular mention since it has a striking classical presentation and a specific pathology.

Clinical: Classically, an adolescent complains of well localised, increasingly severe pain in a lower limb long bone.

Pathological: The essential lesion is a small focus of newly formed irregular trabeculae of osteoid or poorly calcified woven bone in a highly vascular stroma.

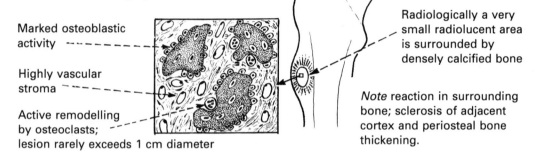

Marked osteoblastic activity

Highly vascular stroma

Active remodelling by osteoclasts; lesion rarely exceeds 1 cm diameter

Radiologically a very small radiolucent area is surrounded by densely calcified bone

Note reaction in surrounding bone; sclerosis of adjacent cortex and periosteal bone thickening.

GIANT CELL TUMOUR (osteoclastoma)

This is not a common tumour but presents characteristic histological appearances. The tumour arises in adult life (age 20–40 years), usually at the end of a long bone – especially adjacent to the knee. The basic pathological process is essentially destructive of bone so that the cortex, gradually expanded by the tumour, becomes egg-shell thin and may be ruptured. Pathological fracture is common.

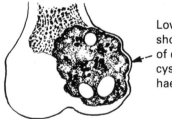

Lower end of femur showing expansion of cortex by partly cystic, partly solid haemorrhagic tumour

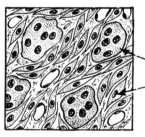

Numerous osteoclast-like giant cells and ovoid tumour cells in a vascular stroma

Behaviour: 50% of tumours are *benign* and are cured by thorough removal: 30% recur: about 10% are malignant or become malignant after radiotherapy and metastasise to the lungs.

In general terms, a tumour showing cellular pleomorphism and abnormal mitotic activity can be expected to behave as a sarcoma, but unfortunately behaviour cannot always be certainly assessed from histological appearances.

TUMOURS IN BONE

MALIGNANT TUMOURS

Primary malignant tumours of bone are not common, but they assume importance because some arise in young people and are highly malignant and in a few, specific pre-existing bone disorders are known precursors, e.g. Paget's disease, multiple enchondromatosis.

Osteosarcoma (Osteogenic sarcoma)

This highly malignant tumour is the commonest primary malignant tumour of bone (excluding myelomatosis). It affects two distinct age groups and there is a preponderance of males over females.

Young age group – majority of cases (10–25 years)
The tumour usually arises near the end of a limb long bone (particularly around the knee).

Elderly subjects (over 60 yrs.)
In 50% of this group, Paget's disease is associated. Vertebrae, pelvis and skull are often affected, and tumours may be multicentric in origin.

The classical tumour in a young man will be described: tumour growth begins in the medullary cavity and is latent. Clinical signs present relatively late, i.e. when the cortex has been destroyed and penetrated.

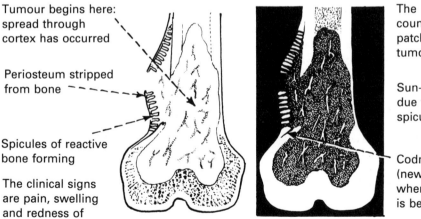

Tumour begins here: spread through cortex has occurred

Periosteum stripped from bone

Spicules of reactive bone forming

The clinical signs are pain, swelling and redness of the lower thigh

The radiological counterpart is a patchily radiolucent tumour

Sun-ray appearance due to new bone spicules

Codman's triangle (new bone forming where periosteum is being stripped)

NB at this stage lung metastases may be present.

The tumour arises from primitive cells which retain to a varying extent the ability to form bone. Histologically, varying amounts of osteoid, irregularly woven bone and sometimes islands of primitive cartilage are seen in a vascular sarcomatous matrix of which the cells are pleomorphic.

793

TUMOURS IN BONE

Chondroscarcoma

This shows a much slower growth pattern and affects the age group 40–70 years. Multiple enchondromatosis pre-exists in a number of cases. The tumours arise particularly in the spine, limb girdles and proximal long bones and consist of primitive cartilage. Progressive local destruction is usual. Metastases to the lung are rare.

Ewing's tumour

This rare malignant tumour affects young subjects (age 5–20 years): it arises in long bones, pubis, ribs and scapulae. The tumour is very aggressive, metastasising early to lungs and other bones.

The tumour cells are small and uniform with pale, open nuclei: the cytoplasm contains glycogen. The histological appearances may mimic lymphoma.

Histogenesis and Aetiology

It is considered to be a primitive neuro-ectodermal tumour and is associated with translocation and fusion of genes on chromosomes 11 and 22 (85% of cases) and chromosomes 21 and 22 (15% of cases).

Lymphoid tumours

Lymphoid tumours, including myelomatosis (see p.592), arise in bone, causing osteolysis.

SECONDARY TUMOURS IN BONE

This is the most common type of tumour in bone. Metastases are usually multiple: occasionally latent renal and thyroid cancers present as single bony metastases with pathological fracture. Tumours which show a predilection for spread to bone are carcinoma of the PROSTATE, BREAST, LUNG, KIDNEY and THYROID particularly. The incidence of bone secondaries ESPECIALLY IN THE SPINE is very high when these tumours become widespread.

The effects of metastatic growth are essentially osteolytic with extensive destruction of bone. In a minority of cases, osteoblastic activity is stimulated by the presence of the tumour so that dense reactive bone is formed. Osteosclerotic secondaries of this type are seen particularly in cancers of the PROSTATE and BREAST.

JOINTS

The diagram illustrates the important components of a **diarthrotic joint**.

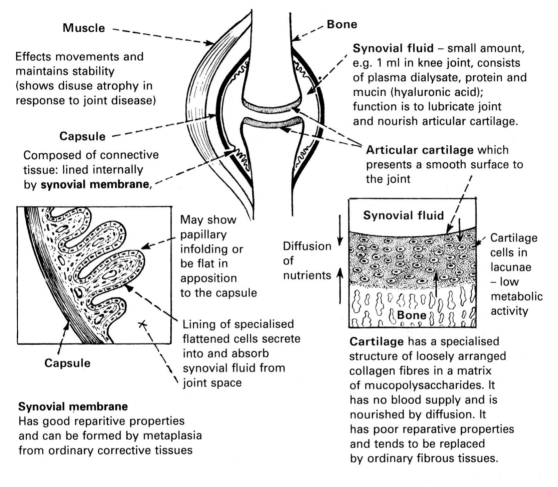

Muscle

Effects movements and maintains stability (shows disuse atrophy in response to joint disease)

Capsule

Composed of connective tissue: lined internally by **synovial membrane,**

Bone

Synovial fluid – small amount, e.g. 1 ml in knee joint, consists of plasma dialysate, protein and mucin (hyaluronic acid); function is to lubricate joint and nourish articular cartilage.

Articular cartilage which presents a smooth surface to the joint

May show papillary infolding or be flat in apposition to the capsule

Diffusion of nutrients

Synovial fluid

Cartilage cells in lacunae – low metabolic activity

Bone

Capsule

Lining of specialised flattened cells secrete into and absorb synovial fluid from joint space

Synovial membrane
Has good reparitive properties and can be formed by metaplasia from ordinary corrective tissues

Cartilage has a specialised structure of loosely arranged collagen fibres in a matrix of mucopolysaccharides. It has no blood supply and is nourished by diffusion. It has poor reparative properties and tends to be replaced by ordinary fibrous tissues.

The two most common joint diseases illustrate how individual components of a joint may be initially affected:

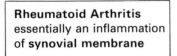

| **Rheumatoid Arthritis** essentially an inflammation of **synovial membrane** | **Osteoarthritis** essentially a degeneration of **articular cartilage** |

As the diseases progress, other secondary effects are added and may obscure the basic pathology.

JOINTS

Trauma is very variable in its severity and effects.

At one end of the scale a single incident of 'sprain or strain' involves only minor soft tissue damage with minimal associated haemorrhage – in these circumstances the healing capacity of joints is rapid and complete.

In contrast, many modern road traffic accidents involve serious damage to joints.

These include:

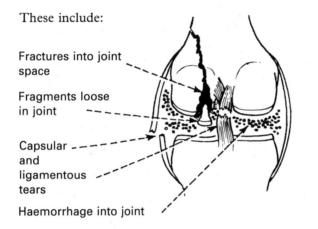

Fractures into joint space

Fragments loose in joint

Capsular and ligamentous tears

Haemorrhage into joint

Possible sequels are:
1. The articular surface is permanently deformed (ineffective repair of cartilage).
2. Loose body continues to cause traumatic damage to synovium.
3. Ligaments may not heal or are united by poor scar tissue.
4. Haemorrhagic exudate may not be resorbed – adhesions form within the joint.

With lesser degrees of trauma, particularly if repeated, the synovial membrane shows non-specific reactive changes which include **HYPERAEMIA** and **MILD CHRONIC INFLAMMATORY CELLULAR INFILTRATE**. There is often a joint **effusion**.

The knee joint is susceptible to a particular type of injury in which one (particularly the medial) of the fibrocartilagenous menisci is torn.

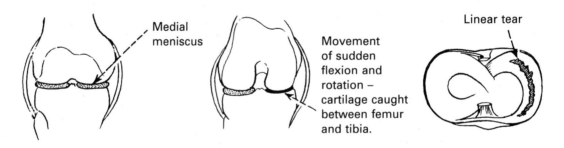

Medial meniscus

Movement of sudden flexion and rotation – cartilage caught between femur and tibia.

Linear tear

Repair of the tear is by poor scar tissue; recurrence with locking of the joint and effusion is common.

Apart from damage directly attributable to trauma, the most important sequel is that the scene is set within the joint for the more rapid development of **DEGENERATIVE DISEASE**.

JOINTS

OSTEOARTHRITIS (OA)

This is the commonest disorder of joints and, by causing pain and stiffness, is the commonest cause of chronic disability after middle age. The basic pathological progress is degenerative and is similar to that seen in lesser degree in simple ageing. The suffix 'itis' is really inappropriate since any inflammatory changes are secondary.

The disorder is divided into two main groups:

1. In **secondary OA** there is a clear association with some predisposing condition which may be virtually any abnormality of a joint. Of particular importance are:
   (a) alterations to the joint mechanics (e.g. abnormal alignments and angulations); a particularly severe form (Charcot's joint) is seen when the nerve supply to a joint and its adjacent muscles is defective.
   (b) abnormality of the articular surfaces (e.g. following injury).
   (c) abnormal stresses on the joint (e.g. the increased weight-bearing demanded by obesity; association with particular occupations and sports).

2. In **primary OA**, no obvious predisposing cause is evident; there is a presumptive abnormality of chondrocyte metabolism but its essential nature remains obscure. A familial pattern is apparent in some cases.
   In both types of osteoarthritis the basic pathological processes are the same.

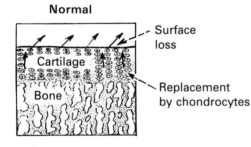

Normal

Surface loss

Cartilage

Replacement by chondrocytes

Bone

The integrity of the articular cartilagenous surface represents a fine balance between 'wear and tear' losses and replacement by chondrocytes of the specialised matrix.

The earliest change in ageing and OA is in the chemical composition of the matrix which becomes softer. This is followed by progressive characteristic morphological changes.

At site of pressure

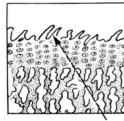

Early

Flaking and fibrillation of surface

Later

Areas of cystic degeneration

Loss of cartilage; exposure of bone – becomes hard and polished (eburnated)

JOINTS

OSTEOARTHRITIS (continued)

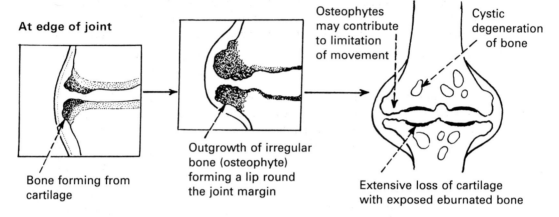

At edge of joint

Bone forming from cartilage

Outgrowth of irregular bone (osteophyte) forming a lip round the joint margin

Osteophytes may contribute to limitation of movement

Cystic degeneration of bone

Extensive loss of cartilage with exposed eburnated bone

The synovial membrane may show mild, non-specific inflammation and effusion may occur but these changes are secondary.

Distribution: secondary OA often affects a single predisposed joint.

In primary OA, the larger weight bearing joints and the spine in particular are susceptible, but interphalangeal joints bear osteophytic outgrowths (Heberden's nodes). Similar lesions (at the proximal interphalangal joints – Bouchard's nodes) superficially mimic the deformities of rheumatoid arthritis; they are, however, not associated with severe disability and muscle wasting is negligible.

Cervical spondylosis. When osteophytes form around the various intevertebral joints, particularly in the cervical spine, neurological complications ranging from compression of individual nerves to actual spinal cord damage are seen.

Note: OA is a local degenerative disease; there is no associated systemic illness.

Gout. The arthritis of gout begins as an acute inflammatory process affecting usually a great toe; with repeated attacks, degenerative arthritis supervenes.

Aetiology: the disease is a disorder of purine metabolism. There is hyperuricaemia (serum uric acid >7mg/dl). Periodically, urate crystals are deposited within the affected joint, at first in the articular cartilage, but later both in the adjacent bone and soft tissues. An acute inflammatory reaction is evoked.

Pseudo-gout. In this condition, crystals of calcium pyrophosphate are deposited in the joint, evoking a similar inflammatory reaction. Larger joints such as the knee tend to be affected; chronic degenerative arthritis supervenes.

RHEUMATOID ARTHRITIS

Rheumatoid arthritis (RA) is a fairly common systemic disease (1–3% of population in Europe). The main target tissue is the synovial membrane of joints (polyarthritis). The typical clinical course is insidious in its onset and progression. In a minority of cases, the onset is acute and the progress rapid. Frequently there are remissions and exacerbations.

Incidence: female > male   *Age of onset:* usually 35–55 years, but also in
          2–3:1   childhood – usually severe.

Typically, the joints of the hands and feet and the knee joints are affected; less commonly there is involvement of the cervical spine and temporomandibular joints.
Pathology: The essential condition is an active chronic inflammation of the synovial membrane.

Early

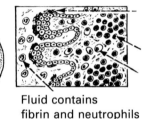

Swollen inflamed synovium

Fibrinous exudate

Intense infiltration with lymphocytes and plasma cells

Fluid contains fibrin and neutrophils

Signs of inflammation with *swelling* over *joints*

A raised ESR and normochromic anaemia are evidence of the systemic illness.

Intermediate

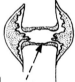

Laxity of capsule and soft tissue – inflammation in periarticular tissues

Destruction of cartilage by enzymatic action and granulation tissue spreading over the articular surface (pannus)

Joints swollen + marked muscle wasting (interosseous and thenar muscles)

Late

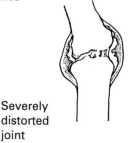

Severely distorted joint

Inflammation usually less marked – fibrous adhesions across joint – may be irregular bony union

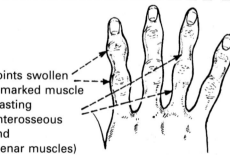

Permanent deformity due to contracture and often subluxation

RHEUMATOID ARTHRITIS

The **aetiology and mechanisms** responsible for the disorder remain unknown. A popular current hypothesis is:

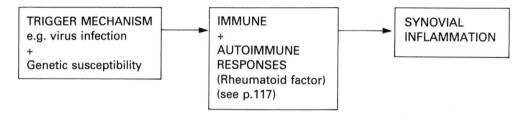

The local condition is aggravated by affection of other synovial tissues – particularly tendon sheaths and bursae.

The systemic nature of the disease is illustrated by inflammatory processes affecting the connective tissues at other sites.

1. **Rheumatoid nodules** occur under the skin at pressure points, particularly in the forearms and elbow joints in 1/5 of cases. They range in size up to a few centimetres in diameter. The histological appearance is striking.

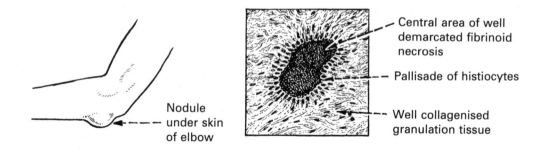

2. The lung may be diffusely affected or, in some cases, lesions similar to rheumatoid nodules are seen. In coal miners, the mixture of coal dust and collagen gives characteristic radiological and pathological appearances – Caplan's nodules.
3. Necrotising arteritis is a serious concomitant in a few cases.
4. A mild interstitial myocarditis, polymyositis or neuritis may be seen in some cases.
5. Lymphoid and splenic reactive enlargements (particularly in juvenile rheumatoid arthritis).

Complications:
1. Amyloid disease.
2. Splenomegaly causing hypersplenism – so-called Felty's syndrome.

SERO-NEGATIVE ARTHRITIS

Ankylosing spondylitis (AS) is an arthritis affecting particularly the sacroiliac, costovertebral and vertebral joints.

Incidence: .05 per cent of population male > female; 8:1

Age of onset: Young adults progressive into middle age. Rheumatoid factor negative

The disorder is, like RA, an active chronic arthritis, but differs in that it may proceed to calcific and osseous ankylosis, so that no movement of the affected joints is possible.

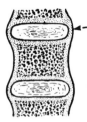

Bony union on the periphery of the intervertebral discs gives the characteristic radiological appearance – bamboo spine.

The aetiology and mechanisms of the disorder are not known – a few cases are associated with Reiter's syndrome or chronic inflammatory bowel disease.

Psoriatic arthritis is very similar to RA, but rheumatoid factor is absent. Typically the distal inter-phalyngeal joints are involved.

Reiter's syndrome (polyarthritis, urethritis and conjunctivitis) has similar chronic inflammatory joint disease, but rheumatoid factor is negative. There is strong evidence that a chlamydial infection is primary, but the detailed mechanisms remain obscure.

HLA association. It is of great interest in that ankylosing spondylitis, psoriatic patients with arthritis and Reiter's syndrome all have a close association with HLA-B27 (90% in AS). This suggests that a genetic susceptibility is an important factor predisposing to the arthritis.

No such association with HLA-B27 is evident with RA, which however shows an association (60%) with HLA-DR4.

Arthritis in acute rheumatic fever

During this stage, arthritis of the knee, ankle and wrist joints is common. The synovial tissues are inflamed and there is an inflammatory cellular infiltrate: the joint fluid contains neutrophils but is sterile. The arthritis is usually self-limiting and without sequelae, in contrast to the cardiac valvular lesions.

OSTEO- AND RHEUMATOID ARTHRITIS – COMPARISON

	OSTEOARTHRITIS	RHEUMATOID ARTHRITIS
Type of disorder	Degenerative	Inflammatory
Site of initial damage	Articular cartilage	Synovial membrane
Age	Late middle age +	3rd decade (any age)
Joints affected	Large weight bearing often single, pre-existing local factors in some cases	Small of hands and feet, multiple
Systemic disease	None ESR – normal Rheumatoid factor – absent	++ ESR ↑ Rheumatoid factor positive Secondary anaemia

INFECTIONS OF JOINTS

1. **Acute infective arthritis**
   (a) Primary pyogenic haematogenous infection is rare nowadays. It remains, however, a serious complication in joints already damaged. S. aureus is the common infecting organism. The essential changes are:

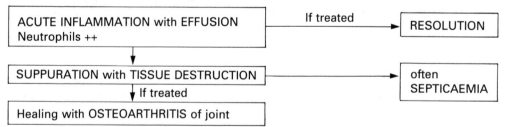

   (b) Arthritis complicating **gonorrhoea** and **brucellosis**.
   In both of these conditions, a polyarthritis may occur in the acute phase and, in a small number, continues as a low grade arthritis. The spine particularly is affected in brucellosis.

2. **Tuberculous arthritis**
   In Western countries the incidence is low: a few cases arise complicating reactivated pulmonary tuberculosis in the elderly. If untreated, there is a low grade chronic inflammation with effusion and progressive destruction of tissues.

   The diagnosis requires culture of joint fluid and/or biopsy when the typical histology of tuberculosis is seen.

PROLIFERATIONS AND TUMOURS OF SYNOVIAL TISSUES

Pigmented villonodular synovitis (PVNS)

This may affect any synovial tissue, but the knee and hip joints are most commonly affected. There is a strong male predominance (age 20–50). The synovial membrane shows a striking proliferation either in the form of brown pigmented large villi or rounded nodules.

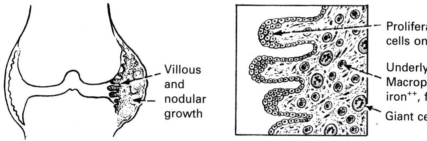

Villous and nodular growth

Proliferating synovial cells on surface

Underlying tissue: Macrophages with iron^{++}, fat^{+}

Giant cells

The exact nature of the lesion is not certain. It may be reactive or neoplastic **but it certainly never metastasises.**

The so-called benign giant cell tumour of tendon sheath is now considered to be a solitary variant of PVNS.

Synovial sarcoma (malignant synovioma)

This is a rare but highly malignant tumour arising in soft tissues often adjacent to a joint (usually the knee or ankle) in young adults: it does not arise in synovium. The histological distinction from other sarcomas requires the demonstration of synovial spaces in the tumour.

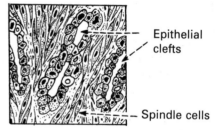

Epithelial clefts

Spindle cells

LOOSE BODIES IN JOINTS

Loose bodies are usually found in diseased or damaged joints and their presence tends to aggravate any existing disease. Clinically, there is often recurrent 'locking' of the joint.

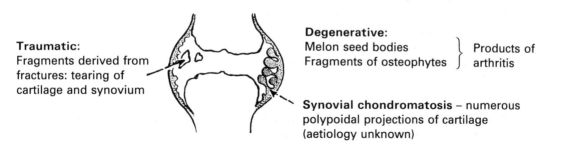

Traumatic:
Fragments derived from fractures: tearing of cartilage and synovium

Degenerative:
Melon seed bodies
Fragments of osteophytes } Products of arthritis

Synovial chondromatosis – numerous polypoidal projections of cartilage (aetiology unknown)

PARA-ARTICULAR TISSUES – MISCELLANEOUS

Bursae

These are synovial-lined spaces usually overlying bony prominences and often connected with adjacent joint spaces. They are subject to traumatic and inflammatory disorders as have been described in joints.

Ganglion

This is a swelling which forms in relation to joint synovium or more usually, tendon sheath. The essential lesion is a myxomatous degeneration of the sheath substance; it is not lined by synovium. Ganglia are classically seen around the wrist.

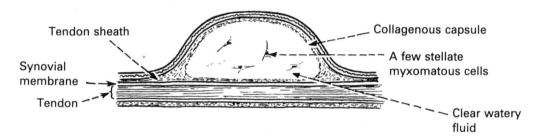

This type of myxomatous cystic degeneration may occur at other less prominent sites, e.g. within the cartilagenous menisci of the knee.

Dupuytren's Contracture. See page 130.

CONNECTIVE TISSUE DISEASES

Some five decades ago, the idea that the collagen component of the connective tissues throughout the body were subject to specific disorders gave rise to the concept of diffuse collagen diseases. Since, in fact, damage to collagen is not usually the primary event, the name was changed to the CONNECTIVE TISSUE DISEASES.

The group includes the 'rheumatic' diseases – rheumatoid arthritis (RA), ankylosing spondylitis (AS) and rheumatic fever; systemic lupus erythematosis (SLE); scleroderma; polyarteritis nodosa (PAN) and dermatomyositis.

Some of these disorders have already been described (RA p.799; AS p.801; rheumatic fever p.270; PAN p.223; dermatomyositis p.774).

CONNECTIVE TISSUE DISEASES

Systemic lupus erythematosis (SLE)

This is a rare disease predominantly affecting young women. The clinical progress varies from acute and rapid to insidious and slow. Most frequently the skin, kidneys, serous membranes and endocardium are damaged and, in a few cases, the central nervous system. The essential lesion is a vasculitis affecting arterioles, capillaries and venules with fibrinoid necrosis and a variable inflammatory cellular infiltrate. In the kidney, the lesion is a glomerulitis (see p.619).

The formation of various autoimmune antibodies is the basic abnormality. Various cell constituents including nuclear DNA are destroyed. Lymphocytotoxic antibodies, by destroying T lymphocytes, further disturb the balances within the immune system, e.g. loss of self recognition and tolerance, and allow unsuppressed B cell proliferation.

Progressive systemic sclerosis

This is a rare, slowly progressive disease in which there is gradual fibrosis of various organs including the skin (face and hands), gastrointestinal tract, heart and lungs. Raynaud's disease is a common concomitant. The basic abnormality is in the small blood vessels, which show sclerosis with intimal thickening. The change is associated with fibrosis of the surrounding tissues by a mechanism as yet undetermined. The evidence for an autoimmune basis is less clear in systemic sclerosis than in the other disorders in this group.

From the descriptions of these various disorders it will be seen that the basic mechanisms are essentially inflammatory and are mediated by autoimmune processes. The inflammatory damage is very variable in its severity, its site of predilection and even in its local effects. Multiple factors, of which inherited susceptibility and resistance are important, are involved. The following diagram illustrates the basic mechanisms:

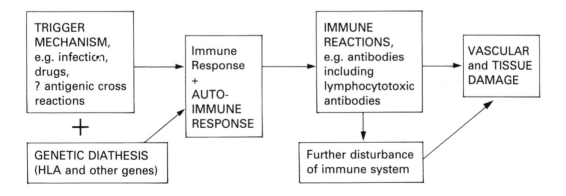

CHAPTER 16

ENDOCRINE SYSTEM

PITUITARY GLAND

The endocrine organs form a control system related to the function and metabolism of the organs and peripheral tissues. In this, the pituitary plays a central role.

Anterior pituitary (Adenohypophysis)

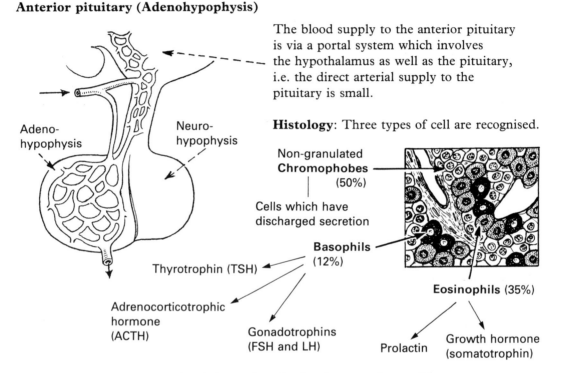

The blood supply to the anterior pituitary is via a portal system which involves the hypothalamus as well as the pituitary, i.e. the direct arterial supply to the pituitary is small.

Histology: Three types of cell are recognised.

Non-granulated **Chromophobes** (50%)

Cells which have discharged secretion

Basophils (12%)

Eosinophils (35%)

Adeno-hypophysis

Neuro-hypophysis

Thyrotrophin (TSH)

Adrenocorticotrophic hormone (ACTH)

Gonadotrophins (FSH and LH)

Prolactin

Growth hormone (somatotrophin)

This histological classification is becoming obsolete because the specific secretory products of all the pituitary cells can now be identified with certainty using immunohistochemical and electron microscope techniques.

CONTROL of ENDOCRINE FUNCTION

A two tier system operates controlling the function of the pituitary and the other endocrines.

1. **Peripheral control**. This can be illustrated by thyroid function.
   The blood level of the peripheral hormone controls the pituitary secretion of the stimulating hormone.

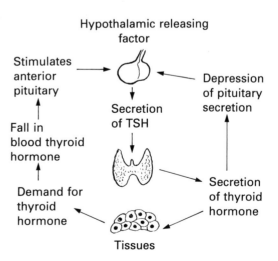

Hypothalamic releasing factor

Stimulates anterior pituitary

Depression of pituitary secretion

Secretion of TSH

Fall in blood thyroid hormone

Demand for thyroid hormone

Secretion of thyroid hormone

Tissues

PITUITARY GLAND

Control of endocrine function (continued)

2. **Central control**. In the hypothalamus (median eminence), peptide substances are produced which are transmitted to the anterior pituitary via the portal system of vessels. These peptides act as permissive hormones, allowing release or inhibition of pituitary hormone secretion. Releasing substances have been identified for TSH, LH/FSH, and GH. An inhibiting substance, somatostatin, has been discovered. It inhibits not only growth hormone secretion, but also secretion of insulin, glucagon and prolactin. It is thought that there is a release-inhibition mechanism for each pituitary hormone. The action of the hypothalamic centres is controlled directly or indirectly (it is not always clear which) by the concentration of hormones in the blood.

Action of anterior pituitary hormones

Growth hormone
1. Stimulates growth.
2. Acts with insulin and thyroid hormone in controlling protein, fat and carbohydrate metabolism. Promotes nitrogen retention and stimulates protein synthesis.

Prolactin
Helps to initiate and maintain lactation.

Gonadotrophins
1. **Follicular Stimulating Hormone (FSH)** — Promotes growth of follicles in ovary
   — Promotes spermatogenesis

2. **Luteinising Hormone (LH)** — Induces ovulation
   — Stimulates testosterone production by testes

Thyroid-stimulating hormone (TSH)
Induces secretion of thyroid hormones and can cause hyperplasia of thyroid epithelium.

Adrenocorticotrophic hormone (ACTH)
Stimulates secretion of glucocorticoids by the adrenal cortex.

PITUITARY GLAND

Inflammations of the pituitary gland

Apart from involvement in acute meningitis inflammation, acute or chronic, is uncommon. Tuberculosis, syphilis and sarcoidosis have been reported.

Lesions of the anterior pituitary generally result in hypofunction or hyperfunction.

ADENOHYPOPHYSEAL HYPOFUNCTION

This produces characteristic syndromes:

IN CHILDHOOD   (a) **Lorain-Levi syndrome (Pituitary dwarfism)**

Growth hormone secretion is deficient. There may also be deficiencies of other pituitary hormones. Attacks of hypoglycaemia occur. Gonadotrophins are usually lacking and puberty does not occur.

In $^2/_3$ of cases, no cause can be found. The condition may be familial and in these circumstances the only deficiency may be of growth hormone. A pituitary tumour or craniopharyngioma is the cause in other cases.

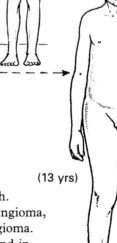

- Skeletal growth diminished
- Retarded sexual development
- Normal intelligence

(13 yrs)

(b) **Frohlich's syndrome**

Stunting of growth
Obesity: feminine distribution of fat.
Arrested sexual development
Mentally subnormal.
Decreased production of growth and other pituitary hormones.

The cause is a lesion affecting the hypothalamus or anterior pituitary or both. Sometimes it is a tumour *e.g.* craniopharyngioma, chromophobe adenoma, glioma or meningioma.

A similar condition is found in adults and in some cases a chromophobe adenoma is present.

(13 yrs)

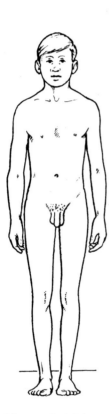

Normal child aged 13 yrs

PITUITARY GLAND

ADENOHYPOPHYSEAL HYPOFUNCTION (continued)

IN ADULTS

Simmond's disease (Sheehan's syndrome)
This occurs in women and is due to ischaemic necrosis of the pituitary following post-partum haemorrhage. The normally low pressure in the pituitary portal vascular supply increases the susceptibility of the gland. The results vary with the extent of necrosis and may include the following:

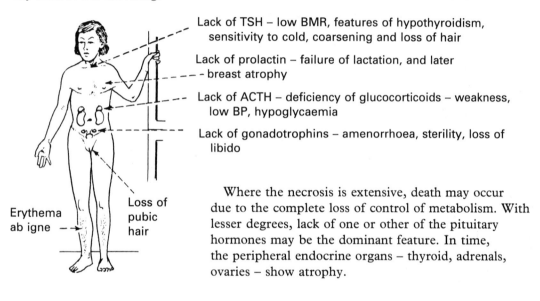

Lack of TSH – low BMR, features of hypothyroidism, sensitivity to cold, coarsening and loss of hair

Lack of prolactin – failure of lactation, and later breast atrophy

Lack of ACTH – deficiency of glucocorticoids – weakness, low BP, hypoglycaemia

Lack of gonadotrophins – amenorrhoea, sterility, loss of libido

Erythema ab igne

Loss of pubic hair

Where the necrosis is extensive, death may occur due to the complete loss of control of metabolism. With lesser degrees, lack of one or other of the pituitary hormones may be the dominant feature. In time, the peripheral endocrine organs – thyroid, adrenals, ovaries – show atrophy.

ADENOHYPOPHYSEAL HYPERFUNCTION
In most cases, this is associated with a PITUITARY ADENOMA.

Giantism and acromegaly
These are both the result of excess production of growth hormone by an eosinophil adenoma. Giantism arises in children before the epiphyses have fused; acromegaly arises in adult life.

Giantism
The excess growth hormone induces skeletal growth, the bones retaining their normal shape and relative proportions. Fusion of epiphyses is delayed, but eventually occurs and the features of acromegaly appear. As in acromegaly, there is initially increase in pituitary secretions and there may be sexual precocity.

PITUITARY GLAND

Acromegaly
The soft tissues increase in thickness. This is followed by periosteal ossification causing thickening of bones.

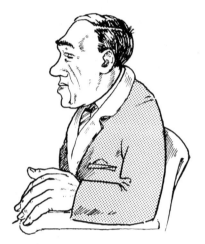

Clinical signs
> Features coarsened: nose enlarged.
> Prognathic (projecting jaw).
> Irregular bone formation – interferes with joint
>   function – leads to osteoarthritis.
> Limbs enlarged.

Pain due to nerve compression is common. Initially, secretion of other pituitary hormones is increased leading to increased strength and increased libido. Glucose tolerance is diminished. Diabetes occurs in 10%. Later, tumour destroys other parts of the pituitary causing weakness, muscle wasting and increased glucose tolerance. High blood pressure with cardiac hypertrophy and extensive atheroma is common, and the patient may die in cardiac failure.

In both giantism and acromegaly, the tumour may compress surrounding structures, *e.g.* optic nerves, leading to hemianopia; or the hypothalamus, leading to diabetes insipidus.

Prolactinoma. Small adenomas, often of chromophobe cells, may secrete prolactin and cause infertility in the female (see p.692).

POSTERIOR PITUITARY (NEUROHYPOPHYSIS)

This is composed of neural tissue and serves as a store for two hormones produced in the hypothalamus.

1. **Vasopressin (antidiuretic hormone, ADH)**
   By altering the permeability of renal collecting tubules and concentrating the urine, vasopressin helps to control water balance. Diabetes insipidus is the condition which results when it is deficient. Absence of the concentrating mechanism results in the loss of large quantities of fluid. Abnormal thirst and polydypsia result. The condition results from damage (injury, tumour or encephalitis) to the hypothalamus.

2. **Oxytocin**
   This hormone causes contraction of smooth muscle and is often used to aid uterine contraction in labour. It also causes expulsion of milk during lactation.

THYROID GLAND

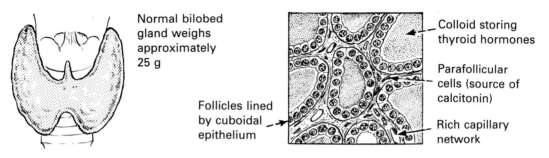

Normal bilobed gland weighs approximately 25 g

Colloid storing thyroid hormones

Parafollicular cells (source of calcitonin)

Follicles lined by cuboidal epithelium

Rich capillary network

The thyroid gland is under the control of the pituitary thyroid-stimulating hormone (TSH).

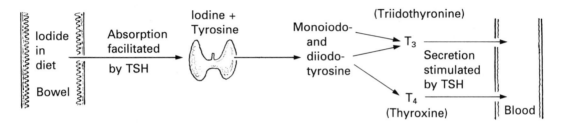

Iodide in diet — Bowel → Absorption facilitated by TSH → Iodine + Tyrosine → Monoiodo- and diiodo-tyrosine → (Triidothyronine) T_3 / T_4 (Thyroxine) → Secretion stimulated by TSH → Blood

The secretion of TSH is determined by the level of T_3 and T_4 in the blood.

THYROID HYPOFUNCTION

Insufficient thyroid hormone is produced, resulting in myxoedema in adults and cretinism in children.

Adults – MYXOEDEMA

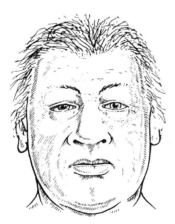

Clinical signs
Basal metabolic rate reduced.
Body temperature falls.
Lethargy and apathy.
Appetite reduced.
Constipation.
Respiratory and heart rates reduced.
Diminished libido.
Lack of ovulation.
Skin thickened, non-pitting oedema due to increase in mucoprotein ground substance.
Hair brittle, dry and falls out.
Blood cholesterol is raised.
TSH secretion is increased.
T_3 and T_4 blood levels low.

THYROID GLAND

Myxoedema (continued)

Causes

1. Autoimmune thyroiditis
   (a) Atrophic form – so-called
   primary myxoedema – the
   commonest cause of hypothyroidism
   (b) Goitrous form –
   Hashimoto's disease.
2. Severe iodine deficiency.

3. Dyshormonogenesis – inborn errors
   in the form of thyroid hormones.
4. Anti-thyroid drugs.
5. Excessive surgical resection of
   thyroid gland.
6. Treatment with radioiodine.
7. Hypopituitarism→reduced TSH.

Pathological changes in primary myxoedema

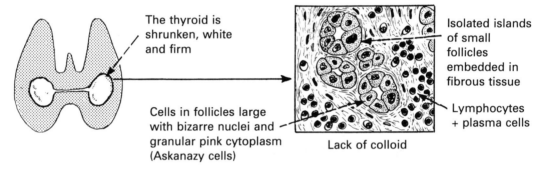

The thyroid is shrunken, white and firm

Cells in follicles large with bizarre nuclei and granular pink cytoplasm (Askanazy cells)

Isolated islands of small follicles embedded in fibrous tissue

Lymphocytes + plasma cells

Lack of colloid

Children – CRETINISM

Infants normal at birth, but abnormality appears within weeks.

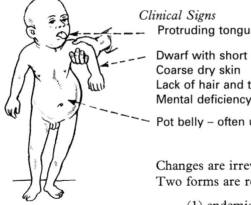

Clinical Signs
Protruding tongue

Dwarf with short limbs
Coarse dry skin
Lack of hair and teeth
Mental deficiency

Pot belly – often umbilical hernia

Changes are irreversible unless treatment is given early.
Two forms are recognised:

(1) endemic and (2) sporadic cretinism.

THYROID GLAND

Endemic cretinism

This occurs in districts where goitre is common due to iodine deficiency. It rarely appears until the 3rd generation of a goitrous family and the mother almost always has a goitre.

The infantile thyroid is usually enlarged and nodular. Histologically, there are hyperplastic foci containing colloid which compress and cause atrophy of the intervening tissue. In some instances the whole gland is atrophic.

Sporadic cretinism

This is due to congenital hypoplasia or absence of the thyroid. The cause is unknown. Deaf mutism is often present.

Dyshormonogenesis

In this condition, cretinism is due to a congenital familial recessive enzyme defect leading to inability to complete the formation of thyroid hormone. The thyroid gland is enlarged and shows epithelial hyperplasia. TSH is increased.

THYROID HYPERFUNCTION

Excessive quantities of circulating thyroid hormone (T_3 and T_4) cause thyrotoxicosis.

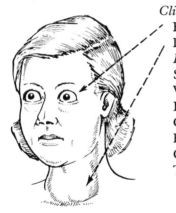

Clinical signs
Exophthalmos – not always present.
Prominent thyroid.
BMR increased.
Skin warm and sweaty: heat intolerance.
Weakness, hyperkinesia and emotional instability.
Loss of weight.
Glucose tolerance diminished, glycosuria.
Rapid Pulse.
Cardiac arrhythmia and failure in older patients.
TSH low.

Three types of thyroid lesion can give rise to thyrotoxicosis.

1. Graves disease (exophthalmic goitre).
2. Toxic adenoma.
3. Toxic nodular goitre.

THYROID GLAND

Graves' disease (exophthalmic goitre)

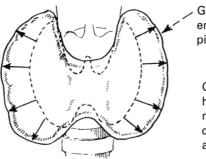

Gland is diffusely enlarged; pale pink in colour

Gland is hyperplastic; numerous closely packed acini of various sizes

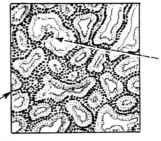

Sometimes intra-acinar papilliform growths

Colloid absent

Cells columnar

In some cases there are foci of thyroiditis with lymphocytes and plasma cells.

Other changes: 1. Thymus is enlarged with increase of lymphocytes. This may be an immune response.
2. Patches of myxoedema – usually on pre-tibial aspect of legs.
3. Exophthalmos, due to auto-immune damage to the eye muscles.

Aetiology: 1. Usually occurs in females.
2. More common in families showing high incidence of autoimmune disease, e.g. thyroiditis, pernicious anaemia.
3. The stimulation of the thyroid is due to an autoantibody (long-acting thyroid stimulator, LATS) which reacts with and activates the surface receptor for TSH on thyroid epithelium. Cyclic AMP is formed and this stimulates hyperplasia of the epithelium and increased formation of thyroid hormone. With the increase in hormone, the blood TSH falls.

Toxic adenoma

Most adenomas are non-active; only a small proportion (1%) give rise to toxic symptoms.

There is usually only one large adenoma present. The histological features are the same as in Graves' disease. Increased production of thyroid hormone by the adenoma, which is autonomous, causes a fall in TSH, and the remainder of the thyroid is inactive.

Toxic nodular goitre

This develops in some cases of non-toxic nodular goitre. Nodules of hyperplasia are interspersed with inactive tissue. The condition is more common over the age of 50. Exophthalmos is absent. Cardiac arrhythmias and failure is common.

THYROID GLAND

Non-toxic goitre

This is a simple enlargement of the thyroid gland, not associated with increased secretion of thyroid hormone.

Two morphological forms are found: (1) parenchymatous and (2) colloid: they are components of a disease spectrum and are separated only on morphological appearances.

1. *Parenchymatous goitre*. The gland is enlarged and pale pink. Two phases can be recognised:

(a) **Diffuse hyperplasia**: The gland consists mainly of small closely packed acini lined by columnar epithelium and containing a small amount of poorly stained colloid. Occasional intra-acinar papilliform epithelial projections may be seen.

(b) **Nodular hyperplasia**: This is a later stage. Areas of marked hyperplasia cause atrophy of intervening parenchyma. It appears to be related to continuing severity of iodine deficiency.

2. *Colloid goitre*. The enlarged gland is translucent and brown due to the large amount of stored colloid.

This is common in women and appears at puberty or during pregnancy.
There are usually no symptoms, but pressure symptoms develop if the thyroid is retrosternal, e.g. pressure on trachea causing stridor, pressure on recurrent laryngeal nerve→hoarseness.

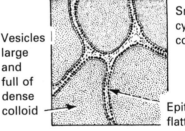

Vesicles large and full of dense colloid

Small cysts common

Epithelium flattened

Aetiology. Goitre is endemic in centre areas of the world, mountainous regions remote from the sea – Switzerland, Himalayas, Andes, etc. There is a lack of iodine in the soil, hence in the food. Sporadic goitre may be induced by other factors.

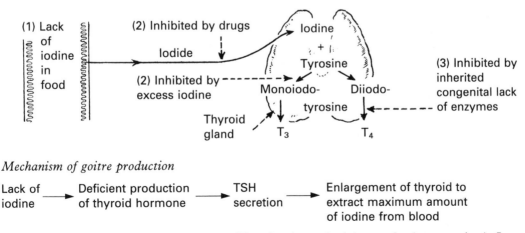

(1) Lack of iodine in food

(2) Inhibited by drugs

Iodide

(2) Inhibited by excess iodine

Iodine
+ I
Tyrosine
Monoiodo-   Diiodo-
tyrosine

Thyroid gland T_3 T_4

(3) Inhibited by inherited congenital lack of enzymes

Mechanism of goitre production

Lack of iodine → Deficient production of thyroid hormone → TSH secretion → Enlargement of thyroid to extract maximum amount of iodine from blood

Where the lack of iodine is severe, proliferation is marked (parenchymatous goitre). In colloid goitre, the process is milder.

817

THYROID GLAND

AUTO-IMMUNE THYROIDITIS
This type of disease is associated with the appearance of thyroid antibodies in the blood and inflammatory changes with lymphocytes and plasma cell reaction in the thyroid gland. The degree of pathological change and the clinical effects tend to form a spectrum, but three conditions can be defined.

1. **Hashimoto's thyroiditis (lymphadenoid goitre)**
   This is the most distinctive type of autoimmune thyroid disease, and the changes are widespread.

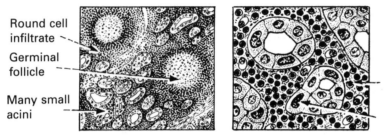

Round cell infiltrate

Germinal follicle

Many small acini

Acini lined by pink cells (Askanazy or Hürthle cells)

Lymphocytes and plasma cells

Nuclei often large and irregular

Clinical effects: While the patient may be euthyroid, it is obvious that the balance is precarious. In 50%, the patient, usually a middle-aged female, develops hypothyroidism. Any attempt to reduce the size of the goitre by surgery inevitably causes hypothyroidism.

The uptake of iodine is reduced and the combination with tyrosine is abnormal. Abnormal thyroid hormone is produced. Antibodies to thyroglobulin and to cytoplasmic microsomes of thyroid epithelium are usually present in high concentration.

2. **Primary Myxoedema**
   Antibodies to thyroid hormones and epithelium are found in this disease (p.813) also, but the plasma concentration is lower than in Hashimoto's disease.

3. **Focal thyroiditis**
   This form of autoimmune disease is usually asymptomatic, but again the balance is disturbed and surgical interference may precipitate hypothyroidism. The concentration of antibodies in the plasma is always low. The thyroid in Graves' disease often shows a form of focal thyroiditis and this may account for the occasional occurrence of hypothyroidism as a late complication in that disease.

Patients with autoimmune thyroiditis are apt to have other organ-specific antibodies, e.g. gastric, adrenal etc., and pernicious anaemia and adrenal insufficiency may occur.

THYROID GLAND

TUMOURS of the THYROID

Follicular Adenoma

This fairly common tumour is usually single and is encapsulated with compression of the surrounding gland. Very occasionally there is hypersecretion with thyrotoxicosis. Degenerative changes including haemorrhage into the tumour are common.

Carcinoma

This is an uncommon condition. Two main forms are recognised:

1. **Papillary carcinoma.** This is the commonest form affecting particularly young women: the tumours are usually small and may be multiple within the thyroid. They metastasise readily to *local lymph nodes* and the first clinical sign may be an enlarged cervical lymph node containing metastatic papillary tumour. Remote spread is unusual.

The histological appearances are typical:

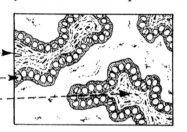

    (1) Small papillary structures

    (2) Uniform, optically clear (Orphan Annie) or grooved nuclei

    (3) Fibro-vascular stroma

2. **Follicular carcinoma.** These tumours have their highest incidence in women over middle age. They present in 2 forms:

(a) As solitary nodules usually well differentiated: some are well encapsulated and can only be differentiated from adenoma by invasion of the capsule and/ or venous venules.

(b) As a tumour of varying degrees of follicular differentiation, which spreads widely in the thyroid and invades venules.

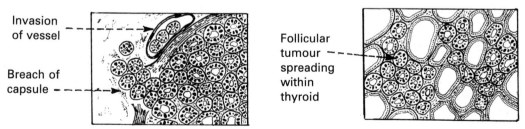

Invasion of vessel

Breach of capsule

Follicular tumour spreading within thyroid

Blood spread particularly to BONES and LUNGS is usual in this type.

Medullary carcinoma

This is a rare tumour arising from the calcitonin-producing cells of the thyroid. Blood calcitonin is high. In addition, there may be production of other hormones resulting in a carcinoid or Cushing's syndrome. There is a familial form in which there are multiple tumours of a number of endocrine organs.

Lymphoma

B cell lymphoma occasionally arises in long-standing auto-immune thyroiditis (particularly Hashimoto's disease).

819

ENDOCRINE PANCREAS

The islets of Langerhans form 1–2% of the pancreatic tissue. Four types of cell make up the islets. The majority are B cells.

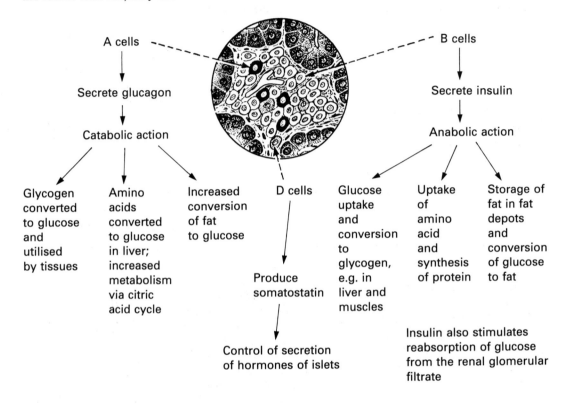

A cells ----→ Secrete glucagon → Catabolic action

B cells ----→ Secrete insulin → Anabolic action

Glycogen converted to glucose and utilised by tissues

Amino acids converted to glucose in liver; increased metabolism via citric acid cycle

Increased conversion of fat to glucose

D cells → Produce somatostatin → Control of secretion of hormones of islets

Glucose uptake and conversion to glycogen, e.g. in liver and muscles

Uptake of amino acid and synthesis of protein

Storage of fat in fat depots and conversion of glucose to fat

Insulin also stimulates reabsorption of glucose from the renal glomerular filtrate

Insulin and glucagon have virtually opposite actions. The action of insulin is also opposed by growth hormone and glucocorticoids.

The fourth type of cell is the pancreatic polypeptide (PP) cell, found in highest concentration in the head of the pancreas.

DIABETES MELLITUS

This condition is due to a lack of insulin activity. Commonly this is the result of diminished production of insulin. In type 2 diabetes there is resistance to the action of insulin i.e. there is a relative insulin deficiency. The condition is a disease complex of mixed aetiology and the manifestations are the result of biochemical abnormalities induced by an inability to control carbohydrate metabolism.

ENDOCRINE PANCREAS

BIOCHEMICAL CHANGES AND CLINICAL EFFECTS
The main results of insulin lack are:

1. **Inability to control carbohydrate metabolism**, causing:

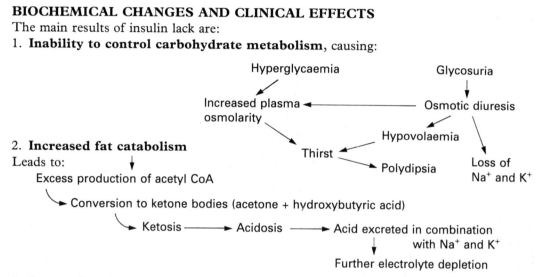

Hyperglycaemia   Glycosuria

Increased plasma ◄——————————— Osmotic diuresis
osmolarity

Hypovolaemia

2. **Increased fat catabolism**
Leads to: Thirst

Excess production of acetyl CoA   Polydipsia   Loss of
Na⁺ and K⁺

Conversion to ketone bodies (acetone + hydroxybutyric acid)

Ketosis ——————► Acidosis ——————► Acid excreted in combination
with Na⁺ and K⁺

Further electrolyte depletion

3. Increased catabolism of amino acids prevents proper protein synthesis and this, together with (1) and (2) above, leads to loss of weight despite polyphagia.

TYPES of DIABETES
Primary forms
TYPE 1 Insulin-Dependent Diabetes (juvenile or early onset diabetes)
This form is due to actual destruction of B cells in the islets of Langerhans.

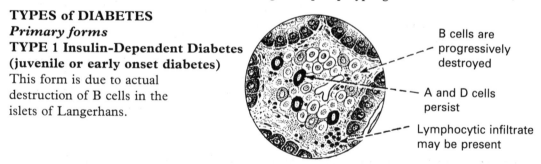

B cells are progressively destroyed

A and D cells persist

Lymphocytic infiltrate may be present

The onset is acute and the peak of incidence is around 13 years. Three factors appear to be of importance in the aetiology

1. There is a familial incidence and in 80% of cases there is an association with Class II HLA antigens (particularly DQ).
2. The onset of the condition is commonest in autumn and winter.
3. Cell-mediated immunity against islet antigens and humoral antibodies are present in at least 50% of cases at onset.

This has given rise to a theory of pathogenesis:

| GENETIC SUSCEPTIBILITY
– inheritance of particular
Class II HLA antigens | **+** | EXTRINSIC FACTORS
– ? virus infection
– ? foods |

Other forms of auto-antibody e.g. gastric, thyroid, adrenal, have been demonstrated. Both sexes are affected and the condition is commoner in lower socio-economic groups.

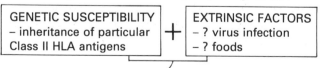

DAMAGE TO B CELLS ——► AUTO-ANTIBODIES ——► TYPE 1 DIABETES

ENDOCRINE PANCREAS

Types of Diabetes (continued)

Primary forms

TYPE 2 Non-Insulin-Dependent Diabetes

This is the commonest form of diabetes affecting 5–7% of adults in Western society and 20–35% in certain groups of South Sea Islanders and North American Indians. It is more frequent in females and the incidence increases with age, peaking at 70 in males and 80 in females. In contrast to Type 1, the onset is slow and the changes in glucose metabolism mild. (Diet restriction to reduce OBESITY and oral hypoglycaemic drugs usually control the blood sugar.) Clinical presentation is often due to complications, particularly vascular, or the disorder is detected at community screening.

Aetiology

This is a multifactorial disorder involving environmental and genetic factors. The basic mechanism is prolonged INSULIN RESISTANCE in the tissues leading eventually to inadequate secretion of insulin by B cells.

The following theory accommodates the known facts:

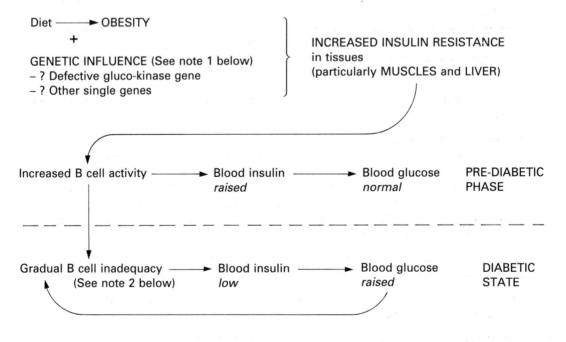

Note 1: In a small group of **children**, Type 2 diabetes has been shown to be inherited as an autosomal dominant trait (defective gluco-kinase gene). In the common Type 2 diabetes other genes are currently being investigated.

Note 2: B cells secrete islet amyloid protein along with insulin. **Amyloid** is deposited in islets in Type 2 diabetes probably reflecting the prolonged B cell activity.

ENDOCRINE PANCREAS

Types of Diabetes (continued)

Gestational Diabetes
This is associated with glycosuria during pregnancy and the birth of overweight babies. Control of the maternal blood sugar reduces birth weight to normal. Permanent diabetes is apt to develop at a later date.

Secondary forms

Diabetes may complicate:
1. A number of endocrine diseases (acromegaly, Cushing's syndrome, Conn's syndrome)
2. Metabolic diseases (haemochromatosis, pancreatic calcification, hypocalcaemia)
3. Drug therapy (steroids, thiazide diuretics)
4. Pancreatic inflammation, etc., (chronic pancreatitis, mumps, cystic fibrosis).

COMPLICATIONS OF DIABETES

1. **Diabetic Coma**. Three forms of coma occur:
   (a) **Keto-acidotic coma**. This is common in Type 1 diabetes. Hyperosmolarity, hypovolaemia, acidosis and loss of electrolytes if unchecked lead to coma.
   (b) **Hyperosmolar non-ketotic coma**. This develops slowly in Type 2 diabetes. Hyperglycaemia builds up and produces profound dehydration.
   (c) **Lactic acidosis coma**. This is uncommon, although increase in lactic acid is frequent in diabetes.

2. **Hypoglycaemic coma**. This occurs when insulin intake is excessive for the amount of food consumed.

3. **Cardiovascular lesions**
   (a) Atheroma develops at an earlier age and with increased severity. Coronary thrombosis is not uncommon.
   (b) Microangiopathy causing occlusion of arterioles and capillaries. These vascular lesions are responsible for many of the clinical lesions e.g. cardiac failure (the commonest cause of death in diabetes) retinopathy, neuropathy, gangrene of limbs, Kimmelstiel-Wilson lesions in the kidney.

4. **Renal failure**. This is the other common cause of death. It may be due to glomerulosclerosis, but pyelonephritis and renal papillary necrosis are other causes.

5. **Infections**. There is an increased susceptibility to sepsis and fungal infections. Tuberculosis is also common.

6. **Neuropathy**. (a) Peripheral ⎫ Possibly due to direct metabolic
                                         damage
                    (b) Autonomic ⎭ ± microvascular occlusion

ADRENAL GLAND

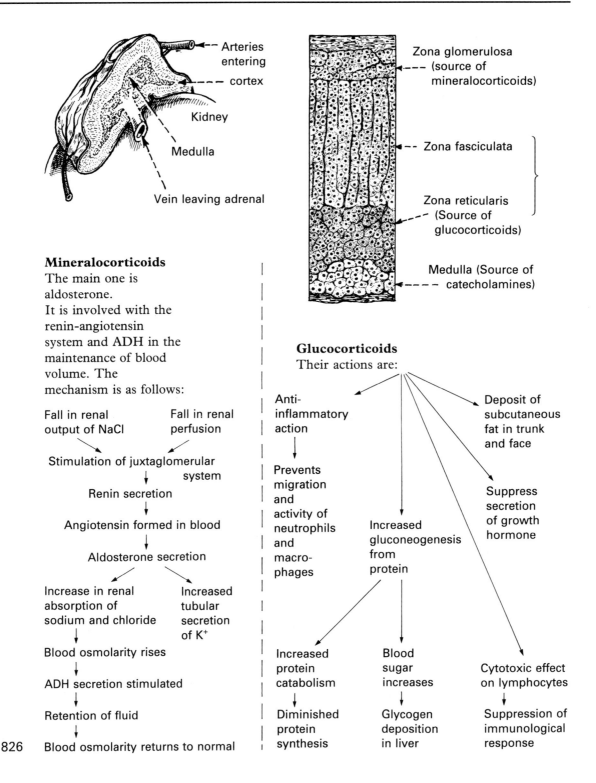

Arteries entering — cortex

Kidney

Medulla

Vein leaving adrenal

Zona glomerulosa (source of mineralocorticoids)

Zona fasciculata

Zona reticularis (Source of glucocorticoids)

Medulla (Source of catecholamines)

Mineralocorticoids
The main one is aldosterone.
It is involved with the renin-angiotensin system and ADH in the maintenance of blood volume. The mechanism is as follows:

Fall in renal output of NaCl   Fall in renal perfusion

↓

Stimulation of juxtaglomerular system

↓

Renin secretion

↓

Angiotensin formed in blood

↓

Aldosterone secretion

Increase in renal absorption of sodium and chloride   Increased tubular secretion of K^+

↓

Blood osmolarity rises

↓

ADH secretion stimulated

↓

Retention of fluid

↓

Blood osmolarity returns to normal

Glucocorticoids
Their actions are:

Anti-inflammatory action

↓

Prevents migration and activity of neutrophils and macro-phages

Increased gluconeogenesis from protein

Deposit of subcutaneous fat in trunk and face

Suppress secretion of growth hormone

Increased protein catabolism

↓

Diminished protein synthesis

Blood sugar increases

↓

Glycogen deposition in liver

Cytotoxic effect on lymphocytes

↓

Suppression of immunological response

ADRENAL GLAND

Control Mechanism

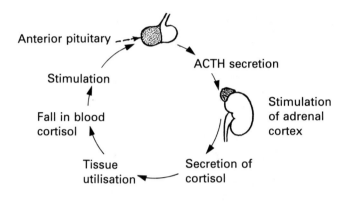

There is also a centre in the hypothalamus which formulates a releasing hormone controlling the secretion of ACTH.

Sex hormones – androgens and oestrogens – are also produced in small quantities.

HYPERACTIVITY

This manifests itself in three ways:

1. **Cushing's syndrome (hypersecretion of cortisol)**

   This condition is commonest in women, but occurs also in men and children.

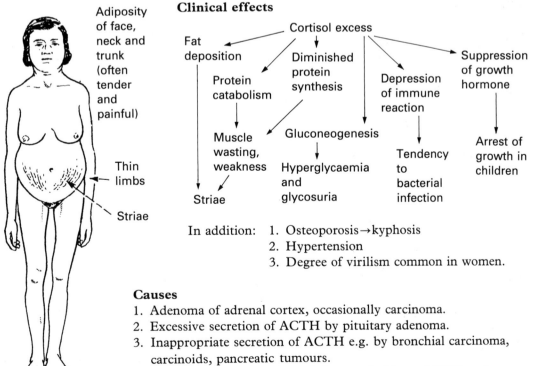

Adiposity of face, neck and trunk (often tender and painful)

Thin limbs

Striae

Clinical effects

In addition:
1. Osteoporosis→kyphosis
2. Hypertension
3. Degree of virilism common in women.

Causes
1. Adenoma of adrenal cortex, occasionally carcinoma.
2. Excessive secretion of ACTH by pituitary adenoma.
3. Inappropriate secretion of ACTH e.g. by bronchial carcinoma, carcinoids, pancreatic tumours.
4. Prolonged administration of glucocorticoids or ACTH as therapy.

827

ADRENAL GLAND

Hyperactivity (continued)

2. Hyperaldosteronism (Conn's syndrome)
This is due to an adenoma or hyperplasia of the zona glomerulosa.

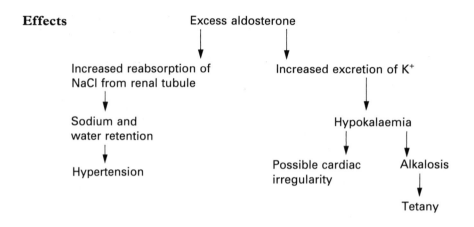

3. **Excessive sex hormone secretion**
   This can occur occasionally with an adrenal cortical adenoma; usually excessive androgens are secreted.
   (a) In males it causes precocious puberty.
   (b) In females – virilism.

HYPOFUNCTION
This results in deficiency of both mineralocorticoids and glucocorticoids.

Acute hypofunction
1. Acute failure to reabsorb Na^+ and excrete K^+.
2. Failure of gluconeogenesis causing hypoglycaemia and increased sensitivity to insulin.

Death is due to:

        1. hypovolaemia causing shock
        2. hyperkalaemia causing cardiac irregularity.

Destruction of the medulla and catecholamine deficiency increase the shock situation.

The cause is usually septicaemia, especially due to meningococci. Endotoxic shock is another cause. These conditions result in necrosis of the cortex and gross haemorrhage in the medulla.

ADRENAL GLAND

Chronic Hypofunction

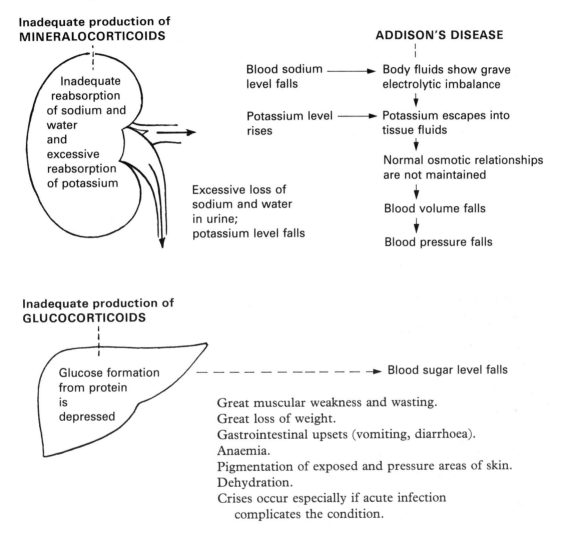

Inadequate production of MINERALOCORTICOIDS

Inadequate reabsorption of sodium and water and excessive reabsorption of potassium

Excessive loss of sodium and water in urine; potassium level falls

ADDISON'S DISEASE

Blood sodium level falls ⟶ Body fluids show grave electrolytic imbalance

Potassium level rises ⟶ Potassium escapes into tissue fluids

Normal osmotic relationships are not maintained

Blood volume falls

Blood pressure falls

Inadequate production of GLUCOCORTICOIDS

Glucose formation from protein is depressed

⟶ Blood sugar level falls

Great muscular weakness and wasting.
Great loss of weight.
Gastrointestinal upsets (vomiting, diarrhoea).
Anaemia.
Pigmentation of exposed and pressure areas of skin.
Dehydration.
Crises occur especially if acute infection complicates the condition.

Administration of adrenal hormones restores individual to normal.

Causes

1. Tuberculous destruction of adrenals.
2. 'Idiopathic' Addison's disease. This is now known to be due to an autoimmune reaction in at least 50% of cases.

Other autoimmune diseases affecting other endocrine glands are commonly associated with this form of Addison's disease.

829

ADRENAL GLAND

Congenital Adrenocortical Enzyme Defects

These are rare, inherited conditions due to autosomal recessive traits.

Each transformation step in the pathways of steroid formation in the adrenal cortex requires the activity of one or more enzymes. Deficiency of any enzyme will interfere with production of the end product.

21 hydroxylase deficiency

This is the commonest type, and the lack of this enzyme prevents the production of cortisol and aldosterone. The low blood cortisol activates ACTH secretion. Adrenal hyperplasia follows and, although cortisol is not formed, other steroids are produced in excess. The resulting clinical syndrome varies with the severity of the defect, e.g:

1. Symptoms of Addison's disease.

2. Lesser degrees of adrenal failure plus symptoms due to excess of sex steroids.
   (a) Pseudohermaphroditism in females;
       precocious puberty in males.
   (b) Virilism in female.

3. No signs of adrenal failure but sex disturbance.

Other variations have been described. Some of these syndromes are also seen with adrenocortical tumours.

ADRENAL MEDULLA

This tissue is composed of chromaffin cells producing two catecholamines – adrenaline and noradrenaline. The first stimulates the cardiorespiratory system, increasing blood sugar and general metabolism; the second raises blood pressure. During stress, they act in concert with the adrenocorticosteroids. Excess production may occur with some tumours of the medulla. Three are described:

1. **Phaeochromocytoma**. This is a benign tumour composed of chromaffin cells. Symptoms are due to paroxysmal overproduction of the amines with hypertension, raised metabolic rate and blood sugar. Arteriosclerosis develops rapidly and cerebral haemorrhage may occur.

2. **Ganglioneuroma**: a benign tumour, composed of well-differentiated ganglion cells (see p.755).

3. **Neuroblastoma**: a very malignant tumour of primitive nerve cells, occurring in children. Catecholamines are occasionally produced by the neurogenic tumours (see p.755).

Coventry University